Pearson's Comprehensive Medical Assisting

STUDENT WORKBOOK FOR

Pearson's Comprehensive Medical Assisting

SECOND EDITION

by

NINA BEAMAN
LORRAINE FLEMING-MCPHILLIPS
KRISTIANA SUE ROUTH
ROBYN GOHSMAN
STACIA REAGAN

with

LORI TYLER

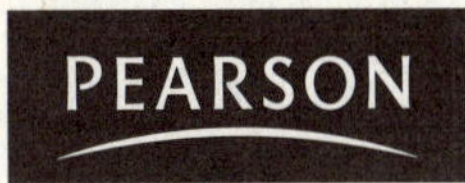

Boston Columbus Indianapolis New York San Francisco Upper Saddle River Amsterdam
Cape Town Dubai London Madrid Milan Munich Paris Montreal Toronto Delhi
Mexico City Sao Paulo Sydney Hong Kong Seoul Singapore Taipei Tokyo

Pearson Education Ltd., London
Pearson Education Singapore, Pte. Ltd.
Pearson Education Canada, Inc.
Pearson Education-Japan
Pearson Education Australia PTY, Limited
Pearson Education North Asia, Ltd., Hong Kong
Pearson Educatión de Mexico, S.A. de C.V.
Pearson Education Malaysia, Pte. Ltd.
Pearson Education Upper Saddle River, New Jersey

10 9 8 7

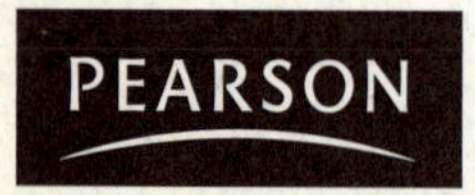

www.pearsonhighered.com

ISBN-13: 978-0-13-507507-4
ISBN-10: 0-13-507507-6

Contents

INTRODUCTION

This student workbook is designed as a study guide and practice tool to accompany the student text, *Pearson's Comprehensive Medical Assisting, Second Edition*. Read the chapter outlines and use the study guide to reinforce what you have learned. Test your knowledge of medical terminology by completing the variety of activities in the Key Terminology Review section. Measure whether you have achieved the learning objectives in each chapter by completing the exercises in the Applied Practice and Learning Activities sections of the workbook. Apply your knowledge to real-life situations by answering the Critical Thinking Questions. Use outside resources to complete the research activity at the end of each chapter.

Each chapter of this student workbook includes the following:

Chapter Outline: This is a list of the major content areas in the chapter. Review each of the topics and refer to your textbook for any topics that remain unclear to you.

Student Study Guide: This is of material presented in the chapter. Fill in the blanks, or answer the questions by following PowerPoint presentations in class, or reading through your text.

Applied Practice: Use the knowledge you learned in the chapter to complete these activities.

Learning Activities: These questions/tasks allow you to measure whether or not you have achieved the learning objectives for the chapter.

Key Terminology Review: This section tests your knowledge of the medical terminology presented in the chapter.

Critical Thinking Questions: These challenging questions allow you to apply your knowledge to real-life situations.

Research Activity: Use outside sources to complete these activities and go beyond the classroom.

Procedure Skill Sheets: These boxed procedures, found in the back of the workbook, correspond to those in the student textbook and allow students to demonstrate the skills needed to become a medical assistant. A space is included for your instructor to document that you have successfully completed the skill. Each step is weighted to better indicate proficiency in the skill.

Mastery of Competency Skills

Procedure Number	Procedure Title	Date Mastered	Instructor's Signature
5-1	Effective Listening Skills		
5-2	Assisting the Hearing-Impaired Patient		
6-1	Handling a Fire in the Medical Office		
6-2	Housekeeping Using OSHA Guidelines		
7-1	Answering the Telephone and Placing Calls on Hold		
7-2	Taking a Telephone Message		
7-3	Taking a Prescription Refill Message		
7-4	Placing a Conference Call		
8-1	Opening the Office		
8-2	Collating Records		
8-3	Registering a New Patient		
8-4	Closing the Office		
9-1	Scheduling Established Patients		
9-2	Scheduling a New Patient Appointment		
9-3	Arranging a Referral Appointment		
9-4	Scheduling Inpatient Surgical Procedures		
9-5	Scheduling Outpatient Surgical Procedures		
11-1	Composing a Business Letter		
11-2	Proofreading Written Documents		
11-3	Opening and Sorting the Daily Mail		
13-1	Adding or Changing Items on a Patient's Record		
13-2	Organizing a Patient's Medical Record		
13-3	Filing a Record Alphabetically		
13-4	Filing a Record Numerically Using the Terminal-Digit Filing System		
13-5	Locating Missing Files		
14-1	Correcting an Entry in the Electronic Medical Record		
15-1	Preparing a Patient Ledger Card		

Procedure Number	Procedure Title	Date Mastered	Instructor's Signature
15-2	Making Collection Calls		
15-3	Writing a Collection Letter		
15-4	Posting a Payment from a Collection Agency		
15-5	Perform Accounts Receivable		
15-6	Using a Pegboard System		
16-1	Prepare a Check		
16-2	Post Nonsufficient Funds (NSF) Checks		
16-3	Prepare a Deposit Slip		
16-4	Reconciling a Bank Statement		
16-5	Generating Payroll in a Medical Office		
17-1	Performing Billing and Collection Procedures		
17-2	Applying Third-Party Guidelines		
17-3	Applying Managed Care Policies and Procedures		
18-1	Completing the CMS-1500 Form		
19-1	ICD-9-CM Coding		
19-2	Assigning a CPT Code		
20-1	Staff Meeting Procedures		
20-2	Developing a Patient Information Booklet		
34-1	Disposal of Infectious Wastes and Substances		
34-2	Performing Hand Washing		
34-3	Applying and Removing Nonsterile Gloves		
34-4	Performing Transmission-Based Precaution: Isolation Techniques		
34-5	Sanitizing Instruments		
34-6	Wrapping and Labeling Instruments for Autoclaving		
34-7	Sterilizing Instruments in an Autoclave		
34-8	Chemically Sterilizing Instruments		

Procedure Number	Procedure Title	Date Mastered	Instructor's Signature
35-1	Measuring Adult Weight and Height		
35-2	Measuring Oral Temperature Using an Electronic or Digital Thermometer		
35-3	Measuring Rectal Temperature Using an Electronic Thermometer		
35-4	Measuring Axillary Temperature		
35-5	Measuring Temperature Using an Aural (Tympanic Membrane) Thermometer		
35-6	Measuring Temperature Using a Heat-Sensitive Wearable Thermometer		
35-7	Measuring Temperature Using a Temporal Artery Thermometer		
35-8	Measuring Radial Pulse		
35-9	Measuring Apical–Radial Pulse (Two Persons)		
35-10	Measuring Respirations		
35-11	Measuring Blood Pressure		
35-12	Measuring Systolic Blood Pressure Using the Palpatory Method		
35-13	Determining the Fat-Fold Measurement in an Adult		
35-14	Calculating Adult Body Mass Index		
36-1	Cleaning the Examination Room		
36-2	Documenting a Chief Complaint During a Patient Interview		
36-3	Interviewing a New Patient to Obtain Medical History Information and Preparing for a Physical Examination		
36-4	Positioning the Patient in the Supine Position		
36-5	Positioning the Patient in the Dorsal Recumbent Position		
36-6	Positioning the Patient in the Lithotomy Position		
36-7	Positioning the Patient in the Fowler's Position		

Procedure Number	Procedure Title	Date Mastered	Instructor's Signature
36-8	Positioning the Patient in the Prone Position		
36-9	Positioning the Patient in the Sims' Position		
36-10	Positioning the Patient in the Knee-Chest Position		
36-11	Assisting with a Complete Physical Examination		
37-1	Performing a Scratch Test		
37-2	Taking a Wound Culture		
37-3	Assisting with a Sigmoidoscopy		
37-4	Administering a Disposable Enema		
37-5	Instructing the Patient in Collecting a Stool Specimen		
37-6	Testing for Occult Blood		
37-7	Performing a Pupil Check on a Patient		
37-8	Assisting with a Neurologic Examination		
38-1	Instructing a Patient on Breast Self-Examination		
38-2	Assisting with a Pelvic Examination and Pap Test		
38-3	Instructing a Male Patient How to Perform a Testicular Self-Examination		
39-1	Testing Visual Acuity Using a Snellen Eye Chart		
39-2	Screening for Near Vision Acuity		
39-3	Screening for Color Vision Acuity		
39-4	Irrigation of the Eye		
39-5	Instilling Eye Medication		
39-6	Irrigation of the Ear		
39-7	Instilling Ear Medication		
39-8	Assisting with Audiometry		
39-9	Instilling Nasal Medications		
40-1	Wrapping an Infant or Small Child		

Procedure Number	Procedure Title	Date Mastered	Instructor's Signature
40-2	Measuring Pediatric Vital Signs		
40-3	Measuring the Weight and Height of an Infant		
40-4	Measuring the Head Circumference of an Infant or Small Child		
40-5	Measuring the Chest Circumference of a Child		
40-6	Calculating Growth Percentiles		
40-7	Perform a Snellen Eye Exam on a Child		
40-8	Applying a Pediatric Urine Collection Device		
41-1	Communicating Effectively with the Elderly		
41-2	Instructing Stroke Patients According to Their Needs		
42-1	Surgical Hand Hygiene/Surgical Scrub		
42-2	Surgical Gloving		
42-3	Opening a Sterile Packet		
42-4	Dropping a Sterile Packet onto a Sterile Field		
42-5	Transferring Sterile Objects Using Transfer Forceps		
42-6	Transferring Sterile Solutions onto a Sterile Field		
42-7	Assisting with Minor Surgery		
42-8	Preparing the Patient's Skin for Surgical Procedures		
42-9	Assisting with Suturing		
42-10	Removing Sutures		
42-11	Changing a Sterile Dressing		
42-12	Applying a Bandage Over a Sterile Dressing		
43-1	Perform Adult Rescue Breathing and One-Rescuer CPR		
43-2	Perform Infant or Young Child Rescue Breathing and One-Rescuer CPR		

Procedure Number	Procedure Title	Date Mastered	Instructor's Signature
43-3	Use an Automated External Defibrillator		
43-4	Respond to an Adult with an Obstructed Airway		
43-5	Administer Oxygen		
43-6	Demonstrate the Application of a Pressure Bandage		
43-7	Demonstrate the Application of Triangular, Figure-Eight, and Tubular Bandages		
43-8	Respond to a Patient Who Has Fainted		
43-9	Demonstrate the Application of a Splint		
43-10	Develop an Environmental Exposure Plan		
44-1	Using and Cleaning the Microscope		
44-2	Completing a Laboratory Requisition and Preparing a Specimen for Transport to an Outside Laboratory		
44-3	Monitoring and Following up on Laboratory Test Results		
45-1	Preparing a Smear		
45-2	Preparing a Wet Mount Slide		
45-3	Performing a Gram Stain		
45-4	Obtaining a Throat Culture		
45-5	Obtaining a Sputum Specimen for Culture		
45-6	Performing a Urine Culture		
45-7	Obtaining a Stool Specimen for Culture and Sensitivity		
45-8	Obtaining a Stool Specimen for Ova and Parasites		
45-9	Obtaining a Stool Specimen for Examination for Pinworms		
46-1	Collecting a 24-Hour Urine Specimen		
46-2	Collecting a Clean-Catch Midstream Urine Specimen		
46-3	Evaluating the Physical Characteristics of Urine		

Procedure Number	Procedure Title	Date Mastered	Instructor's Signature
46-4	Measuring the Specific Gravity of Urine with a Refractometer		
46-5	Testing the Chemical Characteristics of Urine with Reagent Strips		
46-6	Testing for Glucose in Urine Using the Tablet Method		
46-7	Preparing a Urine Specimen for Microscopic Examination		
46-8	Performing a Urine Pregnancy Test Using the Enzyme Immunoassay Method		
47-1	Quality Control for Collecting a Blood Specimen		
47-2	Obtaining Venous Blood with a Sterile Syringe and Needle		
47-3	Performing a Venipuncture Using the Vacutainer Method		
47-4	Performing a Capillary Puncture (Manual)		
47-5	Monitoring Blood Glucose Levels		
47-6	Performing a Microhematocrit		
47-7	Determining Hemoglobin Using the Hemoglobinometer		
47-8	Preparing Slides		
47-9	Performing an Erythrocyte Sedimentation Rate Test Using the Wintrobe Tube Method		
47-10	Performing a PKU Test		
47-11	Performing a Mono Test		
48-1	Procedure for a General X-Ray Examination		
49-1	Recording a 12-Lead Electrocardiograph		
49-2	Preparing and Monitoring the Patient During a Treadmill Stress Test		
49-3	Applying a Holter Monitor		
50-1	Performing a Spirometry Test to Measure Forced Vital Capacity		
50-2	Teaching Peak Flow Measurement		

Procedure Number	Procedure Title	Date Mastered	Instructor's Signature
50-3	Measuring Oxygen Saturation		
51-1	Application of a Hot Compress		
51-2	Application of a Hot Soak		
51-3	Application of a Heating Pad		
51-4	Application of a Cold Compress		
51-5	Application of an Ice Bag		
51-6	Application of a Cold Chemical Pack		
51-7	Instructing a Patient to Use Crutches Correctly		
51-8	Instructing a Patient to Use a Cane or Single Crutch Correctly		
51-9	Teaching a Patient to Correctly Use a Walker		
51-10	Wheelchair Transfer to Chair or Examination Table		
54-1	Administering Oral Medications		
54-2	Administering Sublingual or Buccal Medication		
54-3	Administering a Rectal or Vaginal Suppository		
54-4	Withdrawing Medication from Single-Dose or Multiple-Dose Vials		
54-5	Withdrawing Medication from an Ampule		
54-6	Administering Parenteral, Subcutaneous, or Intramuscular Injections		
54-7	Administering a Z-Track Injection		
54-8	Administering an Intradermal Injection		
54-9	Preparing an Intravenous Tray		
54-10	Reconstituting a Powdered Medication for Administration		
55-1	Creating a Community Resource Brochure		
55-2	Creating a Public Relations Brochure		
55-3	Instructing Patients According to Their Needs for Health Maintenance and Promotion		

Procedure Number	Procedure Title	Date Mastered	Instructor's Signature
57-1	Role-Playing a Situation in Which a Patient Is from Another Culture		
57-2	Role-Playing a Situation in Which a Patient Is Frightened, Angry, or Depressed		
57-3	Develop a Patient Teaching Handout About Stress		
59-1	Conducting a Job Search		
59-2	Preparing Your Resume and References		
59-3	Preparing a Cover Letter		
59-4	Role-Playing an Interview		
59-5	Preparing a Follow-up Letter		

Pearson's Comprehensive Medical Assisting

CHAPTER 1
Medical Assisting: The Profession

CHAPTER OUTLINE

General review of the chapter:

History of Medical Assisting
Education and Training for the Medical Assistant
Role of the Medical Assistant
Characteristics of a Good Medical Assistant
Certifying Professional Organizations
Career Opportunities

STUDENT STUDY GUIDE

Use the following guide to assist in your learning of the concepts from the chapter.

I. The History and Training of Medical Assistants

1. Steps in the History of Trained Medical Assistants
   A. Originally MAs received their training
   ____.
   B. The increase in responsibility and ________________ issues led to the need for medical assistants to be more formally trained.
   C. Prior to the formal training of medical assistants, ________________ were in higher demand to assist physicians.
2. The AAMA
   A. The AAMA as the acronym for the
   ____.
   B. The AAMA was founded by ________________.
   C. In the year _________, the AAMA was organized.
3. AAMA Definition of a Medical Assistant
   A. According to the AAMA's definition of medical assistants, MAs work primarily in ________________ settings.
   B. Medical assistants perform both ________________ and ________________ procedures.
4. Formal Training for the Medical Assistant
   A. Certificate training varies from ________________ weeks to a yearlong program and focuses typically on ________________ skills.
   B. Diploma MA programs are similar to certificate programs but focus on both ________________________________ skills.
   C. Medical assistant degree programs are approximately _________ years in length.

5. Accreditation
   A. Accreditation is a ________________ process.
   B. Accreditation ensures that a program in a school meets or exceeds ________________.
6. Accrediting Agencies for MA Programs
   i. ________________
   ii. ________________
7. Units, Modules, and/or Courses of Instruction Typically Found in an MA Program
   i. ________________
   ii. ________________
   iii. ________________
   iv. ________________
   v. ________________
   vi. ________________
   vii. ________________
   viii. ________________
   ix. ________________
   x. ________________
   xi. ________________
8. The Medical Assistant Externship
   A. Is a ______________ component of an MA program.
   B. Externships take place in ____________, ______________, or __________ settings.

II. Role and Responsibilities of the Medical Assistant
1. Role of the Medical Assistant
   A. The role of the MA is to ______________ the physician.
2. Places of Employment for MAs
   i. ________________
   ii. ________________
   iii. ________________
   iv. ________________
   v. ________________
3. Duties of the Medical Assistant
   A. Duties typically __________ from office to office.
   B. __________ and __________ of setting determine the types of duties the medical assistant will perform.
   C. Duties vary due to __________ and __________ regulations and guidelines.
4. Administrative Duties
   A. ____________ nonpatients and visitors is one example of the MA's administrative duties.
   B. During the physician's absence it is up to the medical assistant to __________ the office.
5. Clinical Responsibilities
   A. Clinical responsibilities of the MA include __________ patients in preparation for physical exams and procedures.
   B. Prior to a physical exam, the MA may need to obtain a patient's __________ history.
   C. Inventory control may involve the ____________ and ____________ of supplies.
6. The Occupational Analysis of the CMA (AAMA) 2007–2008
   A. Defines ________________________________ for medical assisting.
   B. Study used a document called the ________________________.
   C. Study was revised in the year ___________ and again in ___________.

7. General, Clinical, and Administrative Skills of the CMA (AAMA)
   A. Identifies three major categories of competences of entry-level MAs
      i. ____________________
      ii. ____________________
      iii. ____________________
8. General Characteristics of a Good MA
   A. Ability to perform ____________ and ____________ skills.
   B. ____________ cares about others.
   C. Ability to ____________ and get along with others.
9. How to Present a Professional Image
   A. Develop a basic ____________ of human behavior.
   B. Exhibit good daily personal ________ and ________ habits.
   C. Provide ________ care.

III. Certification and Career Opportunities for the MA
1. MA Certifying Organizations
   i. ____________________
   ii. ____________________
   iii. ____________________
   iv. ____________________
2. American Association of Medical Assistants
   A. Headquarters are located in ____________.
   B. Key association in the field of ____________.
   C. Offers ________ credential.
3. AAMA Certification Exam
   A. Offered to graduates of programs accredited by ________ or ________.
   B. Computerized exams are available ________ the year.
   C. ________ indicates that the candidate has met the standards of the AAMA for being an MA.
4. American Medical Technologists
   A. Provides a ____________ certification exam for MAs.
   B. ________ is awarded to candidates who pass the AMT certification exam.
   C. RMA certification exam focuses on three areas:
      i. ____________________
      ii. ____________________
      iii. ____________________
5. AMT Certification Requirements for Applicants
   A. Be of good ________ character.
   B. Graduate must have graduated from an ____________ program/organization.
   C. Applicant must have completed a minimum of ______ clock-hours or ________.
6. General Medical Assisting Knowledge
   i. ____________________
   ii. ____________________
   iii. ____________________
   iv. ____________________
   v. ____________________
   vi. ____________________

7. National Center for Competency Testing
   A. Issues the ______________________________ credential.
   B. Candidate must be a ___________ graduate and have completed an _______ program or provide documentation of 2 years of _______ experience.
   C. Continuation of certification requires ________ hours per year of continuing education.

8. National Certified Medical Office Assistant
   A. Offered by the ____.
   B. To qualify a candidate must have a __________ diploma and must have completed a medical assisting program.
   C. Those who are not graduates of a MA program but are able to provide documentation of _____ years experience working as an MA are eligible to sit for the NCMA exam.

9. National Healthcareer Association
   A. Founded in the year ___________.
   B. Grants the following two credentials: ___________________, _________________.
   C. Qualified applicants must pass a _____________ examination.

KEY TERMINOLOGY REVIEW

Complete the sentences below using the correct key terms found at the beginning of the chapter.

1. One of Juan's greatest qualities as a medical assistant was his ability to show ____________________ to his patients at the oncology clinic where he was employed.
2. The ___________________________________ was previously known as the Kansas Medical Assistant Society.
3. ______________ is the process in which an institution voluntarily completes a process of determining whether or not their school meets or exceeds standards set forth by an accrediting body.
4. Malcolm was scheduled to take a Medical Assistant Review class that would prepare him to enter his ____________________; which was necessary to complete his medical assistant training.
5. Someone with __________ is honest, dependable, dedicated to high standards, and adheres to a code of values.
6. ______________ is the issuance by an official body or professional organization of a certificate and credentials to one who has met the education and experience standards of the organization.
7. ___________________ provides oversight for the registration and testing of medical assistants, medical technologists, and phlebotomists.
8. _________________ is awarded to candidates who pass the AMT certification examination.
9. After becoming certified as an RMA and acquiring additional administrative experience, a medical assistant can apply for the ______________________ credential.
10. Credential issued by the National Center for Competency Testing is the _________________.

APPLIED PRACTICE

Give two examples of each positive quality that a medical assistant should possess.

Quality	Example
Integrity	
Empathy	
Discretion	
Confidentiality	
Thoroughness	
Punctuality	
Congeniality	
Proactivity	
Competence	
Appearance	

LEARNING ACTIVITY: TRUE/FALSE

Indicate whether the following statements are true or false by placing a T or an F on the line that precedes each statement.

_______ 1. Historically, medical assistants were trained on the job by physicians.

_______ 2. An externship is typically a paid position for a period of 160 hours.

_______ 3. A medical assistant can only call him- or herself a nurse if certified by either an ABHES- or a CAAHEP-accredited medical assisting program.

_______ 4. Membership in the AAMA is not necessary to take the certification examination.

_______ 5. For the MA credential to remain current, it must be revalidated every 3 years.

_______ 6. The RMT is a nonprofit certifying body.

_______ 7. Entry-level medical assistants may find work as office managers, medical records managers, hospital unit secretaries, and instructors for medical assistant programs.

_______ 8. A rehabilitation center provides care to patients who need immediate medical treatment.

_______ 9. If you witness behaviors that are unsafe to workers, you must notify OSHA.

_______ 10. As a medical assistant, it is a crime to perform procedures that only nurses or physicians are licensed to do.

CRITICAL THINKING

Answer the following questions to the best of your ability. Utilize the textbook as a reference.

1. Sara Dunn is taking an administrative medical assisting class as part of her training toward earning a medical assisting certificate. She has been assigned the task of writing a paper that outlines the history of medical assisting. Part of the assignment is to include the milestones reached by this profession over the past 50 years. How should Sara outline this paper?

2. Diane Luder, CMA (AAMA), has been working as an administrative medical assistant in a busy pediatric office for 5 years. Diane's job has been in the billing and coding department. Helga, a colleague of Diane's in the billing and coding department, tells Diane about the benefits of joining a professional organization of coders. How might Diane benefit from joining such a group?

RESEARCH ACTIVITY

Utilize Internet search engines to research the following topics and write a brief description of what is found. It is important to utilize reputable websites.

1. Research your state and local chapters of the American Association of Medical Assistants. What information is available? When and where are meetings located? If a chapter does not exist in your area, what are the requirements for starting a chapter?

CHAPTER 2

Medical Science: History and Practice

CHAPTER OUTLINE

General review of the chapter:

History of Medicine
Medical Practitioners
Medical Practice Acts
Health Care Costs and Payments
Types of Medical Practices
Medical and Surgical Specialties
Health Care Institutions
Allied Health Professionals
Centers for Disease Control and Prevention (CDC)

STUDENT STUDY GUIDE

Use the following guide to assist in your learning of the concepts from the chapter.

I. The History of Medicine

1. Code of Hammurabi
   A. Used by ____________ physicians in 3000 B.C.
   B. Laws related to the ________________.
   C. Hammurabi was ___________________________.
2. Early Contributions
   A. Personal hygiene, the sanitary preparation of food, and other matters of public health were pioneered by the practices of the ________ culture.
   B. Some records of early ________ practitioners depict them using nonpoisonous snakes to treat the wounds of patients.
3. The Caduceus
   A. The Caduceus is the recognized symbol for _____________.
4. Other Early Contributions to Medicine
   A. Herbal medical remedies originating from ancient ____________ are recorded as early as 800 B.C.
   B. The _______ culture wrote about human blood pulses around the time of 250 B.C.
5. Early Medicinal Remedies Still Used Today
   A. ______________ used to treat heart patients.
   B. ______________ from the foxglove plant to regulate and strengthen the heartbeat.
   C. ______________ to treat urinary tract infections.

6. Fifth Century to 16th Century

   A. During this time frame ____________ progress was made in medical practices.
   B. ____________ epidemics occurred during this medieval period.
   C. Wealthy individuals were treated by surgeons, others were treated by ______________.

7. Hippocrates

   A. Known as the ________________________________.
   B. Shifted medicine from ___________ to science.
   C. Stressed the body's ____________ nature.

8. The Hippocratic Oath

   A. The oath serves as a widely used __________ guide for physicians.
   B. When taking the oath, physicians pledge to work for the _____ of patients, to __________ no deadly drugs, and to do no __________ to patients.

9. Galen

   A. Stressed the value of _______________.
   B. Founded _________________________.
   C. Known as the ____________________.

10. Other Influential Individuals of Early Medicine

    A. ___________ was the first individual to use a telescope to study the skies, leading to the invention of the microscope.
    B. John Hunter is known as the Founder of _________________________.
    C. The first individual to perform the first vaccination using the smallpox vaccine was ______________.

11. Advancements made in Medicine During the 19th Century

    A. Discovered that certain diseases and wound infections were caused by ______________.
    B. Use of _________ microscopes.
    C. Improved knowledge of the _________ body through accurate documentation.

12. Influential Individuals in Medicine During the 19th Century

    A. ____________ established the science of bacteriology.
    B. Joseph Lister introduced the _____________ system in surgery.
    C. ___________ traced the cause of puerperal sepsis.
    D. One of the original "microbe hunters" was ______________.

13. Other Major Advancements During the 19th Century

    A. ___________ discovered x-rays.
    B. The discovery of radium by ____________ and ____________.
    C. ________________ worked in the field of psychiatry.

14. Contributions from Americans in the 19th Century

    A. Both __________ and ________ discovered the use of ether.
    B. ___________ helped to conquer yellow fever.

15. Influential Women in Medicine

    A. ____________ is known as the founder of modern nursing.
    B. ____________ established the American Red Cross.

II. The Practice of Medicine

1. Title of Doctor

   A. Designates a person who holds a ___________ degree.
   B. Practicing medicine requires a minimum of _________ years of education and training.

2. Doctor of Osteopathy
   A. Learns the skill of ___________ therapy.
   B. Places greater emphasis on the relationship between the _____________ and the _____________.
   C. Attends school of __________.
3. Medical Practice Acts
   A. Indicates who must be _________ to perform certain procedures.
   B. Designates reports that must be made to the ________________.
   C. Denotes ________ associated with a license.
4. Ways a Medical License May Be Granted
   i. ______________________________
   ii. ______________________________
   iii. ______________________________
5. Causes for Suspension or Revoking of a Medical License
   i. ______________________________
   ii. ______________________________
   iii. ______________________________
6. Types of Medical Practices
   i. ______________________________
   ii. ______________________________
   iii. ______________________________
   iv. ______________________________
   v. ______________________________
   vi. ______________________________
7. Categories of Hospitals
   i. ______________________________
   ii. ______________________________
   iii. ______________________________
   iv. ______________________________
8. Outpatient Surgical Centers
   A. Facility where __________ procedures are performed.
   B. Also known as ________________ surgical centers.
   C. Surgeries typically require __________ recovery time.
9. Urgent Care Centers
   A. Offer quick care for non-________ situations.
   B. In some managed care systems, these centers may be designated as a _____________ facility.
10. Types of Long-Term Care Institutions
   i. ______________________________
   ii. ______________________________
   iii. ______________________________
   iv. ______________________________
11. Hospice
   A. Emphasizes improved quality of care for the ________________.
   B. Most hospice care is provided at ________________.
12. National Health Care Skill Standards
   A. Developed to define the body of knowledge and _______ _______ health care workers should possess for entry-level and technical-level positions.

B. ________ standards are used by schools, colleges, and health care facilities to establish curriculum and competencies.
C. ________ cluster careers include those that involve the health care status of the patient.

13. Diagnostic Career Cluster
    A. Careers that involve _________, ____________, and reporting patient information.
    B. Laboratory technicians are skilled in ________ blood, urine, lymph, and body tissue.
    C. Phlebotomists are skilled in _______ blood.
14. Information Services Career Cluster
    A. Careers involved with ____________ patient information.
    B. Health information technologists _________ the permanent records relating to patient's condition and treatment.
    C. The job that entails being responsible for clerical duties and other communications duties in hospitals are those of a __________.
15. Environmental Services Career Cluster
    A. Careers involved with the patient's ______ _______ environment.
    B. Career examples in this cluster include ____________, ______________, ___________, and ____________.
16. Centers for Disease Control and Prevention (CDC)
    A. Division of the ________________________.
    B. Purpose is to safeguard public health by ___________ and __________ disease.
    C. Act as a resource for the ___________ ___________.

KEY TERMINOLOGY REVIEW

Complete the sentences below using the correct key terms found at the beginning of the chapter.

1. The medical specialty __________ treats patients who are obese.
2. ____________ is a medical specialty that treats abnormal responses to acquired hypersensitivity to substances with medical methods, including testing and desensitization.
3. ___________ shows that an individual has met the educational/experience standards in their profession.
4. Malcolm is dying of cancer and is now receiving ________ care.
5. A disease that affects many people in different countries at the same time is called a _________.
6. __________ provides proof that the individual has been authorized by a government agency to perform work in their profession.
7. To numb the pain, Dr. Antolik gave his patient local ________________ prior to the removal of an in-grown toenail.
8. Mrs. Krichko took her anatomy and physiology class to the local morgue to view a ________________ and witness its dissection for pathological study.
9. Rates of disease or illness are called ______________.
10. _________________________ is a hospital payment system that classifies each Medicare patient according to his or her illness.

APPLIED PRACTICE

Match the early contributor of medicine with his or her accomplishment.

a. Hippocrates

b. Galen

c. Laennec

d. Franklin

e. Koch

f. Leeuwenhoek

g. Fleming

h. Salk

i. Semmelweiss

j. Blackwell

1. ______________ Discovered that colds could be passed from one person to another.
2. ______________ First to study bacteria and protozoa using a microscope.
3. ______________ His experiment with hand washing reduced the death rate of women who delivered babies in hospitals.
4. ______________ He practiced and taught medicine on the island of Kos, Greece. He is known as the "Father of Medicine."
5. ______________ Discovered penicillin.
6. ______________ Invented the stethoscope.
7. ______________ Discovered the cause of tuberculosis.
8. ______________ Developed vaccines.
9. ______________ Founded experimental physiology.
10. ______________ First female physician in the United States.

LEARNING ACTIVITY: TRUE/FALSE

Indicate whether the following statements are true or false by placing a T or an F on the line that precedes each statement.

_______ 1. The Hippocratic Oath is no longer used, but it was around for nearly 2,000 years.

_______ 2. During the early part of the 20th century, the main form of medical practice was solo practice.

_______ 3. In a partnership practice, each partner is responsible for the actions of all partners.

_______ 4. Many early and historic plant remedies are still used today for heart conditions, indigestion, bleeding, and urinary tract infections.

_______ 5. An associate practice consists of three or more physicians who share the same facility and practice medicine together.

_______ 6. A group practice is managed by a board of directors.

_______ 7. A technician typically has an associate's degree from a 2-year community college or vocational program.

_______ 8. Registered nurses have more training than nurse practitioners.

_______ 9. Physical therapists develop programs that help restore the patient's ability to manage the activities of daily living.

_______ 10. In nearly every state, a physician's assistant can prescribe medications.

CRITICAL THINKING

Answer the following questions to the best of your ability. Utilize the textbook as a reference.

1. Michelle Manwiller, CMA (AAMA), is working with Harold Chan, a 55-year-old patient. Mr. Chan tells Michelle that he would like to try Chinese medicine treatments instead of taking the

medication the physician has prescribed. He asks Michelle if she is familiar with the philosophy behind Chinese medicine. How might Michelle answer?

2. Robert Bautista is taking an administrative medical assisting course as part of his training to earn a certificate in medical assisting. He has been asked to write a paragraph outlining the contributions the Greek physician Galen made to medicine. Robert has been told to include the reasons why Galen's findings were not completely accurate. What could Robert write on this topic?

3. Willie Harrison is creating a presentation for a history class he is enrolled in. Since he is in a medical assisting program, he wants his history paper to revolve around a medical topic. Willie has chosen to write about the history of the use of anesthesia in medicine. How should he start his outline for this presentation?

4. Marian Reiman, CMA (AAMA), is teaching a night class to medical assisting students. Marian wants to lecture on the different types of hospitals that currently exist in the United States. What are the four categories of hospitals she should talk about and how should Marian describe one of these categories?

RESEARCH ACTIVITY

Utilize Internet search engines to research the following topics and write a brief description of what is found. It is important to utilize reputable websites.

1. Using the Internet, choose and research one of the early contributors to medicine and write a two- to three-paragraph summary regarding your findings.

Chapter 3
Medical Law and Ethics

CHAPTER OUTLINE

General review of the chapter:

Classification of the Law
Professional Liability
Patient and Physician Relationship
Documentation
Public Duties of Physicians
Drug Regulations
Role of the Medical Assistant
Code of Ethics
Medical Ethics
Medical Assistant's Principles of Medical Ethics
Medical Assistant's Standard of Care
The Patient's Bill of Rights
HIPAA and Confidentiality
Ethical Issues and Personal Choice

STUDENT STUDY GUIDE

Fill in the study guide below using both your textbook and notes from your instructor's lecture.

I. Law and Liability

1. Classification of Law

A. ____________ law is made to protect the public as a whole from the harmful acts of others.
B. ____________ law concerns relationships between individuals or between individuals and the government.
C. ____________ law is concerned with a breach or neglect of an understanding between two parties.

2. Civil Law

A. ____________ law falls under civil law and covers acts that result in harm to another.
B. ____________ occurs when the patient is injured as a result of the health care professional not exercising the ordinary standard of care.
C. When an individual is being threatened with imminent bodily harm, the person doing the act could be charged with ____________.
D. A violation of the personal liberty of another person through unlawful restraint is known as ____________ ____________.

3. The Four Ds of Unintentional Torts

i. ____
ii. ____

iii. ______________________________
iv. ______________________________

4. Laws Governing Collection
   i. ______________________________
   ii. ______________________________
   iii. ______________________________
   iv. ______________________________
   v. ______________________________

5. Standard of Care
   A. Asserts that the physician must provide the same ________, ________, and ______ that a similarly trained physician would provide under the same circumstances in the same locality.
   B. Physicians are expected to perform the same acts that ____________ and ___________ physicians would perform.
   C. If the physician violates the standard of care he or she is liable for __________.

II. Patient–Physician Relationship

1. Physician Rights
   A. Both the physician and the patient must agree to ____________ if there is to be a contract for service and treatment. The patient must confide ___________ to the physician in order to receive proper treatment.
   B. Physicians have the right to __________ payment for the treatment given.

2. Patient Rights
   i. ______________________________
   ii. ______________________________
   iii. ______________________________
   iv. ______________________________

3. Patient Obligations
   i. ______________________________
   ii. ______________________________
   iii. ______________________________

4. Common Exceptions to Informed Consent
   A. A physician does not have to inform a patient about risks that are __________ known.
   B. If the physician feels that the disclosure of risks may be __________ to the patient, then he or she is not responsible for disclosing them.
   C. If the patient requests that the physician __________ disclose the risks.

5. Categories of Minors Who Can Give Consent
   i. ______________________________
   ii. ______________________________

6. Legal Implications to Consider When Treating a Minor
   i. ______________________________
   ii. ______________________________
   iii. ______________________________

7. Durable Power of Attorney (DPOA)
   A. Allows an agent or ____________ to act on behalf of the patient.
   B. Agent may be a ________, __________, ________, or an _________.
   C. Used when a patient becomes physically or _________ ____________.

8. Uniform Anatomical Gift Act

   A. Allows a person ______ years or older and of sound mind to make a gift of any or all parts of his or her body for the purposes of organ transplantation or medical research.
   B. A physician who is not involved in the transplant will determine the ___________.
   C. No ______ is allowed to change hands for organ donations.

III. Documentation and Regulations

1. When a Medical Record Is Subpoenaed for Court

   A. Copy only the parts of the record that are __________.
   B. Send a ________ ______ unless the original record is subpoenaed.
   C. Place a _______ for the subpoenaed record in the patient's file.

2. Considerations for Testifying in Court

   i. ____
   ii. ____
   iii. ____
   iv. ____
   v. ____
   vi. ____

3. Childhood Vaccines and Toxoids Required by Law

   i. ____
   ii. ____
   iii. ____
   iv. ____
   v. ____
   vi. ____

4. Drug Regulation Agencies

   A. The ___________________ has jurisdiction over testing and approving drugs for public use.
   B. The ___________________ is a branch of the U.S. Department of Justice.
   C. The ___________________ regulates the sale and use of scheduled drugs.

5. Requirements for Controlled Substances

   A. Controlled drugs must be kept in a ___________ cabinet.
   B. Any theft must be immediately reported to both the regional _______ office and local police.
   C. Federal regulations require a _________ inventory of drug supplies.

6. Role of the Medical Assistant as Related to Controlled Substances

   A. Does not ________ controlled substances.
   B. Must be knowledgeable about the ___________ governing the documentation and control of drugs.
   C. Must always ________ any unusual patient behavior indicating addictive drug use.

7. MA's Role Related to Drug Administration

   A. May administer medication only under the ________ supervision of a physician.
   B. When preparing medications for administration, check the medication ________ times.
      i. ____
      ii. ____
      iii. ____

IV. Medical Ethics

1. Ethics and Medical Ethics

   A. Branch of philosophy related to ________ or _________ principles.
   B. Medical ethics refers to the _________ conduct of people in medical professions.
   C. The members of the medical profession set __________ and _________ for themselves.

2. Areas Covered in the AMA Principles of Medical Ethics
   i. ______
   ii. ______
   iii. ______
   iv. ______
   v. ______
3. Pledge Made Under the AAMA Code of Ethics
   A. Render service with full _____ for the _____ of humanity.
   B. Uphold the honor and high ____________ of the profession and accept its ____________.
   C. Seek to continually improve the __________ and ___________ of medical assistants for the benefit of patients and professional colleagues.
4. As a medical assistant, you are NOT expected to:
   i. ______
   ii. ______
   iii. ______
5. The Patient's Bill of Rights
   A. Developed by the ______.
   B. Describes the ______ relationship.
6. HIPAA
   A. Defined as the ______.
   B. Regulates the _________ of patient health information.

KEY TERMINOLOGY REVIEW

Write a sentence using the selected key terms in the correct context.

1. ***Defamation of character:***

______

______

2. ***Bioethics:***

______

______

3. ***Breach of contract:***

______

______

4. ***Contributory negligence:***

______

______

5. ***Informed consent:***

______

______

6. ***Living Will:***

______

______

7. *Practice of medicine:*

____

____

8. *Reasonable person standard:*

____

____

9. *Tort:*

____

____

10. *Statute of limitations:*

____

____

APPLIED PRACTICE

Provide answers to the following questions.

1. Considering the Latin terms discussed throughout the text, identify which of the Latin terms pertain to the situations below and then translate the term:

   A. A physician is sued because he amputates the wrong leg during surgery.

   ____

   ____

   B. Dr. Lin is being sued because his medical assistant injured a patient while suturing a 3-mm incision on the patient's lower leg, a procedure that is clearly outside the MA's scope of practice.

   ____

   ____

   C. Due to possible negligence by a physician, a child has been injured. When the case goes to court, an individual is appointed to represent the child.

   ____

   ____

LEARNING ACTIVITY: TRUE/FALSE

Indicate whether the following statements are true or false by placing a T or an F on the line that precedes each statement.

_______ 1. Although less serious in nature, misdemeanors may carry a punishment of jail time.

_______ 2. Tort law is an example of contract law.

_______ 3. Libel is the name for an oral defamatory statement.

_______ 4. In the case of unintentional tort, the plantiff must prove proximate cause.

_______ 5. It is harder to prevent negligence than it is to defend it.

_______ 6. Medical malpractice can include medical errors but every mistake or error is not considered malpractice.

_______ 7. Breach of contract can only occur when both parties fail to comply with the terms of the agreement.

_______ 8. Physicians have a duty to issue a legal certificate of death for natural and unnatural deaths.

_______ 9. Physicians have a duty to report all injuries of children.

_______ 10. The requirements of reporting elderly abuse vary by state.

CRITICAL THINKING

Answer the following questions to the best of your ability. Utilize the textbook as a reference.

1. Beth Clark is taking an administrative medical assisting course as part of her medical assisting training. She has been given the assignment of writing a paper that outlines the current ethical standpoints of the AMA. What points should Beth include?

____

____

____

____

2. Mary Alice Durfey, RMA is the administrative manager for Shepard Valley Out-Patient Surgery Clinic. She has been asked to create a checklist for surgeons that will cover the vital information of the Doctrine of Informed Consent. Surgeons will use this as they explain to patients the procedure or surgery that will be performed. What should Mary Alice include on this check list?

____

____

____

____

____

3. Create a medical malpractice scenario in which the statute of limitations defense would apply.

____

____

____

____

____

4. Create a scenario, different from the one listed in the textbook, in which a health care worker would utilize the Good Samaritan Act as a defense in a lawsuit.

____

____

____

____

____

RESEARCH ACTIVITY

Utilize Internet search engines to research the following topics and write a brief description of what is found. It is important to utilize reputable websites.

1. Using the Internet as a research source, search for a medical malpractice case. Describe the case you find and include whether the patient or the physician won the case. Did you feel the case was decided fairly? Why or why not?

CHAPTER 4
Medical Terminology

CHAPTER OUTLINE

General review of the chapter:

Word Parts
Grammar and Medical Terms
Gross Anatomy
Body Structure and Function
Surgical and Diagnostic Terms

STUDENT STUDY GUIDE

Fill in the study guide below using both your textbook and notes from your instructor's lecture.

I. Word Parts and Combining Forms

1. Words for Forming Medical Terms

A. Medical terms also will often contain prefixes and suffixes, both of which add further _____ to the given term. If a word root is used, to prepare the word root for combining with another part, a __________ is sometimes added.

2. Combining Vowels

A. If the suffix begins with a vowel, _____ the combining vowel from the combining form and _____ the suffix. If the suffix begins with a consonant, ***keep*** the combining vowel and _____ the suffix to the combining.

3. Prefix

A. A prefix is a word element that is placed _____, or is ______ to the beginning of the word root.

B. Prefixes are always placed at the _______ of words to alter or modify their meanings or to create new words.

4. Suffix

A. In medical terminology usage, a suffix is a word element that is affixed to the ________ of the word.

B. A suffix could be a _______ or group of ________ attached to the _____ of a word to alter or modify its meaning or to create a new word.

II. Anatomy and Physiology

1. Anatomical Position

A. Used when describing the _________ and __________ of a structure in the human body.

B. Describes the position of the body standing _______ with arms _______ of the body, palms facing _______, eyes looking ______ ahead.

C. Legs are _______ with feet and toes are pointing ______.

2. Body Planes (indicate the position of each of the body planes)

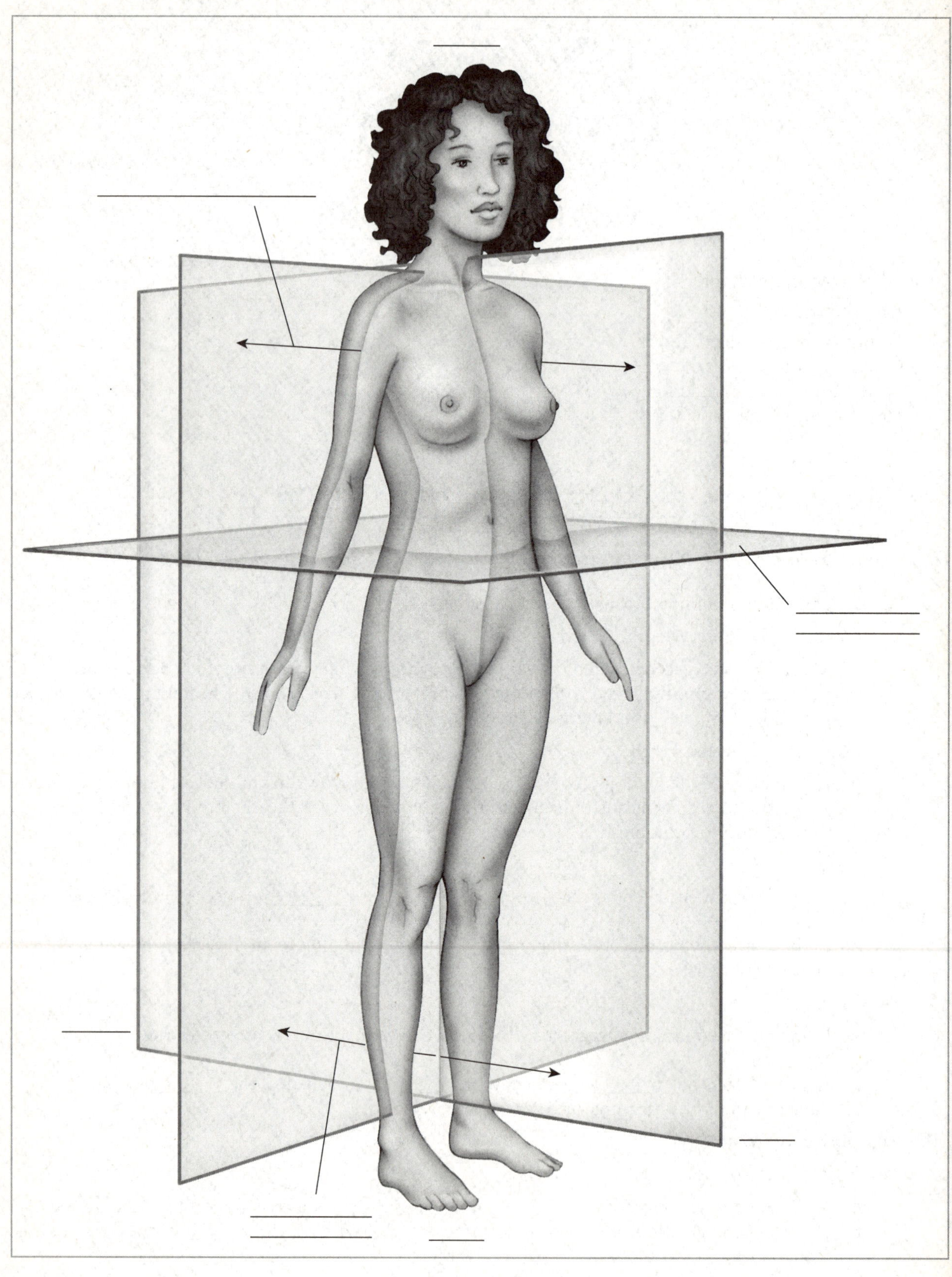

3. Terms for Describing Body Position (explain each)
    A. Superior or cephalic: ____________________
    B. Inferior or caudal: ____________________
    C. Anterior or ventral: ____________________
    D. Posterior or dorsal: ____________________
    E. Medial: ____________________
    F. Lateral: ____________________
    G. Apex: ____________________
    H. Base: ____________________
    I. Proximal: ____________________
    J. Distal: ____________________
    K. Superficial: ____________________
    L. Deep: ____________________
    M. Supine: ____________________
    N. Prone: ____________________

4. Positions
    A. One of the main tasks of the medical assistant is to ____________ the patient in the correct ________ for whatever procedure is to be performed.
    B. The vast majority of examinations require positioning patients on their ______________.
    C. For a pelvic examination, the ____________ position is used, with legs flexed in stirrups.
    D. For a proctological examination, the _________ position is favored.
    E. If a patient has low blood pressure, as is the case when a patient is in shock, the medical assistant should place the patient in the ______________ position.

5. Body Cavities (explain each)
    A. The body's __________ are contained in cavities.
    B. The cranial cavity houses the _________.
    C. The chest, or _______, cavity holds the lungs and heart.
    D. Under the diaphragm, the ____________ cavity holds other vital organs including the intestines, stomach, reproductive organs.

6. Anatomical Divisions of the Abdomen (on the figure provided label each region of the abdomen)

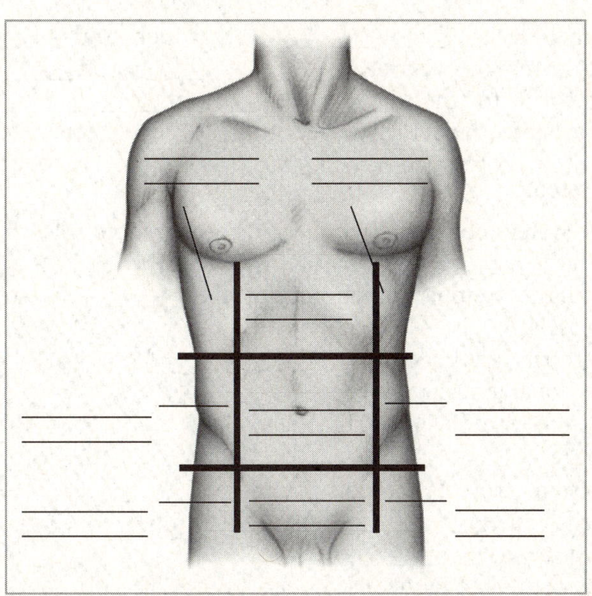

7. The Integumentary System

   A. The integumentary system includes various parts that aid in the protection, exchange of heat and fluids, and absorption. List these components:

      i. ______________________________
      ii. ______________________________
      iii. ______________________________
      iv. ______________________________
      v. ______________________________
      vi. ______________________________

8. The Skeletal System

   A. The skeletal system consists of bones that are used to store ___________, to give the body height and movement, and to __________ and __________ the body organs.
   B. The combining form for bone is __________.
   C. –clast is the combining form for ___________.
   D. cost/o is the combining form for ___________.
   E. Physician specializing in (straightening) bones is an ___________.

9. The Muscular System

   A. Muscles aid bones in _____________.
   B. The combining forms for muscles are ___________ and ___________.
   C. The word part –trophy means _________________.
   D. tax/o is the combining form for _________________.
   E. A medical assistant or physician may perform _____________ activities to assess a muscle's ability to extend, flex, or rotate as necessary.

10. The Nervous System

   A. The nervous system helps the body to sense changes in the __________ and __________ environments.
   B. Pain is referred to with the suffixes __________ and __________.
   C. A frequently used medication that reduces pain is referred to as an __________.
   D. Pain in the diaphragm is known as __________.
   E. *cephal/o* means the __________, and *encephal/o* is ___________.

11. Special Senses

   A. Special senses include ________, ______, taste, touch, and _______.
   B. The combining forms for eye are _______, _______, and _______.
   C. The combining forms for the ear are ________ and ________.
   D. __________ measures the acuity of hearing.

12. The Circulatory System

   A. The circulatory system consists of the heart, the blood vessels, the blood, and the structures that make up the _____________ system.
   B. The cardiovascular system is a subsystem of the _________ system and is comprised of the heart and its vessels.
   C. The combining form for the heart is ________.
   D. Fatty plaque in the arteries is referred to as ________.

13. The Immune System

   A. The immune system protects the body from __________.
   B. White blood cells called __________ defend the body.
   C. Word part bas/o means ___________.
   D. The combining form –phage means ________.

14. The Respiratory System

    A. The respiratory system exchanges oxygen (O_2) in the environment for _______ in the body.
    B. The main organs of respiration are the __________.
    C. A specialist in the respiratory system is a ____________.
    D. __________ is a combining form that means "lung."

15. The Digestive System

    A. The digestive system either _______ or _____ food and drugs for the body.
    B. The ______________ is another term for the mouth.
    C. Key organs of this system are the __________ and __________.
    D. A physician with specialized training in the digestive system is a ____________.

16. The Urinary System

    A. The urinary system rids the body of the toxic byproducts of __________.
    B. The combining form for the kidney is _________.
    C. A physician with specialized training related to the kidney is a _________.
    D. The _______ go toward the bladder, and the ________ goes toward the outside of the body.

17. The Endocrine System

    A. The endocrine system is the ductless glandular system that controls other body systems by secreting _______ within the bloodstream.
    B. *Endo*- means _______ and –*crine* means _______.
    C. The _________ is the master gland of this system.
    D. The word part estr/o means _________.

18. The Reproductive System

    A. The reproductive system aids in reproducing _________.
    B. The physician with specialized training in women's health is a ___________.
    C. The combining forms for the uterus are ______ and _____.
    D. A common abbreviation related to the male reproductive system is ____________.

19. Surgical and Diagnostic Terms (define each of the following word parts)

    A. –graphy: ____________________
    B. –scopy: ____________________
    C. –tome: ____________________
    D. –stomy: ____________________
    E. –tomy: ____________________

KEY TERMINOLOGY REVIEW

Write a sentence using each of the word parts listed. Note the word part by underlining it in your sentence.

1. ***combining form:***

____

____

2. ***combining vowel:***

____

____

3. ***prefix:***

____

____

4. *suffix:*

____

____

5. *word root:*

____

____

APPLIED PRACTICE

For each of the following rules related to forming plurals, write a sentence without the use of the plural ending and then rewrite the sentence using the word with a plural ending.

1. Words ending in *on* will drop *on* and add *a*.

____

____

2. Words ending in *us* will drop *us* and add *I*.

____

____

3. Words ending in *um* will drop *um* and add *a*.

____

____

4. Words ending in *y* will drop *y* and add *ies*.

____

____

5. Words ending in *nx* will change the *x* to *g* and add *es*.

____

____

LEARNING ACTIVITY: TRUE/FALSE

Indicate whether the following statements are true or false by placing a T or an F on the line that precedes each statement.

______ 1. When identifying medical words, if the suffix begins with a consonant, drop the combining vowel from the combining form and add the suffix.

______ 2. The abbreviation for anterioposterior is AP.

______ 3. The root word *ankyl* means stiff or bent.

______ 4. The combining form for vein would be *vein/o*.

______ 5. The prefix *de* means through or apart.

______ 6. Prefixes used in medical terminology have only one meaning.

______ 7. The suffix *drome* means to lead or pull.

______ 8. In a court of law, misspelling and improperly used medical terminology can imply sloppy patient care.

______ 9. The frontal plane divides the body and its parts into left and right positions.

______ 10. The transverse plane is a crosswise plane that runs parallel to the ground.

CRITICAL THINKING

Answer the following questions to the best of your ability. Utilize the textbook as a reference.

1. Andrea Natal has been working as an MA for Dr. Smith for about a month. Andrea has just finished assisting with a patient examination. As Dr. Smith leaves the examination room, he hands Andrea the patient's chart and indicates that he has written down some instructions that need to be given to the patient. After the physician leaves the room, Andrea looks at the patient's chart and discovers that she is unable to decipher some of the information. What should Andrea say to the patient and do to ensure that the patient receives the correct information? What should Andrea not do?

____

____

____

____

____

____

____

____

RESEARCH ACTIVITY

Utilize Internet search engines to research the following topics and write a brief description of what you find. It is important to utilize reputable websites.

1. Select one of the organs of the body described in your textbook. Using your school's library and/or information obtained on the Internet, conduct research on the various conditions that can occur in that system. Prepare a one- to two-page paper on what you learned about the system and the conditions that can occur within the system. Be sure to cite your sources at the end of your paper.

____

____

____

____

____

____

____

____

____

____

____

Chapter 5
Communication: Verbal and Nonverbal

CHAPTER OUTLINE

General review of the chapter:

Interpersonal Dynamics
The Communication Process
Verbal and Nonverbal Communication
Communication Techniques
Assertive versus Aggressive Behavior
Barriers to Communication
Communication in Special Circumstances
Intraoffice Communication
Staff Arrangements
Communication and Patients' Rights

STUDENT STUDY GUIDE

Use the following guide to assist in your learning of the concepts from the chapter.

I. The Communication Process

1. The Holistic Approach to Medicine
   - A. Means caring for the ________ patient.
   - B. Addresses the social, ___________, and ___________ needs, as well as the physical treatment of the patient.
   - C. Means treating everyone with _________ and _________.

2. Importance of Self-Awarenss
   - A. Leads to more effective _______________.
   - B. Terms to self-awareness include:
     - i. ______________________________
     - ii. ______________________________
     - iii. ______________________________
     - iv. ______________________________
     - v. ______________________________

3. The Learning Styles of Our Patients (list and explain each)
   - i. ______________________________
   - ii. ______________________________
   - iii. ______________________________

4. Units of the Communication Process (Fill in the blanks)

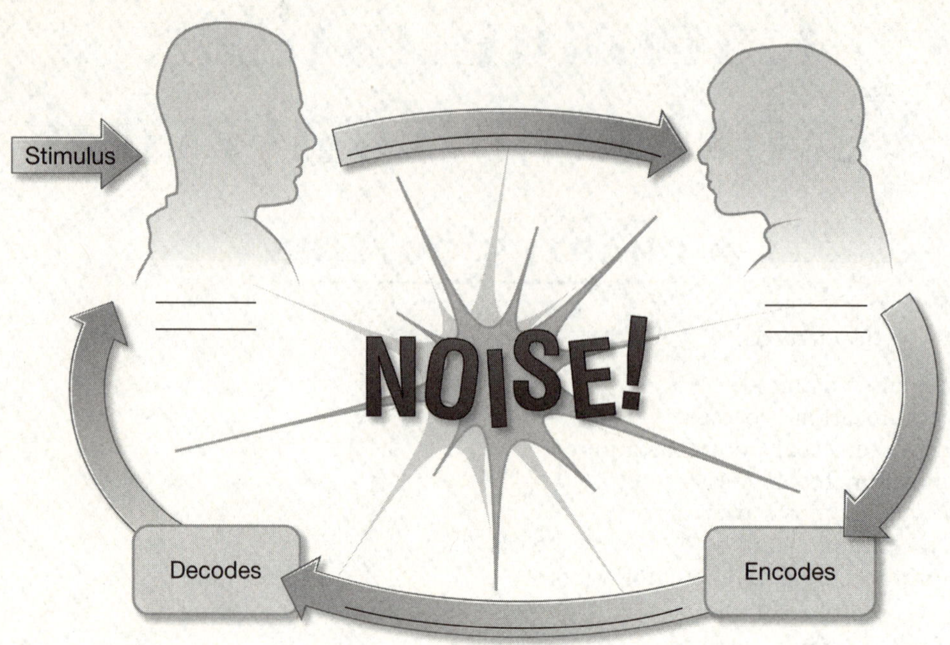

5. Factors Affecting Verbal Communication
   i. ____________________
   ii. ____________________
   iii. ____________________
   iv. ____________________
   v. ____________________
   vi. ____________________

6. Factors in Nonverbal Communication
   i. ____________________
   ii. ____________________
   iii. ____________________
   iv. ____________________
   v. ____________________
   vi. ____________________

II. Communication Techniques

1. Considerations When Communicating
   A. __________ of the communication.
   B. __________ to be given.
   C. __________ skills to be used.
   D. __________ clarification and feedback.
   E. __________ if goal was met.

2. Barriers to Communication
   i. ____________________
   ii. ____________________
   iii. ____________________

iv. ______
v. ______
vi. ______
vii. ______
viii. ______
ix. ______

3. Avoiding Prejudging and Stereotyping (list the ways to avoid)
   i. ______
   ii. ______
   iii. ______
   iv. ______
   v. ______
   vi. ______

III. Communicating with Patients and Staff

1. Fears that Can Cause Patient Anger
   i. ______
   ii. ______
   iii. ______
   iv. ______

2. The "White Coat" Syndrome
   A. Patients who are fearful of anyone in a ______ ______.
   B. Patients with this syndrome experience ______ ______.

3. Methods for Communicating with Anxious Patients
   i. ______
   ii. ______
   iii. ______
   iv. ______
   v. ______

4. Communicating with the Mentally Ill
   A. Determine the level of ______ that is possible.
   B. Speak ______ and ______.
   C. Keep messages ______.

5. Steps for Addressing Conflict
   A. Communicate your needs in ______ terms.
   B. Know when to express your ______.
   C. Do not ______ you know the other person's feelings.
   D. Look at the issue from the other person's ______.

6. Elements of Critical Thinking
   A. ______ questions.
   B. ______ the problem.
   C. ______ the evidence.
   D. ______ emotional reasoning.
   E. ______ assumptions and bias.
   F. ______ oversimplification.
   G. ______ other interpretations.
   H. ______ ambiguity.
   I. ______ about one's own thinking.

7. Staff Meetings
   A. Should be _________ scheduled.
   B. The success of staff meetings is due to:
      i. Presence of an _________.
      ii. Adhering to _________ and _________ times.
      iii. Avoiding _________ sessions.

IV. Patient Education

1. HIPAA Privacy Rule
   A. Protects _________ ___________.
   B. Allows patients to have better access to _________ _________.
   C. Provides patients with _______ control over who can release medical information and how it will be done.

2. The MA's Role in Advising Patients
   A. ___________ empathetically and establish rapport.
   B. Ask __________ or _________ questions.
   C. ___________ the information the physician has related to the patient.
   D. Keep all matters related to the patient's personal health information ___________.

KEY TERMINOLOGY REVIEW

Choose the term that best represents each statement below.

a. kinesthetic
b. active listening
c. risk management
d. close-ended question
e. character
f. empathy
g. leading questions
h. feedback
i. values
j. open-ended question
k. bias
l. prejudice
m. ethnocentric
n. passive listening
o. stereotyping
p. sympathy

1. _____________ Identification with another person's feelings.
2. _____________ Questions that contain part of the answer.
3. _____________ Unfair preference or dislike of something.
4. _____________ Involves completely paying attention to the speaker, concentrating on the verbal message, watching for nonverbal cues, and offering a response.
5. _____________ Feeling sorry for or pitying someone.
6. _____________ "Do you have a headache?"
7. _____________ A set of standards a person uses to measure the worth or importance of someone or something.
8. _____________ An opinion that is based on race, gender, or economic status.
9. _____________ Refers to planning and implementing strategies for reducing the physician's risk of a lawsuit in the medical setting.
10. _____________ The sum of the values, attitudes, and behaviors.
11. _____________ The belief which some individuals have that their cultural background is better than any other.

12. ______________ "Can you describe your headache?"
13. ______________ Listening to someone without offering a reply.
14. ______________ Learner assimilates knowledge better through hands-on activities.
15. ______________ A preformed and unfavorable belief or attitude toward a certain culture or group with little or no information about the culture or group.
16. ______________ Information that is reflected in an interpersonal exchange.

APPLIED PRACTICE

1. *Without using the examples in the textbook, for each of the following defensive behaviors provide your own example of how a patient may exhibit this behavior.*
   i. Compensation
   ____
   ____
   ii. Denial
   ____
   ____
   iii. Displaced anger
   ____
   ____
   iv. Introjection
   ____
   ____
   v. Projection
   ____
   ____
   vi. Rationalization
   ____
   ____
   vii. Regression
   ____
   ____
   viii. Repression
   ____
   ____
   ix. Sublimation
   ____
   ____

2. A patient has arrived at the office for a yearly physical. After reviewing the steps for listening to obtain a patient's chief complaint, write a script that outlines your interactions with the patient and how the steps illustrate your understanding of how to demonstrate effective listening skills when obtaining the patient's chief complaint.
____
____

LEARNING ACTIVITY: MULTIPLE CHOICE

Circle the correct answer to each of the questions below.

1. Assertive behavior:
   a. Is imposing one's viewpoint on another.
   b. Can result in resentment by others.
   c. Is trusting one's own ideas or instincts.
   d. All of the above.

2. Which of the following would be an open-ended question?
   a. Mrs. Knight, would you explain to me how you are feeling today?
   b. Mrs. Knight, how are you feeling today?
   c. Mrs. Knight, do you need help?
   d. None of the above.

3. Which of the following would be a barrier to communication?
   a. Eye contact
   b. Use of meaningful statements
   c. Noise
   d. None of the above

4. An example of a probing question would include:
   a. "You say your head hurts?"
   b. "Where on your head do you feel pain?"
   c. "Do you have pain anywhere else?"
   d. All of the above.

5. Mr. Marlon Jones has come to the office due to an ear infection. Which of the following would be an example of the use of reflecting to ensure good communication?
   a. Mr. Jones states that he hurts. You ask him where it hurts.
   b. Mr. Jones states that he is feeling very scared. You ask him what he is scared about.
   c. Mr. Jones states that he has recently been feeling very tired. You repeat back to him that recently he has been feeling very tired.
   d. Any of the above.

CRITICAL THINKING

Answer the following questions to the best of your ability. Utilize the textbook as a reference.

1. Mrs. Jean Smith has come into the office to address a concern that she has. How can you make sure that you are actively listening to what Mrs. Smith is saying?

____

____

____

____

____

2. A patient has just walked into the office and begins to yell at the front desk medical assistant about the bill. Consider and outline the methods that the MA should use to communicate with the angry patient.

____

____

____

____

____

3. A hearing-impaired patient has come into the office. What methods might you use to communicate with this patient?

____

____

____

____

____

4. Now consider a visually impaired patient. What methods might you use to communicate with this patient?

____

____

____

5. As an MA, you may encounter patients who are terminally ill. What skills might you employ when communicating with a terminally ill patient?

6. Write a scenario (either real or imagined) where a problem occurs with a patient or staff member and the steps that you would take to solve the problem. If you choose to describe a real-life situation, you do not have to use real names or any personal information.

RESEARCH ACTIVITY

Utilize Internet search engines to research the following topics. It is important to utilize reputable websites.

1. Use the Internet to find information regarding the aspects of a professional, well-developed policy and procedures manual. Answer the following questions:
   a. What website would you recommend to an office manager that may help guide him or her in the development of the manual?
   b. What did you learn from your research about what makes a successful policy and procedures manual?

Chapter 6
The Office Environment

CHAPTER OUTLINE

General review of the chapter:

General Safety Measures
Employee Safety
Proper Body Mechanics
Office Security
Quality Medical Care
What Is Quality Assurance?

STUDENT STUDY GUIDE

Use the following guide to assist in your learning of the concepts from the chapter.

I. Safety in the Medical Office

1. Occupational Safety and Health Administration
   A. Concerned with any ___________ hazard.
   B. Sets __________ standards for workplaces.
   C. ___________ are levied against employers who fail to comply with regulations.
2. General Safety Guidelines
   A. ____________, don't run, during an emergency.
   B. Walk on the ______________ side of the hallway.
   C. Use ____________ when using stairways.
   D. Never carry _______________ syringes or sharp objects.
   E. Report _____________ any unsafe conditions.
   F. Use different _____________ for lab specimens and medications.
   G. Store ____________ substances in locked cabinets.
3. Disasters in a Medical Office
   i. ______________________________
   ii. ______________________________
   iii. ______________________________
   iv. ______________________________
   v. ______________________________
   vi. ______________________________
4. Disaster Plan in the Medical Office
   A. All employee training on the disaster plan must be ___________ to demonstrate OSHA compliance.
   B. Further regulations are required for sites with ___________ equipment.
   C. All employees must be ___________ on the steps to follow in any emergency.

5. Guidelines for Fire Safety
   A. Floor plans should indicate ___________, _____________, and __________.
   B. Portable ____________ fire extinguishers should be placed no more than _________ feet from any employee area.
   C. Fire drills should be conducted at least ____________.
   D. ___________ cabinets should be used to protect records.
   E. Emergency numbers should be placed in ____________ areas.
6. Steps for Handling a Fire
   i. ______________________________
   ii. ______________________________
   iii. ______________________________
   iv. ______________________________
   v. ______________________________
   vi. ______________________________
   vii. ______________________________
7. Necessary Items in Case of a Fire
   A. Fire extinguishers with proper documentation of ____________________.
   B. Clearly marked ___________ and ___________ that are free of debris.
   C. _______ of all exits.
8. Guidelines for Electrical Safety
   A. All equipment should be ___________.
   B. ___________ protectors should be used for all electronic equipment.
   C. Use of ___________ outlets for "wet" areas.
9. Material Safety Data Sheets
   A. Written materials on ______________ chemicals.
   B. Provides information on the ___________ of the ___________ and what to do in order to be protected.
   C. Must be filed in a _____________ binder.
10. Types of Medical Waste
    i. ______________________________
    ii. ______________________________
    iii. ______________________________
    iv. ______________________________
11. Exposure Control Plan
    A. A written document required by ____________.
    B. Assists in _____________ employee exposure to infectious materials.
    C. Reviewed by all employees, with _____________ kept for ___________ years after termination of employment.
    D. Updated ____________.
12. Universal Precautions
    A. Issued by the ____.
    B. Treats all blood and body fluids as contaminated with ______________ pathogens.
    C. Emphasizes the use of a ______ ______ when infectious material has been spilled.
13. OSHA Guidelines Regarding the Use of PPE
    A. Employer must supply the PPE and provide __________ or ___________.
    B. PPE must be of a strength to act as a ___________ to infectious materials.
    C. _____________ gloves may not be reused.

D. Protective eye equipment must have ___________ sides to prevent infectious material from entering the area.
E. All PPE must be ___________ and placed in a ___________ container before leaving the office.

14. Guidelines for Housekeeping Department Personnel
    A. Must be ___________ trained.
    B. Housekeeping should only empty _________________, NOT _______________ and ___________ containers.

15. Housekeeping Guidelines for Medical Personnel
    A. Wear appropriate ___________.
    B. For wet spills, use prepared ______________ according to package directions.
    C. Immediately clean and disinfect contaminated surfaces with ___________ bleach/water solution after exposure to infectious materials.
    D. ______________ all surfaces on a regular schedule.
    E. Properly bag contaminated clothing and laundry in ___________, labeled biohazard bags.
    F. Have biohazardous waste removed by a ___________ waste disposal service.
    G. Use ___________, ___________, biohazardous sharps containers for all needles and sharps.
    H. Replace the sharps container when ___________ full.
    I. ___________ and ___________ the sharps container before placing with the biohazardous waste.
    J. Perform hand hygiene __________ and __________ using gloves.

16. Steps for Securing the Medical Office
    A. Ensure that doors and windows have ________ ________ .
    B. Provide only a few keys to ___________ personnel for opening and closing the office.
    C. Change ________ ________ if a key is missing.
    D. ___________ the electronic security system after the last person leaves the office.

17. Incident Reports
    A. Protect ___________ and ___________ against lawsuits.
    B. Must be written in ___________ ink.
    C. Should contain only ___________ information.

II. Quality Assurance

1. The AMA's Eight Essentials of Quality Care
    A. Emphasize ___________ detection and treatment.
    B. Encourage the patient's ______________ in the decision-making process regarding his or her treatment.
    C. Demonstrate ___________ for the patient and the patient's family.
    D. Achieve the ___________ goal through the wise use of technology and other resources.
    E. Provide adequate _____________ in the patient's medical record to facilitate ___________ evaluation and ___________ of care.

2. Major Areas of Health Care Regularly Examined to Determine Quality
    i. ______________________________
    ii. ______________________________
    iii. ______________________________
    iv. ______________________________
    v. ______________________________

3. Components of a Quality Assurance Program
    A. Review of all ___________ and ___________ services and procedures.
    B. Structure set up to ___________ items for review.

C. ___________ all issues such as number of errors and "needle sticks."
D. Emphasis is placed on areas where ___________ actions should be taken.

4. Medical Assistant's Role in Quality Assurance

A. _____________ patient complaints.
B. _____________ patient education.
C. _____________ laboratory tests done in the office.
D. _____________ with the physician regarding patient complaints.

5. CLIA

A. CLIA stands for _______________________________.
B. Mandates __________ control of __________ tests by category and documentation.
C. Categories include _____________, _______________, and ______________.

KEY TERMINOLOGY REVIEW

Choose the term that best represents each statement below.

a. incident
b. quality assurance (QA)
c. National Committee for Quality Assurance (NCQA)
d. ground fault circuit interrupter (GFCI)
e. ergonomics
f. body mechanics
g. personal protective equipment (PPE)
h. OSHA
i. biohazards
j. MSDS

1. ______________ Process of gathering and evaluating information about the services provided.
2. ______________ Contains printed material concerning a hazardous chemical.
3. ______________ Gloves, fluid-resistant lab coats, safety glasses, and a surgical mask, shield, or respirator.
4. ______________ Evaluates the quality of health plans.
5. ______________ Provides very specific regulations regarding chemical hazards and hazardous waste.
6. ______________ A prescription pad is missing.
7. ______________ Coordination of body alignment, balance, and movement.
8. ______________ Biological substances, such as medical waste and samples of a virus or bacterium, that pose a threat to human beings and are potentially infectious.
9. ______________ Applies scientific information and data regarding human body mechanics to the design of objects and overall environment for human use.
10. ______________ Designed to protect people from severe or fatal electrical shocks.

APPLIED PRACTICE

1. *Provide two examples of when the use of each of the following PPEs would be important:*

   i. Gloves

   ____

   ____

ii. Mask

____

____

iii. Eye and face shield

____

____

iv. Gowns or lab coats

____

____

LEARNING ACTIVITY: TRUE/FALSE

Indicate whether the following statements are true or false by placing a T or an F on the line that precedes each statement.

______ 1. The proper way to clean up a wet spill is to use the closest item, which is usually paper towels or wash rags.

______ 2. Front office equipment to be considered biohazards in a medical office includes printer and copier ink.

______ 3. All back office equipment is considered to be a biohazard.

______ 4. Employees cannot refuse to get the Hepatitis B vaccine if they choose to work in a clinical environment.

______ 5. The best way to prevent exposure to bloodborne pathogens is to wear personal protective equipment.

______ 6. To be safe, gloves must be worn at all times when working with a patient.

______ 7. Face masks are typically not worn if eye shields are being used.

______ 8. When moving an object, be sure to create a base of support by keeping your feet 6 to 8 inches apart.

______ 9. When moving heavy objects, keep your back and knees slightly bent.

______ 10. An incident report should be completed if a patient has misplaced or lost personal property while at the office.

CRITICAL THINKING

Answer the following questions to the best of your ability. Utilize the textbook as a reference.

1. What is the main premise of Standard/Universal Precautions? What impact on patient discrimination do you think this could have?

____

____

____

____

____

____

2. In your clinic, one of the laundry receptacles has a biohazardous label and another is for regular laundry without visible blood or body fluids. Your manager tells you that the laundry services will

be a day late due to snow and asks you to wash the regular laundry at home and bring it back tomorrow. Would you do this? Explain why or why not.

RESEARCH ACTIVITY

Utilize Internet search engines to research the following topics and write a brief description of what you find. It is important to utilize reputable websites.

1. Research the website for the Occupational Safety and Health Administration, *www.osha.gov*.

    What information can be found for health care facilities?
    List some facts found within the website:

CHAPTER 7
Telephone Techniques

CHAPTER OUTLINE

General review of the chapter:

Telephone Techniques
Typical Incoming Calls
Prescription Refill Requests
Telephone Triage
Handling Difficult Calls
Using a Telephone Directory
Telephones Used for Patient Education
Long Distance Calls
Using an Answering Service
Handling an Emergency Telephone Call

STUDENT STUDY GUIDE

Use the following guide to assist in your learning of the concepts from the chapter.

I. Telephone Techniques

1. Guidelines for Answering the Office Telephone

   i. ____
   ii. ____
   iii. ____
   iv. ____
   v. ____

2. Elements of a Professional Greeting

   i. ____
   ii. ____
   iii. ____

3. Guidelines for Making Calls

   A. Access ________ line as required.
   B. Dial ________ code if necessary.
   C. Identify the ________ to ensure that you are speaking with the intended person.
   D. Do not disclose ________ information to an unauthorized person.
   E. Know the ________ of the office with regard to personal calls.

4. Guidelines for Using the Hold Button

   A. An individual should not be left on hold for more than about ____________ seconds.
   B. When taking a second call, ask the ____________ caller if he or she may be placed on hold. Ensure that the ____________ caller is not an emergency, and then return to finish

the call with the ____________ caller prior to handling issues with the ____________ caller.

C. If information must be retrieved for the caller, ____________ to place the caller on hold.

5. Steps for Transferring Calls

   i. ____
   ii. ____
   ____.
   iii. ____
   iv. ____
   v. ____

6. Items Required When Taking a Message

   i. ____
   ii. ____
   iii. ____
   iv. ____

7. Guidelines for Taking a Message

   A. Have _________ and _________ ready.
   B. Obtain the necessary __________.
   C. _________ the message with the caller.
   D. _________ the telephone number for a return call.
   E. Pull the patient's medical record, if required, for the return call. Attach the message to the front of the _________.
   F. Ensure that the telephone message is placed in the patient's chart as _________ of the call.
   G. Follow _________ rules with regard to patient information.

8. Pagers and Cell Phones

   A. Know the office policy with regard to _________ use.
   B. Obtain the necessary _________ and codes for contacting the physician by pager and/or cell phone.
   C. Follow hospital building policies on _________ of pagers and cell phones.

9. Prescription Refill Requests

   A. Due to a high volume of calls, __________ __________ systems are often used.
   B. The MA is often responsible for __________ and __________ to messages.
   C. Messages should be checked at least __________ a day.
   D. A prescription refill request must be __________ on by a physician.
   E. A message may need to be attached to the __________ prior to obtaining a physician's approval.

10. Steps for Taking a Prescription Refill Message

   i. ____
   ii. ____
   iii. ____
   iv. ____
   v. ____
   vi. ____
   vii. ____
   viii. ____
   ix. ____

11. Purposes for Using a Telephone Log

   A. Typically used to keep track of _______ _______ calls.
   B. Helps to identify any _______ _______ calls that are not _______ related.

12. Purposes for Using an Answering Service
    i. ____________________
    ii. ____________________
    iii. ____________________

13. Handling Emergency Calls
    A. Every office should have a __________ protocol.
    B. Immediately get caller's __________ and __________.
    C. If it is an emergency, alert the __________ and/or __________.
    D. Try to __________ the individual.

KEY TERMINOLOGY REVIEW

Use the key terms found at the beginning of the chapter to finish the sentences below. Key terms may be more than one word in length.

1. Dr. Adamson at the local hospital would like to conduct a meeting by phone with his patient and the referring physician. The best way to facility this would be to set up a __________.
2. __________ refers to the changes in pitch and tone of your voice and the way you utter your words and phrases.
3. Before seeing a specialist, Mrs. Smith has been told that she must get a __________.
4. When the office is closed, the __________ will typically handle all emergency calls.
5. A __________ allows messages (voice mail) to be left or recorded when the medical assistant is unavailable to answer the telephone.
6. Most medical offices will use some form of a multi-line telephone. Some may have separate lines, where you must press a particular line's button to answer it, or a system that will feed calls to you from a __________ or waiting line.
7. __________ refers to the quality or state of being understandable.
8. Being careful not to speak too rapidly will help with word __________.
9. When calling a patient, it is important for the medical office to set up a system to block the office number from showing up on the patient's __________.
10. A medical assistant is on the phone with a patient; the process she uses to determine the order in which patients should be treated is called __________.
11. Have you ever noticed that when you ask a question your voice tends to rise at the end of the phrase? This is an example of the __________ of your voice.
12. When calling the office, Ms. Perez encounters an __________ that helps direct her call to the appropriate person with whom she should speak regarding her concerns.

APPLIED PRACTICE

Using your textbook, complete the activity or answer the questions below.

1. Using the box below, create a message pad template that could be used in a medical office to take telephone messages. Consider the important information to be obtained from callers when they call the office.

2. Manuel Vargas is an administrative medical assistant. He receives a phone call from a patient requesting a refill for one of her prescription medications. How should Manuel handle this call? What information must Manuel obtain from the patient? What should he do with the message after the call has ended?

____

____

____

____

____

LEARNING ACTIVITY: MULTIPLE CHOICE

Circle the correct answer to each of the questions below.

1. Which of the following would be appropriate to play for callers who are on hold?
   a. A local radio station
   b. Prerecorded music
   c. A message about seasonal allergies
   d. All of the above

2. Which of the following might be offensive or irritating for callers to listen to while they are on hold?
   a. Religious music
   b. Prerecorded music
   c. A message about seasonal allergies
   d. A local radio station

3. How long is an acceptable period of time to leave a caller on hold?
   a. Less than 10 seconds
   b. 20–30 seconds
   c. 45–60 seconds
   d. 1–2 minutes

4. What items should a medical assistant have available before answering the office telephone?
   a. Pen or pencil
   b. Paper
   c. Telephone message pad
   d. All of the above

5. The medical office telephone should be answered within how many rings?
   a. On the first ring
   b. By the second ring
   c. By the third ring
   d. No more than five rings

6. What rule are you violating if a patient's private information is thrown into the trash?
   a. OSHA's privacy rule
   b. HIPAA's privacy rule
   c. HIPPA's privacy rule
   d. AMA's privacy rule

7. Which of the following telephone calls should be taken care of first?
   a. A patient who says she needs to schedule her yearly mammogram
   b. An angry patient who is calling about her bill
   c. A patient who says he is having chest pains
   d. A patient who is calling to find out his laboratory results

8. What information would you expect to find in a telephone triage notebook?
   a. Driving directions to the medical office
   b. The hours the clinic is open
   c. The questions to ask a patient who complains of chest pains
   d. All of the above

9. In the event of a medical emergency in the office, what information should the medical assistant have available before calling for emergency services?
   a. The patient's name
   b. The patient's age
   c. The patient's gender
   d. All of the above

10. Which of the following emergency telephone numbers should the medical assistant have readily available at the front desk?
   a. Poison control
   b. The local police department
   c. The local fire department
   d. All of the above

CRITICAL THINKING

Answer the following questions to the best of your ability. Utilize the textbook and other resources such as the Internet in considering the following questions.

1. Rosie Sanchez, CMA (AAMA), has been working as an administrative medical assistant in an internal medicine clinic for the past year. A large part of her day is spent answering the office telephone and scheduling appointments. She would like the office to provide her with a hands-free headset for the telephone system. The clinic director has asked Rosie to create a list that outlines the benefits of having a hands-free headset over a conventional telephone headset. What should Rosie list?

2. Ron Douglas is a student in an administrative medical assisting class. He has been given an assignment to create an office policy that discusses how the speakerphone function of the front desk telephone system can be used without violating patient confidentiality. What should Ron write?

3. Martin Taylor, RMA, is working in an audiology clinic. The clinic is researching the possibility of purchasing a new telephone system that will include an automatic routing unit where callers can dial an extension to reach the desired party. Martin has been asked to create a list of pros and cons for this type of system. What should Martin include on his list?

RESEARCH ACTIVITY

Utilize Internet search engines to research the following topics. It is important to utilize reputable websites.

1. Search the Internet for on-call, after-hours answering services that are provided for medical offices. What types of services are offered by these companies? What is the general cost for on-call answering services?

CHAPTER 8
Patient Reception

CHAPTER OUTLINE

General review of the chapter:

Duties of a Receptionist
Personal Characteristics and Physical Appearance
Opening the Office
Collating Records
Greeting the Patient upon Arrival
Registering New Patients
Charge Slips
Consideration for the Patient's Time
Escorting the Patient into the Examination Room
Patient Education
Managing Disturbances
No-Shows
Closing the Office

STUDENT STUDY GUIDE

Use the following guide to assist in your learning of the concepts from the chapter.

I. Opening the Office and Receiving Patients

1. The Duties of a Receptionist

   A. ______________ patients upon arrival.
   B. Assisting new patients with ______________ of proper forms.
   C. ______________ copayments.
   D. Maintaining a ______________ and ______________ environment in the reception area.
   E. ______________ any disturbances in the reception room.
   F. ______________ return appointments.
   G. Making ______________ calls for upcoming appointments.

2. The Reception Room

   A. The term __________ is to be avoided.
   B. Often, it is the MA's job to keep the reception room _________ and _________ of hazards.
   C. The reception room provides the __________ impression of the office.

3. The Image of the Medical Assistant

   A. Image is important because the MA is often the _________ person the patient meets.
   B. Attention should be paid to good _________ and _________ habits.
   C. Make-up, hairstyle, and jewelry should reflect _________.
   D. Name __________ should always be visible.

4. Responsibilities in Opening the Office
   A. Arrive __________ minutes prior to office hours.
   B. Ensure that the day's charts have been __________ and __________.
   C. Ensure that __________ slips have been printed in advance for each patient.
   D. Print out __________ lists of patient appointments and distribute them.
5. The Task of Collating Records
   A. This is usually done the day __________ patients are seen.
   B. All necessary information should be received and in the record __________ to the patient's visit.
   C. In some offices, patients' records are organized in the __________ in which patients will be seen.
   D. A __________ appointment list is placed on top of the collated records.
   E. As patients arrive, the __________ should be verified on the schedule.
6. Steps for Collating Records
   i. __________
   ii. __________
   iii. __________
   iv. __________
   v. __________
   vi. __________
7. General Guidelines for Greeting Patients
   A. Make a good impression by being __________ and __________.
   B. If possible, have emergency or __________ patients enter through a private entrance.
   C. Place __________ ahead of other visitors.
   D. Follow __________ guidelines.
8. Patient Sign-in Sheet
   A. The sheet is maintained at the __________ desk.
   B. The sheet provides a __________ record of all patients who come to the office.
   C. The sheet should be checked for __________ and __________ of information.
   D. In order to be HIPAA compliant, all efforts should be made to protect __________ __________.
9. Patient Registration Forms
   A. Forms are sometimes sent to patients __________ to their first appointment.
   B. Some offices request that patients arrive __________ minutes early to complete the forms.
   C. Forms contain __________ information.
   D. Forms should be __________ marked to indicate areas that patients need to complete.
   E. Patients should be provided __________ as needed to ensure the completeness of the forms.
10. Registering New Patients
   A. Office billing and payments policies should be __________ explained to new patients.
   B. Obtain the patient's signature on an __________ form.
   C. Ensure that forms are filled out __________ and __________, including signatures.
   D. Verify information with the patient's __________ card.
   E. Photocopy __________ __________ of the insurance card.
   F. Determine if a __________ is required.
11. Payment for Services
   A. Should be documented on the __________ slip.
   B. The charge slip contains a list of the most common __________ for procedures and diagnoses at that office.
   C. Payment or __________ should be made prior to the patient leaving the office.
12. Consideration for the Patient's Time
   A. Inform the patient when the wait for his or her appointment will be longer than __________ minutes.

B. Listen and do not __________ to a patient's anger.
C. Remain calm and be ______________.
D. Tell the patient if a longer wait time is due to an _____________ emergency.
E. Addressing both the patient's and the physician's time issues is ___________ to successful scheduling.

II. Completing a Patient Visit

1. Escorting the Patient to the Examination Room
   A. When calling the patient, verify the patient's ___________ with the record and with the patient.
   B. Offer ____________ to those who need it.
   C. Walk at a ____________ pace.
2. The Patient and the Examination Room
   A. Enter the room with the patient and _____________ explain what clothing the patient should remove.
   B. _____________ patients in disrobing if necessary.
   C. Make every effort to protect the patient's ____________.
   D. Once the physician has completed the exam, return to the examination room and _________ before entering.
   E. ____________ ask the patient if he or she has any additional questions.
3. Ensuring Effective Patient Education
   A. Ensure that patient education is adapted and provided at a __________ that the patient understands.
   B. Assess the patient's level of understanding by asking the patient to __________ what he or she heard.
   C. If a misunderstanding is apparent, _________ the information to an appropriate level and ask the patient to repeat again.
   D. Provide _____________ information to which the patient can refer.
   E. Do not ____________ to ask the physician or another individual in the office to help clarify information for the patient.
4. Electronic Educational Materials
   A. Education is easily accomplished if the office has ___________ medical records.
   B. Software can target patients with certain conditions and then provide __________ with educational materials that are related to those conditions.
   C. E-mail can be a __________ -effective way to inform patients of various treatment options and procedures.
5. Guidelines for Dealing with Disturbances
   A. If possible, move angry or loud patients into a ___________ office area.
   B. Handle the situation as ___________ and ___________ as possible.
   C. Using a quiet, calm manner, ___________ respond to the patient's complaint.
   D. Ask the patient to ___________ the issue.
   E. Discuss _____________ with the patient.
   F. Know office policy regarding when the ___________ must be called.
6. Dealing with Children
   A. The children of adult patients are allowed in the examination room unless ____________ is required.
   B. If a child does not follow the adult to the examination room, the MA must ensure the child's ____________ while left alone.
   C. Rarely are children seen by physicians without the presence of a ____________.
7. Handling Medical Emergencies in the Reception Room (list the steps)
   i. ____
   ii. ____

iii. ______________________________

iv. ______________________________

v. ______________________________

vi. ______________________________

8. Steps for Closing the Office
   A. Allow for ______________ minutes at the end of the day to close the office.
   B. Check records for any missing ____________ and ensure that visits have been posted for billing.
   C. ________, ________, and ________ all records for patients who will be seen the next day.
   D. Place the collated records with _______ _______ attached and the _______ _______ of the next day's scheduled patients together in the appropriate place.
   E. Make a copy of the ________ ________ of patients for each physician.
   F. Deposit in the bank or place in the office safe, all money received from ________ payments.
   G. Lock all ________ and file rooms, as well as _________ offices and any other individual offices within the medical practice.
   H. Turn off all ____________ equipment and appliances.
   I. Ensure that all ____________ rooms are clean and ready for the next day.
   J. Straighten and ____________ the reception room.
   K. ____________ the answering service.
   L. Double-check to ensure that ____________ are locked and the alarm system is activated.

KEY TERMINOLOGY REVIEW

Choose the term that best represents each statement below.

a. Receptionist
b. Copayments
c. Demographic
d. Medical emergency
e. Overbooking
f. Collating
g. Fax
h. No-show

1. ______________ Machine used to send reports between facilities.
2. ______________ When more than one patient is scheduled for the same time slot.
3. ______________ Designated amounts that some medical insurance plans require patients to pay for medical services.
4. ______________ May be responsible for providing and explaining instructions regarding tests and procedures such as fasting before a particular blood test.
5. ______________ Information, such as age, gender, ethnic background, education, and Social Security number.
6. ______________ Patient condition that requires the immediate attention of a physician.
7. ______________ Patients who do not keep their appointment and do not call to cancel.
8. ______________ Refers to collecting all records, test results, and information pertaining to a patient who is scheduled to be seen by the physician.

APPLIED PRACTICE

Using information from your textbook and other sources you may find on the topic, complete the following applied practice.

1. Aubrey Cody is a CMA (AAMA) who has been hired as a medical assistant for a new pediatric practice that is being built. The physicians within the practice have asked her to design and decorate

the reception area. In the practice, there are three physicians who can see up to four patients each hour. How could Aubrey design the medical office reception area? What is the minimum amount of seating that should be in the reception area? What theme, toys, and reading materials would be appropriate for the reception area? Explain your answer after you have designed the reception area.

LEARNING ACTIVITY: MULTIPLE CHOICE

Circle the correct answer to each of the questions below.

1. If the medical assistant is on the telephone when a patient arrives at the office what should she do to let the patient know that she is aware of their presence?
   a. Continue looking down at the desk so that the patient realizes that she is on the telephone and will not be able to offer help right away.

b. Make eye contact with the patient, smile, and hold up an index finger to indicate that she'll be with them in just a moment.
c. Turn her back to the patient in order to keep the telephone conversation more private.
d. Any of the above

2. When mentioning another patient's name over the telephone or to another staff member within hearing distance of any patients in the reception room
   a. use caution and speak in a low voice.
   b. be sure that the glass partition at the reception desk is closed so that others in the reception room are not able to hear the conversation.
   c. step into a private area where other patient's are unable to hear the conversation.
   d. Any of the above

3. When established patients check in at the front desk, what information should the receptionist first confirm with the patient?
   a. That the patient's marital status has not changed since their last visit
   b. The type of medications that the patient is taking
   c. Current contact information
   d. All of the above

4. When using a sign-in sheet, HIPAA allows the following information to be requested:
   a. Patient's name
   b. Time of arrival
   c. Physician's name
   d. All of the above

5. Patient information forms should contain which of the following pieces of information?
   a. Patient's home address
   b. Patient's insurance information
   c. Patient's contact telephone numbers
   d. All of the above

6. A charge slip is also known as
   a. a checklist.
   b. superbills or encounter forms.
   c. a patient booklet.
   d. Any of the above

7. In general, patients should not be made to wait longer than ______ minutes for their appointment.
   a. 10
   b. 15
   c. 20
   d. None of the above

8. Overbooking
   a. is when more than one patient is scheduled for the same time slot.
   b. should only be done in an emergency.
   c. is an acceptable practice as long as patients are informed ahead of time.
   d. All of the above

9. When escorting a patient into the examination room,
   a. the receptionist will typically escort the person.
   b. the patient should be called by his or her first name unless instructed otherwise.
   c. making pleasant conversation with the patient may help ease the patient's anxieties.
   d. All of the above

10. How should the receptionist respond when confronted with an angry patient?
    a. Move the patient out of the front desk area.
    b. Ask the patient to sit down in the reception room until they have calmed down.
    c. Walk away from the front desk until the patient calms down.
    d. Any of the above

CRITICAL THINKING

Answer the following questions to the best of your ability. Utilize the textbook as a reference.

1. Marcus Winston, RMA, has been hired to work as an administrative medical assistant at the front desk in a small, one-physician medical office. Dr. Quan has been using a paper sign-in sheet for his patients for many years. Marcus has recently completed his medical assisting education and remembers learning that sign-in sheets must be HIPAA compliant. What can Marcus tell Dr. Quan about the paper sign-in system that he is currently using?

   ____

   ____

   ____

2. Sara Womack, CMA (AAMA), is the medical office manager in a women's clinic. She has two employees who share the job of front desk receptionist. Aaron Shelley, CMA (AAMA), doesn't like to work at the front desk. He is often short with the patients, some of whom have complained to the physician. Michael Sulley, RMA, is the other front desk receptionist. Michael has a sunny personality and thoroughly enjoys the fast pace at the front desk. Would Sara be better serving the patients at the women's clinic if she moved Aaron out of that position and had Michael work there full-time? Why or why not? What sort of ramifications might occur if Sara leaves Aaron in the front desk position?

   ____

   ____

   ____

   ____

3. Marjorie Sorensen, CMA (AAMA), has just been hired to work as the office manager for Dr. Rodriguez. The doctor tells Marjorie that she has noticed that many tasks are being skipped by the front desk staff when opening the office in the morning. Dr. Rodriguez believes that the front desk staff is forgetting these tasks and has asked Marjorie to come up with a solution to this problem. What might Marjorie suggest?

   ____

   ____

   ____

   ____

4. Isaiah Chung is taking an administrative medical assisting course as part of his training to become a medical assistant. His instructor has assigned the task of creating an office policy for opening the medical office. How might Isaiah's policy read?

RESEARCH ACTIVITY

Utilize Internet search engines to research the following topics and write a brief description of what you find. It is important to utilize reputable websites.

1. Using the information and décor theme of the reception area that you designed in the applied practice activity, search the Internet and obtain figures and estimates regarding the cost of decorating a reception area. Take into consideration paint, accessories, seating, tables, and so forth. Be sure to cite the websites that you use to find your information.

Chapter 9
Appointment Scheduling

CHAPTER OUTLINE

General review of the chapter:

Appointment Schedules
Scheduling Systems
Patient Scheduling Process
Established Patient Appointments
New Patient Appointments
Maintaining the Schedule
Future Appointments
Patient Referrals
Hospital Admission Scheduling
Scheduling Surgery and Outpatient Procedures
Appointment Exceptions
Telephone and E-mail Scheduling
Scheduling Other Types of Appointments

STUDENT STUDY GUIDE

Use the following guide to assist in your learning of the concepts from the chapter.

I. Scheduling Systems

1. Factors to Be Considered in Selecting a Scheduling System

   i. ______________________________
   ii. ______________________________
   iii. ______________________________
   iv. ______________________________
   v. ______________________________
   vi. ______________________________
   vii. ______________________________

2. Purpose of a Scheduling System

   A. Assists in the __________ of the office.
   B. Provides __________ management.
   C. __________ efficiency.
   D. Helps to ensure the __________ of patient care.

3. Variations in Appointment Schedules

   i. ______________________________
   ii. ______________________________
   iii. ______________________________
   iv. ______________________________

v. ____
vi. ____

4. Specified Times
   A. Length of appointment is determined by ________ needs.
   B. Up to each staff member to reduce ________ time.
   C. Important for office to build in ________ time.
5. Wave Scheduling
   A. Provides ________ for unforeseen events.
   B. Purpose is to ________ and ________ each hour on time.
   C. Each hour is divided into ________ amounts of time.
   D. Three ________ -minute or four ________ -minute appointments could be seen in an hour.
   E. Patients are seen in the ________ in which they arrive.
6. Open Office Hours
   A. ________ structured of all systems.
   B. Patients may arrive at ________ during business hours.
   C. This method is ________ by some because it avoids the disruption caused by missed appointments.
7. Advantages of Computerized Scheduling Systems
   A. Completed in a ________ -time environment.
   B. Provides the ability to ________ appointment information with ease.
   C. Maximizes office process ________ and patient ________.
   D. Provides the ability to track ________ in the medical practice.
8. Manual Scheduling Systems
   A. Consists of a ________ schedule book.
   B. Book is selected based on practice ________ and ________.
9. Requirements for Both Computerized and Manual Systems
   A. The appointment book is a legal document that can be ________ by the court.
   B. Appointment books should be ________ for future reference and kept for several years in the event of a court case.
   C. If there are any changes in the scheduled patients in the appointment book, these should be noted both in the ________ and in the ________.

II. Patient Scheduling Process

1. Steps for Scheduling the Patient
   i. ____
   ii. ____
   iii. ____
   iv. ____
   v. ____
   vi. ____
   vii. ____
   viii. ____
2. Steps for Manually Scheduling Established Patients
   A. Use a ______ so that appointments can be erased to make changes as needed.
   B. Set up a ______ by blocking out all time periods when the physician is not available for appointments.
   C. Print the patient's ______ first and last names next to the appropriate time on the schedule.
   D. Add ______ for *junior* and ______ for *senior* if there are two patients with the same name in a family.

E. Ask the patient for _________ work and home telephone numbers, including the area codes.
F. Write these numbers next to the _________.
G. Record the _________ for the visit on the schedule.

3. Additional Steps Related to Scheduling Patients Electronically
   A. Ensure that the scheduling system is _________.
   B. Search for the _________ patient.
   C. _________ that the telephone numbers in the system are correct.

4. Steps for Scheduling New Patients
   A. _________ the necessary appointment scheduling equipment.
   B. Obtain the patients full _________ name.
   C. Record the patient's chief _________ and _________.
   D. Request the name of the patient's insurance _________ and policy _________.
   E. Attempt to _________ the new patient's request for his or her preferred appointment time.
   F. Provide the new patient with _________ to the office.
   G. Welcome and thank the new patient by _________ for selecting your medical office.
   H. _________ new patient information in a new medical record.

5. Addressing Missed Appointments and No-Shows
   A. Charge the patient according to office _________.
   B. _________ the patient and reschedule.
   C. _________ the missed appointment and rescheduled date.
   D. Write _________ or _________ on the appointment schedule and in the patient chart.

6. Advance Bookings and Follow-up
   A. Advance bookings are done for _________ scheduled appointments.
   B. Ensure that the patient receives an _________ card.
   C. Follow-ups can be made in _________, by _________, or via _________.

7. Issues Related to Arranging a Referral Appointment
   A. Information required for an outgoing or incoming referral includes
      i. _________________________
      ii. _________________________
      iii. _________________________
      iv. _________________________
      v. _________________________
      vi. _________________________
      vii. _________________________
   B. Depending on the insurance, _________ may be necessary before scheduling the appointment.

8. Steps for Arranging a Referral Appointment
   A. Before providing the patient's name, etc., _________ that the practice accepts the patient's medical insurance.
   B. Record the referral appointment information in the _________, as well as on an appointment _________ for the patient.
   C. Record the name of the individual with whom you spoke in the _________, as well as on the _________.
   D. Notify the patient of the _________ and _________ of the appointment.

9. Considerations for Scheduling a Direct Admission to a Hospital
   A. Contact the patient's _________ for pre-admissions approval.
   B. Verify the _________ of the patient's first and last names.
   C. Obtain the patient's social security number from the _________.
   D. Ask patient for _________ phone number and area code.

E. Give the physician's statement from the _______________ as the reason for the admission.
F. Document the patient's name with the insurance company that gave _______________.

10. Steps for Scheduling an Inpatient Surgical Procedure
   i. ______________________________
   ii. ______________________________
   iii. ______________________________
   iv. ______________________________
   v. ______________________________
   vi. ______________________________
   vii. ______________________________
   viii. ______________________________
   ix. ______________________________
   x. ______________________________

11. Steps for Scheduling an Outpatient Procedure
   i. ______________________________
   ii. ______________________________
   iii. ______________________________
   iv. ______________________________
   v. ______________________________
   vi. ______________________________
   vii. ______________________________
   viii. ______________________________
   ix. ______________________________
   x. ______________________________
   xi. ______________________________
   xii. ______________________________

12. Considerations for Handling Nonscheduled Patients
   A. Determine the __________ of the patient's condition.
   B. Ask the patient for his or her telephone number and where he or she is calling from, and determine whether the patient is __________.
   C. Follow office __________ and __________ regarding handling emergency situations.
   D. Inform the __________ immediately regarding a potential emergency.

KEY TERMINOLOGY REVIEW

Match the correct medical term with the definition listed below.

a. Acute conditions
b. Advance bookings
c. Archived
d. Catch-up
e. Cycle time
f. Double-booking
g. Established patient
h. Matrix
i. Modified wave scheduling
j. Open-ended questions
k. Privacy screen
l. Real time
m. Scheduling system
n. Subpoena
o. Time patterns
p. Triage
q. Wave scheduling

1. _______________ Block others from viewing the computer screen.
2. _______________ Also known as assigning priority.

3. _______________ Allows patients to book their next appointment 3 to 6 months ahead of time.

4. _______________ Requires more than a *yes* or *no* answer and are used to gather pertinent information.

5. _______________ A time when appointments are not scheduled.

6. _______________ Facilitates the coordination of appropriate time segments for staff, patients, and the practice's available equipment.

7. _______________ Illnesses or injuries that patients suddenly experience and that require treatment but may not be life threatening.

8. _______________ A patient who has been seen by a practitioner within the past 3 years.

9. _______________ Process of blocking out times in the appointment schedule when the provider is unavailable or out of the office.

10. _______________ Information requested by the courts.

11. _______________ The length of time the average patient spends in the medical office.

12. _______________ Another term for "stored."

13. _______________ To have three patients scheduled at intervals during the first half hour with none scheduled for the second half hour.

14. _______________ Refers to automatically placing the appointment, patient needs, and information within the appropriate areas of the computer program versus the manual system.

15. _______________ Patients are scheduled only during the first half hour and are served on a first come, first served basis.

16. _______________ Similar to matrixing off time within the schedule to allow for catch-up time or unscheduled appointments.

17. _______________ Scheduling more than one patient for the same appointment time.

APPLIED PRACTICE

Follow the directions as instructed for each question below.

1. Using the information below and the manual schedule on the following pages, create a matrix for the medical office. *(Remember to use a pencil.)*
   a. The medical offices open at 8:30 A.M. every day.
   b. The last appointment for the day is scheduled no later than 3:30 P.M.
   c. The office is closed for appointments for lunch starting at 12:00 P.M.; it reopens at 1:15 P.M.
   d. Dr. Cho has hospital rounds every Wednesday from 7:30 A.M.–10:00 A.M.
   e. Dr. Jackson has hospital rounds every Thursday from 7:45 A.M.–10:15 A.M.
   f. On February 3, Dr. Cho has a meeting at Alliance Assisted Living that starts at 3:30 P.M.
   g. On February 2, Dr. Jackson has a meeting with a pharmaceutical representative that is scheduled for 12:45–1:30 P.M.

2. Schedule the following patients on the appointment schedule.
   a. LaToya Atwater is a new patient to see Dr. Cho. Wednesdays work best for LaToya.
   b. Sujin Dalywhal wants to see Dr. Jackson on Thursday afternoon for an abdominal suture removal.
   c. Jose Alvarez calls on Wednesday morning because he has had a terrible headache for the past 2 days.
   d. Anna Maria DeCamillo is a diabetic patient who wants to see Dr. Jackson for her 3-month diabetic check-up on Wednesday afternoon.
   e. Mark Tomlinson wants to see Dr. Cho for his annual check-up on Thursday.
   f. Aiden Taylor needs to be seen on Thursday morning for his 3-year well-child visit with Dr. Jackson.
   g. Dr. Cho requests that an appointment be made on Wednesday morning with her patient, Lydia Pazmino, regarding her blood test results.

Pearson Family Clinic

Wednesday, February 2, 20xx

	Dr. S. Cho	Dr. A. Jackson
7:30		
7:45		
8:00		
8:15		
8:30		
8:45		
9:00		
9:15		
9:30		
9:45		
10:00		
10:15		
10:30		
10:45		
11:00		
11:15		
11:30		
11:45		
12:00		
12:15		
12:30		
12:45		
1:00		
1:15		
1:30		
1:45		
2:00		
2:15		
2:30		
2:45		
3:00		
3:15		
3:30		
3:45		
4:00		

Thursday, February 3, 20xx

	Dr. S. Cho	Dr. A. Jackson
7:30		
7:45		
8:00		
8:15		
8:30		
8:45		
9:00		
9:15		
9:30		
9:45		
10:00		
10:15		
10:30		
10:45		
11:00		
11:15		
11:30		
11:45		
12:00		
12:15		
12:30		
12:45		
1:00		
1:15		
1:30		
1:45		
2:00		
2:15		
2:30		
2:45		
3:00		
3:15		
3:30		
3:45		
4:00		

LEARNING ACTIVITY: MULTIPLE CHOICE

Circle the correct answer to each of the questions below.

1. How many minutes do most patients consider to be an acceptable wait time prior to seeing the doctor?
   a. 10
   b. 15
   c. 20
   d. None of the above

2. Which of the following is an acceptable way to note a missed appointment in a hardcopy appointment book?
   a. Use white correction fluid to cover the patient's name.
   b. Use a black marker to obliterate the patient's name.
   c. Use an eraser to remove the patient's name.
   d. Write no-show (NS) both on the appointment schedule and in the patient's chart.

3. What is one way to remind patients of their upcoming appointment in the medical office?
   a. Send out a reminder card to the patient just prior to the appointment.
   b. Call the patient to remind him or her of the appointment.
   c. Send an e-mail to the patient to remind him or her of the appointment.
   d. Any of the above.

4. The __________ method of scheduling is where two or three patients are scheduled at the beginning of each hour, followed by single patient appointments every 10 to 20 minutes for the rest of that hour.
   a. wave
   b. modified wave
   c. open hours
   d. fixed appointment

5. The __________ method of scheduling is where patients are scheduled only for the first half of each hour. The first patient to arrive is seen first.
   a. wave
   b. modified wave
   c. open hours
   d. fixed appointment

6. The __________ method of scheduling is most commonly used in walk-in clinics, laboratories, and x-ray facilities where patients are typically seen on a first come, first served basis.
   a. wave
   b. modified wave
   c. open hours
   d. fixed appointment

7. To eliminate the need to "squeeze in" an emergency or unscheduled appointment, the medical assistant should integrate __________ into the office schedule, if office policy allows.
   a. more time
   b. time patterns
   c. wave scheduling
   d. None of the above

8. Examples of emergency conditions that require patients to be seen immediately include
   a. Skin rash
   b. Pain or burning on urination
   c. Chest pain
   d. All of the above

9. When confirming an appointment with a patient on the telephone, the patient should be asked to repeat the following information:
   a. Location of the appointment
   b. Date of the appointment
   c. Time of the appointment
   d. All of the above

10. Triage
    a. Becomes necessary when more than one seriously ill patient is waiting to see the patient.
    b. Takes place each time a patient visits the office.
    c. Is only done in a hospital setting.
    d. A skill performed only by the physician.

CRITICAL THINKING

Answer the following questions to the best of your ability. Utilize the textbook as a reference.

1. Dylan Reilly, CMA (AAMA), is working in a busy family practice office. The physicians and staff all agree that the appointment scheduling system is not working and patients are frequently waiting long periods of time for appointments. How should Dylan go about creating a new scheduling procedure for this office?

   ____

   ____

   ____

   ____

2. Armando Alonso is taking an administrative medical assisting course as part of his medical assisting training. He has been given an assignment to create a list of the information patients should be given when scheduling the patient in order to help prepare the patient for medical procedures. What sort of information should Armando list?

   ____

   ____

   ____

   ____

3. Anna Simonenko, CMA (AAMA), is working at the front desk in a family practice clinic. Anna has been asked to schedule Roger Edetsberger for a procedure to be performed in the hospital. Anna tells Roger that she will need to call his insurance company before she can schedule the procedure. Roger asks, "Why do you need to do that? Can't you just schedule the procedure now and call the insurance company some other time?" What can Anna say to Roger?

   ____

   ____

   ____

   ____

RESEARCH ACTIVITY

Utilize Internet search engines to research the following topics and write a brief description of what you find. It is important to utilize reputable websites.

1. Research various appointment scheduling software programs for medical offices.
   What products are available?
   What must be considered prior to purchasing medical office software?
   What type of technical support is available?

Chapter 10
Office Facilities, Equipment, and Supplies

CHAPTER OUTLINE

General review of the chapter:

Medical Office Facility
Office Layout
Office Equipment
Supplies

STUDENT STUDY GUIDE

Use the following guide to assist in your learning of the concepts from the chapter.

I. Medical Office Facility and Equipment

1. Desirable Characteristics of a Medical Facility

A. Presents a ________ and ________ environment.
B. Is clean, neat, and well ________.
C. Makes a good ________ impression.
D. Generates positive employee ________.

2. Aspects to Be Considered in the Medical Office

i. ____________________
ii. ____________________
iii. ____________________
iv. ____________________
v. ____________________
vi. ____________________
vii. ____________________
viii. ____________________
ix. ____________________
x. ____________________
xi. ____________________

3. Americans with Disabilities Act

A. Protects the rights of the disabled regarding access to ______________, ______________, ______________, ______________, ______________, and ______________.

4. Lighting and Colors

A. ____________ colors are typically used.
B. ____________ art should hang on the walls.
C. Fish tanks are ____________ for children and adults.

5. Reception Room Safety
   A. Prevent fires by eliminating sparks from __________, and __________ and __________ equipment.
   B. Ensure that staff members understand their __________ during a fire.
   C. Post __________ plans in a central location within the office.
6. Equipment Typically Found in Administrative Areas
   i. ______________________________
   ii. ______________________________
   iii. ______________________________
   iv. ______________________________
   v. ______________________________
   vi. ______________________________
   vii. ______________________________
   viii. ______________________________
   ix. ______________________________
7. Factors Promoted by an Effective Office Flow
   i. ______________________________
   ii. ______________________________
   iii. ______________________________
   iv. ______________________________
   v. ______________________________
8. Considerations for the Patient Entrance
   A. It provides the ________ impression.
   B. High steps should be ________.
   C. Push and pull indicators should be placed on ________.
9. Considerations for the Reception Area
   A. Desk area should provide __________ and the confidentiality of information.
   B. Desk area should allow for ease of __________ to patient records but at the same time protect patient privacy.
   C. Waiting area should contain seats that can be __________ and that provide good __________.
   D. Toys in the waiting area should be __________ and __________.
10. Assisting Patients in Understanding the Office Layout
   A. Provide __________ that indicate the location of the various areas in the office.
   B. The use of __________ indicators on the floor or walls may be helpful.
   C. Ensure that __________ and __________ are clear of obstructions.
11. Considerations for Office Bathrooms
   i. ______________________________
   ii. ______________________________
   iii. ______________________________
   iv. ______________________________
   v. ______________________________
   vi. ______________________________
   vii. ______________________________
12. Uses of Word Processing in the Medical Office
   A. Makes creating and retrieving documents more ____________.
   B. Allows the ability to ____________ and ____________ text without having to cut and paste a paper document.
   C. Allows for making ____________ copies.

13. Use of Voice Recognition Software
    A. Allows the physician to speak into a ____________ connected to a computer program that transcribes the physician's dictated office notes into a ________ report.
    B. Due to the set-up ____________, few physicians have adopted this system.
    C. It is used in some hospital ________ ________ departments.
14. Electronic Postage
    A. Requires the user to apply for and receive approval from the ______________________ prior to use.
    B. User is required to determine the __________ of postage required for letters and packages and then a computer interfaces with the postal system to print the appropriate postage.
    C. Method may be used in offices with a lot of ________ mail.
15. Considerations for Purchasing Equipment
    i. ____
    ii. ____
    iii. ____
    iv. ____
16. Purposes of an Equipment Log
    A. Used to ___________ pieces of equipment that require regular maintenance.
    B. Helps prove that the ____________ has been well maintained.
    C. May be a required document for ____________ purposes.

II. Supplies and Inventory
1. Factors Affecting the Selection of Vendors
    i. ____
    ii. ____
    iii. ____
    iv. ____
    v. ____
    vi. ____
    vii. ____
    viii. ____
    ix. ____
    x. ____
2. Considerations for Supply Inventory Control
    A. Mark the ___________ sheet whenever an item is removed from the supply cabinet.
    B. Assign a staff member the responsibility for ___________ all supplies.
    C. Ensure that reordering occurs in a ___________ manner so that the supply is never totally depleted.
    D. Consider the ___________ with which supplies are used and the amount of ___________ necessary for having the order processed and delivered when reordering supplies.
3. Establishing an Ordering System
    A. It is important to determine when ___________ of the supply will have been used and how long an order takes to arrive.
    B. Use of ___________ reminders or ___________ reminder cards may be useful.
    C. ___________ scanning systems can be purchased as an ordering system.
4. Drug Samples
    A. These are small packages of drug samples for physicians to distribute to _________.
    B. The are provided by _________ representatives.
    C. The discarding of samples must be done according to _________ and _________ regulations.

KEY TERMINOLOGY REVIEW

Use the key terms found at the beginning of the chapter to complete the sentences below.

1. The ________________________ is the legislation that protects the rights of the disabled regarding access to employment, public buildings, transportation, housing, schools, and health care facilities.
2. Dr. Sabol chose to purchase an extended ________________________ that would cover repair and maintenance for an additional 7 years.
3. Supplies that are used up quickly and have a relatively inexpensive unit cost are called ____________ supplies.
4. The distinguishing factor between capital equipment and general office supplies is the ____________ of the product.
5. ________________________ equipment refers to items that require a large dollar amount to purchase (generally more than $500) and have a relatively long life.
6. The medical facility generally has a flow that lends itself easily to teamwork, time management, organized and efficient office equipment usage, and patient flow. This is known as ________________________.
7. Dr. Linn asked his clinical manager to create a/an ________________________ of all the supplies located in the supply closet.
8. ________________________ is the length of time that the average patient spends in the medical office.
9. ________________________ refers to the positive or negative state of mind of employees with regard to their work or work environment.
10. An ________________________ can be purchased to cover some period of time after the warranty has expired.
11. Capital equipment also has a ________________________, which is referred to as depreciation.
12. ________________________ is a loss in the value of the product resulting from normal aging, use, or deterioration.
13. In general, it takes multiple ________________________ to provide all of the supplies for a medical practice.

APPLIED PRACTICE

Read the scenario and answer the questions that follow.

Scenario

Javier Gomez, CMA (AAMA), is working in the front office of a busy family practice. His manager, Chris, has asked him to create a detailed inventory list of all of the supplies needed for his station at the patient check-out desk. Below is a list that Javier has started.

Item Name	Company	Amount on Hand
Pens	Office Supplies R Us	14
Message pad	Office Supplies R Us	2 tablets
Ink pad	Office Supplies R Us	2 pads

1. Based on the inventory list, what additional important information should Javier include before submitting his list to Chris?

____

____

____

2. Considering that Javier is working at a patient check-out desk, where patients pay co-payments and schedule follow-up appointments as needed, what additional items would Javier be likely to add to his inventory list? Name at least five additional items.

____

____

____

____

____

LEARNING ACTIVITY: MULTIPLE CHOICE

Circle the correct answer to each of the questions below.

1. ADA regulations ensure that every public facility
   a. is made easily accessible to the handicapped.
   b. provides unrestricted hallways.
   c. has elevators or ramps available.
   d. All of the above

2. When addressing safety issues in the medical office, concerns noted may include
   a. the use of throw rugs.
   b. the culture of the office.
   c. the tone of the office.
   d. All of the above

3. Issues to be considered when setting up a medical office include the
   a. employees who work in the office.
   b. office design and layout.
   c. other offices in the building.
   d. None of the above

4. The first element of office flow is the
   a. restrooms.
   b. patient entrance.
   c. placement of examination rooms.
   d. staff offices.

5. Which of the following is considered to be capital equipment?
   a. Copy machine
   b. EKG paper
   c. Medications
   d. All of the above

6. Uses and advantages of using a postal meter include which of the following?
   a. Metered mail does not have to be stamped when it arrives at the post office.
   b. A postal meter will calculate the exact postage required and either print it directly onto the letter or print out a strip to be affixed to the package.
   c. A postal meter allows for postage to be printed directly onto an envelope or onto an adhesive-backed strip that is placed directly on an envelope or package.
   d. All of the above

7. Examples of expendable supplies include
   a. scanners.
   b. the telephone system.
   c. clinical supplies such as catheters.
   d. All of the above

8. An inventory list of all sample drugs must be maintained to adhere to ____________ regulations.
   a. Drug Enforcement Administration (DEA)
   b. Americans with Disabilities Act (ADA)
   c. Food and Drug Administration (FDA)
   d. None of the above

9. Which of the following guidelines should be followed with regard to drug samples?
   a. Must be placed in a secure location.
   b. Should be kept all together by category.
   c. All samples should be rotated like other supplies, with newer samples placed in the back behind samples of the same medication and strength with earlier expiration dates.
   d. All of the above

10. A warranty
    a. is a manufacturer's guarantee in writing that its product will perform correctly under normal conditions.
    b. can be purchased to cover a period of time after the original warranty has expired.
    c. will state in detail what is actually covered by the contract.
    d. provides for replacement of defective parts but for an additional charge.

CRITICAL THINKING

Answer the following questions to the best of your ability. Utilize the textbook as a reference.

1. Corey Steinberg, CMA (AAMA), has recently been hired to work as an administrative medical assistant in a busy cardiology practice. Corey has been given the task of creating a manual that outlines the warranty information, as well as the maintenance schedule for each piece of medical office equipment. How should Corey go about beginning this task?

   ____

   ____

   ____

   ____

2. Monte Beaton, RMA, is the office manager in a gastroenterology practice. Monte has recently hired three new medical assistants and wants to ensure that they are properly trained to use each piece of equipment in the medical office. How can Monte ensure that the training is done properly?

3. Krystle Shawger is taking an administrative class as part of her medical assisting training. She has been given an assignment to write an essay describing how an equipment maintenance log would be useful in the medical office. What might Krystle include in her paper?

4. Marian Harrison, RMA, is the administrative office manager in a family practice clinic. She is writing an office policy for the inventory of administrative office equipment. What might her policy include?

5. Joanne Felmer, CMA (AAMA), works in a walk-in clinic. At the weekly office staff meeting, the office manager mentioned the need for purchasing a new EKG machine. The office manager has asked Joanne to research the various options available. How should Joanne handle this task?

RESEARCH ACTIVITY

Utilize Internet search engines to research the following topics and write a brief description of what you find. It is important to utilize reputable websites.

1. Conduct an Internet search for office and medical supply companies. Which companies supply products at competitive prices? What are the shipping charges? Which company seems to have the best variety of products? How could this information be useful for medical offices?

Chapter 11
Written Communication

CHAPTER OUTLINE

General review of the chapter:

Letter Writing
Word Choice
Composing Letters
Letter Styles
Interoffice Memoranda
Proofreading
Editing
Abbreviations
Reference Materials
Preparing Outgoing Mail
Classifications of Mail
Size Requirements for Mail
Mail Handling Tips
Electronic Mail
Reflection on the Medical Practice

STUDENT STUDY GUIDE

Use the following guide to assist in your learning of the concepts from the chapter.

I. Written Communication in the Medical Office

1. How Professionalism Is Reflected in Written Communication

   A. Physical __________ of the letter.
   B. __________ of the message being sent.
   C. Use of grammar and __________.

2. Elements to Be Included in a Professional Letter

   A. Message should be __________ and to the point.
   B. Expected outcome should be __________.
   C. Threats or derogatory comments should __________ be made.
   D. Negative __________ should be avoided.

3. Usage to Be Avoided

   i. ______________________________
   ii. ______________________________
   iii. ______________________________
   iv. ______________________________
   v. ______________________________
   vi. ______________________________

4. Ways to Improve Sentences and Paragraphs
   A. Ensure that the sentence length never exceeds __________ words.
   B. Eliminate all words that are _______________.
   C. Cover __________ point in each paragraph.
   D. Avoid use of the _____________ pronoun.
   E. Avoid redundancy and ___________.
   F. Eliminate inflated ___________.
5. Active vs. Passive Voice
   A. When using the active voice, the subject of the sentence does the ____________.
   B. The use of the active voice is considered to be more effective because it is _________ and more _________ than the use of the passive voice.
   C. When using the passive voice, the _________ receives the action.
6. Rules for Writing Numbers
   A. Numbers _________ through _________ are spelled out.
   B. Only Arabic ____________ are used in tables, statistical data, dates, measurements, money, percentages, and time.
   C. When placing numbers in columns, align them as follows: Arabic integers are aligned on the _________. Decimal numbers are aligned on the ___________ point. Roman numerals are aligned on the _________.
   D. Do not use __________ when writing on-the-hour time.
7. Eight Parts of Speech
   i. ______________________________
   ii. ______________________________
   iii. ______________________________
   iv. ______________________________
   v. ______________________________
   vi. ______________________________
   vii. ______________________________
   viii. ______________________________
8. Standard Components of a Business Letter
   i. ______________________________
   ii. ______________________________
   iii. ______________________________
   iv. ______________________________
   v. ______________________________
   vi. ______________________________
   vii. ______________________________
   viii. ______________________________
   ix. ______________________________
   x. ______________________________
9. Address of the Recipient
   A. Address is typed along the __________ margin and is __________-spaced.
   B. Company name is typed exactly as shown on the company's own ____________.
   C. Name of the city is followed by a __________.
   D. Two-letter state abbreviation is followed by __________ spaces and then the ZIP code.
10. Guidelines for Using Courtesy Titles
   A. ________ is always an appropriate title for men.
   B. If there is a professional title, such as MD or PhD, this is used instead of the ________ title.
   C. ________ is used when the marital status of a woman is unknown.

D. ________ is appropriate for unmarried women who prefer that title and is also used for young girls.

11. Body of the Letter

A. Contains the _______ of the letter.
B. Begins _______ lines below the salutation.
C. The body is _______-spaced, with _______-spacing between each paragraph.
D. Paragraphs are either _______ or indented on the first line.
E. Most letters bearing a single message are usually _______ or _______ paragraphs in length and are confined to a _______ page.

12. Signature Line

A. Typed _________ lines below the complimentary close.
B. If the name and title are on the same line, they are separated by a _________.

13. Steps for Composing a Business Letter

i. ____________________
ii. ____________________
iii. ____________________
iv. ____________________
v. ____________________
vi. ____________________

14. Developing a Two-Page Letter

A. _________ stationary is used only for the top sheet.
B. A _________-inch margin is used at the bottom of the page.
C. All pages following the first page must begin with the _______ and the _______ _______ of the letter.

15. Letter Styles

i. ____________________
ii. ____________________
iii. ____________________
iv. ____________________
v. ____________________

16. Editing

A. When editing medical reports, do not change the _______ of the report or _______ the meaning in any way.
B. If the meaning seems to be unclear, check with the writer of the report before any _______ changes are made.
C. When editing material that you have composed, changes can be made to increase _______.

17. Medical Abbreviations

A. _________ medical abbreviations can be used in medical reports and when filing insurance documents.
B. The ______________________________ has released a list of abbreviations that should never be used.

18. Reference Tools for Writing

i. ____________________
ii. ____________________
iii. ____________________
iv. ____________________

II. Handing Mail in the Medical Office

1. Tasks Related to the Handling of Incoming Mail

   i. ______________________________

   ii. ______________________________

   iii. ______________________________

2. Sizes of Letterhead Stationary

   A. __________ letterhead is used for most office correspondence.

   B. __________ or __________ style is used by some physicians for their social correspondence.

   C. __________ letterhead is a half-sheet used for brief letters and memoranda.

3. Folding and Inserting Letters into a No. 10 Envelope

   A. Fold the bottom __________ of the letter upward and crease the fold.

   B. Fold the top of the letter downward to __________ inch from the previous crease and crease this fold.

   C. Place this edge into the envelope __________.

4. Folding and Inserting Letters into a No. 6¾ Envelope

   A. Bring the bottom edge up to __________ inch from the top edge.

   B. Fold the right edge __________ __________ the width of the paper and crease this fold.

   C. Fold the left edge to __________ inch from the previous crease and insert this edge into the envelope first.

5. Guidelines for Optimal Efficiency of OCR Scanning

   A. The address must be typed on the envelope using __________-spacing and capital letters with no __________.

   B. The last line in the address must include the city, the two-digit state code, and the ZIP code. The line must not exceed __________ characters.

6. Considerations When Typing an Envelope

   A. The bottom margin of the No. 10 envelope should be __________ inch with __________ -inch margins on the left and right sides.

   B. No. 6¾ envelopes should have a __________-inch margin on the left side, with the address __________ lines from the top of the envelope.

   C. The return address for the sender should always be placed in the upper-__________ corner of the envelope.

7. ZIP Codes

   A. ZIP codes start on the East Coast with the number __________, increasing to the number __________ on the West Coast and in Hawaii.

   B. The first __________ numbers identify the city and all five digits combine to identify the individual post office and __________ within the city.

   C. __________ additional digits have been added to the ZIP code by the USPS. These represent the addressee's __________ location.

8. Common Types of Mail

   i. ______________________________

   ii. ______________________________

   iii. ______________________________

   iv. ______________________________

   v. ______________________________

   vi. ______________________________

9. Size Requirements for Mail

   A. Domestic mail must be at least ________ inch thick.
   B. Mail that is ________ inch or less in thickness must be ________ inches in height and at least ________ inches long. All mail not meeting this requirement is considered to be ___________.
   C. Items that are bulky and lightweight require a ______________-pound balloon rate surcharge.

10. Guidelines for Preparing Mail That Is to Be Metered

   A. Separate all _________ mail from the _________ mail.
   B. Separate all mail destined to either _________ or _________ from the rest of the international mail.
   C. When mailing letter-size envelopes, flaps must be _________, ________, or ________.
   D. Envelopes larger than a _________ size envelope must be sealed before being sent.

11. Issues Related to Electronic Mail

   A. Electronic mail cannot be used if the original __________ on the document must be sent.
   B. The __________ of the message should remain as professional as if you were typing a letter to be sent through the USPS.
   C. E-mail is not efficient for use in ____________.
   D. It is imperative to adhere strictly to all _____________confidentiality laws when using e-mail.

12. Issues Related to Instant Messaging

   A. Instant Messaging is a way to communicate with another person in _________ _________.
   B. Instant messages are not ____________ documents and cannot be attached to a person's ____________ records or be used in a court of law.
   C. Abbreviating words when instant messaging is not acceptable for electronic messages sent from within the ____________ .

13. Steps in Opening and Sorting Mail

   i. ______________________________
   ii. ______________________________
   iii. ______________________________
   iv. ______________________________
   v. ______________________________
   vi. ______________________________
   vii. ______________________________
   viii. ______________________________
   ix. ______________________________
   x. ______________________________
   xi. ______________________________
   xii. ______________________________

14. Guidelines for Sending a Fax

   A. __________ document is inserted into the fax machine.
   B. __________ sheet should be sent first.
   C. All fax cover sheets must be __________ compliant.

15. Contents of a Fax Cover Sheet

   i. ______________________________
   ii. ______________________________
   iii. ______________________________
   iv. ______________________________
   v. ______________________________

KEY TERMINOLOGY REVIEW

Without using your textbook, write a sentence using the selected key terms in the correct context.

1. *active voice*

2. *block letter style*

3. *complimentary close*

4. *constant information*

5. *electronic mail*

6. *enclosure*

7. *gender bias*

8. *homophones*

9. *letterhead*

10. *memos*

11. *modified block letter style*

12. *optical character recognition*

13. *passive voice*

____

____

14. *proofreading*

____

____

15. *redundant*

____

____

16. *reference initials*

____

____

17. *salutation*

____

____

18. *signature line*

____

____

19. *thesaurus*

____

____

20. *variables*

____

____

APPLIED PRACTICE

Follow the directions for each assignment below.

1. Using proofreader's marks, make the necessary corrections to the body of the business letter. (Refer to Figure 11-5 in your textbook.)

Mr. SUSAN Rowe (8-12-1877 was seen in my office today. She presents with complaints of uper right quadrant pain times too weeks. Mrs. rowe states that alon g with the pain, she is experiencing nausea and vomitting. Upon palpation the abdomen appears bloted and is sensitive to the touch

2. Using word processing software, create an interoffice memo. Andrew Edwards, CMA (AAMA), is the sender of the memo and all clinical staff members are intended to be the recipients. The purpose of the memo is to inform the clinical staff that a pharmaceutical sales representative will be presenting information on a new cardiac drug that Dr. Sheila Tyrone is considering using for patient therapy. The presentation will occur on Friday during the lunch hour.

LEARNING ACTIVITY: MULTIPLE CHOICE

Circle the correct answer to each of the questions below.

1. Which of the following is the size of a standard business envelope?
   a. 3½" × 8½"
   b. 4⅛" × 9½"
   c. 4¼" × 9¼"
   d. None of the above

2. How much postage is required to mail an interoffice memo?
   a. $0.31
   b. $0.23
   c. $0.20
   d. None of the above

3. In order to catch all of the errors in a written document, how many times should the medical assistant read a letter before sending it out?
   a. Once
   b. Twice
   c. Three times
   d. Four times

4. The __________ of a professional letter typically appears two lines down from the ending portion of the body.
   a. closing
   b. subject line
   c. salutation
   d. letterhead

5. Which of the following pieces of information are typically included in the office letterhead?
   a. Office name
   b. Office address
   c. Office e-mail address
   d. All of the above

6. Which of the following statements is written correctly?
   a. The patient is taking five milligrams of the medication every hour.
   b. The patient is taking 5 milligrams of the medication every hour.
   c. The patient is taking five (5) milligrams of the medication every hour.
   d. All of the above are correct.

7. Which of the following words is misspelled?
   a. foriegn
   b. occurrance
   c. liason
   d. All of the above are misspelled

8. The closing appears __________ spaces below the end of the body of the letter.
   a. one
   b. two

c. three
d. four

9. Which of the following parts of speech modifies a noun or a pronoun?
   a. Verb
   b. Adverb
   c. Adjective
   d. Preposition

10. Which of the following style of letters is spaced with all lines flush with the left margin except for the first line of each paragraph?
    a. Modified block
    b. Simplified letter block
    c. Semi-simplified letter block
    d. None of the above

CRITICAL THINKING

Answer the following questions to the best of your ability. Utilize the textbook as a reference.

1. Missy Hurst, RMA, is working as an administrative medical assistant with a gastroenterology practice. Dr. Brown has asked Missy to annotate the laboratory reports that come back from the lab. What is he asking Missy to do?

____

____

____

____

____

2. Henry Connelly, CMA (AAMA), has just been hired to work at the front desk in a family practice clinic. Part of his job is to open and sort the mail. There is no written office policy about this task currently on file in the office so Henry decides to create one. How should Henry proceed and what might his policy look like?

____

____

____

____

____

3. Willie Rachenko, RMA, has been working with Dr. Stuart for several years. Dr. Stuart asks Willie to contact Mr. Brocheer regarding his lab results from earlier this week. Willie looks into Mr. Brocheer's chart and sees that the patient has listed his work e-mail address. Willie isn't able to reach Mr. Brocheer by telephone and instead of leaving a voice mail message asking the patient to return his call, Willie decides to e-mail the patient with his lab results. Later that day, Mr. Brocheer calls the office very upset. He tells Willie that his boss intercepted the e-mail and now knows that his employee was screened for a possible sexually transmitted disease. What did Willie do wrong?

____

____

____

4. Mallory Valdez is taking an administrative medical assisting class. She has been given the assignment of writing a short paper that outlines the various mailing services offered by the U.S. Postal Service. What should Mallory include in her paper?

RESEARCH ACTIVITY

Utilize Internet search engines to research the following topics and write a brief description of what you find. It is important to utilize reputable websites.

1. Visit www.usps.com and research information regarding certified mail, rates, and extra services available. When could some of the "extra services" be useful when dealing with written correspondence between the medical office and patients?

CHAPTER 12
Computers in the Medical Office

CHAPTER OUTLINE

General review of the chapter:

Use of Computers in Medicine
Types of Computers
Basic Computer Components
Security for the Computer System
Selecting a Computer System
The Internet
Electronic Signatures
Computers and Ergonomics

STUDENT STUDY GUIDE

Use the following guide to assist in your learning of the concepts from the chapter.

I. Computers in the Medical Office

1. Functions of Computers in the Medical Office (List six general functions.)

   i. ______________________________
   ii. ______________________________
   iii. ______________________________
   iv. ______________________________
   v. ______________________________
   vi. ______________________________

2. Microcomputers

   A. Contains a small piece of electronic hardware called a __________.
   B. Allows the __________ of information in a very small amount of space.

3. Central Processing Unit

   A. The CPU contains the main __________ of a computer.
   B. The CPU acts as a traffic controller, directing the computer's __________ and sending electronic signals to the right place at the right time.
   C. The transmission speed of these electronic signals is measured in __________.
   D. One __________ equals one __________ cycles per second.
   E. The higher the __________, the faster the __________.

4. Random Access Memory (RAM)

   A. RAM is available only as long as the computer is __________.
   B. Once the computer is turned off, or powered down, all information stored in RAM is __________.

5. Read-Only Memory (ROM)
   A. Once data is recorded, it cannot be removed, only _______.
   B. ROM is used to _______ information that is not actively being used by the computer.
   C. ROM is used primarily to _______ permanent data.
6. The Computer Monitor
   A. Allows the user to __________ what the computer has been told to do.
   B. Monitors are available in a variety of __________ and __________.
   C. The screen size is measured in __________ inches.
7. Types of Monitors
   A. A _____________ monitor displays two colors—one for the background and one for the foreground.
   B. A _____________ monitor is a special type of monochrome monitor that is capable of displaying different shades of gray.
   C. A _____________ monitor displays anywhere from 16 to more than 1 million different colors.
8. Hard-Disk Drive
   A. A hard-disk drive is the ___________ storage media inside the computer.
   B. It is controlled by the ___________.
   C. ___________ and information can be stored on a hard-disk drive.
   D. The more visual the software, the ___________ the amount of storage space that is required.
9. CD-ROM
   A. Stands for ____.
   B. Computer programs, databases, and other large amounts of information on CD-ROM are _______________ encoded and may not be changed by the user.
   C. It is capable of holding or storing more information than _______________ floppy disks.
10. DVD
   A. Stands for ______________ or ______________.
   B. Used most often to record presentations that combine ______________ and ______________.
11. Removable Disk Drive
   A. Uses disks mounted in _________.
   B. Comes in a variety of sizes ranging from _________ megabytes to _________ gigabytes.
12. Portable Universal Serial Bus Drive
   A. Also known as a _________ drive, a _________ drive, or a _________ drive.
   B. This small portable storage device can hold up to _________ GB of data.
13. Microsoft Office Application Programs (List three commonly used applications.)
   i. ____
   ii. ____
   iii. ____
14. Computer Office Security Considerations
   A. Position the computer __________ so that it cannot be easily seen by patients.
   B. Use a __________ screen around the computer workstation.
   C. Use a screen __________.
   D. Use computer __________.
15. Uses of the Internet in the Medical Office (List three common uses.)
   i. ____
   ii. ____
   iii. ____

16. Chair Ergonomics When Working on the Computer
    A. Push your hips as _______ back in the chair as possible.
    B. Adjust the seat height so that your feet are _______ on the floor and your knees are _______, or _______ than, your hips.
    C. Adjust the back of the chair to a _______ to _______ reclined angle.
    D. Make sure that your upper and lower back are _______.
17. Ergonomics When Working on the Keyboard
    A. If possible, adjust the keyboard height so that your shoulders are _______, your elbows are in a slightly _______ position, and your wrists and hands are _______.
    B. Wrist rests can help maintain a _______ posture and pad hard surfaces.
    C. Wrist rests should only be used to rest the _______ of the hands between keystrokes.
18. The Monitor and Ergonomics
    A. Adjust the monitor and source documents so that your __________ is in a neutral, relaxed position.
    B. Position the top of the monitor approximately __________ to __________ inches above your seated eye level.
    C. To reduce glare, place the screen at a __________ angle to windows and adjust curtains or blinds.
19. Body Ergonomics When Working on the Computer
    A. Take short ______ or ______ -minute stretch breaks every ______ to ______ minutes.
    B. After each hour of work, take a break or change tasks for at least ______ to ______ minutes.
    C. Avoid eye fatigue by resting and ______ your eyes periodically.
    D. Rest your eyes by covering them with your palms for ______ to ______ seconds.

KEY TERMINOLOGY REVIEW

Match the term to the correct definition below.

a. bandwidth
b. central processing unit (CPU)
c. clock speed
d. computer
e. input devices
f. Internet
g. Internet service provider (ISP)
h. kilobytes (KB)
i. main memory
j. mass storage device
k. memory
l. output devices
m. random access memory (RAM)
n. read-only memory (ROM)
o. software
p. universal serial bus (USB)
q. World Wide Web (WWW)

1. ______________ A programmable machine or system of hardware that responds to a specific set of instructions and performs a list of instructions in programmed language.
2. ______________ Provides access to the Internet.
3. ______________ Set of instructions by means of which the computer performs its functions.
4. ______________ Makes it possible for a computer to temporarily store data and programs.
5. ______________ Internal storage area in the computer that can be accessed randomly.
6. ______________ The amount of data that can be transmitted in a fixed amount of time.
7. ______________ The speed at which the CPU can process instructions.

8. ______________ Makes it possible for a computer to permanently retain large amounts of data even when the computer is off.
9. ______________ Allow the user to see what the computer has accomplished.
10. ______________ The brain of the computer, which executes the specific set of instructions.
11. ______________ An internal storage area in the computer where data have been recorded.
12. ______________ Computer network of thousands of interfacing networks worldwide.
13. ______________ Acts as a traffic controller, directing the computer's activities and sending electronic signals to the right place at the right time.
14. ______________ Feed data and instructions into a computer.
15. ______________ A system of Internet servers.
16. ______________ One thousand units of storage or memory
17. ______________ A small portable storage device that can hold up to 64 GB or more of data.

APPLIED PRACTICE

Read the scenario and answer the questions that follow.

Scenario

Shane Eiler, RMA, is an office manager for Inner Harbor Sports Medicine. His office computer has had a recent attack from a malware program. This attack has left his computer unusable.

1. Shane has been asked to research the cost of purchasing a new computer for the medical office. Create a list of the steps he should take to determine the type of system that is best for the office.

____
____
____
____

2. The physicians have also asked Shane to create a list of suggestions for securing the office computers from unauthorized access. What suggestions should Shane make?

____
____
____
____

LEARNING ACTIVITY: MULTIPLE CHOICE

Circle the correct answer to each of the questions below.

1. ______________ are devices that allow documents to be copied and transferred to the computer.
   a. Thumb drives
   b. Personal digital assistants

c. Printers
d. Scanners

2. _____________ is the computer equipment.

a. The hardware
b. The software
c. The peripheral
d. The USB

3. _____________ are typically used in a medical office.

a. Supercomputers
b. Mainframe computers
c. Minicomputers
d. Microcomputers

4. The computer's CPU is considered to be the computer's _____________.

a. brain
b. memory
c. keyboard
d. mouse

5. An articulating keyboard is used to _____________.

a. connect to the computer via a wireless connection
b. reduce typing stress by supporting the hands and wrists comfortably
c. type faster than when using a conventional keyboard
d. maintain patient privacy when using the keyboard

6. As computer technology advances, _____________ are becoming obsolete.

a. floppy disk drives
b. CD drives
c. DVD drives
d. Thumb drives

7. _____________ makes it possible for a computer to temporarily store data and programs.

a. Mass storage device
b. Memory
c. Software
d. CPU

8. Laptops are also known as _____________.

a. Palm pilots
b. PDAs
c. Notebooks
d. CPUs

9. The hard-disk drive, a magnetic storage media inside the computer, is usually called the _____________.

a. A drive
b. B drive

c. C drive
d. D drive

10. An/A ____________ printer works by forming dots when the ink is blown onto the paper.
    a. dot matrix
    b. laser
    c. deskjet
    d. inkjet

CRITICAL THINKING

Answer the following questions to the best of your ability. Utilize the textbook and other resources such as the Internet in considering the following questions.

1. Marcia Dukat is taking a computer applications class in the medical assisting program. She has been given an assignment to create a list of steps that medical office staff can take in order to protect the office computers from viruses. What should Marcia's list include?

____

____

____

____

2. Rolf Von Trapp, RMA, is discussing the need for a new computer system with the physician. Dr. Nyrse has asked Rolf to describe the difference between the hardware, the software, and the peripherals that go with the various computer systems. How might Rolf define these three components?

____

____

____

____

3. George El Fashir, CMA (AAMA), has been asked to describe the various computer drives that might be used to store information from the computer systems in his office. What information should George prepare?

____

____

____

____

4. Riley Gaddum is taking a computer class as part of his medical assistant training. He has been given an assignment to describe the difference between ROM and RAM. What might Riley write for this assignment?

____

____

____

____

RESEARCH ACTIVITY

Utilize Internet search engines to research the following topics and write a brief description of what you find. It is important to utilize reputable websites.

1. Use the Internet to research medical office software programs. What software program do you like the most? What features does it have? Why would you recommend its use?

CHAPTER 13
Managing Medical Records

CHAPTER OUTLINE

General review of the chapter:

The Medical Record
Documentation of Patient Medical Information
Components of the Medical Record
Filing
Quality Assurance for Quality Medical Care
Releasing Medical Records
Storing Medical Records
Medical Transcription
Ownership of the Medical Record
Retention and Destruction of Medical Records

STUDENT STUDY GUIDE

Use the following guide to assist in your learning of the concepts from the chapter.

I. Managing Medical Records

1. Categories and Reports Found in a Medical Record

i. ______________________________
ii. ______________________________
iii. ______________________________
iv. ______________________________
v. ______________________________
vi. ______________________________
vii. ______________________________
viii. ______________________________
ix. ______________________________
x. ______________________________
xi. ______________________________
xii. ______________________________
xiii. ______________________________
xiv. ______________________________
xv. ______________________________
xvi. ______________________________

2. The Chronological Medical Record

A. Follows the patient __________.
B. Each visit consists of a new entry by __________ rather than by __________ or __________.
C. This record can sometimes makes it more difficult to "catch" __________.

3. The Problem-Oriented Medical Record
   A. Used to identify patient problems and chart by those ______.
   B. The functional aspect of this type of charting is that the patient ______ list is found at the ______ of the chart.
   C. As new problems and diagnoses are identified, they are noted on the ______ list.
   D. Helps health care providers who do not already know a specific patient to obtain a ______ regarding previous visits and problems at a glance.
4. Sections of the Problems-Oriented Medical Record
   i. ______________________________
   ii. ______________________________
   iii. ______________________________
   iv. ______________________________
5. SOAP Charting
   A. "S" identifies the __________ information gathered from the patient.
   B. "O" stands for __________, the data gathered during the visit.
   C. "A" is for __________, the physician's __________ diagnosis.
   D. "P" indicates the __________ of the chart where __________ for the care of this patient are discussed.
6. The Source-Oriented Medical Record
   A. Patient information is placed in the medical record in __________ __________ order and is organized in different sections.
   B. Each office determines which __________ to be used and in what order they are to appear in the medical chart.
   C. The sections commonly include medical history and physical, insurance, __________ notes, __________, laboratory reports, and __________.
7. Information that SHOULD NOT BE INCLUDED in a Patient's Chart
   i. ______________________________
   ii. ______________________________
   iii. ______________________________
8. Information that SHOULD BE INCLUDED in the Medical Record
   A. _______ statements.
   B. Everything that is done during a _______ _______ visit.
   C. Legible writing in _______ ink.
9. Correcting Errors Made When Documenting Care in an Electronic Medical Record
   A. When documenting care in an EMR, prior to saving the entry, errors may be corrected by _______ as you would with any other type of computer program.
   B. If an error is discovered after the entry is saved, an _______ entry, called an _______, will be required.
   C. When using an EMR, the entry will be automatically _______ and _______ electronically when saved.
10. Steps for Adding Items to a Patient's Record
   i. ______________________________
   ii. ______________________________
   iii. ______________________________
   iv. ______________________________
   v. ______________________________
   vi. ______________________________
   vii. ______________________________

11. Guidelines for Changing Items in a Patient's Record
    i. ____________________
    ii. ____________________
    iii. ____________________
    iv. ____________________
    v. ____________________
    vi. ____________________
    vii. ____________________
12. Responsibilities of the MA
    A. Document information _________ in the medical record.
    B. Ensure that the information added to the medical record is _________.
    C. _________ that patients' records are kept up to date.
    D. Make files as easily _________ as possible.
13. Contents of Medical Records
    i. ____________________
    ii. ____________________
    iii. ____________________
    iv. ____________________
    v. ____________________
    vi. ____________________
    vii. ____________________
    viii. ____________________
    ix. ____________________
    x. ____________________
    xi. ____________________
    xii. ____________________
    xiii. ____________________
    xiv. ____________________
    xv. ____________________
    xvi. ____________________

II. Filing
1. Categories of Medical Records
    i. ____________________
    ii. ____________________
    iii. ____________________
2. The Vertical File Cabinet
    A. Set up ______ to ______ stacked pull-out drawers holding up to ______ files per drawer.
    B. A drawback of this method is that the files are _________ and consume _________ .
3. The Lateral File Cabinet
    A. Set up with ___________ allowing for easy access to files by pulling them off the ___________.
    B. Use a ___________ method for visual recognition of files.
4. The Movable File Cabinet
    A. Set up with ______________ powered or __________ controlled file units that move on tracks in the floor.
    B. This method is a type of ___________ filing system.
    C. This method is ___________ saving since the file units can be moved close together when they are not in use.
    D. Useful for ______ and ______ since the floor can be reinforced when the track is installed.

5. Traditional Hard-copy Patient Record

   A. The patient's file typically has tabs on the __________ or __________ edge.
   B. These tabs are marked with __________ labels.
   C. It is easier to read the labels in the file drawer if the files have __________ tab cuts.
   D. File folders may be ____________ to indicate the primary care physician.

6. Outguide

   A. Inserted where a file has been __________ to indicate the place to which the file should be __________.
   B. Can be used to indicate who has __________ the file and when it was __________.
   C. Especially helpful in a large office when trying to __________ charts.
   D. Usually a distinctive color, such as __________, to indicate that a file is missing.

7. The Purposes of Labels on File Folders

   A. The main purpose is to __________ what is in the file.
   B. The label can include a __________ stripe that can be used for other purposes, such as identifying the __________ __________ physician.
   C. Offices use special labels on charts to bring attention to patient __________, required __________, and the year of the last visit.
   D. Special labels help the staff find __________ information at a glance.

8. Rules for an Alphabetical Filing System

   A. A name with only an __________ in place of the first name is filed before a __________ name.
   B. Hyphenated names are treated as __________ unit.
   C. Apostrophes are __________.
   D. Titles and initials are __________, but placed in __________ after the name.
   E. Married women are to be indexed using their __________ name.
   F. Seniority units are filed __________.

9. Numerical Filing or Patient Identification System

   A. Used in __________ and many larger clinics.
   B. A number is assigned to each patient's __________ __________.
   C. The number is generally a __________ -digit number divided into __________ sections of __________ digits each.

10. Straight Numerical Filing

    A. This is the __________ numerical method.
    B. Each record is filed __________ based on its assigned number.
    C. Numbers used in this system begin at __________ and continue upward.

11. Terminal Digit Filing

    A. Based on the last digits of the __________ number.
    B. Evenly distributes the files within the entire filing system, eliminating the need for frequent __________ of files.
    C. Requires dividing the files into __________ primary sections, starting with __________ and ending with __________.
    D. Three sections of numbers assigned to each file are designated as __________, __________, and __________ sections, respectively.

12. Unit Numbering

    A. Assigns a number to patients the __________ time that they are seen or admitted to a hospital.
    B. All other hospitalizations or hospital visits use the __________ number.
    C. Requires that all of the records be kept at the __________ location.

13. Serial Numbering
    A. With this system, the patient receives a different medical record number for each _________ visit.
    B. The patient acquires _________ records that are stored at _________ locations.
    C. The assigned numbers are kept in an _________ record in which numbers in sequential order have a _________ placed next to them as each new _________ is entered.
14. Subject Matter Filing
    A. Used for _________ files.
    B. The method is adequate as long as the files are relatively _________.
15. Color-Coding Systems
    A. Assigns a _________ for each number from _________.
    B. _________ bars on files correspond to the medical record number.
    C. Typically, the _________ primary digits are color-coded.
    D. The system allows for misfiles to be _________ seen.
16. The Alpha-Z System
    A. The system is based on _________ colors using _________ letters on a _________ background for the first half of the alphabet, with the addition of a white stripe on the _________ background for the second half of the alphabet.
    B. Uses _________ _________ to denote the patient's name and a colored label with the letter of the alphabet to indicate the _________ unit.
    C. In large practices with several physicians, each physician may have a _________ assigned to him or her.
17. Advantages of Cross-Referencing Files
    i. ____
    ii. ____
    iii. ____
18. Guidelines for Locating Missing Files
    i. ____
    ii. ____
    iii. ____
    iv. ____
    v. ____
    vi. ____
    vii. ____
19. Tickler Files
    A. A tickler file is a _________ for future events
    B. Should be reviewed _________.
    C. Contents may include _________, _________, _________, and _________.

III. Releasing, Retaining, and Storing Medical Records

1. Quality Assurance Programs
    A. The _________ is to improve the quality of care.
    B. Implementation requires developing _________ criteria.
    C. One method for documenting problem areas is the use of _________ reports.
2. The Incident Report
    A. A report should be completed whenever there is an _________ occurrence.
    B. The purpose is to document exactly what happened, with the goal of _________ another similar episode.

C. Details on completing an incident report are usually included in every office's __________ __________.

3. The Joint Commission
   A. The Commission is a private, __________ agency.
   B. Establishes guidelines to address the __________ of care provided by __________ and __________ agencies.
   C. Conducts __________ and __________ programs to ensure that institutions are following the guidelines for __________.
   D. Works with facilities to correct __________.

4. The Occupational Safety and Health Administration
   A. OSHA's purpose is to ensure a __________ __________ environment for employees.
   B. Sets basic __________ standards that all institutions must follow.
   C. Violators of OSHA standards must __________ __________.

5. Authorizing the Release of Records
   A. The __________ owns the medical record.
   B. The patient has the __________ right to access the record.
   C. A __________ __________ must be signed to authorize the release of a patient's record.

6. The Skills of a Medical Transcriptionist
   i. ______________________________
   ii. ______________________________
   iii. ______________________________
   iv. ______________________________
   v. ______________________________
   vi. ______________________________

7. Ownership of X-rays
   A. X-rays are the property of the __________.
   B. Physicians are able to loan their films to other physicians for further examination; however, the __________ must sign a __________.
   C. The films should always be returned to the __________.

8. Ownership of Medical Records
   A. If a patient requests to view his or her own medical records, access must be allowed, unless the physician determines that it may be __________ to the patient.
   B. Prior to allowing the patients to view their records, the MA must first check with the __________ or __________ for approval.
   C. Never leave patients __________ with their records.

9. Guidelines for Retaining Medical Records
   A. To be absolutely safe, medical records should be retained __________.
   B. The standard set by most states is to keep records __________ to __________ years after the last treatment or __________ years after the patient reaches the age of __________.
   C. The AMA recommends keeping the records for __________ years.

KEY TERMINOLOGY REVIEW

Match the correct medical term with the definition listed below.

a. active records
b. addendum
c. alphabetical filing
d. chronological medical records
e. closed records
f. electronic medical records

g. inactive records
h. medical record
i. microfiche
j. microfilm
k. numerical filing
l. POMR
m. SOMR
n. SOAP
o. terminal-digit filing

1. ______________ The key to this type of filing is to divide the names and titles into units (first, second, and third).
2. ______________ Source of all documentation related to the patient.
3. ______________ Used to identify patient problems and chart by those problems.
4. ______________ Miniaturized photographs of records.
5. ______________ Patients who have been seen within the past 3 years and are currently being treated.
6. ______________ Based on the last digits of the ID number; evenly distributes the files within the entire filing system.
7. ______________ A computerized means of gathering, documenting, and storing information about the patient and the care received in the medical setting.
8. ______________ A charting method that is distinct because of the four parts of the approach.
9. ______________ Follows the patient over a period of time, with each visit consisting of a new entry by date, rather than by symptoms or diagnosis.
10. ______________ Patients who have not been seen within the past 3 years or another period determined by office policy.
11. ______________ Organizes patient information in the medical record in reverse chronological order.
12. ______________ Patients who have actively terminated their contact with the physician.
13. ______________ Patient identification system used in hospitals and many larger clinics.
14. ______________ Sheets of microfilm.
15. ______________ An addition to an original document.

APPLIED PRACTICE

Follow the instructions with each question below.

1. Indicate if the following patients would be considered active, inactive, or closed patient files?
   a. Lori Hughes, a patient who has moved out of the state
      Patient file status: ______________________________
   b. Quin Tao, a patient who has not been seen in the office for 5 years
      Patient file status: ______________________________
   c. Gloria Sanchez, a patient who was in the office for care last week
      Patient file status: ______________________________
   d. Sara Womack, a patient who died last year
      Patient file status: ______________________________
2. Using the progress note below, accurately place the statements below into SOAP format. Mario Reynolds, born August 12, 1990, presents to the office with the following:
   - T: 100.3°
   - Positive Rapid Strep Test
   - "My throat is sore."
   - Pharyngitis and Strep Throat
   - Throat appears red and white spots present on tonsils.

- Penicillin V 250mg BID × 10 days
- BP: 118/86
- Wt: 192#
- Patient has been sick with a fever for 3 days.

PROGRESS NOTE

Patient: ______________________________ **DOB:** ______________

	S O A P

LEARNING ACTIVITY: MULTIPLE CHOICE

Circle the correct answer to each of the questions below.

1. Which of the following techniques is the appropriate way to correct an error in the patient's medical record?
   a. Use white correction fluid to obliterate the error.
   b. Use a black marker to obliterate the error.
   c. Draw a single line through the error; initial and date the correction.
   d. Any of the above

2. Under which of the following circumstances can the patient's medical record be copied and released?
   a. When the patient's spouse comes to the office to request a copy
   b. When the patient's employer calls the office to request a copy
   c. When the patient has signed a release form
   d. When the patient's brother sends a letter asking for a copy

3. The American Medical Association recommends keeping medical records for __________.
   a. 2 years
   b. 5 years
   c. 10 years
   d. Indefinitely

4. Once an office is out of room for storing patient medical records, which of the following is an appropriate way to store records?
   a. On a separate backup system
   b. In computer database files
   c. On microfilm
   d. Any of the above

5. Which of the following is true about retaining patient medical records?
   a. The record should be kept for 3 years from the date of the last service.
   b. The length of time that the record is kept is determined by the statute of limitations in any particular state.
   c. The record should be kept until the patient reaches age 18.
   d. All of the above are true.

6. __________ patient files are the files of patients who have moved and will not be continuing to receive treatment by the physician or facility.
   a. Open
   b. Closed
   c. Inactive
   d. None of the above

7. __________ patient files are the files of patients who have not been seen within the past 3 years or another period determined by office policy.
   a. Open
   b. Closed
   c. Inactive
   d. None of the above

8. __________ patient files are the files of patients who have been in to see the physician recently.
   a. Open
   b. Closed
   c. Inactive
   d. None of the above

9. The simplest numerical method of filing is __________.
   a. straight numerical filing
   b. terminal-digit filing
   c. middle-digit filing
   d. unit-number filing

10. __________ is a type of medical charting that tracks a patient's problems throughout medical care by assigning a number to each of the patient's medical problems.
   a. Narrative notes
   b. SOAP notes
   c. POMR notes
   d. None of the above

CRITICAL THINKING

Answer the following questions to the best of your ability. Utilize the textbook and other resources such as the Internet in considering the following questions.

1. Chris Nichols, CMA (AAMA), has been given the task of deciding which patient files to purge from the clinic in order to create more storage space. How should Chris proceed with this project?

____

____

2. Michael Manson, RMA, has just been hired to work in a family practice clinic. On his first day in the office, he notices that many patients' records have words such as "problem" and "talker" listed on them. He asks the MA who is training him about these words and is told that it is the office's way of noting those patients who are difficult to work with or who talk excessively during their visit. What kinds of problems might this facility encounter when using these notations?

3. Susan Haufe, RMA, is working with a small, one-doctor internal medicine clinic. The physician, Dr. Chentow, is unable to retain his patient records indefinitely. What considerations must Susan give to the method of destruction?

RESEARCH ACTIVITY

Utilize Internet search engines to research the following topics and write a brief description of what you find. It is important to utilize reputable websites.

1. Using the Internet as a research source, research the types of filing systems that may be found in a medical setting. Describe the pros and cons of each system.

CHAPTER 14
Electronic Medical Records

CHAPTER OUTLINE

General review of the chapter:

Electronic Medical Records Are Easily Accessible
How Does Paper Charting Differ from Electronic Charting?
Making the Conversion from Paper to Electronic Medical Records
Electronic Medical Records and HIPAA Compliance
Using Personal Digital Assistants with Electronic Medical Records
Benefits of Electronic Medical Records
Making Corrections in the Medical Record

STUDENT STUDY GUIDE

Use the following guide to assist in your learning of the concepts from the chapter.

I. Electronic Medical Records

1. Electronic Medical Records (EMRs)
   A. EMRs are sometimes called ___________ ___________ ___________.
   B. The EMR is a means of ___________, ___________, and ___________ information about the patient and the care received in the medical setting.

2. Advantages of the EMR—Accessibility!
   i. ______________________________
   ii. ______________________________
   iii. ______________________________
   iv. ______________________________
   v. ______________________________
   vi. ______________________________
   vii. ______________________________
   viii. ______________________________

3. Converting from Paper to Electronic Medical Records
   A. Some clinics are able to use a __________ to __________ the patient's paper medical record for use in the EMR system.
   B. Other clinics may need to enter information from the paper medical record to the EMR ___________.
   C. Once the information from the paper medical record has been transferred to the EMR, the clinic staff may choose to __________ the paper record by __________ the documents.
   D. Some offices may choose to __________ the paper record in a secure location rather than __________ it.

4. Training Staff on the EMR
   A. Training should be attended by __________ in the office who will be using the software.
   B. A training __________ should be supplied for use in training future staff members.
   C. A technical support person from the __________ should be available to answer questions or concerns related to the software.
5. Ensuring Patient Privacy with the EMR
   A. All computer users must have their own __________ to access patient medical records.
   B. With each person having login information, the software can __________ each entry or deletion and who made it.
   C. Each station must be __________ __________ when the user is away from the desk.
   D. Computer screens must not be __________ by other patients while private patient information is displayed on the screen.
6. Data Backup System
   A. Mandated by __________.
   B. Must be used on a __________ basis.
7. Personal Digital Assistants in the Medical Office
   A. A PDA is a lightweight, __________, usually pen- or stylus-based computer that is used as a personal __________.
   B. A PDA offers the benefit of being __________ enough for physicians to carry with them from patient to patient.
   C. Most EMR systems can be __________ to work according to an office's specific needs.
8. Benefits Gained Through Using the EMR
   i. ______________________________
   ii. ______________________________
   iii. ______________________________
   iv. ______________________________
   v. ______________________________
   vi. ______________________________
9. Electronic Signatures
   A. Most electronic medical records provide an electronic signature component that is based on the individual's __________ via his or her user name and __________.
   B. Once the entry is made into the patient's chart, the staff member or physician clicks __________ and the entry is electronically __________.
10. Avoiding Medical Errors
    A. EMR software typically has a __________ mechanism built in that alerts the prescribing physician to any __________ medications that a particular patient may be taking.
    B. Studies have found that medical errors are caused by __________ or __________ handwriting, a problem that would be eliminated if providers made their entries electronically.
11. Saving Time
    A. Time saved by the use of an EMR system may be better invested in __________ .
    B. Many EMR systems include lists of possible __________ for the physician to choose from based on the symptoms that the patient lists.
    C. EMRs allow medical staff to easily transmit __________ information to a patient's health insurance provider when requested.
12. Availability of Medical Records Online
    A. Some clinics allow patients to look up portions of their EMR via the __________.
    B. Using a __________-__________ system, patients can access a company's network or intranet for their laboratory results, dates of immunization, or history of medications prescribed.

13. Steps for Correcting an Error in the EMR
    i. ______
    ii. ______
    iii. ______
    iv. ______
    v. ______
    vi. ______

KEY TERMINOLOGY REVIEW

Without using your textbook, write a sentence using the selected key terms in the correct context.

1. *Electronic medical record:*

2. *Electronic signature:*

3. *Indecipherable:*

4. *Electronic health record:*

5. *Health Insurance Portability and Accountability Act (HIPAA):*

6. *Personal digital assistant (PDA):*

APPLIED PRACTICE

Read the scenario and then answer the questions that follow.

Scenario

Jeffery Cody, RMA, is the office manager for Foothills Family Medicine. The office has slowly been transferring from paper medical records to electronic medical records.

1. In the final stages of this process, how will the medical office include written reports and consultations from other facilities?

2. Jeffery is writing a memo to the office staff regarding making corrections to medical records. What information should he include in his memo?

____

____

____

____

LEARNING ACTIVITY: TRUE/FALSE

Indicate whether the following statements are true or false by placing a T or an F on the line that precedes each statement.

_______ 1. Electronic medical records offer enhanced ease, efficiency, and accessibility.

_______ 2. Using electronic medical records, a medical office can send reminder postcards to patients more easily than performing this task using paper medical records.

_______ 3. Using electronic medical records, a medical office is able to perform many tests in the office and have the results shown immediately in the electronic medical record.

_______ 4. It is much more difficult to remain HIPAA-compliant with patient medical records if the office is using electronic medical records instead of paper medical records.

_______ 5. Once a paper medical record has been converted to an electronic version, the paper record may be kept in secure storage or may be shredded.

_______ 6. Most electronic medical records programs have drop-down menus that allow the user to choose information from a list.

_______ 7. As a result of a study released in 1999, the Institute of Medicine suggested that some medical errors are caused by indecipherable handwriting.

_______ 8. Using electronic medical records, health care providers may be alerted to possible medication errors.

_______ 9. In medical offices where electronic signatures are used, an original version of the user's signature does not need to be kept on file in the office.

_______ 10. All medical facilities use the same software for electronic medical records.

CRITICAL THINKING

Answer the following questions to the best of your ability. Utilize the textbook as a reference.

1. Rosa Valdez, CMA (AAMA), is working in the billing office of a urology practice. The office uses electronic medical records for patient charting. Rosa frequently finds that she needs to alert other staff members of her need to speak with a patient about their account. How might Rosa devise a way to alert her coworkers of her need to see a patient when that patient comes into the office?

____

____

____

____

2. Chris Hernandez, RMA, is the office manager of a busy family practice clinic. Chris has been asked by the physicians to come up with some ideas for using the electronic medical records

software to create a marketing program. What kinds of ideas could Chris suggest for this project?

3. Mickey Cape is taking a course on electronic medical records. Mickey has been given an assignment to write a policy on how to dispose of paper medical records once the record has been converted to electronic form. What might Mickey come up with?

4. Barret Risenhour, RMA, is the office manager in a women's clinic. The physicians in the clinic are considering moving to electronic medical records from the paper records that they have been using for years. Barret has been asked to create a list of the pros and cons of using electronic medical records versus paper records. What might Barret's list contain?

5. Dr. Shawn Hagen has been using paper medical records in his practice for more than 20 years. He is reluctant to change to electronic medical records because he feels that his computer skills are poor. What sort of information can his office manager give him about the ease of converting from paper to electronic medical records?

RESEARCH ACTIVITY

Utilize Internet search engines to research the following topics and write a brief description of what you find. It is important to utilize reputable websites.

1. Using the Internet as a research source, locate three companies that sell electronic medical records software. Create a list of the pros and cons of each system.

Chapter 15
Fees, Billing, Collections, and Credit

CHAPTER OUTLINE

General review of the chapter:

Professional Fees
Billing
Credit Policy
Collections
Accounting Systems
Bookkeeping Systems
Computerized Systems
Professional Courtesy

STUDENT STUDY GUIDE

Use the following guide to assist in your learning of the concepts from the chapter.

I. Fees, Billing, Collections, and Credit

1. Factors Used to Determine Physician's Fees
    i. ____________________
    ii. ____________________
    iii. ____________________
2. Informing Patients of Fees and Payment Policies
    A. Information should include __________, __________, and __________ procedures.
    B. Information can be conveyed during the __________ phone call with the patient and then a __________ can be mailed to the patient.
    C. Fees and payment __________ should be posted in the office.
3. Methods for Securing Payment
    A. Collect payment at the time that the __________ is provided.
    B. __________ the patient.
    C. Use an outside __________ __________.
4. Truth in Lending Form
    A. The form clearly states the __________ of the __________ charge and the __________ payments.
    B. Where there are no finance charges, this is to be stated on the __________ form.
    C. The original form is given to the __________ and a copy is retained by the __________.
5. Consent Form for Billing
    A. Allows the medical office to bill the __________ on behalf of the patient for the services provided.

B. Grants the office permission to forward information regarding the patient's visit, including __________ and __________, to the insurance carrier if requested.
C. Should be placed in the file and updated __________.

6. Billing Methods

A. __________ internally.
B. Generated by the __________ __________.
C. Generated externally through the use of a __________ service.

7. Superbill

A. Also known as an __________ form.
B. Can be used as a __________ slip, statement, and insurance reporting form.
C. Provides a __________ list of patient services with __________ and __________.

8. Ledger Card and Mailing Statements

A. __________ ledger card is created for each patient.
B. Used to record __________, __________, and __________ for the patient.
C. When mailing a statement to the patient, the ledger card can be __________ and used as the __________.

9. Information Required for Billing

i. ______________________________
ii. ______________________________
iii. ______________________________
iv. ______________________________
v. ______________________________
vi. ______________________________
vii. ______________________________

10. Billing Third-Party Payers and Minors

A. Third-party payers are individuals other than the patient who have agreed to pay the __________ __________.
B. Assignment of benefits ensures __________ payment to the __________ .
C. __________ minors can be billed.

11. Steps for Preparing a Ledger Card

i. ______________________________
ii. ______________________________
iii. ______________________________
iv. ______________________________
v. ______________________________

12. Making Credit Arrangements with Patients

A. Remind patients during the __________ reminder call about their obligation to pay.
B. Try to obtain payment at the time of __________.
C. Provide a billing statement to patients when they leave the office with a __________ for payment.
D. If credit arrangements are necessary, make them during the patient's __________ visit.

13. Guidelines for Collections

i. ______________________________
ii. ______________________________
iii. ______________________________
iv. ______________________________
v. ______________________________
vi. ______________________________

vii. ______________________________
viii. ______________________________
ix. ______________________________

14. Reasons for Outstanding Bills
    A. The patient does not feel that the bill is ____________.
    B. The patient is ____________ to pay.
    C. The patient does not ____________ the bill.

15. Effects of Having Delinquent Accounts
    A. Patients stay away from the office because they are ____________ about their financial situation.
    B. There is a possible implication of ____________ on the part of the physician as to the ____________ of care that the patient received.
    C. Loss of ____________.

16. Account Age Analysis
    A. Computerized systems provide reports that indicate accounts which are ____________, ____________, and ____________ days overdue.
    B. The collection step needed is determined by the ____________ of the account.
    C. Manual systems utilize ____________ systems with various colors or flags attached to ____________ cards to indicate the age of the accounts.

17. Collection Techniques
    i. ______________________________
    ii. ______________________________
    iii. ______________________________
    iv. ______________________________
    v. ______________________________

18. Guidelines for Making Collection Calls
    A. Avoid placing calls earlier than ____________ A.M. or later than ____________ P.M. and on Sundays and holidays.
    B. Do not call the patient's ____________.
    C. ____________the person prior to discussing the account.
    D. Be ____________ regarding who you are and the intent of the call.
    E. Do not ____________ or intimidate the patient.
    F. Ask the patient when payment should be expected and ____________ this information in the patient's record.
    G. Politely ____________ the patient for his or her time and repeat back to the patient the terms agreed upon.

19. Guidelines for Sending a Personalized Letter
    A. Insert the letter with the ____________ statement.
    B. The letter should inquire ____________ the bill has not been paid.
    C. In the letter, an offer should be made to assist the patient with making payment ____________.
    D. The letter must convey the message that ____________ will be taken to resolve the payment obligation.

20. Basic Guidelines for Drafting a Collection Letter
    i. ______________________________
    ii. ______________________________
    iii. ______________________________
    iv. ______________________________
    v. ______________________________
    vi. ______________________________

vii. ___
viii. ___
ix. ___
x. ___
xi. ___

21. "Skips"
    A. Steps for finding skips:
        i. Check the ___ form to confirm the information.
        ii. Call the telephone numbers and ___ to try to locate the individual.
        iii. Ensure that ___ has been indicated on the billing envelope.

22. Claims Against Estates
    A. When a patient dies, a bill should be sent to the ___ of the deceased.
    B. Contact the next of kin to obtain information regarding who is the ___ of the estate.
    C. It is important to follow up on the collection of bills to prevent any impression that the physician was at ___ with regard to the medical care of the deceased patient.

23. Posting a Payment from a Collection Agency
    A. After verifying the correct patient account to which the payment is to be applied, ___ the patient's ledger card to the next line on the ___ sheet.
    B. Enter the ___ name and previous balance in the appropriate ___.
    C. Enter the ___ of the payment, the ___ of the collection agency, and the ___ of the payment in the appropriate ___.
    D. Enter the amount of the payment on the ___ portion of the ___ sheet in the check's ___.
    E. Subtract the payment from the ___ patient balance and record the new balance on the patient's ___ card.
    F. If an adjustment is to be made to the account because of the collection agency's fee, record the amount in ___ in the ___ column of the ___ card. Enter the description ___.
    G. Subtract the amount of the adjustment from the previous patient ___ and record the new ___ on the patient's ___ card.

II. Accounting Systems

1. Key Points for Bookkeeping
    A. Use ___ ink and write clearly. Do not use a ___ .
    B. Keep the ___ straight with the decimal points aligned.
    C. Check all arithmetic carefully for errors such as ___ decimal points and errors in ___ and ___ .
    D. Do not ___, write over, or use ___ ___ fluid.
    E. ___-check every entry.

2. Steps for Performing Accounts Receivable
    i. ___
    ii. ___
    iii. ___
    iv. ___

3. Defining Credit
    A. To credit an account means to ___ the payment from the account.
    B. A patient has a credit balance when an ___ occurs.
    C. A credit balance may be noted on the patient's account either in ___ or by enclosing the amount in ___ .

4. Single-Entry Bookkeeping
   A. Information is entered __________.
   B. The tools required include a __________ sheet, a cash payment __________, and an accounts receivable __________.
   C. A payroll record and __________ __________ voucher may also be included.
5. Double-Entry Bookkeeping
   A. This system requires financial transactions to be recorded in __________ places.
   B. A __________ bookkeeper is required for this system.
   C. The __________ system forces a balance.
6. The Philosophy of Accounting
   A. Accounting is based on the premise that the __________ of the business, less the __________ of the business, equal the net worth of that business.
   B. This concept is expressed by the following standard accounting equation: __________ = __________ + __________.
   C. Assets include everything owned by the medical practice, such as __________, bank accounts, and __________.
   D. Liabilities are __________ that the medical practice owes to its __________.
7. The Pegboard System
   A. Used to document patient __________ and __________.
   B. Also called the __________ method.
8. Components of the Pegboard System
   i. ______________________________
   ii. ______________________________
   iii. ______________________________
9. The Receipt Form
   A. Used when a patient's payment is made but __________ __________ is provided on that day.
   B. Use carbonless paper to allow the entering of __________, __________, and __________ onto the master day sheet, the superbill, and the patient's __________ card at the same time.
10. Recording Payments
   A. When the superbill is received at the front desk, the MA or the receptionist will enter the correct charge next to every __________ or __________ and place the total on the front of the superbill.
   B. The superbill is then placed back on the __________, using care to line it up on top of the correct patient's name.
   C. The ledger card is then placed under the last page of the __________ slip, aligning the first blank line of the ledger card with the carbonized entry strip on the __________.
11. Posting Adjustments
   A. When an adjustment is made, the MA or the receptionist enters the correct __________ amount into the computer system or __________ it from the balance due from the insurance company.
   B. If the adjustment is for __________ funds, __________ the check amount and service fee charged by the bank to the patient's balance.
12. Posting Collection Agency Payments
   A. If the patient pays a collection agency and the collection agency forwards the money, __________ that payment to the patient's account and write __________ next to it.
   B. If a credit balance exists and the physician or the office manager approves, issue a __________ check to the patient.

13. Balancing the Day Sheet
    A. To ensure that the accounts and entries are correct, the day sheet(s) need to be balanced __________.
    B. Use a calculator to balance the day sheets, and always __________ each total.
    C. When errors in posting are corrected, the corrections should be made in the same __________ as the original posting.
14. Steps for Performing Accounts Receivable
    i. ______________________________
    ii. ______________________________
    iii. ______________________________
    iv. ______________________________
15. Considerations for Selecting Practice Management Software
    i. ______________________________
    ii. ______________________________
    iii. ______________________________
    iv. ______________________________
16. Issues Related to Backing Up Data
    A. Always back up data and information onto a __________ disk, such as a CD-ROM that is then stored __________ in a __________ box.
    B. A paper backup copy of the computer files is not necessary, but a __________ backup file or an off-premises __________ backup file is necessary.
    C. The process by which the backup files can or should be accessed should be written into the office's __________ __________, along with the reasons and circumstances for granting access.

KEY TERMINOLOGY REVIEW

Match the selected key terms with their appropriate definitions.

a. accounting
b. accounts payable (AP)
c. age analysis
d. assignment of benefits
e. bad debt
f. bookkeeping
g. charge slip
h. copayment
i. day sheet
j. encounter form
k. Fair Debt Collection Practices Act
l. ledger card
m. posted
n. professional courtesy (PC)
o. statute of limitations
p. subscriber
q. superbill
r. third-party payer
s. Truth in Lending Form
t. usual, customary, and reasonable (UCR)

1. ____________ Physician opts not to charge other physicians, staff, family members, or clergy.
2. ____________ Process of determining how long an account has been past due and then instituting the necessary collection procedures.
3. ____________ Refers to the fees charged for medical services.
4. ____________ The person who holds the insurance.
5. ____________ An amount owed and not collected.
6. ____________ Federal law that protects debtors from harassment.

7. __________ Contains all of the charges and payments made by both the patient and the insurance company.
8. __________ The system of reporting the financial results of a business.
9. __________ A component of the pegboard system, used to list or post each day's financial transactions—charges, payments, adjustments, and credits.
10. __________ The document generated by the medical office that is a record of services for billing and for insurance processing.
11. __________ A party or person other than the patient, such as an insurance company, who is responsible for paying the patient's bill.
12. __________ Refers to the amount of time a legal collection suit may be brought against a debtor.
13. __________ Ensure that insurance payments are made directly to the physician.
14. __________ If credit is extended and it is determined that the patient will make set payments to the physician over four or more installments, the patient must sign this document.
15. __________ A predetermined amount of money that the patient must pay for medical services at every visit, as determined by the insurance company.
16. __________ Recording an insurance payment.
17. __________ Also known as the encounter form or the charge slip.
18. __________ The amounts that the physician owes to others for supplies, equipment, and services.
19. __________ Also known as the charge slip.
20. __________ The process of managing the accounts for a business.

APPLIED PRACTICE

Complete the activities and answer the questions that follow.

1. Call a local medical office in your area and ask to speak to someone in the billing office. Interview this person about his or her job function. Ask the person the following questions:
   a. What type of system does the person's office use for billing (manual or computerized)?
   ____
   ____
   b. If the office uses a computer system for billing, what is the name of the software used?
   ____
   ____
   c. What functions does the computer system have that helps the billing office staff better perform their jobs?
   ____
   ____
2. Read the scenario below and answer the questions that follow.

Scenario

Kaley McManus, RMA, works for Havensburg Audiology. The payment policy for the audiology practice states that all copayments are expected at the time of service. The patient, Arturo Alamos, is responsible for paying 20% of all services and his insurance company, Healthy Care, will reimburse the physician the remaining 80%.

Mr. Alamos was seen today by Dr. Lynst. Two procedures were performed: a comprehensive audio examination and a tympanography. Following is the fee schedule for the office.

AUDIOLOGY SERVICES		
Screening audio air only	92551	$ 38.00
Pure tone air	92552	$ 37.00
Pure tone air and bone	92553	$ 50.00
Comprehensive audio	92557	$101.00
Loudness balance test	92562	$ 38.00
Tone decay	92563	$ 41.00
Tympanography	92567	$ 40.00
Acoustic reflex	92568	$ 42.00
Reflex decay	92569	$ 43.00
Visual reinforced audio	92579	$ 78.00
Brain stem audiogram	92585	$327.00

a. How much will Kaley collect from Mr. Alamos today?

b. How much will Healthy Care be billed for the services provided to Mr. Alamos?

c. As Mr. Alamos gets ready to pay for his office visit, he realizes that he has only a $20 bill. What should Kaley do?

LEARNING ACTIVITY: MULTIPLE CHOICE

Circle the correct answer for each of the questions below.

1. ______________ are documents that detail the money owed to the medical practice and how long the account has been outstanding.
   a. Accounts payable
   b. Aging reports
   c. Superbills
   d. None of the above

2. The fee is determined by the physician or the practice's partners as a result of taking into consideration the _______________________.

   a. services involved
   b. economic level of the community
   c. prevailing fees in the community
   d. All of the above

3. The customary fee refers to ____.

   a. what a physician usually charges for a procedure or service
   b. the fee charged for the same procedure by the majority of physicians with the same or similar training
   c. what a physician charges for a modified procedure or service that is more difficult and requires more time and effort than a standard procedure
   d. None of the above

4. When should fees be discussed with patients?

   a. Before care is provided
   b. While care is being provided
   c. After care is provided
   d. Never

5. When using a Truth in Lending form, the original form is given to the patient and a copy is retained by the doctor and must be kept on file for ____________________.

   a. 1 year
   b. 2 years
   c. 3 years
   d. 5 years

6. Database programs are used to collect and maintain ____________________.

   a. patient information
   b. procedure and diagnosis codes
   c. insurance company information
   d. All of the above

7. Cycle billing requires that ____.

   a. statements leave the office in time to reach the patient no later than the last day of the month
   b. certain portions of the accounts receivable (AR), or money owed to the practice, are billed at given times during the month
   c. offices have a software medical billing program
   d. All of the above

8. A *skip* is ____.

   a. an individual who has missed his or her appointment.
   b. a bookkeeping procedure
   c. a collection problem that requires immediate action
   d. None of the above

9. If a patient has filed for bankruptcy, ________________________________.
   a. the patient is still obligated to address his or her payment issues with the collection agency hired by the medical office
   b. the medical office must file a claim for payment with the courts
   c. no payment will be obtained
   d. All of the above

10. The accounting term "debit" indicates ________________________________.
   a. that a payment has been received on an account.
   b. that a charge has been entered into the account record
   c. the difference between the money owed and the credit
   d. that a charge has been entered and added to the account balance

CRITICAL THINKING

Answer the following questions to the best of your ability. Utilize the textbook and other resources such as the Internet in considering the following questions.

1. Dr. Roger Dominguez operates a single-physician practice. Dr. Dominguez employs one medical assistant, Garrick Sinclair, CMA (AAMA). The clinic has been using a manual accounting system for many years and Dr. Dominguez has asked Garrick to research the pros and cons of moving to a computerized system versus keeping the manual system. What might Garrick list as pros and cons for using a manual system versus a computerized system?

   ____
   ____
   ____
   ____
   ____

2. Margaret Larson, RMA, is working in the billing office of a family practice clinic. The clinic uses a superbill for physicians to indicate the charges assigned to each patient on each patient visit. The superbill used by this clinic was designed nearly 5 years ago and contains several codes that are no longer used by the clinic. Also, there are several codes that the physicians use which are not on the printed superbill, forcing the physicians to write in these codes by hand. What might Margaret suggest that the facility do to solve this problem and make the superbill more accurate for use in this office?

   ____
   ____
   ____
   ____
   ____

RESEARCH ACTIVITY

Utilize Internet search engines to research the following topics and write a brief description of what you find. It is important to utilize reputable websites.

1. Using the Internet as a research source, look up three collection agencies that offer their services in your area. List the pros and cons for using each of these three companies.

CHAPTER 16
Financial Management

CHAPTER OUTLINE

General review of the chapter:

Function of Banking
Checks
Paying Bills
Deposits
Accepting Cash
Cash Disbursements
Bank Hold on Accounts
Bank Statement
Saving Documentation
Petty Cash
Payroll

STUDENT STUDY GUIDE

Use the following guide to assist in your learning of the concepts from the chapter.

I. Online Banking and Writing Checks

1. Basic Banking Functions (List six general functions.)
   - i. ______________________________
   - ii. ______________________________
   - iii. ______________________________
   - iv. ______________________________
   - v. ______________________________
   - vi. ______________________________
2. The MA's Responsibility with Regard to Banking
   - A. Ensure ________ when accomplishing accounting and bookkeeping tasks.
   - B. Act as an ________ for the physician when dealing with the business's financial matters.
3. Types of Bank Accounts
   - i. ______________________________
   - ii. ______________________________
   - iii. ______________________________
4. Checking Account
   - A. Allows the owner of the account to ________ money from the account.
   - B. It is not usually an ________ account.
   - C. Some accounts earn interest only if there is a ________ balance in the account.

5. Savings Account
   A. This is an ________ account where funds that are not needed for daily expenses are placed.
   B. Interest is earned ________ or ________.
   C. Cash can be withdrawn or transferred in to a ________ account.
6. Money Market Account
   A. Used more as an ________ tool; usually pays a ________ ________ rate.
   B. Typically requires a minimum balance of ________ to ________.
7. Online Banking
   A. The functions that customers can perform include ________ the account, comparing the account with the bank's records, paying bills, and ________ data from the bank.
   B. This is a ________ system that requires notations to be entered into the ________ ________ records.
8. Checks
   A. A check is a document that orders a bank to ________ or ________ money.
   B. It is ________ on demand.
   C. It is a ________ instrument.
9. Preprinted Information on Checks
   i. ________
   ii. ________
   iii. ________
   iv. ________
   v. ________
   vi. ________
   vii. ________
   viii. ________
   ix. ________
   x. ________
10. Advantages of Checks
   i. ________
   ii. ________
   iii. ________
   iv. ________
   v. ________
11. Types of Checks
   i. ________
   ii. ________
   iii. ________
   iv. ________
   v. ________
   vi. ________
   vii. ________
   viii. ________
12. Cashier's Check
   A. Written using the bank's own check or form; issued by the ________.
   B. Funds to pay the check are ________ against the payer's account when the check is issued to the bank.
   C. Can be requested from a bank by ________ ________ holders who do not have a checking account.

13. Bank Draft and Limited Check
   A. A bank draft is a check that is drawn up by a bank against funds that are ________ into its account in another bank.
   B. A limited check is issued on a ________ ________ form that indicates a preprinted ________ dollar amount for which the check can be written.
   C. A ________ limit may exist for a limited check.
   D. Limited checks are used for ________ checks and ________ payments.

14. Money Order
   A. Purchased for the ________ value embossed on the check.
   B. Can be purchased from ________, the ________, and other authorized agents.
   C. Frequently used by individuals who do not have ________ accounts and who do not want to send cash by mail.
   D. Considered safe to accept as payment since they are ________ at the value embossed on the check.

15. Traveler's Check
   A. ________ and ________ in certain dollar amounts.
   B. Considered a safe means for carrying money when ________.
   C. Contains ________ spaces for the signature of the ________ one space that is signed upon purchase of the check, the other for when the check is presented in payment.

16. Voucher Check
   A. Contains ________ detachable sections for transaction information.
   B. Frequently used for ________ checks since additional information can be supplied to the payee.
   C. ________ portion of the check contains the actual check.
   D. ________ portion provides details about the transaction.

17. Magnetic Ink Character Recognition
   A. It is a form of identification for the ________ and the ________.
   B. The first series of numbers identifies the ________ and its ________.
   C. The second series of numbers identifies the ________ ________.

18. Guidelines for Writing Checks
   i. ____
   ii. ____
   iii. ____
   iv. ____
   v. ____
   vi. ____
   vii. ____
   viii. ____
   ix. ____

19. The Write-It-Once System
   A. Allows a record to be kept of the ________, ________ ________, ________, and net amount of the check.
   B. The ________ system, the check ________ sheet, and the checks with a ________ writing strip on the back are used for this method.
   C. A check ________ sheet is placed over the pegs of the ________.
   D. Checks must be ________ when using this method.
   E. The check register has space for ________ checks to be recorded on one page.

20. Steps for Preparing a Check
    i. ______
    ii. ______
    iii. ______
    iv. ______
    v. ______
    vi. ______
    vii. ______
    viii. ______
    ix. ______
    x. ______
    xi. ______
    xii. ______
    xiii. ______
    xiv. ______

21. Errors in Writing Checks
    A. Do not ________ on checks.
    B. For checks with major errors, ________ a ________ through the check and write ________ in ink across the check.
    C. If the error is minor, ________ the information and ________ the change.

22. Risky Checks
    i. ______
    ii. ______
    iii. ______
    iv. ______

23. Third-Party Check
    A. The first party is the person who ________ the check.
    B. The second party is the ________ who has received a check from another person to pay the ________ own medical bill.
    C. The third party is the MA or other office staff who is ________ the money.

24. Overpayment-of-Account Checks
    A. This can happen accidentally if a patient has not maintained adequate records or if the patient's ________ ________ has also made a payment to the patient's account at the medical office.
    B. If the check has not been deposited, the check can be ________ to the patient and a request for a new check for the ________ amount can be made.

25. "Paid in Full" Checks
    A. Checks written with the statement ________ added are to be avoided.
    B. If the check is deposited, you are ________ that this is correct, making it difficult to collect any further payments.

26. Considerations for Endorsing a Check
    A. Place the endorsement on the ________ of the check within the top ________ inches on the left-hand side of the check as it is turned over.
    B. An endorsement can either be a payee's written signature or a ________.
    C. To prevent theft, checks should be endorsed for ________ as soon as they are received.
    D. Endorsements are regulated by the ________________.

27. Types of Check Endorsements (List and explain each.)
    i. ______
    ii. ______
    iii. ______

28. Reasons for Returned Checks

i. ______________________________
ii. ______________________________
iii. ______________________________

29. Steps for Posting Non-Sufficient Funds Checks

i. ______________________________
ii. ______________________________
iii. ______________________________

30. Guidelines for Paying Bills

i. ______________________________
ii. ______________________________
iii. ______________________________
iv. ______________________________
v. ______________________________

31. Guidelines for Handling Deposits

i. ______________________________
ii. ______________________________
iii. ______________________________
iv. ______________________________
v. ______________________________
vi. ______________________________

32. Steps for Completing a Deposit Slip

i. ______________________________
ii. ______________________________
iii. ______________________________
iv. ______________________________
v. ______________________________
vi. ______________________________
vii. ______________________________
viii. ______________________________
ix. ______________________________
x. ______________________________
xi. ______________________________
xii. ______________________________
xiii. ______________________________

II. Bank Statements and Payroll

1. Bank Statement

A. Provides ________ of the funds in an account.
B. Assists in ________ errors made by the office or bank bookkeeping system.
C. Includes all ________ and ________ processed.

2. Information Included on a Bank Statement

i. ______________________________
ii. ______________________________
iii. ______________________________
iv. ______________________________
v. ______________________________
vi. ______________________________
vii. ______________________________
viii. ______________________________

ix. ____
x. ____

3. Instructions for Reconciling a Bank Statement
   A. Compare the ________ balance of the current statement with the ________ balance of the previous statement.
   B. Write the current ________ balance in the appropriate space on the reverse side of the bank statement.
   C. Compare the ________ noted on the statement against your records or ________ by making a check mark next to each correct number.
   D. List ________ all outstanding deposits.
   E. Add these together, and place the total on the ________ side of the statement in the space provided.
   F. Add the ________ balance to the total of the deposits not already included, and write this amount on the ________ line.
   G. Compare the value of the checks listed on the statement with the value listed in the ________ or check subs, and place a check mark next to each correct number.
   H. Note all numbers missing from the ________ list of check numbers.
   I. List all ________ checks.
   J. Add the total for the ________ checks and place that figure on the line indicated on the back of the statement.
   K. Subtract the total for the checks outstanding from the ________ total on the ________ of the statement to determine the current balance.
   L. The current balance should ________ with the amount in your checkbook or stub balance.
4. Documents Used to Verify Banking Procedures
   i. ____
   ii. ____
   iii. ____
   iv. ____
   v. ____
5. Petty Cash
   A. Must be ________ and recorded in a ________ financial log.
   B. A ________ is used to replenish petty cash.
   C. Typically handled by ________ individual in the office.
   D. Kept under ________ and ________ for security purposes.
6. Payroll Periods
   i. ____
   ii. ____
   iii. ____
7. Payroll Information That Employers Must Maintain
   i. ____
   ii. ____
   iii. ____
   iv. ____
   v. ____
   vi. ____
8. Steps for Manually Generating Payroll
   i. ____
   ii. ____
   iii. ____
   iv. ____

v. ____

vi. ____

vii. ____

viii. ____

ix. ____

x. ____

xi. ____

xii. ____

xiii. ____

xiv. ____

xv. ____

xvi. ____

xvii. ____

xviii. ____

9. Information to Be Included on the W-4 Form

   A. Employee's name and ________.
   B. Employee's ________ number.
   C. Employee's ________ status.
   D. The number of ________ that the employee is claiming.

KEY TERMINOLOGY REVIEW

Match the vocabulary term to the correct definition below.

a. accounts payable (AP)
b. accounts receivable (AR)
c. American Bankers Association (ABA)
d. audit
e. canceled checks
f. cash disbursement
g. cashier's check
h. certified check
i. credits
j. debits
k. deposits
l. embezzlement
m. gross annual wage
n. magnetic ink character recognition (MICR)
o. negotiable instrument number
p. non-sufficient funds (NSF)
q. payee
r. payer
s. reconciliation
t. stale check
u. stop-payment order
v. tax withholding
w. third-party check
x. warrant

1. ____________ Amount of money the employee earns in a year before deductions.
2. ____________ Guarantees payment because it is written on a check drafted by a bank.
3. ____________ Refers to the comparison of the figures on the bank statements with the records maintained in the medical office and the adjustment of banking records so that both are in agreement.
4. ____________ A check that has not been presented for payment within the time suggested on the check.
5. ____________ Refers to an official inspection of an individual's or organization's accounts, typically by an independent body.
6. ____________ A system of combining characters and numbers located at the bottom left-hand side of checks and deposit slips.

7. ____________ Identifies the area where the bank issuing the check is located, as well as identifying the individual bank.
8. ____________ The unauthorized taking of funds; involves a breach of trust.
9. ____________ If a ____________ has been issued by the payer, then the bank will not allow the funds to be disbursed.
10. ____________ One that actualizes or permits the transfer of money to another person.
11. ____________ Checks that have been processed and paid to the medical practice's creditors by the bank.
12. ____________ Refers to money (cash, checks, and money orders) placed in a bank account; can be made to either checking or savings accounts.
13. ____________ Additions to an account.
14. ____________ Money owed to the physician or medical practice.
15. ____________ Charges against an account.
16. ____________ Statements issued to indicate that debts should be paid.
17. ____________ Similar to cashier's checks because the bank guarantees that the money is available.
18. ____________ When the payer's account does not have enough money to cover the amount of the check.
19. ____________ When money is withheld from an employee's paycheck.
20. ____________ The holder of the check.
21. ____________ Refers to a check written by a party unknown to you.
22. ____________ One that actualizes or permits the transfer of money to another person.
23. ____________ Refers to a payment made to creditors.
24. ____________ Money that is owed to vendors, suppliers, utility companies, and others for services rendered.

APPLIED PRACTICE

Read the scenario and answer the questions that follow.

Scenario

Daniel Evans, CMA (AAMA), works as the administrative medical assistant for Happy Valley Medical Center. Handling payroll, accounts payable, and banking procedures are part of his work responsibilities. It is Thursday and he must perform these duties.

1. Daniel must calculate the gross earnings for the two clinical medical assistants who work in the back office. The office pays its employees every week, for the previous week's work. For every hour over 40 hours worked, employees get paid time and a half. Last week, Shelby Coleman worked 43.5 hours. She earns $13.00 per hour. Chantal Jefferson worked 45 hours last week. Chantal earns $13.75 per hour.

   a. What are Shelby's gross earnings?

   ____

   b. What are Chantal's gross earnings?

   ____

2. Daniel Smith has received an invoice from a vendor that supplied the physician with new business cards. The invoice reads as follows:

SELECT STATIONERY UNLIMITED

Bill to: Happy Valley Medical Center
1129 Felicity Road
Springfield, PA 00010
Account #: 288901HVMC

Remit Payment to: Select Stationery Unlimited
PO Box 588
New York, NY 11110

Item Number	Description	Price	Total
0123	250 Business Cards	32.99	32.99
		Tax (5%)	1.65
		Shipping and Handling	4.95
		Total	$ 39.59

a. Complete the check according to how Daniel should pay this bill.

Happy Valley Medical Clinic
1129 Felicity Road
Springfield, PA 00010

13003
Date ____________ 20___

Pay to the order of: ____ ________________

____

____dollars

MEMO: ______________________________ ______________________________

LEARNING ACTIVITY: MULTIPLE CHOICE

Circle the correct answer to each of the questions below.

1. Which of the following would be considered deductions for the purposes of employee payroll?
   a. Federal tax withholding
   b. Vacation pay
   c. Overtime pay
   d. All of the above

2. Petty cash is available for incidentals such as ________________.
   a. small purchases
   b. reimbursements
   c. miscellaneous expenses
   d. All of the above

3. In order to have a negotiable instrument, the check must ________________.
   a. be written and signed by an authorized payer of the check.
   b. state a sum of money to be paid.

c. be payable on demand or at a fixed date in the future.
d. be payable to the holder (the payee) of the check.
e. All of the above

4. Types of checks include ________________.
   a. bank drafts
   b. warrants
   c. money orders
   d. All of the above

5. The American Bankers Association (ABA) number is always located ________________.
   a. in the phone book
   b. in the upper right-hand corner of a printed check
   c. in the lower left-hand corner of a printed check
   d. None of the above

6. What are check stubs used for?
   a. As a permanent record of the date, amount, payee, and purpose of the check
   b. As a bookmark
   c. As an example of the correct way to write a check
   d. The quarterly form

7. How much is typically paid to employees as overtime wages?
   a. Twice the employee's normal rate of pay
   b. 1.5 times the employee's normal rate of pay
   c. Three times the employee's normal rate of pay
   d. None of the above

8. The ________________ IRS form is used to calculate the correct amount of federal withholding tax for an employee.
   a. quarterly report
   b. W-2
   c. Circular E
   d. None of the above

9. A money market account ________________.
   a. is an interest-bearing account
   b. is used more as an investment tool
   c. typically requires a minimum balance of $500
   d. All of the above

10. Banking is one of the critical office procedures because ________________.
    a. it requires careful handling of money and records
    b. many offices do not have a bookkeeper or medical assistant assigned to perform this duty
    c. it requires specialized training
    d. All of the above

CRITICAL THINKING

Answer the following questions to the best of your ability. Utilize the textbook and other resources such as the Internet in considering the following questions.

1. Ronnie Nguyen, CMA (AAMA), is the office manager for Dr. Hyun Kim. Ronnie has been handling the office payroll, using a manual system for several years. Dr. Kim has asked Ronnie to research the possibility of buying software for the payroll function. Dr. Kim wants Ronnie to provide her with a list of pros and cons for manual and computerized systems for the payroll function. What should Ronnie include?

2. Francie Crook, RMA, has been newly hired to work in a busy family practice clinic. When Francie looks at her first paycheck, she notices that a tax has been taken out for something called FICA. She asks her office manager to explain what this tax is. How might the office manager explain this tax to Francie?

3. Linnea Wagner is responsible for training new employees in the correct way to write checks. In order to do this, she must also explain the parts of the check. What might Linnea include in her instructional sessions?

RESEARCH ACTIVITY

Utilize Internet search engines to research the following topics and write a brief description of what you find. It is important to utilize reputable websites.

1. Using the Internet as a research source, look up three different software programs that can perform the payroll function. Create a list of the pros and cons of these three programs, as well as manual versus computerized payroll systems.

CHAPTER 17
Medical Insurance

CHAPTER OUTLINE

General review of the chapter:

The Purpose of Health Insurance
Health Insurance and the Availability of Health Insurance
Managed Care Organizations
Group-Sponsored or Individual Policies
Government Programs
Types of Health Insurance Benefits
Payment of Benefits
Verification of Insurance Benefits
Fee Schedules
Health Care Cost Containment
The *Federal Register*

STUDENT STUDY GUIDE

Use the following guide to assist in your learning of the concepts from the chapter.

I. Health Insurance and Managed Care

1. Why Learn About Insurance as an MA?
   - A. To assist the physician in maintaining a ____________ strong business.
   - B. To assist the patient in ____________ the patient's financial responsibility to the practice.
2. The Basics of Insurance
   - A. Provides protection from ____________ and ____________ loss.
   - B. Money is paid to the ____________.
   - C. Premiums are paid for by the ____________.
3. The Purposes of Medical Insurance
   - A. Assists patients in covering costs incurred for ____________.
   - B. Expenses that are covered by insurance include the following:
     - i. ____
     - ii. ____
     - iii. ____
     - iv. ____
4. Coverage Offered Through Hospitalization Insurance
   - i. ____
   - ii. ____
   - iii. ____
   - iv. ____
   - v. ____

5. Insurance Coverage for Surgery
   A. Coverage is typically based on __________ and __________ charges.
   B. Costs vary by __________.
   C. Copays and __________ may apply.
6. Fixed Payment Plan
   A. The payment of a fixed fee provides __________ coverage.
   B. The fixed fee is known as a __________.
   C. Reimbursement is available once the __________ has been paid.
7. Managed Care Organization
   A. The payment of a __________ __________ provides monthly coverage.
   B. Reimbursement is available once the __________ has been paid.
   C. These plans are referred to as __________ plans.
8. Prepaid Plan
   A. Physicians contract to provide services for a __________ fee.
   B. __________ __________ providers may be assigned.
9. The Advantages of Managed Care
   i. ______________________________
   ii. ______________________________
   iii. ______________________________
   iv. ______________________________
   v. ______________________________
   vi. ______________________________
   vii. ______________________________
10. The Disadvantages of Managed Care
   i. ______________________________
   ii. ______________________________
   iii. ______________________________
   iv. ______________________________
   v. ______________________________
   vi. ______________________________
   vii. ______________________________
   viii. ______________________________
11. Health Maintenance Organization (HMO)
   A. An HMO is a type of __________ __________ plan.
   B. The original intent was to __________ health care costs.
   C. Membership is limited to certain __________.
   D. Services are provided for a __________ fee.
   E. Patients must see the plan's __________ physicians.
   F. Emphasizes the __________ of health.
12. Preferred Provider Organization (PPO)
   A. The purpose is to __________ costs.
   B. Patients must use __________ providers.
   C. Members are not restricted to designated __________ or __________.
13. Point-of-Service Plan (POS)
   A. A POS is a type of __________ __________ plan.
   B. Offers more __________ than some HMOs and PPOs.
   C. An out-of-network or __________ provider may be seen.

14. Exclusive Provider Organization (EPO)

    A. An EPO is a __________ __________ system.
    B. Patients select physicians from a __________.
    C. __________ are reimbursed on a modified fee-for-service basis.

15. Integrated Delivery System (IDS)

    A. An IDS is an organization of provider sites __________ to offer services to subscribers
    B. Examples include the following:
        i. ______________________________
        ii. ______________________________
        iii. ______________________________
        iv. ______________________________
        v. ______________________________

II. Group-Sponsored or Individual (Commercial) and Government Plans

1. Commercial Insurance Carriers

    A. These are typically __________ organizations.
    B. Often offer both traditional __________ service plans and __________ __________ plans.
    C. Require subscribers to pay a __________ for membership.

2. Contents of a Health Insurance Card

    i. ______________________________
    ii. ______________________________
    iii. ______________________________
    iv. ______________________________
    v. ______________________________
    vi. ______________________________
    vii. ______________________________

3. Blue Cross/Blue Shield

    A. This is the largest __________ medical insurance system in the United States.
    B. Exists in __________ state.
    C. Operates __________ under state laws.
    D. Provides coverage for medical __________ and __________.
    E. Offers various types of health care __________.

4. Medicare

    A. Medicare is health coverage provided by the __________.
    B. Available to persons who are age __________ and older and those who are __________ __________.
    C. Operated by the __________ __________ Administration.
    D. Medicare is funded through __________ __________.

5. Medicare Parts A and B

    A. Part A provides coverage for __________ expenses.
    B. No __________ is paid for Part A.
    C. A __________ deductible must be met for Part B.

6. The Resource-Based Relative Value Scale

    A. This is a formula used to determine Medicare's __________ reimbursement rate.
    B. Developed with the use of values that consider the following:
        i. ______________________________
        ii. ______________________________
        iii. ______________________________
        iv. ______________________________

7. Medicare Coverage

   A. Pays all expenses for the first __________ days of hospitalization.
   B. Pays a portion of hospitalization costs for an additional __________ days.
   C. Coverage does not include __________ nursing home care or costs for __________ or __________ illnesses.

8. Medicare Part D

   A. Implemented in __________.
   B. Offered as a __________ plan for Medicare recipients.
   C. Covers a __________ list of prescription drugs at participating pharmacies.
   D. Includes __________ deductibles, applicable __________ or coinsurance, and __________ benefits.

9. Medicare Supplements

   A. Paid by the __________ individual, not by __________.
   B. May require __________ forms to be submitted prior to paying the insured individual.

10. Medicaid

   A. Medicaid is insurance for individuals who are medically __________.
   B. Paid for by __________ and __________ governments.
   C. Administered by __________ __________.
   D. The rules of eligibility and payment __________ by state.
   E. Typically, individuals must qualify on a __________ basis.

11. Workers' Compensation

   A. Also known as __________ __________.
   B. This is one of the first __________ insurance programs.
   C. Employers pay the __________; employees pay __________.

12. Disability Insurance

   A. Usually begins paying the insured individual after he or she has been disabled for a __________.
   B. The benefit period is the amount of time that the __________ individual will receive a monthly check after the policy begins to pay.
   C. Insurance is not used for the purpose of paying __________ bills, but instead is used to replace the __________ that the patient has lost due to his or her disability.

III. Payment of Benefits

1. Coverage Provided by Basic Insurance Policies

   i. __________
   ii. __________
   iii. __________
   iv. __________
   v. __________

2. Major Medical Insurance

   A. Provides coverage for __________ __________ or __________ and __________ __________.
   B. It is typically a __________ policy.
   C. Usually increases the __________ paid by the insured individual.

3. Dental Insurance

   A. Typically provides coverage for the following:
      i. __________
      ii. __________
      iii. __________

iv. ______________________________

v. ______________________________

B. Often requires a __________.

C. Plans generally offer __________ to __________ coverage.

4. Coverage Provided by Vision Insurance

i. ______________________________

ii. ______________________________

iii. ______________________________

iv. ______________________________

v. ______________________________

5. The UCR Method

A. UCR stands for __________, __________, and __________.

B. Used to determine the portion that an __________ __________ is obligated to pay.

C. Takes into consideration the following:

i. ______________________________

ii. ______________________________

iii. ______________________________

6. Indemnity Schedules

A. These are another method used to determine the __________ __________ payment.

B. Based on the __________ amount charged for a specific service.

C. The payment is determined on the basis of the __________ charge submitted by the physician or by the physician's fee schedule.

7. Relative Value Studies (RVS)

A. RVS is a method to determine __________ factors in reimbursement.

B. Areas considered in the accounting include the __________, the __________, and the __________.

8. Filing Requirements

A. Claims must be filed in a __________ manner.

B. If a deadline is not met, then __________ __________ can be retrieved from the insurance carrier.

C. Filing deadlines __________ by insurance carrier.

9. Steps for Filing Primary and Secondary Claims

i. ______________________________

ii. ______________________________

iii. ______________________________

iv. ______________________________

10. Steps for Manually Recording Payments

i. ______________________________

ii. ______________________________

iii. ______________________________

iv. ______________________________

v. ______________________________

vi. ______________________________

vii. ______________________________

11. Preauthorization

A. Preauthorization is also called __________.

B. Must be acquired prior to the patient's appointment, unless it is an __________.

C. Failure to obtain preauthorization may __________ treatment.

D. If service is provided without preauthorization, the insurance carrier may __________ to pay.

12. Calling the Insurance Carrier for Precertification
    A. If possible, obtain precertification at least __________ hours prior to the provision of patient services.
    B. Gather all pertinent __________ information prior to calling the insurance carrier.
13. Pertinent Information for Precertification
    i. ______________________________
    ii. ______________________________
    iii. ______________________________
    iv. ______________________________
    v. ______________________________
14. Steps for Obtaining Approval
    i. ______________________________
    ii. ______________________________
    iii. ______________________________
    iv. ______________________________
    v. ______________________________
15. Steps to Take When Preauthorization Is Denied
    i. ______________________________
    ii. ______________________________
    iii. ______________________________
16. Referrals
    A. Requires paperwork to be sent to the __________ physician.
    B. The referral recommendation must be made __________ __________.
    C. Documentation must be placed in the __________ __________.
17. Materials Needed to Request a Referral
    i. ______________________________
    ii. ______________________________
    iii. ______________________________
    iv. ______________________________
    v. ______________________________
    vi. ______________________________
    vii. ______________________________
18. Why Verify Patient Insurance?
    A. Minimizes __________ and __________ problems.
    B. Ensures that the practice will be paid for __________ rendered.
19. Steps for Verifying Information
    i. ______________________________
    ii. ______________________________
    iii. ______________________________
    iv. ______________________________
    v. ______________________________

KEY TERMINOLOGY REVIEW

Match the selected key terms to their definitions below.

a. benefit period

b. capitation rate

c. claim

d. closed-panel HMO

e. coordination of benefits (COB)
f. crossover claim
g. deductible
h. exclusive provider organization (EPO)
i. fee-for-service
j. fee schedule
k. formulary
l. gatekeeper
m. health maintenance provider organization (HMO)______(PCP)
n. integrated delivery system (IDS)
o. medical foundation
p. open-panel HMO
q. point-of-service plan (POS)
r. preauthorization
s. preferred provider organization (PPO)
t. premium
u. prepaid plan
v. primary care
w. referral
x. self-referral

1. ____________ The type of claim that is submitted if an individual has both Medicare and Medicaid.
2. ____________ A nonprofit IDS.
3. ____________ Determines the medical necessity of services provided by specialists.
4. ____________ Period of time that payments for Medicare hospital benefits are available.
5. ____________ Lists the amount to be paid by the insurance company for each procedure or service subject to the managed care contract.
6. ____________ Also known as a primary care physician, this is the provider who is responsible for the overall management of the patient's health.
7. ____________ The portion the patient must pay before the insurance company will pay any benefits.
8. ____________ An HMO enrollee chooses to see an out-of-network provider without authorization.
9. ____________ Obtaining permission from the insurance carrier before performing a procedure or providing certain services to subscribers.
10. ____________ A predetermined fee.
11. ____________ A plan in which patients may choose to use the panel of providers within the HMO network or to utilize the services of non-HMO providers.
12. ____________ An approved list of medications specific to each insurance carrier.
13. ____________ A managed care system that allows the patient to select only from a defined panel of providers.
14. ____________ Involves a group of providers who have a contractual agreement to provide services to subscribers on a negotiated fee-for-service basis.
15. ____________ An organization of provider sites (e.g., ambulatory centers, clinics, or hospitals) with a contracted relationship that offer services to subscribers.
16. ____________ Used to send a patient for treatment to another facility or physician.
17. ____________ A type of HMO where the clinic is owned by the HMO and the providers are employees of the HMO.
18. ____________ A fixed monthly fee or semimonthly fee.
19. ____________ A separate charge or fee set up by individual physicians for every service.
20. ____________ A type of HMO where the health care providers are not employees of the HMO and do not belong to a medical group owned or managed by the HMO.
21. ____________ A system that insurance carriers have in place to prevent payment by more than one carrier.

22. ____________ Requires the patient to use a provider under contract with the insurance company. The provider is reimbursed at a discounted rate.

23. ____________ A type of managed care plan in which a range of health care services performed by a limited group of providers is made available to plan members for a predetermined fee.

24. ____________ A written and documented request for reimbursement.

APPLIED PRACTICE

Complete the activity and answer the questions that follow. Select and complete Activity 1 if you currently have health insurance. Select and complete Activity 2 if you currently do not have health insurance.

1. If you have health insurance, do you know everything about your plan? Conduct research either through the Internet or by calling your insurance company to find out the following information:
   a. What conditions does the insurance plan not cover?

   ____

   ____

   b. For conditions not covered, is it possible to receive coverage for an additional fee?

   ____

   ____

   c. When is preauthorization required and who typically should perform this activity?

   ____

   ____

2. If you do not have health insurance, begin to research the types of health insurance plans that may be affordable for you in your area.
   a. Does your school offer health insurance for students? If so, what is the cost and what type of coverage is offered?

   ____

   ____

   b. List two other types of insurance plans you found in your area that may be affordable for you. If your school offers health insurance, what is the difference between these two other plans and the plan offered by the school?

   ____

   ____

   c. When is preauthorization required for the plans you researched and who typically should perform this activity?

   ____

   ____

LEARNING ACTIVITY: TRUE/FALSE

Indicate whether the following statements are true or false by placing a T or an F on the line that precedes each statement.

______ 1. Children of veterans with total or permanent service-related disabilities are currently not covered under CHAMPVA; only spouses and widows are covered.

_______ 2. Most insurance carriers require a deductible.

_______ 3. Insurance is considered a two-party contract between the insured (the patient or the patient's family) and the insurance company.

_______ 4. Most patients are completely aware of what their insurance covers.

_______ 5. The most basic insurance policies cover office visits, hospitalization, emergency room visits, surgical procedures, and wellness examinations.

_______ 6. To reduce unnecessary patient visits to the provider's office, insurance companies typically do not require a copayment.

_______ 7. Managed care organizations (MCOs) offer options that are available through public insurance carriers and through some government programs.

_______ 8. Before HMOs became so widespread, insurance companies reimbursed providers for all of their charges without questioning whether or not the services were medically necessary.

_______ 9. Health care insurance providers determine fees on the basis of three main components.

_______10. Most insurance plans have lifetime maximum benefits.

CRITICAL THINKING

Answer the following questions to the best of your ability. Utilize the textbook and other resources such as the Internet in considering the following questions.

1. Monica Swinger is taking an administrative medical assisting course. She has been given the assignment of writing an essay describing how health insurance began in the United States. What information should Monica include?

____

____

____

____

____

2. Erica Owsley, CMA (AAMA), is working with Charles Wong, a patient in the clinic where Erica works. Charles tells Erica he has the option of buying into the group insurance plan that his employer offers or he can buy an individual policy on his own. He isn't sure which option to choose and asks Erica if she can tell him the differences between individual and group insurance plans. What should Erica tell Charles?

____

____

____

____

____

RESEARCH ACTIVITY

Utilize Internet search engines to research the following topics and write a brief description of what you find. It is important to utilize reputable websites.

1. Using the Internet as a research source, find your state's Medicaid website and research the criteria for being covered under Medicaid in your state. Write an essay describing the persons who may be covered under Medicaid in your state.

CHAPTER 18
Medical Insurance Claims

CHAPTER OUTLINE

General review of the chapter:

Types of Health Insurance and Claim Forms
Types of Claims
The Claim Form
Claims Processing
Claims Security
Tracking Claim Forms

STUDENT STUDY GUIDE

Use the following guide to assist in your learning of the concepts from the chapter.

I. Insurance Claim Forms

1. Purpose of the Health Insurance Claim Form
   A. Reports patient __________ and __________ to the insurance carrier.
   B. Helps __________ reporting.
   C. Improves communication between the __________ and the __________.
2. Guidelines for Improving the Communication Process
   i. ____
   ii. ____
   iii. ____
3. Submitting a Medicare Claim
   A. Staying current with their knowledge regarding __________.
   B. The __________ form is used for Medicare claims
   C. Knowing the __________ and __________ is critical to successful claims submission.
4. Submitting a Medicaid Claim
   A. Claims submission __________ from state to state.
   B. Eligibility is not __________.
   C. __________ is required for some services.
5. Submitting a Medicaid Claim
   A. __________ claims are filed for patients with both Medicare and Medicaid.
   B. Claims are submitted on a __________ form.
6. Submitting a Workers' Compensation Claim
   A. The claim form to be used depends on the state and the __________ in that state.
   B. Typically, the __________ form is acceptable.
   C. The patient does not pay for __________ and __________ covered by workers' compensation.

II. Types of Claims

1. Methods for Submitting Claims

   A. No matter which method is used, the __________ information is provided.
   B. The method used is dependent upon the __________.

2. Paper Claims

   A. Claims are completed __________.
   B. Problems that occur with this method often include __________, leading to the claim being __________ or time being lost because claims must be __________.

3. Requirements for Paper Claims

   A. All claims must be on an __________ claim form.
   B. Claims must be __________.
   C. __________ ink must be used.
   D. __________ letters should be used when appropriate.
   E. The use of correction tape is __________.
   F. Documentation must be submitted in the __________ envelope as the paper claim.

4. Electronic Claims

   A. Electronic claims are sent directly to the __________ or the __________.
   B. All medical offices were required to have the ability to submit electronic claims by __________.

5. The National Supplier Clearinghouse

   A. Charges for the __________ provided.
   B. Eliminates the need for different carriers to have specific __________.
   C. Checks the claim for __________, thereby reducing the number of claims that are __________.

6. Steps for Sending Claims Electronically

   i. ______________________________
   ii. ______________________________
   iii. ______________________________
   iv. ______________________________
   v. ______________________________
   vi. ______________________________

7. Three Ways That Claims Are Transmitted

   i. ______________________________
   ii. ______________________________
   iii. ______________________________

III. The CMS-1500 Form

1. Information Needed to Complete the CMS-1500 Form

   i. ______________________________
   ii. ______________________________
   iii. ______________________________
   iv. ______________________________
   v. ______________________________

2. Prior to Submitting a Claim

   A. Check the __________ of the claim form.
   B. If you are submitting a paper claim, make a __________ for the patient's file.
   C. Enter the data on the __________ log.
   D. Send the completed CMS-1500 form and the required documentation to the __________.

3. Confidentiality and the CMS-1500 Form

   A. As with all patient data, information must remain __________.
   B. Release of information must be authorized by the __________.
   C. A signed standard __________ form must be used.
   D. The form must be placed in the __________ file.

4. Assignment of Benefits

   A. Assignment of benefits is allowed by __________ and other carriers.
   B. A __________-time form must be signed by the patient.
   C. This form __________ the __________ of patient information.
   D. Once signed, use __________.
   E. The form must be kept __________ in the patient's file.

5. Materials Needed to Complete the CMS-1500 Form

   i. ______________________________
   ii. ______________________________
   iii. ______________________________
   iv. ______________________________
   v. ______________________________

6. The Superbill

   A. Contains the __________, __________, __________, and __________.
   B. Originally created to allow patients to file __________ claims.
   C. Accepted by some insurance companies as a substitute __________.
   D. Provides detailed information on the __________ received.

7. The Birthday Rule

   A. Used only for parents who are __________ married.
   B. The primary plan is the plan held by the parent whose birthday falls __________ in the year.
   C. If both parents' birthdays are on the same day, the parent with the __________ date of inception would hold the primary plan.
   D. The primary plan of divorced parents is determined by the __________.

8. Prior to Submitting a Claim

   i. ______________________________
   ii. ______________________________
   iii. ______________________________
   iv. ______________________________

IV. Claims Security and Tracking Claims

1. Maintaining the Confidentiality of Patient Information

   A. Maintaining confidentiality is the responsibility of __________ health care workers.
   B. A breach of confidentiality occurs when information is provided to individuals who have not been __________ to __________ the information.

2. How to Keep Patient Information Secure

   i. ______________________________
   ii. ______________________________
   iii. ______________________________
   iv. ______________________________

3. Documentation of Permission

   i. ______________________________
   ii. ______________________________
   iii. ______________________________

4. The Most Common Reasons for Rejection of Claims
   i. ______________________________
   ii. ______________________________
   iii. ______________________________
   iv. ______________________________
   v. ______________________________
   vi. ______________________________
   vii. ______________________________
   viii. ______________________________
   ix. ______________________________

5. Resubmitting Claims
   A. Information must be __________ and resubmitted.
   B. The use of patient data and other resources is important for ensuring __________.
   C. Refiling must occur within the specified __________ limits.

KEY TERMINOLOGY REVIEW

Match the selected key terms to their definitions below.

a. Assignment of Benefits Form
b. The Birthday Rule
c. breach of confidentiality
d. clean claim
e. The National Supplier Clearinghouse
f. CMS-1500 Form
g. denied claim
h. dirty claim
i. invalid claim
j. nonparticipating provider
k. participating provider
l. primary insurance
m. secondary insurance
n. write-off

1. ____________ The failure to keep patient information confidential.
2. ____________ The most common health insurance claim form.
3. ____________ Has a contractual agreement with an insurance plan to render care to eligible beneficiaries and then bill the insurance carrier directly.
4. ____________ A health insurance claim form that has been completed but has some type of incorrect information.
5. ____________ Form that allows the insurance carrier to pay the physician directly for billed charges.
6. ____________ Applies if the patient has primary insurance and also has coverage available through the spouse's employer.
7. ____________ Bills the patient directly. The patient is expected to pay the charges and then submit the claim to the insurance company.
8. ____________ A health insurance claim form that has been completed correctly without any errors or omissions.
9. ____________ Term used to indicate that the physician has agreed to forfeit the amount that the insurance company does not authorize.
10. ____________ Can occur when procedures or services are not covered by the patient's insurance policy or when the patient has not met his or her deductible.
11. ____________ When a health insurance claim form is incorrect because it has missing data or errors.
12. ____________ The coverage provided by the patient's employer.

13. ____________ Used by insurance claims administrators to determine which parent's benefit plan will be the primary insurance plan of a dependent child who is covered by the employer-sponsored insurance plans of both parents.

14. ____________ An independent entity that reviews claims.

APPLIED PRACTICE

Complete the CMS-1500 form (Figure 18-1) using the patient registration form, the encounter form, and the fee schedule that is provided.

(1500)

HEALTH INSURANCE CLAIM FORM

APPROVED BY NATIONAL UNIFORM CLAIM COMMITTEE 08/05

PICA ☐☐☐ PICA ☐☐☐ CARRIER

1. MEDICARE MEDICAID TRICARE CHAMPUS CHAMPVA GROUP HEALTH PLAN FECA BLK LUNG OTHER
☐(Medicare #) ☐(Medicaid #) ☐(Sponsor's SSN) ☐(Member ID#) ☐(SSN or ID) ☐(SSN) ☐(ID)

1a. INSURED'S I.D. NUMBER (For Program in Item 1)

2. PATIENT'S NAME (Last Name, First Name, Middle Initial)

3. PATIENT'S BIRTH DATE MM | DD | YY SEX M☐ F☐

4. INSURED'S NAME (Last Name, First Name, Middle Initial)

5. PATIENT'S ADDRESS (No., Street)

6. PATIENT RELATIONSHIP TO INSURED Self☐ Spouse☐ Child☐ Other☐

7. INSURED'S ADDRESS (No., Street)

CITY STATE

8. PATIENT STATUS Single☐ Married☐ Other☐

CITY STATE

ZIP CODE TELEPHONE (Include Area Code) ( )

Employed☐ Full-Time Student☐ Part-Time Student☐

ZIP CODE TELEPHONE (Include Area Code) ( )

9. OTHER INSURED'S NAME (Last Name, First Name, Middle Initial)

10. IS PATIENT'S CONDITION RELATED TO:

11. INSURED'S POLICY GROUP OR FECA NUMBER

a. OTHER INSURED'S POLICY OR GROUP NUMBER

a. EMPLOYMENT? (Current or Previous) ☐YES ☐NO

a. INSURED'S DATE OF BIRTH MM | DD | YY SEX M☐ F☐

b. OTHER INSURED'S DATE OF BIRTH MM | DD | YY SEX M☐ F☐

b. AUTO ACCIDENT? PLACE (State) ☐YES ☐NO

b. EMPLOYER'S NAME OR SCHOOL NAME

c. EMPLOYER'S NAME OR SCHOOL NAME

c. OTHER ACCIDENT? ☐YES ☐NO

c. INSURANCE PLAN NAME OR PROGRAM NAME

d. INSURANCE PLAN NAME OR PROGRAM NAME

10d. RESERVED FOR LOCAL USE

d. IS THERE ANOTHER HEALTH BENEFIT PLAN? ☐YES ☐NO *If yes,* return to and complete item 9 a-d.

READ BACK OF FORM BEFORE COMPLETING & SIGNING THIS FORM.

12. PATIENT'S OR AUTHORIZED PERSON'S SIGNATURE I authorize the release of any medical or other information necessary to process this claim. I also request payment of government benefits either to myself or to the party who accepts assignment below.

SIGNED ____________ DATE ____________

13. INSURED'S OR AUTHORIZED PERSON'S SIGNATURE I authorize payment of medical benefits to the undersigned physician or supplier for services described below.

SIGNED ____________

PATIENT AND INSURED INFORMATION

14. DATE OF CURRENT MM | DD | YY ◀ ILLNESS (First symptom) OR INJURY (Accident) OR PREGNANCY (LMP)

15. IF PATIENT HAS HAD SAME OR SIMILAR ILLNESS, GIVE FIRST DATE MM | DD | YY

16. DATES PATIENT UNABLE TO WORK IN CURRENT OCCUPATION FROM MM | DD | YY TO MM | DD | YY

17. NAME OF REFERRING PHYSICIAN OR OTHER SOURCE

17a.

17b. NPI

18. HOSPITALIZATION DATES RELATED TO CURRENT SERVICES FROM MM | DD | YY TO MM | DD | YY

19. RESERVED FOR LOCAL USE

20. OUTSIDE LAB? ☐YES ☐NO $ CHARGES

21. DIAGNOSIS OR NATURE OF ILLNESS OR INJURY (Relate Items 1,2,3 or 4 to Item 24E by Line)

1. ____ . ____

2. ____ . ____

3. ____ . ____

4. ____ . ____

22. MEDICAID RESUBMISSION CODE ORIGINAL REF. NO.

23. PRIOR AUTHORIZATION NUMBER

24. A. DATE(S) OF SERVICE From MM DD YY To MM DD YY	B. PLACE OF SERVICE	C. EMG	D. PROCEDURES, SERVICES, OR SUPPLIES (Explain Unusual Circumstances) CPT/HCPCS MODIFIER	E. DIAGNOSIS POINTER	F. $ CHARGES	G. DAYS OR UNITS	H. EPSDT Family Plan	I. ID. QUAL	J. RENDERING PROVIDER ID. #
1								NPI	
2								NPI	
3								NPI	
4								NPI	
5								NPI	
6								NPI	

PHYSICIAN OR SUPPLIER INFORMATION

25. FEDERAL TAX I.D. NUMBER SSN EIN ☐☐

26. PATIENT'S ACCOUNT NO.

27. ACCEPT ASSIGNMENT? (For govt. claims, see back) ☐YES ☐NO

28. TOTAL CHARGE $

29. AMOUNT PAID $

30. BALANCE DUE $

31. SIGNATURE OF PHYSICIAN OR SUPPLIER INCLUDING DEGREES OR CREDENTIALS (I certify that the statements on the reverse apply to this bill and are made a part thereof.)

SIGNED DATE

32. SERVICE FACILITY LOCATION INFORMATION

a. b.

33. BILLING PROVIDER INFO & PH. # ( )

a. b.

SECOND FOLD — FIRST FOLD WHCF-10-ENV / WHCF-10-ENV-SS

NUCC Instruction Manual available at: www.nucc.org

WCMS-1500CS

APPROVED OMB 0938-0999 FORM CMS-1500 (08/05)

Capital City Medical—123 Unknown Boulevard, Capital City, NY 12345-2222 (555)555-1234	Patient Information Form
Phil Wells, MD, Mannie Mends, MD, Bette R. Soone, MD	Tax ID: 75-0246810
	Group NPI: 1513171216

Patient Information:

Name: (Last, First) Colich, Guy ☒ Male ☐ Female Birth Date: 04/23/1958

Address: 872 Hickory Pl, Capital City, NY 12345 Phone: (555) 555-9069

Social Security Number: 142-86-2078 Full-Time Student: ☐ Yes ☒ No

Marital Status: ☐ Single ☒ Married ☐ Divorced ☐ Other

Employment:

Employer: None Phone: ( ) ____________

Address: ____________

Condition Related to: ☐ Auto Accident ☐ Employment ☐ Other Accident

Date of Accident: ____________ State ____________

Emergency Contact: ____________ **Phone: ( )** ____________

Primary Insurance: Aetna Phone: ( ) ____________

Address: 1625 Healthcare Bldg, Capital City, NY 12345

Insurance Policyholder's Name: Same ☐ M ☐ F DOB: ____________

Address: ____________

Phone: ____________ Relationship to Insured: ☒ Self ☐ Spouse ☐ Child ☐ Other

Employer: ____________ Phone: ____________

Employer's Address: ____________

Policy/ID No: 9567305 Group No: 511669 Percent Covered: ___%, Copay Amt: $ 35.00

Secondary Insurance: ____________ Phone: ( ) ____________

Address: ____________

Insurance Policyholder's Name: ____________ ☐ M ☐ F DOB: ____________

Address: ____________

Phone: ____________ Relationship to Insured: ☐ Self ☐ Spouse ☐ Child ☐ Other

Employer: ____________ Phone: ( ) ____________

Employer's Address: ____________

Policy/ID No: ____________ Group No: _____ Percent Covered: _____%, Copay Amt: $_____

Reason for Visit: I am here for a recheck on my manic depression

Known Allergies: ____________

Were you referred here? If so, by whom?: ____________

Patient Name Guy Colich

Capital City Medical
123 Unknown Boulevard, Capital City, NY 12345-2222

Date of Service
10-07-20XX

New Patient					Laboratory	
Problem Focused	99201		Arthrocentesis/Aspiration/Injection		Amylase	82150
Expanded Problem, Focused	99202		Small Joint	20600	B12	82607
Detailed	99203		Interm Joint	20605	CBC & Diff	85025
Comprehensive	99204		Major Joint	20610	Comp Metabolic Panel	80053
Comprehensive/High Complex	99205		**Other Invasive/Noninvasive**		Chlamydia Screen	87110
Well Exam Infant (up to 12 mos.)	99381		Audiometry	92552	Cholesterol	82465
Well Exam 1–4 yrs.	99382		Cast Application		Diqoxin	80162
Well Exam 5–11 yrs.	99383		Location Long Short		Electrolytes	80051
Well Exam 12–17 yrs.	99384		Catheterization	51701	Ferritin	82728
Well Exam 18–39 yrs.	99385		Circumcision	54150	Folate	82746
Well Exam 40–64 yrs.	99386		Colposcopy	57452	GC Screen	87070
			Colposcopy w/Biopsy	57454	Glucose	82947
			Cryosurgery Premalignant Lesion		Glucose 1 HR	82950
			Location (s):		Glycosylated HGB A1C	83036
Established Patient			Cryosurgery Warts		HCT	85014
Post-Op Follow Up Visit	99024		Location (s):		HDL	83718
Minimum	99211		Curettement Lesion		Hep BSAG	87340
Problem Focused	99212		Single	11055	Hepatitis panel, acute	80074
Expanded Problem Focused	99213	×	2–4	11056	HGB	85018
Detailed	99214		>4	11057	HIV	86703
Comprehensive/High Complex	99215		Diaphragm Fitting	57170	Iron & TIBC	83550
Well Exam Infant (up to 12 mos.)	99391		Ear Irrigation	69210	Kidney Profile	80069
Well exam 1–4 yrs.	99392		ECG	93000	Lead	83655
Well Exam 5–11 yrs.	99393		Endometrial Biopsy	58100	Liver Profile	80076
Well Exam 12–17 yrs.	99394		Exc. Lesion Malignant		Mono Test	86308
Well Exam 18–39 yrs.	99395		Benign		Pap Smear	88155
Well Exam 40–64 yrs.	99396		Location		Pregnancy Test	84703
Obstetrics			Exc. Skin Taqs (1–15)	11200	Obstetric Panel	80055
Total OB Care	59400		Each Additional 10	11201	Pro Time	85610
Injections			Fracture Treatment		PSA	84153
Administration Sub. / IM	90772		Loc		RPR	86592
Drug			w/Reduc w/o Reduc		Sed. Rate	85651
Dosage			I & D Abscess Single/Simple	10060	Stool Culture	87045
Allergy	95115		Multiple or Comp	10061	Stool O & P	87177
Cocci Skin Test	86490		I & D Pilonidal Cyst Simple	10080	Strep Screen	87880
DPT	90701		Pilonidal Cyst Complex	10081	Theophylline	80198
Hemophilus	90646		IV Therapy—To One Hour	90760	Thyroid Uptake	84479
Influenza	90658		Each Additional Hour	90761	TSH	84443
MMR	90707		Laceration Repair		Urinalysis	81000
OPV	90712		Location Size Simp/Comp		Urine Culture	87088
Pneumovax	90732		Laryngoscopy	31505	Drawing Fee	36415
TB Skin Test	86580		Oximetry	94760	Specimen Collection	99000
TD	90718		Punch Biopsy		**Other:**	
Unlisted Immun	90749		Rhythm Strip	93040		
Tetanus Toxoid	90703		Treadmill	93015		
Vaccine/Toxoid Admin <8 Yr Old w/ Counseling	90465		Trigger Point or Tendon Sheath Inj.	20550		
Vaccine/Toxoid Administration for Adult	90471		Tympanometry	92567		

Diagnosis/ICD-9: **296.80**

I acknowledge receipt of medical services and authorize the release of any medical information necessary to process this claim for healthcare payment only. I do authorize payment to the provider.

Patient Signature Guy Colich

Total Estimated Charges: __________

Payment Amount: __________

Next Appointment: __________

New Patient Examinations		
Office Visit, Level 1	99201	$ 55.00
Office Visit, Level 2	99202	$110.00
Office Visit, Level 3	99203	$154.00
Office Visit, Level 4	99204	$226.00
Office Visit, Level 5	99205	$299.00
Established Patient Examinations		
Office Visit, Level 1	99211	$ 45.00
Office Visit, Level 2	99212	$ 60.00
Office Visit, Level 3	99213	$ 80.00
Office Visit, Level 4	99214	$123.00
Office Visit, Level 5	99215	$199.00

Note: This activity has been adapted from Vines/Comprehensive Health Insurance: Billing, Coding, and Reimbursement Student CD.

LEARNING ACTIVITY: TRUE/FALSE

Indicate whether the following statements are true or false by placing a T or an F on the line that precedes each statement.

_______ 1. Many Blue Cross/Blue Shield plans provide their own type of health insurance claim form.

_______ 2. Depending on the type of service, the CMS-1500 form or the CMS-1450 form may also be used.

_______ 3. The CMS-1500 form was previously known as the UB-04 form.

_______ 4. Most patients are well aware of what their insurance covers.

_______ 5. Medicaid is a state-run insurance program for those individuals who are considered medically indigent.

_______ 6. When working with Medicaid patients, the medical assistant must verify coverage prior to each and every visit.

_______ 7. The most frequently used claim form for workers' compensation is the DD Form 2642.

_______ 8. The electronic filing of claims speeds the processing time for both the provider and the insurance carrier.

_______ 9. It is improper for insurance companies to make special incentives available to physicians who choose to become participating providers.

_______ 10. It is against the law to talk to a patient about his or her condition anywhere but in a professional setting.

CRITICAL THINKING

Answer the following questions to the best of your ability. Utilize the textbook and other resources as needed.

1. Josie Svien, CMA (AAMA), is working in the billing office of a family practice clinic. Josie is new to the job and is just beginning the process of filing insurance claims. To what areas should Josie pay particular attention in order to avoid the rejection of claims?

2. Erica Miller, CMA (AAMA), has just completed a claim form. Explain the use of the insurance claims log. What information is entered into the log for each step of the reimbursement process? What is the purpose of such documentation?

RESEARCH ACTIVITY

Utilize Internet search engines to research the following topics and write a brief description of what you find. It is important to utilize reputable websites.

1. Using the Internet as a research source, write an essay on the advantages and disadvantages of electronic medical records and the electronic submission of claims. Cite your sources.

CHAPTER 19
Medical Coding

CHAPTER OUTLINE

General review of the chapter:

Insurance Coding
History of Coding
Understanding the ICD-9-CM
Procedural Coding
Getting to Know the CPT
Insurance Fraud
Compliance Plan

STUDENT STUDY GUIDE

Use the following guide to assist in your learning of the concepts from the chapter.

I. Introduction to Coding and the ICD-9-CM Coding Manual

1. The Purposes of Codes
   A. Provide information to the __________ regarding patient __________ and __________.
   B. Assist in the communications process to ensure __________ and __________ reimbursement.
2. The Superbill
   A. Used as a __________, a statement, and an __________ reporting form.
   B. Must be updated __________ to reflect the most current diagnostic and procedural codes
   C. Can be used as a reference base for traditional __________ insurance forms and __________ insurance forms.
3. The History of Coding
   i. ______________________________
   ii. ______________________________
   iii. ______________________________
   iv. ______________________________
   v. ______________________________
4. Contents of Volume II of the ICD-9-CM Coding Manual
   A. Contains the __________ index.
   B. Lists __________ and __________ found in the __________ list.
   C. Provides information on __________ and the adverse effects of __________ and __________.
   D. Contains an index of injuries resulting from __________ causes.
5. The ICD-9-CM Codes
   A. Each diagnosis is given a _________-digit code.
   B. The _________ and _________ digits are added to the main code to provide more _________.

C. If __________ digits are applicable for describing the patient's condition, then the __________ -digit code must be used.

6. The Uses of Tables in the ICD-9-CM Coding Manual

A. The __________ table is used to code a diagnosis of high blood pressure.
B. The __________ table is used to code __________, both benign and malignant.
C. The __________ table is used to code the behavior of the neoplasm.

7. Abbreviations and Symbols Used in the ICD-9-CM Coding Manual (List each that is used.)

i. ______________________________
ii. ______________________________
iii. ______________________________
iv. ______________________________
v. ______________________________
vi. ______________________________
vii. ______________________________
viii. ______________________________
ix. ______________________________
x. ______________________________

8. Comparing ICD-10 Codes with ICD-9 Codes

A. ICD-10 has __________ codes, as well as __________ and content modifications.
B. In the ICD-10, identification is from the __________ versus from the __________.
C. Conversion to use of the ICD-10 codes has been pushed back to __________.

9. Expectations for the ICD-10 Codes

A. Support __________ purchasing and Medicare's __________ and __________ activities.
B. Support __________ reporting of quality data.
C. Ensure more __________ payments for new procedures and fewer rejected claims.
D. Improve __________ management, __________ of disease monitoring, and reporting worldwide.
E. Allow the United States to compare its data with __________ data to track the incidence and spread of __________ and __________ outcomes.

10. HCPCS

A. Stands for ______________________________.
B. Used to report services and procedures for __________ and __________ patients.
C. Consists of __________ coding levels.

11. Contents of HCPCS Level I

A. Contains codes for __________ and __________.
B. Provides additional codes not found in the __________.
C. Contains __________ sections.
D. Codes are for items covered under Medicare, such as __________, __________, and __________.

12. HCPCS Level II and Modifiers

A. Level II contains codes that begin with a __________ and then __________.
B. Modifiers consist of __________ letters.
C. Modifiers can be used in addition to the modifiers found in the __________ Manual.

II. Getting to Know the CPT Manual

1. Sections in the CPT Manual

i. ______________________________
ii. ______________________________

iii. ____________________

iv. ____________________

v. ____________________

vi. ____________________

2. Evaluation and Management Section
   A. Beginning section in the __________ Manual.
   B. Includes codes for __________ visits and __________.
   C. Codes link the __________ or __________ with the __________ needed for treatment.

3. Factors Affecting Code Selection
   i. ____________________
   ii. ____________________
   iii. ____________________
   iv. ____________________

4. Four Levels of Decision Making
   i. ____________________
   ii. ____________________
   iii. ____________________
   iv. ____________________

5. Use of Modifiers
   A. Provides further classification of __________ and __________.
   B. Follows the __________ -digit __________ code.
   C. Contains a __________ -digit code preceded by a __________.
   D. The most common modifier is __________.
   E. Use of multiple modifiers requires the use of the modifier __________ first.

6. Codes Found in the Medicine Section
   A. Codes for __________ procedures and treatment procedures.
   B. Codes for many __________ tests.

7. Items Needed for Proper Coding
   i. ____________________
   ii. ____________________
   iii. ____________________
   iv. ____________________
   v. ____________________

8. Steps for Proper Coding
   i. ____________________
   ii. ____________________
   iii. ____________________
   iv. ____________________
   v. ____________________
   vi. ____________________
   vii. ____________________

III. Insurance Fraud

1. Tips for the Patient for Preventing Insurance Fraud from the Centers for Medicare & Medicaid Services
   A. Look at your Medicaid bill __________ to ensure that Medicaid has been billed for __________ services and goods that you actually __________. Check that the __________ of service is correct.

B. DO NOT give your Medicaid ___________ to anyone except your doctor, clinic, hospital, or other health care provider.
C. DO NOT let anyone ___________ your Medicaid card.
D. DO NOT ___________ your name on a blank form.
E. Ask for a ___________ of everything that you sign.
F. If you are offered free tests or screenings in exchange for your Medicaid card number, be ___________.
G. Give your Medicaid ___________ card only to those individuals who have provided you with ___________.
H. NEVER allow a medical services provider to ___________ for ___________ rendered without ___________ you first.

2. The Most Common Forms of Medicare Fraud

i. ___________
ii. ___________
iii. ___________
iv. ___________
v. ___________
vi. ___________

3. Suspicious Office Practices that Should Alert Consumers to Improper Behavior

A. Routinely ___________ copayments without checking on the patient's ability to pay.
B. Advertise ___________ consultations to Medicare beneficiaries.
C. Claiming that they ___________ Medicare.
D. Using ___________ or ___________ tactics to sell high-priced medical services or diagnostic tests.
E. Bill Medicare for services that the patient ___________ recall receiving.
F. Use ___________ and ___________ selling as marketing tools.

4. Information Requested by the National Fraud Hotline

i. ___________
ii. ___________
iii. ___________
iv. ___________
v. ___________
vi. ___________

5. The Benefits of Having a Compliance Plan

A. The medical office is at a ___________ risk for liability.
B. Demonstrates to the physicians, fraud investigators, and insurance carriers that the medical office is making every effort to ___________ and ___________ errors.
C. Gives the office staff a process for ___________, ___________, and ___________ practices that are illegal.

6. Basic Components of a Compliance Plan

A. Conducting ___________ audits of billing and coding practices.
B. ___________ written standards and procedures for compliance.
C. Training and educating office staff on ___________.
D. Investigating ___________ and disclosing ___________ to the appropriate government agencies.

KEY TERMINOLOGY REVIEW

Match the selected key terms to their definitions below.

a. Current Procedural Terminology (CPT) Manual
b. Established patient
c. Evaluation and Management (E/M)
d. ICD-9-CM
e. ICD-10
f. Kickback
g. Modifier
h. New patient
i. Principal diagnosis
j. Procedural coding
k. Symbols
l. Upcoding
m. World Health Organization (WHO)

1. ______________ Based on the following criteria: the history of the patient, the complexity of the examination, and the degree of difficulty in medical decision making.
2. ______________ Used in circumstances in which the procedure code does not accurately describe the procedure.
3. ______________ Publishes the International Classification of Diseases, 9th Revision, Clinical Modification (ICD-9-CM).
4. ______________ Used in the CPT Manual to distinguish changes or give instructions to be used when coding.
5. ______________ The process of translating a narrative description of procedures into numbers.
6. ______________ Provides a comprehensive list of procedure and service codes.
7. ______________ One who has never been seen by anyone in the practice or has not been seen by anyone in the practice for more than 3 years.
8. ______________ Contains numeric and alphanumeric diagnostic codes.
9. ______________ An incentive provided by another physician, laboratory, hospital, or pharmaceutical representative for using their services.
10. ______________ Billing for a service at a higher level than was actually provided.
11. ______________ The reason that the patient sought care on a particular date.
12. ______________ Contains increased specificity and includes recently discovered or diagnosed diseases.
13. ______________ One who has been seen within the past 3 years by any practitioner in the practice.

APPLIED PRACTICE

Follow the directions that apply to each section.

Section A: Provide the correct modifier for each of the following descriptions.

1. Bilateral procedure: ______________
2. Discontinued procedure: ______________
3. Unusual procedural service: ______________
4. Preoperative management only: ______________
5. General anesthesia provided by the surgeon: ______________

Section B: Code the following using the CPT Manual:

1. Debridement of 10 nails by any method: ______________
2. Chemical peel, facial; dermal: ______________
3. Mastectomy, subcutaneous: ______________
4. Incision and draining (I&D) of hematoma, soft tissue of neck: ______________
5. Manipulation, elbow, under anesthesia: ______________

6. Endoscopy, surgical; operative tissue ablation and reconstruction of atria, without cardiopulmonary bypass: _______________
7. Laparoscopy, surgical, appendectomy: _______________
8. Vaginal delivery only, including postpartum care: _______________
9. Mammography, bilateral: _______________
10. Spirometry, including graphic record, total and timed vital capacity, expiratory flow rate measurement with or without maximal voluntary ventilation: _______________

Section C: Using Volumes I and II of the ICD-9-CM Coding Manual, identify the diagnostic code for each of the following diagnoses.

1. Diabetes with ketoacidosis: _______________
2. Acute idiopathic pericarditis: _______________
3. Acute lymphadenitis: _______________
4. Pneumococcal meningitis: _______________
5. Acute pharyngitis: _______________
6. Hirsutism: _______________
7. Chest pains, unspecified: _______________
8. Special Screening for Diabetes Mellitus: _______________
9. Cushing's Syndrome: _______________
10. Glycosuria: _______________

LEARNING ACTIVITY: MULTIPLE CHOICE

Circle the correct answer for each of the questions below.

1. The CPT Manual has ___________ major sections.
   a. three
   b. four
   c. five
   d. six

2. All CPT codes are ___________ digits long.
   a. four
   b. five
   c. six
   d. All of the above

3. Within the CPT Manual, ___________ indicate(s) that this is a new code.
   a. a black circle
   b. a triangle
   c. two triangles
   d. a circle with an inner dot

4. Within the CPT Manual, ___________ indicate(s) that this is a revised code.
   a. a black circle
   b. a triangle
   c. two triangles
   d. a circle with an inner dot

5. Within the CPT Manual, __________ indicate(s) a new or revised description.

   a. a black circle
   b. a triangle
   c. two triangles
   d. a circle with an inner dot

6. When physicians perform procedures that are not listed in the CPT Manual, what must the medical assistant do?

   a. Choose the code for the procedure that most closely approximates the actual procedure.
   b. Not bill for the service.
   c. Ask the physician to choose an appropriate code.
   d. Use an unlisted procedure code and submit copies of the procedure report with the claim.

7. Which volume of the ICD-9-CM Coding Manual contains a tabular list of diseases?

   a. Volume I
   b. Volume II
   c. Volume III
   d. Volume IV

8. Which volume of the ICD-9-CM Coding Manual contains a list of diagnosis codes used for hospital billing?

   a. Volume I
   b. Volume II
   c. Volume III
   d. Volume IV

9. Appendix __________ contains a list of the morphology of neoplasms.

   a. A
   b. B
   c. C
   d. D

10. Volume I of the ICD-9-CM Coding Manual has __________ appendices.

   a. four
   b. five
   c. six
   d. seven

CRITICAL THINKING

Answer the following questions to the best of your ability. Utilize the textbook as a reference.

1. Teresa Clymer is taking a course in medical insurance billing as part of her medical assistant training. She has been asked to write a paper describing how proper diagnostic coding is linked to proper reimbursement from insurance carriers. What information should Teresa include in her paper?

____

____

____

____

____

2. Mavis Raschenko, RMA, has been asked by her office manager to explain the difference between volumes I and II of the ICD-9-CM Coding Manual. How might Mavis explain the differences?

3. Marc Alaimo, RMA, has been newly hired to work in the billing office in a family practice clinic. Marc has been asked to explain to the physicians how V codes are to be used. What should Marc include in his explanation?

4. Kira Stansfield, CMA (AAMA), is working with Dr. Ramey in an internal medicine clinic. Dr. Ramey is unsure of which evaluation and management code to choose for certain patients whom she has seen. How can Kira advise Dr. Ramey in choosing the appropriate code?

5. Gloria Heritage, RMA, is working in the billing office of a pediatric practice. One of the physicians in the practice frequently chooses a high-level E/M code when billing for his patients. When Gloria consults the patient's charts, she finds that there is not sufficient information to use the higher billing codes and determines that a lower code would be more appropriate. What can Gloria do in this situation?

RESEARCH ACTIVITY

Utilize Internet search engines to research the following topics and write a brief description of what you find. It is important to utilize reputable websites.

1. Using the Internet as a research source, go to your state's website for the Department of Health. Research the laws that apply to billing for medical services in your state. Create a list of the laws that are relevant to the issue of fraudulent practices in billing and coding.

CHAPTER 20

Medical Office Management

CHAPTER OUTLINE

General review of the chapter:

Systems Approach to Office Management
The Office Manager
Leadership Styles
Creating a Team Atmosphere
Hiring Procedures: Selecting the Right Staff Members
Orientation and Training
Using Performance Evaluation Effectively
Time Management
Personnel Policy Manual
Office Policies and Procedures Manual
Medical Meetings and Speaking Engagements
Patient Information Booklet
Medical Practice Marketing and Customer Service

STUDENT STUDY GUIDE

Use the following guide to assist in your learning of the concepts from the chapter.

I. Managing the Medical Office

1. General Skills for Office Management
   i. ______________________________
   ii. ______________________________
   iii. ______________________________
2. General Duties of the Office Manager
   i. ______________________________
   ii. ______________________________
   iii. ______________________________
3. Critical Resources Used in Managing a Medical Office
   i. ______________________________
   ii. ______________________________
   iii. ______________________________
4. Personnel Management Responsibilities
   A. Hiring new employees and establishing __________ training.
   B. Performing __________ reviews.
   C. Disciplinary measures should occur as soon as they are warranted and not be held over until an __________.

5. Employee Records
   A. Federal law requires records to be maintained for __________ employee.
   B. Payroll records must include the following:
      i. ______________________________
      ii. ______________________________
      iii. ______________________________
      iv. ______________________________
6. Elements of Financial Management
   i. ______________________________
   ii. ______________________________
   iii. ______________________________
   iv. ______________________________
7. Effective Scheduling
   A. Can contribute to the __________ level of the practice.
   B. If the office staff is continuously scheduled inappropriately, it affects __________ and may cause __________ among the physicians and patients.
   C. __________ must be built into the staff schedule to allow for __________ occurrences such as sick days and business appointments.
8. Elements of Facility and Equipment Management
   i. ______________________________
   ii. ______________________________
   iii. ______________________________
   iv. ______________________________
   v. ______________________________
   vi. ______________________________
9. Communications
   A. To be effective, one must be able to communicate at __________ __________.
   B. Contributes significantly to the __________ of the staff.
   C. Includes __________ and __________ materials.
10. The Basic Duties of the Office Manager
   A. Acts as a liaison between the __________ and the __________.
   B. Conducts __________ and __________ reviews.
   C. __________ responsibilities to staff.
   D. Maintains the office procedures __________.
   E. Oversees HIPAA __________.
   F. Plans and __________ staff meetings.
   G. Prepares __________ educational materials.
   H. Supervises employees on a __________ basis.
   I. Supervises the purchase and __________ of equipment and supplies.
11. Qualities of a Good Manager
   i. ______________________________
   ii. ______________________________
   iii. ______________________________
   iv. ______________________________
   v. ______________________________
   vi. ______________________________
   vii. ______________________________
   viii. ______________________________
   ix. ______________________________

x. ____________________

xi. ____________________

xii. ____________________

xiii. ____________________

12. Managing the Monthly Planning Calendar

   A. Develop a system in which the schedule for the __________ is laid out on a calendar.
   B. List __________ vacations on a calendar because it helps to prevent overlapping of vacations, which can leave an office __________.
   C. Note all physicians' __________, __________, __________, accountant meetings, and vendor visits.
   D. Ensure that all vacations have been __________.
   E. Compare the office's calendar with the __________ calendar on a periodic basis and update the office's __________ calendar as necessary.

13. Staff Meetings

   A. Facilitate communications between __________ and the __________.
   B. Time, date, and agenda are created by the __________ with input from the __________.
   C. Ensure that staff meetings are __________ to help minimize wasted time.
   D. The minutes and the __________ of attendees should be recorded.

14. Equipment Needed for a Staff Meeting

   i. ____________________
   ii. ____________________
   iii. ____________________
   iv. ____________________

15. Preparing for the Staff Meeting

   A. __________ week before the meeting, request agenda items from the __________.
   B. Before the meeting, create a meeting __________ which includes all topics that need to be discussed.
   C. On the agenda, include the following:
      i. ____________________
      ii. ____________________
      iii. ____________________

16. Ensuring the Success of Staff Meetings

   A. Start the meeting __________.
   B. Begin by __________ reviewing the last meeting.
   C. Address each topic within its __________ amount of __________.
   D. Allow for time at the end of the meeting to have __________ of any new business.
   E. After the meeting, the __________ of the meeting should be distributed to __________.

17. The Staff's Expectations of Management

   i. ____________________
   ii. ____________________
   iii. ____________________
   iv. ____________________
   v. ____________________
   vi. ____________________
   vii. ____________________
   viii. ____________________
   ix. ____________________
   x. ____________________
   xi. ____________________
   xii. ____________________

18. Ways to Show Respect
    A. Greet employees in a __________ manner.
    B. Always __________ employees' hard work.
    C. Never __________ employees in front of their peers.
    D. Be __________ and listen to employees when they need to talk.
    E. Take employees' suggestions into __________.
    F. Work toward having __________ employees.
    G. When possible, provide __________ space for each employee.
    H. Create a sense of __________ with the medical office.
    I. Ensure that employees feel that they have been __________ for the amount of work that they accomplish.
    J. Provide employees with __________ beyond pay.
    K. Maintain a cohesive work environment by ensuring that communication is __________ and __________.

II. Leadership and Team Accountability

1. Attributes of Good Leaders
    i. ______________________________
    ii. ______________________________
    iii. ______________________________
    iv. ______________________________
    v. ______________________________

2. Attributes of Authoritarian Leaders
    A. Make most decisions on their own without the __________ of others.
    B. Are not as likely to be team __________ as are solid __________.
    C. Want __________ and __________ from their staff.
    D. Use __________ to achieve obedience from their staff.
    E. Are motivated by __________ and __________ authority.
    F. Work best under great __________ and in __________.

3. Attributes of Democratic Leaders
    A. Concentrate more on the relationships among __________ and emphasize __________ in the office.
    B. Are motivated from __________ to provide a comfortable work environment for all employees.
    C. Leadership style often results in a __________ staff.

4. Attributes of Permissive Leaders
    A. Are not strict with regard to __________ and __________.
    B. Leadership style may result in __________ and even __________ conditions in the work environment.
    C. Are self- __________.

5. Attributes of Bureaucratic Leaders
    A. Very strongly __________ rules.
    B. Are motivated by __________ factors.
    C. Rely on __________ management methods for office matters.
    D. Are __________ because they do not trust themselves when making decisions that affect the office.
    E. Are very __________ and formal.

6. Types of Power (*List and briefly describe each type.*)
    i. ______________________________
    ii. ______________________________

iii. ______________________________
iv. ______________________________
v. ______________________________
vi. ______________________________

7. Task-Oriented Roles That Team Members May Assume
   i. ______________________________
   ii. ______________________________
   iii. ______________________________
   iv. ______________________________
   v. ______________________________
   vi. ______________________________

8. Nurturing Roles That Team Members May Assume
   i. ______________________________
   ii. ______________________________
   iii. ______________________________
   iv. ______________________________

9. Holding Team Members Accountable
   A. The team must come together to locate and __________ the problem.
   B. The team should not __________ or try to __________ a problem on any one member.
   C. The team members must decide together how they got off track and how they can __________ a reoccurrence.

10. Methods for Providing the Job Application
   A. Send to the applicant by __________ and have him or her bring the application to the interview.
   B. Provide a __________ to the online version.
   C. Have the applicant fill out the form at the time of the __________.

11. The Benefits of Having the Application Completed at the Interview
   A. You will see how the applicant handles filling out forms under __________.
   B. You will obtain a visual of the applicant's __________.
   C. You will learn how __________ the applicant is at completing a required task.

12. Areas for Consideration During the Interview
   i. ______________________________
   ii. ______________________________
   iii. ______________________________

13. The Contents of Questions Prohibited by the Equal Employment Opportunity Act
   i. ______________________________
   ii. ______________________________
   iii. ______________________________
   iv. ______________________________
   v. ______________________________

14. Information to Be Obtained About an Applicant
   A. Past office __________.
   B. Types of __________ with whom the applicant has worked.
   C. The applicant's ability to __________ on his or her feet.

15. Possible Office Requirements for an Applicant
   i. ______________________________
   ii. ______________________________

iii. ____________________
iv. ____________________
v. ____________________

16. The Purpose of the Probationary Period
    A. Allows the supervisor to __________ the new employee at work and to __________ if he or she is suited to the position.
    B. During the probationary period, an employee can be __________ without cause.
    C. After __________ days, the employer must show just cause, or reason, to dismiss an employee.

17. The Contents of an Orientation Checklist
    i. ____________________
    ii. ____________________
    iii. ____________________
    iv. ____________________
    v. ____________________
    vi. ____________________
    vii. ____________________
    viii. ____________________
    ix. ____________________
    x. ____________________
    xi. ____________________
    xii. ____________________
    xiii. ____________________

18. Types of Reviews (*Explain each type.*)
    A. Orientation or training: ____________________
    B. Routine performance review: ____________________
    C. Poor performance review: ____________________
    D. Salary review: ____________________

19. Actions that Require Disciplinary/Probationary Measures
    i. ____________________
    ii. ____________________
    iii. ____________________
    iv. ____________________
    v. ____________________

20. Possible Disciplinary Actions
    A. Giving a __________ and/or __________ warning.
    B. __________ the employee while the incident is being investigated.
    C. Placing the employee on __________ and telling the employee that if the situation occurs again within a set period of time, the employee will be __________.

21. Steps for Creating a Time Management System
    A. Define the office __________ in consultation with the __________.
    B. Create a __________ list of __________.
    C. Incorporate the __________ list into a __________ list.

22. Information Found in an Employee Handbook
    i. ____________________
    ii. ____________________
    iii. ____________________
    iv. ____________________
    v. ____________________

23. The Office Procedures Manual
    A. Contains detailed descriptions of ________________________ and how to perform both _____________ and _____________ tasks.
    B. The terms "policy" and "procedure" are used _________________ in many offices.
24. The Primary Functions of a Procedures Manual
    i. ____________________
    ii. ____________________
    iii. ____________________
25. The Benefits of an Effective Patient Information Booklet
    A. Reduces the number of __________ by telephone from __________.
    B. Enhances the office's __________.
    C. Reduces the number of patients who __________ to remember instructions.
    D. Useful either for __________ with __________ or for teaching methods of __________ prevention.

III. Marketing the Medical Practice
1. Steps to Take After Determining the Services to Be Offered
    A. Look for any _________ or _________ that may arise during the conduct of a marketing plan.
    B. A marketing plan should describe _________ steps that need to be implemented, who is __________ for these steps, and a reasonable _________ for completion.
    C. A marketing plan must be thought through and in place before you begin to _________ and _________ it.
2. Opportunities for Free Marketing
    i. ____________________
    ii. ____________________
3. Questions to Be Asked When Establishing a Practice Website
    i. ____________________
    ii. ____________________
    iii. ____________________
    iv. ____________________
    v. ____________________
4. Considerations for Operating a Website
    A. Ensure that patient __________ is maintained.
    B. Keep the site __________ to use.
    C. Graphics need to be __________ and colors need to be __________.
5. The Impact of Good Customer Service
    A. Word of mouth can bring you __________ customers.
    B. It can also drive customers __________ if poor services are provided
    C. All patients must be treated with __________ and __________.

KEY TERMINOLOGY REVIEW

Without using information from the textbook, write a sentence using the selected key terms in the correct context.

1. ***Colleagues***

____

____

2. ***Discriminatory***

____

____

3. ***Grievance***

____

____

4. ***Itinerary***

____

____

5. ***Probationary period***

____

____

6. ***Seniority***

____

____

7. ***Solvent***

____

____

APPLIED PRACTICE

Complete the following activity.

1. Develop a patient information booklet as described in Procedure 20-2 in Chapter 20 of your textbook. Your booklet will be graded on accuracy, completeness, and appearance. In addition to other items that may be considered, the following items should be part of the booklet.
   a. Regular office hours
   b. Special services offered by the practice or clinic, such as patient education classes or blood pressure screening
   c. Written procedures for handling prescription refills
   d. Written procedures for how medical insurance forms are processed
   e. General statement about the payment of fees, especially if payment is expected at the time of the delivery of services
   f. Information about the physician and the staff
   g. Written procedures on how emergencies are handled

LEARNING ACTIVITY: TRUE/FALSE

Indicate whether the following statements are true or false by placing a T or an F on the line that precedes each statement.

_______ 1. Personnel management usually requires a performance review every 6 months for each employee.

_______ 2. The clinical aspects of office management are separate from the administrative aspects.

_______ 3. The office manager's time is generally spent on employee and administrative issues.

______ 4. A good office manager strives to become the boss.

______ 5. Many office managers are promoted based on seniority.

______ 6. The office manager creates and updates the physician's own calendar.

______ 7. Staff vacations should be included on the physician's calendar.

______ 8. If a staff meeting is held outside of normal working hours, staff must be compensated.

______ 9. Bureaucratic leaders are very open with the staff.

______ 10. Democratic leaders are typically more receptive to new ideas from staff.

CRITICAL THINKING

Answer the following questions to the best of your ability. Utilize the textbook as a reference.

1. Teresa Clymer, CMA (AAMA), has just been promoted to office manager. In order to create a team atmosphere, what factors should Teresa consider to ensure the building of a successful team?

____

____

____

____

____

2. Mavis Raschenko, RMA, must fill an open medical assistant position. What methods might Mavis choose and why?

____

____

____

____

____

3. When hiring individuals, what cultural considerations need to be considered?

____

____

____

____

____

RESEARCH ACTIVITY

Utilize Internet search engines to research the following topics and write a brief description of what you find. It is important to utilize reputable websites.

1. Using the Internet as a research source, determine the importance of conducting performance evaluations and explore the tools used to perform this task. Write an essay explaining what you have learned through your research. Cite your sources at the end of your essay.

____

____

Chapter 21
Body Structure and Function

CHAPTER OUTLINE

General review of the chapter:

The Human Body: Levels of Organization
Chemistry
Genetics and Heredity

STUDENT STUDY GUIDE

Use the following guide to assist in your learning of the concepts from the chapter.

I. Organization of the Human Body

1. Organization of the Human Body (Diagram the organization of the body.)

2. Atom

A. ___________ and ___________ constitute the majority of the anatomic mass and reside within the nucleus.

B. ___________, ___________, and ___________ combine to create elements.

3. Elements Found in the Human Body

i. ______________________________
ii. ______________________________
iii. ______________________________
iv. ______________________________
v. ______________________________
vi. ______________________________
vii. ______________________________
viii. ______________________________
ix. ______________________________
x. ______________________________
xi. ______________________________
xii. ______________________________
xiii. ______________________________
xiv. ______________________________
xv. ______________________________
xvi. ______________________________
xvii. ______________________________
xviii. ______________________________
xix. ______________________________

4. Molecules
   A. Can take the form of ___________, ___________, or ___________.
   B. Water contains ___________ of molecules.
5. Components of a Cell
   i. ___________
   ii. ___________
   iii. ___________
6. Cell Membrane
   A. Helps maintain the ___________ shape.
   B. Allows some substances to pass into and out of the cell while ___________ the passage of other substances.
7. Cilia
   A. ___________ the overall surface area of a cell.
   B. Propels substances along a cell's surface, which increases the cell's ability to absorb ___________ and ___________.
8. Cytoplasm
   A. ___________ percent water; generally ___________ in color, resembling a ___________.
   B. Provides ___________ and work areas for the cell.
9. Organelles
   A. Each organelle has a specific function and purpose in maintaining the vitality of the ___________.
   B. Organelles include ___________, ___________, ___________, ___________, ___________, and ___________.
10. Nucleus
    A. The nucleus is the ___________ of the cell.
    B. Within the nucleus are the cell's ___________.
11. Nucleic Functions
    i. ___________
    ii. ___________
    iii. ___________
    iv. ___________
    v. ___________
12. Organs
    A. Composed of several types of ___________.
    B. Perform ___________ functions.
13. Passive and Active Transport
    A. Passive transport involves a number of processes, including ___________, ___________, and ___________.
    B. Through active transport, ___________ are able to obtain what they need through ___________ fluid.
14. Electrolytes
    A. An electrolyte is an electrically charged ___________ that moves to either a ___________ or a ___________ electrode.
    B. Used to carry ___________ impulses to other cells.
    C. Electrolytes must be ___________ to keep their concentrations in the body fluids constant.
15. Electrolytes in the Human Body
    i. ___________
    ii. ___________

iii. ______________________________
iv. ______________________________
v. ______________________________
vi. ______________________________
vii. ______________________________
viii. ______________________________

II. Genetics and Heredity

1. Natural Selection Versus Artificial Breeding
   A. Natural selection occurs when the __________ chooses the __________ that are best suited to the current __________ and allows animals with those __________ to reproductively mature and reproduce.
   B. Artificial breeding is human interaction within the process of __________ selection.
2. Heredity
   A. Heredity is the transmission of genes from __________ to __________.
   B. Individuals carry __________ genes for each __________.
3. Genetic Disorders
   A. Mutations are changes in the __________ sequence of a __________.
   B. Genetic mutations can occur at any time during __________.
4. Albinism
   A. Albinism is a common __________ disorder.
   B. It is a congenital but __________ disorder.
   C. A mutation in a recessive gene causes a hereditary lack of pigment in the __________, __________, and eyes.
   D. The patient may complain of __________ and is prone to __________ because protective melanin is not present.
5. ADHD
   A. ADHD stands for ______________________.
   B. It is characterized by a person having difficulty __________ and completing a task.
   C. May be caused by __________ factors. It is __________ times more prevalent in __________ than in __________.
6. Cleft Palate
   A. Cleft palate is a __________ defect in the roof of the mouth that occurs when the __________ bones of the skull do not close properly.
   B. The cleft causes a __________ between the mouth and the nasal cavities.
   C. This defect also may be accompanied by a cleft __________.
   D. Affects __________ more often than __________.
7. Color Deficiency
   A. This disorder was previously called __________.
   B. Often entails difficulty in distinguishing between __________ and __________.
   C. This condition is an __________, sex-linked disorder, usually passed from mother to __________.
   D. With total color deficiency, a person is unable to perceive any color at all because of a defect in or absence of __________ in the __________.
8. Cystic Fibrosis
   A. Cystic fibrosis is a chronic and __________ disease, usually diagnosed in __________.
   B. This disease causes mucus to become __________, __________, and sticky.
   C. Mucus builds up and clogs passages, primarily in the lungs and the __________.

9. Down Syndrome

A. Down syndrome occurs when a person has an ___________ copy of ___________ 21.
B. A mother who gives birth after age ___________ has a higher risk of delivering an infant with Down syndrome.
C. ___________ is generally used as a tool for diagnosing this disorder.

10. Fragile X Syndrome

A. Fragile X syndrome also is known as ___________ syndrome, ___________ syndrome, and ___________ syndrome.
B. This condition is the most common form of inherited ___________.
C. Generally, ___________ are affected with moderate mental retardation and ___________ with mild mental retardation.

11. Hemochromatosis

A. Hemochromatosis is an inherited disorder in which the body accumulates an excessive amount of ___________.
B. Common among the ___________ population, affecting approximately ___________ in ___________ individuals of ___________ ancestry.
C. ___________ deposits in the skin will eventually cause ___________ of the skin.

12. Hemophilia

A. Hemophilia is a ___________, ___________ disorder in which the time it takes for blood to coagulate is greatly increased.
B. Caused by a ___________ gene mutation in the ___________ chromosome.
C. Females carry the ___________ gene and transmit the disorder to their ___________ offspring.

13. Klinefelter's Syndrome

A. Klinefelter's syndrome is a congenital ___________ disorder.
B. Primary ___________ failure occurs, which usually is not evident until puberty.
C. This disorder also can lead to ___________ intelligence.

14. Muscular Dystrophy

A. Muscular dystrophy is a genetic disease that is characterized by a gradual ___________ and ___________ of the muscles.
B. Occurs most frequent in ___________.
C. The most common type is ___________ muscular dystrophy, which accounts for ___________ of all cases.
D. Death often occurs within ___________ to ___________ years after the onset of symptoms.

15. PKU

A. PKU stands for ___________.
B. Caused by a recessive gene ___________.
C. If the condition is not treated early, ___________ occurs because of brain damage.

16. Spina Bifida

A. Spina bifida is a congenital ___________ tube defect.
B. The posterior vertebral arch has a ___________ anomaly.
C. Most often the abnormality occurs in the ___________ region.

17. Tay-Sachs Disease

A. Tay-Sachs disease is an inherited disorder that tends to affect people of ___________ and ___________ European Jewish or French-Canadian ancestry.
B. Caused by a faulty gene that targets the ___________.

C. Symptoms first appear at around ___________ months of age in an otherwise healthy baby.

18. Turner's Syndrome

A. Turner's syndrome is a congenital disorder caused by the failure of the ___________ to respond to the stimulation of ___________ hormones.

B. ___________ may be impaired.

C. The patient is usually ___________ in stature.

KEY TERMINOLOGY REVIEW

Match the selected key terms to their definitions below.

a. Active transport
b. Anatomy
c. Atom
d. Cell
e. Cell membrane
f. Chromosomes
g. Cilia
h. Congenital disorder
i. Cytokinesis
j. Cytoplasm
k. Deoxyribonuleic acid (DNA)
l. Diffusion
m. Electrolyte
n. Filtration
o. Flagella
p. Gametes
q. Genetics
r. Heredity
s. Homeostasis
t. Meiosis
u. Mitosis
v. Molecule
w. Negative feedback
x. Neurons
y. Nucleus
z. Organelles
aa. Organs
bb. Osmosis
cc. Passive transport
dd. Pathophysiology
ee. Physiology
ff. Positive feedback
gg. Ribonucleic acid (RNA)
hh. Striated muscle tissue
ii. Systems
jj. Tissue

1. ______________ Hairlike projections that cover the surface of some cells.
2. ______________ Requires mechanical pressure to diffuse dissolved particles through membranes.
3. ______________ Requires cellular energy to carry materials from an area of lesser concentration to an area of greater concentration.
4. ______________ The body and its systems work together to maintain a constant balance.
5. ______________ A jellylike substance found between the cell membrane and the nuclear membrane.
6. ______________ The body's reaction to either internal or external stimuli.
7. ______________ A form of diffusion whereby water is pulled through a semipermeable membrane.
8. ______________ The outer covering of the cell.

9. ______________ Tail-like structures that enable a sperm cell to move through the reproductive tract.

10. ______________ The study of diseases and disorders within the body.

11. ______________ This process forms gametes, such as ova and sperm.

12. ______________ Involves moving dissolved particles from an area of greater concentration to an area of lesser concentration until they are evenly distributed.

13. ______________ Encourages the stimuli to continue, or even accelerate, which also results in homeostasis.

14. ______________ Formed during the process of meiosis in which cells reduce their chromosomal number from 46 to 23.

15. ______________ A chemical combination of two or more atoms that forms a specific chemical compound.

16. ______________ Does not require the cell to use energy; however, it does involve a number of processes, including diffusion, osmosis, and filtration.

17. ______________ During this process, the cytoplasm divides into two identical daughter cells.

18. ______________ The study of the structure of an organism.

19. ______________ Nerve cells.

20. ______________ Voluntary muscle tissue.

21. ______________ Microscopic bodies that carry the genes that determine hereditary characteristics.

22. ______________ The genetic transmission from parent to child.

23. ______________ Formed by similarly functioning tissues.

24. ______________ Formed by a group of cells that have similar functions.

25. ______________ The most basic unit of life; often considered building blocks of the human body.

26. ______________ Responsible for the cell's metabolism, growth, and reproduction.

27. ______________ A single chain of chemical bases.

28. ______________ The study of the makeup of animals or plants.

29. ______________ Formed by organs that make up the human body.

30. ______________ Provides the cell's blueprint or genetic makeup.

31. ______________ Structures found within cytoplasm.

32. ______________ During this process, the nucleus of the cell divides.

33. ______________ The study of the function of an organism.

34. ______________ A genetic disorder that is present at birth.

35. ______________ A molecule that conducts electricity.

36. ______________ Consists of at least one proton.

APPLIED PRACTICE

1. Label the various cells found in this image.

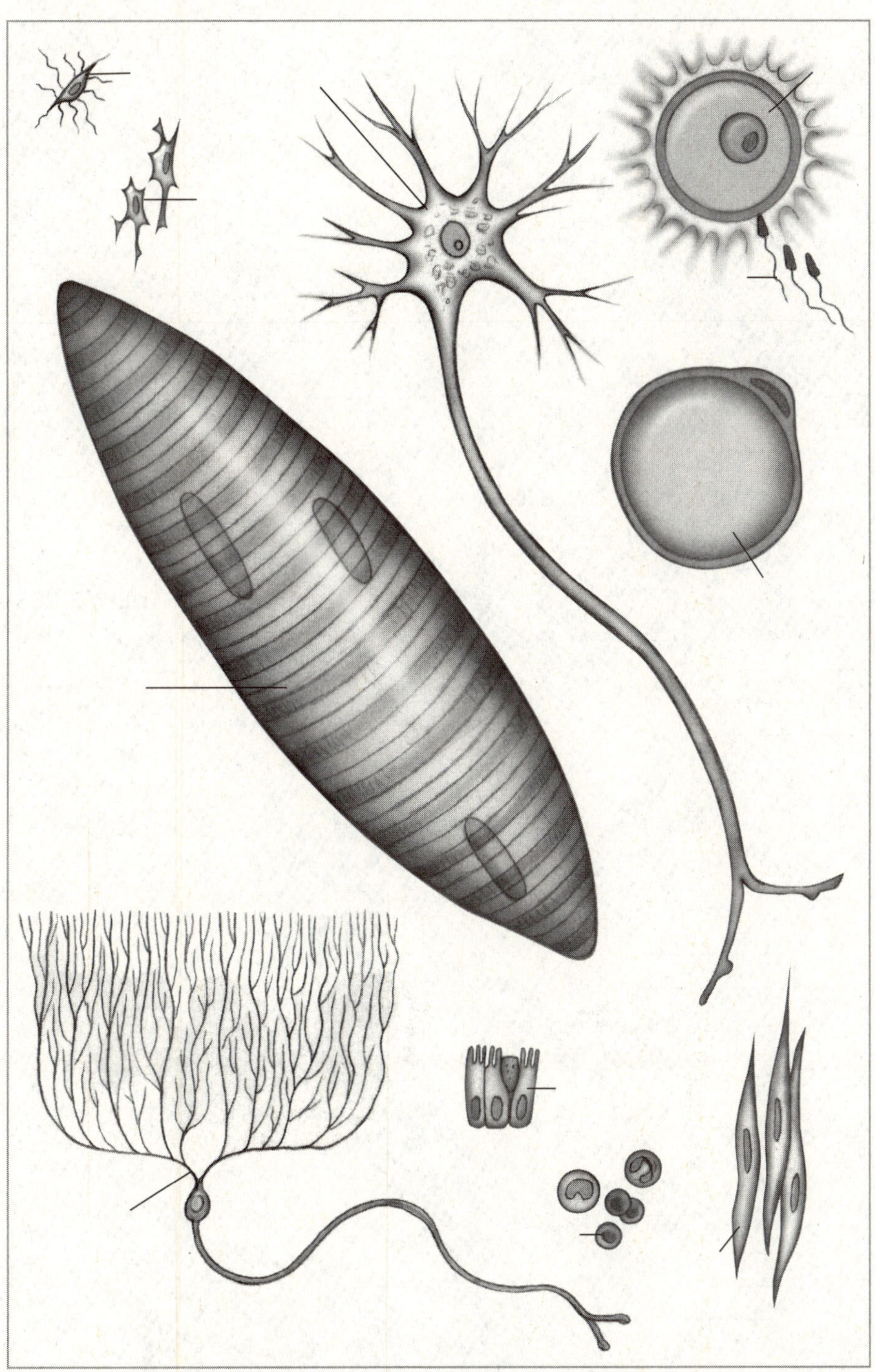

2. Label the types of tissue found in this image.

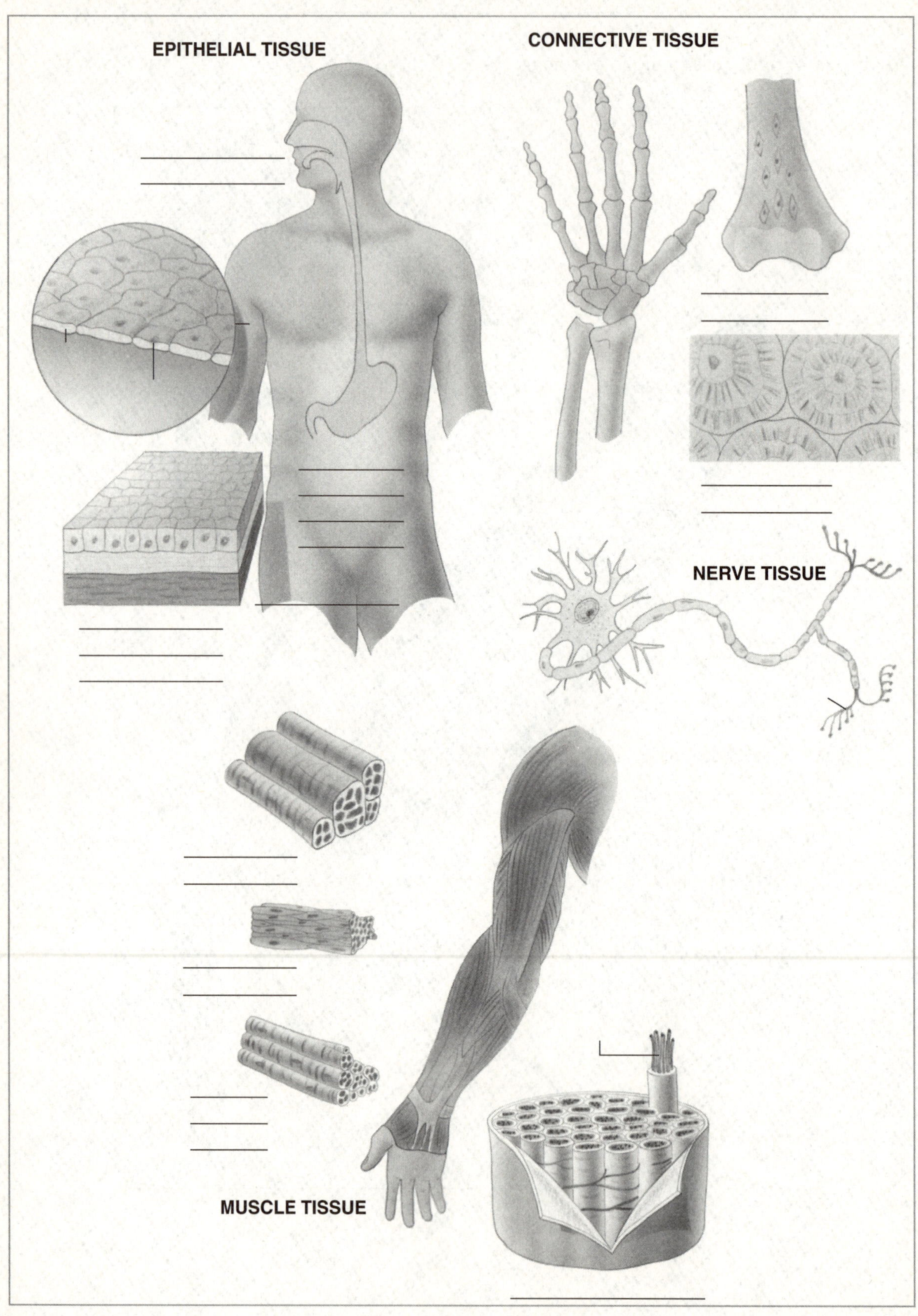

LEARNING ACTIVITY: TRUE/FALSE

Indicate whether the following statements are true or false by placing a T or an F on the line that precedes each statement.

_______ 1. Atoms are found at the most basic level of organization.

_______ 2. Molecules cannot move and thus take the form of solids, liquids, or gases.

_______ 3. DNA is shaped in a single helix.

_______ 4. The golgi apparatus is the location for the production of protein that is essential to the vitality of the cell.

_______ 5. Epithelial tissue is found on the outer layer of skin.

_______ 6. Involuntary or smooth muscle tissues are controlled by the autonomic nervous system.

_______ 7. In the phagocytosis method, the cell "drinks" the fluid required.

_______ 8. The muscular system transmits impulses, responds to change, is responsible for communication, and exercises control over all parts of the body.

_______ 9. Cells utilize electrolytes to maintain voltage or electrical force across their cell membranes.

_______ 10. Genetic disorders are considered medical conditions.

CRITICAL THINKING

Answer the following questions to the best of your ability. Utilize the textbook as a reference.

1. Why is it important for a medical assistant to understand the structures and functions of the human body?

____

____

____

____

____

2. When documenting a patient's treatment, why should documentation always take place after the procedure has been performed?

____

____

____

____

____

RESEARCH ACTIVITY

Utilize Internet search engines to research the following topics and write a brief description of you find. It is important to utilize reputable websites.

1. Using the Internet as a research source, conduct further research on genetic engineering. Discover more about this fascinating topic and write a brief essay to explain what you learned through your research. Be sure to cite your sources.

CHAPTER 22

The Integumentary System

CHAPTER OUTLINE

General review of the chapter:

Functions of the Integumentary System
Structure of the Skin
Accessory Structures of the Skin
Common Disorders of the Integumentary System
Skin Care Treatments

STUDENT STUDY GUIDE

Use the following guide to assist in your learning of the concepts from the chapter.

I. The Integumentary System

1. The Skin and the Accessory Organs, Known as the Integumentary System

   A. Weighs more than _______ (in adults).
   B. Covers _______ of the body.
   C. Its purpose is as follows:
      i. ______________________________
      ii. ______________________________
      iii. ______________________________
      iv. ______________________________
      v. ______________________________

2. The Functions of the Integumentary System

   i. ______________________________
   ii. ______________________________
   iii. ______________________________
   iv. ______________________________
   v. ______________________________

3. Temperature Regulation

   A. Aids in the ____________ of body temperature.
   B. To ____________ heat, superficial blood vessels in skin ____________, bringing more blood to the surface of the skin.
   C. To ____________ heat, superficial blood vessels ____________, keeping warm blood away from the surface.
   D. A continuous layer of ____________ fat acts as insulation.

4. Sensory Receptors

   A. Detect temperature, pain, ________, and ________.
   B. They are located in the ________.
   C. Nerve endings in the ________ layer of skin convey ________ to the brain and spinal cord.

5. The Three Layers of Skin
   A. The epidermis is the ________, ________ membrane layer.
   B. The dermis ("true skin") is the ________, ________ connective tissue layer.
   C. The subcutaneous tissue is the ________ layer.

6. The Layers of the Epidermis: Stratum corneum
   A. The stratum corneum is the ________ layer of skin that consists of dead cells filled with a protein called ________.
   B. Forms a protective ________ for the body.
   C. The ________ of the layer depends on the part of the body.

7. The Layers of the Epidermis: Stratum lucidum
   A. The stratum lucidum is the ________ layer lying directly beneath the ________ ________.
   B. In thinner skin, it is often ________.
   C. Cells in this layer are either ________ or ________.

8. The Layers of the Epidermis: Stratum granulosum
   A. The stratum granulosum consists of several layers of ________ cells that become part of the ________ lucidum and stratum ________.
   B. Cells actively become ________, or hardened, after they lose their ________.

9. The Layers of the Epidermis: Stratum germinativum
   A. Made of several layers of living cells that are still capable of ________, or cell division.
   B. Most responsible for the ________ of the epidermis.

10. The Dermis
   A. The ________ layer of the skin.
   B. Composed of ________ tissue containing nerves and nerve endings, blood vessels, sebaceous and ________ glands, hair follicles, and ________ vessels.
   C. Further divided into two layers: the ________ layer and the ________ layer.

11. The Subcutaneous Layer
   A. Composed of ________ tissue.
   B. Tissue helps support, nourish, insulate, and ________ the skin.

12. Accessory Organs: Hair
   A. Hair fibers are composed of the ________ keratin.
   B. ________ gives hair its color.
   C. Sebaceous glands release ________ into hair follicles.

13. Accessory Organs: Nails
   A. The nails are flat ________ of keratin.
   B. Connected to tissue by the ________ ________.
   C. Grow longer from the ________.
   D. Covered and protected by ________.
   E. The light-colored, half-moon area at the base is the ________.

14. Accessory Organs: Fluid-Producing Glands
   A. Sweat glands assist the body in maintaining its ________ temperature.
   B. Sweat glands create a ________ effect when ________ evaporates.
   C. Sebaceous glands are ________ glands.

15. Summary of the Integument: Label the structure of the integument.

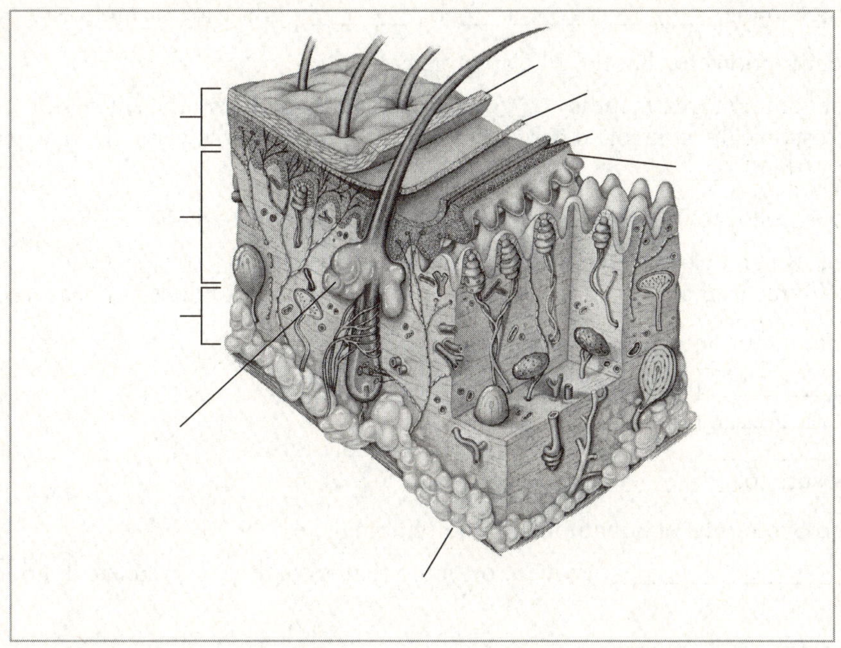

II. Pathology of the Integumentary System

1. Facts About Skin Cancer

   A. Skin cancer is the most ________ of all cancers.
   B. Affects more than ________ people each year in the United States.

2. How Skin Cancer Occurs

   A. Occur when normal skin cells undergo a change during which they ________ and ________ without the normal controls.
   B. As the cells multiply, they form a mass called a ________.
   C. Tumors of the skin are often referred to as ________.
   D. Malignant tumors encroach on neighboring tissues, especially ________, because of their uncontrolled growth.

3. Basal Cell Carcinoma

   A. Basal cell carcinoma is the most ________ form of skin cancer.
   B. Most often caused by ________ to the sun.
   C. May often appear as a change in the skin, such as a ________, an irritation or ________ that does not heal, or a change in a ________ or mole.
   D. Although the ________ is the most common site, it may affect the head, neck, back, chest, or shoulders.
   E. Exposure to ________ is the most common cause of this type of cancer.

4. Signs and Symptoms of Basal Cell Carcinoma

   A. Firm, ________ ________, including tiny blood vessels with a spiderlike appearance (telangiectasias).
   B. Red, tender, ________ ________ that bleeds easily.
   C. Small, fleshy bump with a smooth, pearly appearance, often with a __________ center.
   D. Smooth, shiny bump that may look like a ________ or ________.
   E. ________ patch of skin, especially on the face, that is firm to the touch.

F. Bump that itches, bleeds, ________ ________, and then repeats the cycle, and has not healed in ________ ________.
G. Change in the ________, ________, or ________ of a wart or mole.

5. Treatment Options for Basal Cell Carcinoma
   A. Most common treatment is ________ to destroy or remove the entire skin growth.
   B. Microscopically controlled surgery to remove skin cancer is very effective, with cure rates of higher than ________.

6. Squamous Cell Carcinoma: Indicators
   A. Changes in an existing wart, mole, or other ________ ________.
   B. Development of a ________ ________ that ulcerates and does not heal well.

7. Risks Factors for Squamous Cell Carcinoma
   A. ____________ predisposition.
   B. ____________ pollution.
   C. ____________ to X-rays or other forms of radiation.
   D. Exposure to ____________.

8. Signs and Symptoms of Squamous Cell Carcinoma
   A. A ________ ________, growth, or bump that is small, firm, reddened, nodular, coned, or flat.
   B. A ________ or ________ lesion or growth that is located on the face, ears, neck, hands, or arms.
   C. Occasionally, the growth may occur on the ________, ________, ________, or ________.

9. Treatment Options for Squamous Cell Carcinoma
   A. Surgical removal of the tumor, which may include ________ of the ________ around the tumor.
   B. ________ ________ (Mohs' micrographic surgery) may remove small tumors.
   C. ________ ________ may be needed if broad areas of skin are removed.
   D. ________ treatment.

10. Malignant Melanoma
    A. Originates in the ________ of the skin.
    B. Develops when the cells do not respond to the normal control mechanisms of ________ growth.
    C. The primary tumor begins in the ________.

11. Signs and Symptoms of Malignant Melanoma (List the signs and symptoms.)
    i. ____
    ii. ____
    iii. ____
    iv. ____
    v. ____
    vi. ____
    vii. ____

12. Acne Vulgaris
    A. Occurs when oil and ________ ________ cells clog the skin's pores.
    B. Most often affects ________, with more than 85% of them developing at least a mild form of this condition.
    C. While mild acne is merely annoying, severe acne can lead to ________ and ________ scars.
    D. Most people outgrow acne by the time they are in their ______ and ______.

13. Signs and Symptoms of Acne Vulgaris

    A. Skin blemishes are often ________ and ________.
    B. With a mild case of acne, only __________ and __________ may be present.
    C. Severe acne can mean hundreds of ________ or ________ that can cover the face, neck, chest, and back.
    D. ________ ________ are pimples that are large and deep. These lesions are often painful and can leave scars on the skin.

14. Treatment Options for Acne Vulgaris

    A. The ________ of the acne will determine the most useful and beneficial treatment.
    B. Sometimes treatments will be combined to get the best results and to avoid the development of ________ bacteria.

15. Alopecia

    A. The condition of ________ or ________ of hair.
    B. The most common form is ________ ________, also known as androgenic alopecia.

16. Alopecia Areata

    A. Affects about ________ in ________ people, mostly teenagers and young adults.
    B. Causes patches of baldness that are about the size of a ________ ________, usually appearing on the ________ but can occur anywhere on the body, including the beard, eyebrows, and eyelashes.

17. Male-Pattern Baldness

    A. Tends to follow a ________.
    B. The first stage is usually the ________ of the ________.
    C. The second stage is thinning of the hair on the ________ and ________.
    D. When these two areas meet in the middle, the hair around the back and sides of the head resembles a ________.
    E. Eventually the person may become ________ ________.

18. Treatments for Addressing Baldness

    A. There are drugs that treat both ________ and ________ baldness.
    B. ________ can be rubbed on the scalp.
    C. Shampoos and formulas are available for __________ __________ to the scalp.

19. Contact Dermatitis

    A. An ________ ________ of the skin caused by irritating substances.
    B. Causes include exposure to ________ ________, ________ ________, ________ (especially on jewelry or jeans snaps), lotions, detergents, or other chemicals.

20. Signs and Symptoms of Contact Dermatitis

    A. ________ and ________ skin.
    B. Vesicles (________________) and a rash may appear.
    C. ________ and ________ may be present.
    D. Serious allergic reactions may result in ________.

21. Treatment Options for Contact Dermatitis

    A. ____________ (anti-allergy medicines)
    B. ____________ ____________ creams to reduce inflammation
    C. ____________ ____________ (oral medications)

22. Calluses and Corns

    A. Excessive growth of the ________ ________ layer of the epidermis that often occurs on the hands and feet.
    B. Can be caused by ________ ________ ________ or by other factors such as ill-fitting shoes and unprotected hands during manual labor.

23. Signs and Symptoms of a Callus

A. An area of ________ ________ that does not have an identifiable border.
B. May appear ______________, ________, or even ________ while being painless, or may feel tender, throb, or burn.

24. Signs and Symptoms of a Corn

A. A corn has a ________ ________ with various textures; appears most often on the feet.
B. May be hard or soft; they are ________ ________.

25. Decubitus Ulcer

A. Also called a ________ ________ or a ________.
B. Refers to an area of skin and tissue that ________ ________.
C. Typically occurs when ________ ________ is maintained on a specific area of the skin.
D. The constant pressure on the area __________ the blood supply, causing the ________ of the affected tissue.
E. Common locations include the ________, ________, ________, ________, ________, and the back of the head.

26. The Four Stages of the Decubitus Ulcer

A. Stage I: ________ area on the skin that does not blanch (turn white) when pressed.
B. Stage II: The skin has a ________ or an ________ ________. The area around the site may be red and irritated.
C. Stage III: The skin looks like a ________ with damage to the tissue below the skin.
D. Stage IV: The wound becomes so deep that there is damage to the tissue beneath the ________ ________, including damage to ________ and muscle.

27. Eczema

A. Called ________ ________.
B. Chronic skin condition caused by an ________ ________ on the skin.
C. ________ tends to play a role.
D. Most common in infants; about half of the cases disappear by ________.
E. Signs and symptoms include ________, ________, and ________.
F. Lesions may appear dry or scaly, as well as have a ________ appearance.

28. Treatment Options for Eczema

A. Weeping lesions are treated with ________ ________ and dressings.
B. Severe cases and dry, scaly lesions may be treated with mild, _______ ________ or low-potency topical _______.
C. Very severe cases may require ________ _________ and ________ ________ (TIMs).
D. Sometimes, short exposures in a ________ ________ are useful to dry up the lesions.

29. Folliculitis

A. An infection or inflammation of the ________ ________.
B. Can occur anywhere that there is ________ ________.
C. Most often appears in areas that become irritated by shaving, the rubbing of clothes, or where follicles and pores are blocked by ________ and ________.
D. Common sites include the ________, the ________, ________, and on the legs.

30. Signs and Symptoms of Folliculitis

A. A ________ ________
B. Raised, red, often __________ lesions around hair follicles
C. ________ that occur in areas with a high concentration of hair follicles, such as the face, under the arms, on the scalp, and in the groin area, and eventually crust over
D. ________ at the site of the rash and pimples

31. Treatment Options for Folliculitis
    A. Generally involves taking steps to ________ ________ to the hair follicles by avoiding clothes that rub against the skin.
    B. Shaving with an ________ ________ instead of a razor blade.
    C. Keeping the skin clean using soap and water and ________ ________.
    D. Application of ________ ________.
32. Treatment Options for Shingles
    A. Early treatment can help shorten a shingles ________ and reduce the risk of complications.
    B. Oral antiviral medications are generally prescribed within _____ to _____ hours after the first sign of the rash.
    C. ________ are sometimes prescribed in order to reduce swelling and pain.
    D. When pain is severe, ________ ________ or a skin patch that contains a pain-relieving medication may be required.
33. Keloids
    A. Often referred to as ________ ________.
    B. Typically appear following ________ or an ________.
    C. ________ and ________ have been known to cause keloids.
34. Pediculosis
    A. An ________ by eggs, larvae, or adult lice.
    B. Forms of pediculosis include *Pediculus humanus capitis* (________ ________), *Pediculus humanus corporis* (________ ________), and *Pthirus pubis* (________ ________).
35. Signs and Symptoms of Pediculosis
    A. The most common symptom among all types of lice is ________.
    B. Head lice tend to cause itching on the back of the ________ or around the ________.
    C. Itching around the ________ is an indication of pubic lice.
    D. Body lice tend to travel to the body to feed on ________ and then return to ________.
36. Psoriasis
    A. Affects an estimated ________ Americans.
    B. Most commonly affects persons between ages _____ and _____.
    C. The condition has ________ and ________ characteristics.
    D. Thought to be caused by a buildup of ____________.
37. Signs and Symptoms of Psoriasis
    A. Episodes of redness, itching, and ________, ________ ________ on the skin.
    B. ________ can be gradual or abrupt.
    C. ____________ have been attributed to infection, obesity, and lack of sunlight, as well as sunburn, stress, poor health, and cold climate.
    D. When the case is severe and widespread, large quantities of ________ can be lost, causing ________ and severe secondary infections that can be serious.
38. Treatment Options for Psoriasis
    A. Analgesics, sedation, ________ ________, retinoids, and antibiotics.
    B. Mild cases are treated at home with topical medications such as prescription or nonprescription ________ ________, ________, or other corticosteroids, and antifungal medications.
    C. Severe lesions may require ________ for proper treatment.
39. Rosacea
    A. A disorder primarily of the ________ ________.
    B. Often characterized by ________ and ________.
    C. Affects an estimated ____________ Americans.

40. Signs and Symptoms of Rosacea
    A. ________ on the cheeks, nose, chin, or forehead.
    B. Small visible ________ ________ on the face, ________ on the face, and watery or irritated eyes.
    C. Over time, the ________ becomes ruddier and more persistent.
41. Scabies
    A. A ________ ________ disorder of the skin.
    B. Caused by the scabies mite or human ________ ________.
    C. Spread by ________ ________, such as shaking hands; sleeping together; or close contact with infected articles such as clothing, bedding, or towels.
    D. Common among schoolchildren, roommates, and sexual partners, scabies is usually found where people are ________ ________.
    E. The sides of the ________, the backs of the ________, wrists, heels, elbows, armpits, inner thighs, and the waistline are common locations for scabies.
42. Signs and Symptoms of Scabies
    A. A very small ________ blister
    B. Intense ________ and a red ________ that occurs around the area
43. Treatment Options for Scabies
    A. Application of a lotion or cream with a 6%–10% concentration of ________.
    B. ________ and ________ are often used to relieve itching.
44. Seborrheic Dermatitis
    A. An ___________ condition of the sebaceous or oil glands caused by an increase in sebum.
    B. Most common in infants and children; frequently known as _________.
45. Signs and Symptoms of Seborrheic Dermatitis
    A. Yellow or white scales that attach to the ________ ________.
    B. Thick or patchy crusts on the ________.
    C. Itching or soreness, as well as ________.
46. Treatment Options for Seborrheic Dermatitis
    A. Application of low-strength ________________.
    B. Shampooing the scalp daily with ________ ________.
47. *Tinea corporis*
    A. Sometimes called ________.
    B. Not actually a worm, but instead an integumentary disorder caused by a ________.
    C. Can appear ________ on the body.
    D. If the fungus is on the head, it is called ________ ________.
    E. On the feet, it is known as ________ ________, or athlete's foot.
    F. When found in the genital area, it is referred to as ________ ________.
    G. *Tinea cruris* is more commonly known as ________ ________.
    H. Elsewhere on the body, the fungus is called ________ ________.
48. Urticaria
    A. Better known as ________.
    B. Causes severe ________ because of an acute hypersensitivity to medications or environmental stimuli.
    C. A major concern is that it can obstruct the ________ ________.
    D. Because of the possibility of ________ ________, it is important to observe all patients after an injection or allergy test.
49. Signs and Symptoms of Urticaria
    A. ________ areas of pink, itchy, swollen patches of skin.
    B. ________ or ________ sensations are common.

C. Hives may vary in size from the diameter of a ________ ________ to the diameter of a cereal bowl.
D. Many times, the hives may ________, forming an even larger area of irritation and swelling.

50. Treatment Options for Urticaria
  A. Removal of ________ ________.
  B. Treatment with ___________ and ___________.

51. Vitiligo
  A. Also known as ________.
  B. A disorder that causes white patches and large areas of decreased ___________ to form on the skin.
  C. Patches form because of the destruction of ________, which are the cells that produce ________.
  D. Often linked to immune system disorders such as ________ ________ or pernicious anemia.
  E. Affects persons with ________ disorders.

52. Treatment Options for Vitiligo
  A. Often aimed at ________ skin tone and color.
  B. Accomplished through ________, ________, or ________ means.
  C. Avoiding tanning and using sunscreen help make the _____________ less noticeable.
  D. ________ and ________ lotions may also be used to even out the skin tone.
  E. Medical treatments may include the use of _____________________, as well as topical ultraviolet therapy.
  F. ________ ________, as well as a form of tattooing called ____________, may also be successful.

53. Warts (Verruca)
  A. An infection caused by viruses in the ________ ________ (HPV) family.
  B. There are at least _____ types of HPV viruses that cause warts.
  C. Warts can grow on all parts of the body, including the ________, the inside of the mouth, the genitals, and the ________ ________.
  D. A common wart is the ________ wart, which occurs on the soles of the feet.

54. Signs and Symptoms of Warts
  A. The ________ and ________ of a wart will vary with its location.
  B. Warts may appear ________ or ________, and may vary in color from flesh-toned to red, pink, or white.
  C. Warts may also appear as raised or ________ ________ ________.

55. Treatment Options for Warts
  A. Over-the-counter topical medications that contain ________ ________
  B. ________, which freezes the wart
  C. Various __________ __________
  D. In severe cases, _______ __________ may be an option.

III. Skin Care Treatments
  1. Botox
    A. Popular procedure that is indicated for reducing ________ ________.
    B. A very small, diluted amount of the toxin ________ ________ is injected into the wrinkle lines.
    C. The procedure is usually repeated every _____ to _____ months.
    D. Temporary side effects include headaches, bruising, and ________ ________.

2. Light Chemical Peel

   A. The purpose of this treatment is to reduce the size of ________, make the skin appear ________, and produce more ________ in the skin.
   B. During a light chemical peel, only the ________ layer of the skin is stripped.
   C. The procedure is completed in about an hour and it leaves the skin ____________, which disappears over time.

3. Medium Chemical Peel

   A. The purpose of this treatment is to ________ ________, resulting in a much smoother skin than that achieved with the light chemical peel.
   B. This treatment will strip the ________ ________ and some underlying cells, causing collagen and elastin to be stimulated.
   C. Recovery from a medium chemical peel can take up to _____ days because of the peeling, swelling, and redness that occur after treatment.

4. Deep Chemical Peel

   A. An aggressive treatment that can affect the layers of skin down to the ________ layer.
   B. Results are aimed at reducing all ________ in the face, with the exception of certain areas.
   C. This level of treatment can improve conditions such as ____________ ____________ and remove precancerous lesions.
   D. The healing process includes ________ ________, often felt up to 12 hours after surgery.
   E. ________ medications are required.
   F. It may take ________ for additional peeling, swelling, and redness to subside.

5. Laser Resurfacing

   A. Short, pulsated ________ ________ are used to vaporize damaged or troublesome areas of the skin.
   B. Full-face laser resurfacing takes approximately ______ hours.
   C. Partial-face resurfacing takes ______ minutes.
   D. Resurfacing results in the stimulation and production of new ________ and skin cells.
   E. Immediately following the procedure, ________ ________ and sterile ________ are applied to reduce the incidence of infection.

6. Microdermabrasion

   A. Involves removing the top layer of ________ ________ ________.
   B. ________ ________ are used with abrasion and suction devices to produce healthier-looking skin.
   C. This non- ________ and non- ________ approach is appealing to many patients who do not wish to pursue more aggressive skin-freshening treatments.

KEY TERMINOLOGY REVIEW

Match the vocabulary term to the correct definition below.

a. Acne vulgaris
b. Albinism
c. Alopecia
d. Bacteremia
e. Basal cell carcinoma
f. Callus
g. Carbuncle
h. Cellulitis
i. Contact dermatitis
j. Corn
k. Decubitus ulcer
l. Dermis
m. Dysplastic nevus
n. Eczema
o. Epidermis
p. Erythema

q. Folliculitis
r. Furuncle
s. Herpes simplex
t. Herpes zoster
u. Hirsutism
v. Impetigo
w. Keloid
x. Lunula
y. Malignant melanoma
z. Matrix
aa. Melanin
bb. Melanocytes
cc. Pediculosis
dd. Psoriasis
ee. Rosacea
ff. Scabies
gg. Sebaceous glands
hh. Seborrheic dermatitis
ii. Squamous cell carcinoma
jj. Sudoriferous glands
kk. Sweat glands
ll. *Tinea capitis*
mm. *Tinea corporis*
nn. *Tinea cruris*
oo. *Tinea pedis*
pp. Urticaria
qq. Vesicles
rr. Vitiligo
ss. Warts

1. ____________ An erosion or ulcer that is eating or gnawing away tissue.
2. ____________ An infection or inflammation of the hair follicles.
3. ____________ A condition that causes a burning or tingling sensation followed by the development of genital lesions.
4. ____________ An abnormal mole.
5. ____________ A common skin condition that occurs when oil and dead skin cells clog the skin's pores.
6. ____________ Produces sebum, which acts to protect the body from dehydration and the possible absorption of harmful substances.
7. ____________ A highly aggressive cancer that tends to spread to other parts of the body.
8. ____________ An inherited disorder that causes the absence of melanin in the skin, hair, and eyes.
9. ____________ A highly contagious disorder of the skin caused by the scabies mite or human itch mite.
10. ____________ Sometimes called ringworm.
11. ____________ The most common form of skin cancer; most often caused by overexposure to the sun.
12. ____________ Coiled, ball-shaped structures that are located in the dermis or subcutaneous layers.
13. ____________ A protective pigmentation that guards the body against the sun's ultraviolet rays.
14. ____________ Also known as the nail bed.
15. ____________ The middle layer of the skin; often referred to as the "true skin."
16. ____________ Excessive growth of the stratum corneum layer of the epidermis.
17. ____________ Bacteria arriving from a distant source via the bloodstream.
18. ____________ Cells that produce melanin, the pigment that gives the skin its color.
19. ____________ The crescent-shaped white area at the base of the nail.
20. ____________ A boil that is actually an abscess of a hair follicle and the adjacent subcutaneous tissues.
21. ____________ More commonly referred to as jock itch.
22. ____________ An inflammatory condition of sebaceous or oil glands caused by an increase in sebum.
23. ____________ An allergic reaction of the skin caused by irritating substances.

24. ____________ A chronic skin condition caused by an allergic reaction on the skin.

25. ____________ Also known as athlete's foot.

26. ____________ A skin infection caused by bacteria.

27. ____________ Small blisters associated with contact dermatitis.

28. ____________ The redness associated with cellulitis.

29. ____________ A fungus found on the head.

30. ____________ Also known as shingles.

31. ____________ A collection of furuncles.

32. ____________ Divided into four layers or strata.

33. ____________ Also known as hives.

34. ____________ Thought to be caused by a buildup of dead skin cells.

35. ____________ An area of thickened skin that does not have an identifiable border.

36. ____________ A malignant tumor that affects the middle layer of the skin.

37. ____________ Also known as leukoderma.

38. ____________ A type of infection caused by viruses in the human papillomavirus (HPV) family.

39. ____________ Often referred to as a hypertrophic scar.

40. ____________ A disorder primarily of the facial skin, often characterized by flare-ups and remissions.

41. ____________ Baldness or loss of hair.

42. ____________ Also known as sweat glands.

43. ____________ An infestation of lice in the form of eggs, larvae, or adult lice.

44. ____________ A condition of thick abnormal hair growth that affects men and women, although women are more commonly affected by and diagnosed with the disorder.

45. ____________ An acute spreading bacterial infection below the surface of the skin.

APPLIED PRACTICE

1. Using information found in the textbook, fill out the table below regarding infectious skin disorders.

Disorder	Symptoms	Diagnosis	Treatment
Furuncles/Carbuncles			

Herpes Simplex			
Herpes Zoster (Shingles)			

(*continue*)

Disorder	Symptoms	Diagnosis	Treatment
Impetigo			

2. Label the structure of the nail bed.

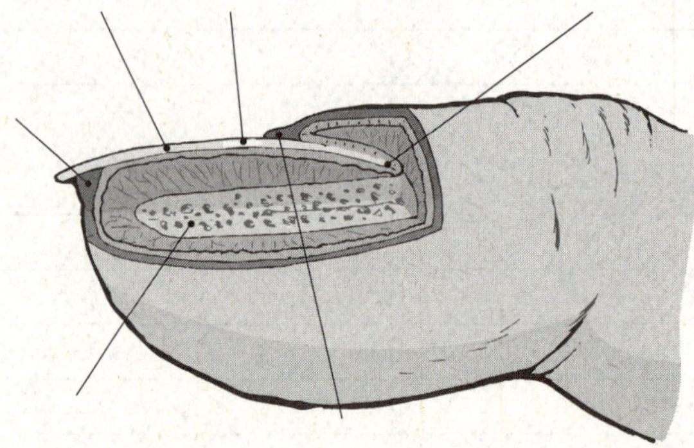

LEARNING ACTIVITY: FILL IN THE BLANK

Using words from the list below, fill in the blanks to complete the following statements

ABCD rule
appearance
blood and lymphatic
common
connective tissue
curable
cushions
dehydration
dermis
diagnosed early
fat cells
generalized illness
hair growth
heat and cold
inflammation and infection
insulation
irritations or lesions
microorganisms
nails
nerve
polycystic
Staphylococcus
subcutaneous
subcutaneous tissue
support
sweat and sebaceous
toxins
temperature
tumors
vitamin D

1. Skin cancers are initially diagnosed according to their _______________. Malignant melanoma is identified by the _______________.
2. The integumentary system includes the _______________, hair, and _______________ glands.
3. Skin cancers are the most _______________ type of cancer, as well as the most _______________ when _______________.
4. The skin serves as a barrier to prevent _______________ and other foreign bodies from entering; regulates _______________; protects against _______________; acts as an environmental sensor for pain, temperature, and touch; synthesizes _______________ from sunlight; and excretes _______________ in perspiration.
5. The dermis contains _______________ vessels, _______________ cell endings, and skin _______________ organs.
6. Hirsutism is a condition of excessive _______________, which may be caused by _______________ ovaries or _______________ of the adrenal glands and ovaries.
7. A break in the defense system of the skin may result in _______________, as well as localized _______________.
8. Cellulitis is a disease of the skin and subcutaneous tissue that presents as _______________. It is commonly caused by _______________.
9. Sweat glands are located in the _______________ and the _______________.
10. The innermost layer of skin, the _______________ tissue, is made up of _______________ and _______________. This layer acts as _______________ for the body, provides protection against extreme _______________ and against heat loss, and _______________ and protects underlying structures.

CRITICAL THINKING

Answer the following questions to the best of your ability. Utilize the textbook as a reference.

1. As you are assisting a geriatric patient get into a gown for an examination, you notice that she has a dime-sized mole with an irregular border on her back. You realize that the patient likely cannot see it and may be unaware of it. Would you mention it to the patient or only to the physician? State the reason for your answer.

____

____

____

____

____

2. Utilize Internet search engines to locate a reputable site that provides pictures of various skin conditions, including lice. Draw a picture of head lice and state how this condition is treated.

____

____

____

____

____

3. What possible advice could you give to a patient who has had a skin cancer removed today and works daily as a lifeguard in the sun?

____

____

4. A female patient comes in for an examination for excessive dark hair that she has developed in the last 6 months or so. She asks you what it is and what can be done for it, but she has not seen the physician yet. What would you say to this patient at this time? Hint: The answer is not specifically in the book and will require your current knowledge and critical thinking skills regarding the medical assistant's scope of practice.

5. Although not specifically stated in the text, what precautions would you recommend to a patient who has an infectious skin disorder to prevent it from spreading?

RESEARCH ACTIVITY

Utilize Internet search engines to research the following topics and write a brief description of what you find. It is important to utilize reputable websites.

1. Visit the Skin Cancer Foundation at www.skincancer.org. After reviewing the website, answer the following questions:
   a. What "Prevention" information do you find most interesting. Why?
   b. After reading "Skin Cancer Facts," which facts do you find most surprising?
   c. What can you do to further reduce your risk of developing skin cancer?

CHAPTER 23
The Skeletal System

CHAPTER OUTLINE

General review of the chapter:

Bones and Their Classification
Joints and Movement
The Axial Skeleton
The Appendicular Skeleton
Common Disorders Associated with the Skeletal System

STUDENT STUDY GUIDE

Use the following guide to assist in your learning of the concepts from the chapter.

I. The Skeletal System

1. Bone Classification

   i. ______________________________
   ii. ______________________________
   iii. ______________________________
   iv. ______________________________
   v. ______________________________
   vi. ______________________________
   vii. ______________________________

2. The Six Main Functions of Bones

   A. Provide __________, __________, and the framework of the body.
   B. Provide __________ for the body's internal organs.
   C. Serve as a storage place for __________, __________, and __________.
   D. Play an important role in the formation of blood cells as __________ takes place in the __________.
   E. Provide an area for the attachment of __________ muscle.
   F. Help to make movement possible through __________.

3. Bone Markings

   i. ______________________________
   ii. ______________________________
   iii. ______________________________
   iv. ______________________________
   v. ______________________________
   vi. ______________________________
   vii. ______________________________

4. Joints
   A. The positioning of the bones at the joint determines the __________ that the joint performs.
   B. Joints are always classified according to the __________ that they provide.

5. The Rib Cage
   A. Ribs form a protective cage that houses the __________, __________, and other vital components of the human body.
   B. Consists of __________ pairs of ribs.

II. The Pathology of the Skeletal System

1. Scoliosis
   A. Often diagnosed early in __________, __________ and __________.
   B. Persons who have scoliosis may often appear as if either their __________ or __________ are uneven.

2. Lordosis
   A. Lordosis is an __________ curvature of the __________ spine.
   B. When diagnosed in adults, may be commonly found in persons who are __________ and in __________ women.
   C. When diagnosed in children, the most common symptom is a prominently protruding __________ and __________.

3. Kyphosis
   A. Kyphosis is an exaggeration of the __________ curvature.
   B. The normal __________ curvature may become exaggerated because of a __________ defect.

4. Arthritis
   A. Causes include __________ injury, __________ disorders, and normal to __________ wear and tear on the joints.
   B. Can occur at any age; however, it most commonly develops in __________ adults.

5. Treatment for Arthritis
   A. Depends on the __________, __________, and __________ of the patient.
   B. Modification of daily activities and low-impact __________ exercise are helpful.

6. Osteoarthritis
   A. Most frequently occurs in the __________, __________, and finger joints of __________ patients.
   B. Obesity, a history of __________, and various genetic and __________ diseases increase the risk of osteoarthritis.

7. Carpal Tunnel Syndrome
   A. Caused when pressure is placed on the __________ __________.
   B. Certain conditions increase the risk of carpal tunnel syndrome, including __________, __________, and __________ arthritis.
   C. Treatment of carpal tunnel syndrome includes the use of proper __________ when engaging in computer use and other activities.

8. Treatment for Fractures
   A. Generally casted by a __________.
   B. At times, with severe fractures, __________ intervention must be performed.
   C. Pain and __________ medications are often prescribed for patient comfort.

9. Treatment for Dislocations

   A. Treat in an __________ department.
   B. Reduction is used to __________ and __________ the joint.
   C. Administer pain relievers and __________ medications.

10. Osteoporosis

   A. Affects more than __________ Americans, mostly women ages __________ to __________ years old.
   B. Persons with osteoporosis are subject to increased __________ potential, especially in the __________, __________, and __________.

11. Individuals at Higher Risk for Osteoporosis

   i. ____
   ii. ____
   iii. ____
   iv. ____
   v. ____
   vi. ____

12. Signs, Symptoms, and Treatment for Osteoporosis

   A. The most common sign is decreased __________ and a __________ posture.
   B. Additional signs and symptoms include __________ pain and frequent __________.
   C. Treatment includes __________ and __________ supplements.

13. Signs, Symptoms, and Treatment for Gout

   A. A __________ joint is often very warm and very sore to the touch.
   B. After joints have been persistently affected by gout, they may become __________.
   C. Treatment includes a diet rich in colorful __________ and __________.

14. Hallux Valgus

   A. The enlargement of the inner portion of the __________ joint at the base of the __________ toe.
   B. Signs and symptoms include __________ skin around the inflamed joint of the __________ toe.
   C. The joint may be filled with __________ and feel __________ to the touch.

15. Treatment for Hallux Valgus

   A. Properly __________ __________ should be worn.
   B. Proper __________ and __________ of the joint should be considered.
   C. __________ surgery and pain medications may be required for severe cases.

16. Hammer Toe

   A. Signs and symptoms include __________ and visible joint __________.
   B. Treatment includes wearing specially designed __________.

17. Rickets

   A. Results in bone __________, especially __________ legs.
   B. Signs and symptoms include __________ and __________ of the bones.
   C. Treatment includes increasing __________ and __________ intake.

18. Osteomalacia

   A. Caused by deficiencies in __________ and __________.
   B. Symptoms include __________ pain, __________ legs, and __________ fractures.
   C. Treatment is similar to the treatment for __________.

KEY TERMINOLOGY REVIEW

Match the selected key terms to their definitions below.

a. Abduction
b. Adduction
c. Amphiarthrotic joint
d. Appendicular skeleton
e. Arthritis
f. Articulation
g. Atlas
h. Axial skeleton
i. Axis
j. Bursa
k. Bursitis
l. Cancellous bone
m. Chondrocytes
n. Circumduction
o. Compact bone
p. Diaphysis
q. Diarthrotic joint
r. Dislocation
s. Dorsiflexion
t. Endosteum
u. Epiphysis
v. Etiology
w. Eversion
x. Extension
y. Flexion
z. Gout
aa. Hallux valgus
bb. Hammertoe
cc. Inversion
dd. Kyphosis
ee. Lordosis
ff. Medullary canal
gg. Orthopedic physician
hh. Osteoarthritis
ii. Osteomalacia
jj. Osteoporosis
kk. Periosteum
ll. Pronation
mm. Protraction
nn. Reduction
oo. Retraction
pp. Rheumatoid arthritis
qq. Rickets
rr. Rotation
ss. Scoliosis
tt. Supination
uu. Synarthrotic joint

1. ____________ The second cervical vertebra.
2. ____________ A disease caused by the formation and accumulation of urate crystals in the joints
3. ____________ A joint that permits very slight movement.
4. ____________ The process of straightening a flexed limb or the spine.
5. ____________ Inflammation of the bursa.
6. ____________ The toe bends upward like a claw because of the abnormal flexion of the proximal interphalangeal joint.
7. ____________ Occurs when a bone slips out of a joint.
8. ____________ The process of moving a body part forward.
9. ____________ The first cervical vertebra.
10. ____________ The cause or source of the patient's disease or disorder.
11. ____________ The most common type of arthritis, resulting from years of wear and tear on joints.
12. ____________ The dense, hard layer of bone tissue.

13. ____________ Often called swayback.

14. ____________ The process of bending (or curving) a flexed limb or the spine.

15. ____________ The process of moving a body part *away* from the midline.

16. ____________ The reticular tissue that makes up most of the volume of bone.

17. ____________ The adult onset of rickets.

18. ____________ The process of bending a body part backward.

19. ____________ The procedure used to align and reposition a joint.

20. ____________ Also called a bunion.

21. ____________ Inflammation of one or more joints.

22. ____________ The process of lying prone, or face down.

23. ____________ An early childhood disease caused by a deficiency in calcium, vitamin D, and phosphate.

24. ____________ The ends of a developing bone.

25. ____________ Characterized by a progressive loss of bone density and the thinning of bone tissue.

26. ____________ The process of moving a body part in a circular motion.

27. ____________ An abnormal lateral curvature of the spine.

28. ____________ The process of turning outward.

29. ____________ A joint that produces no movement.

30. ____________ A joint located at the place where two bones connect.

31. ____________ A physician who treats musculoskeletal conditions.

32. ____________ An autoimmune disorder causing joints to become deformed because of inflammation.

33. ____________ The shaft of the long bone.

34. ____________ Most often known as humpback.

35. ____________ The process of lying supine, or face upward.

36. ____________ The process of moving a body part around a central axis.

37. ____________ A small sac of fluid that cushions and lubricates an area where joint-related tissues rub against one another.

38. ____________ The membrane that forms the covering of bones, except at their articular surfaces.

39. ____________ The process of moving a body part *toward* the midline.

40. ____________ The central portion of the skeleton.

41. ____________ The tough, connective tissue membrane lining the medullary canal that contains the bone marrow.

42. ____________ The process of turning inward.

43. ____________ The process of moving a body part backward.

44. ____________ A joint that allows for free movement in a variety of directions.

45. ____________ The narrow space or cavity throughout the length of the diaphysis.

46. ____________ Consists of 126 bones.

47. ____________ Cartilage-forming cells.

APPLIED PRACTICE

1. Label the bones found on the images of the anterior and posterior views of the skeletal system.

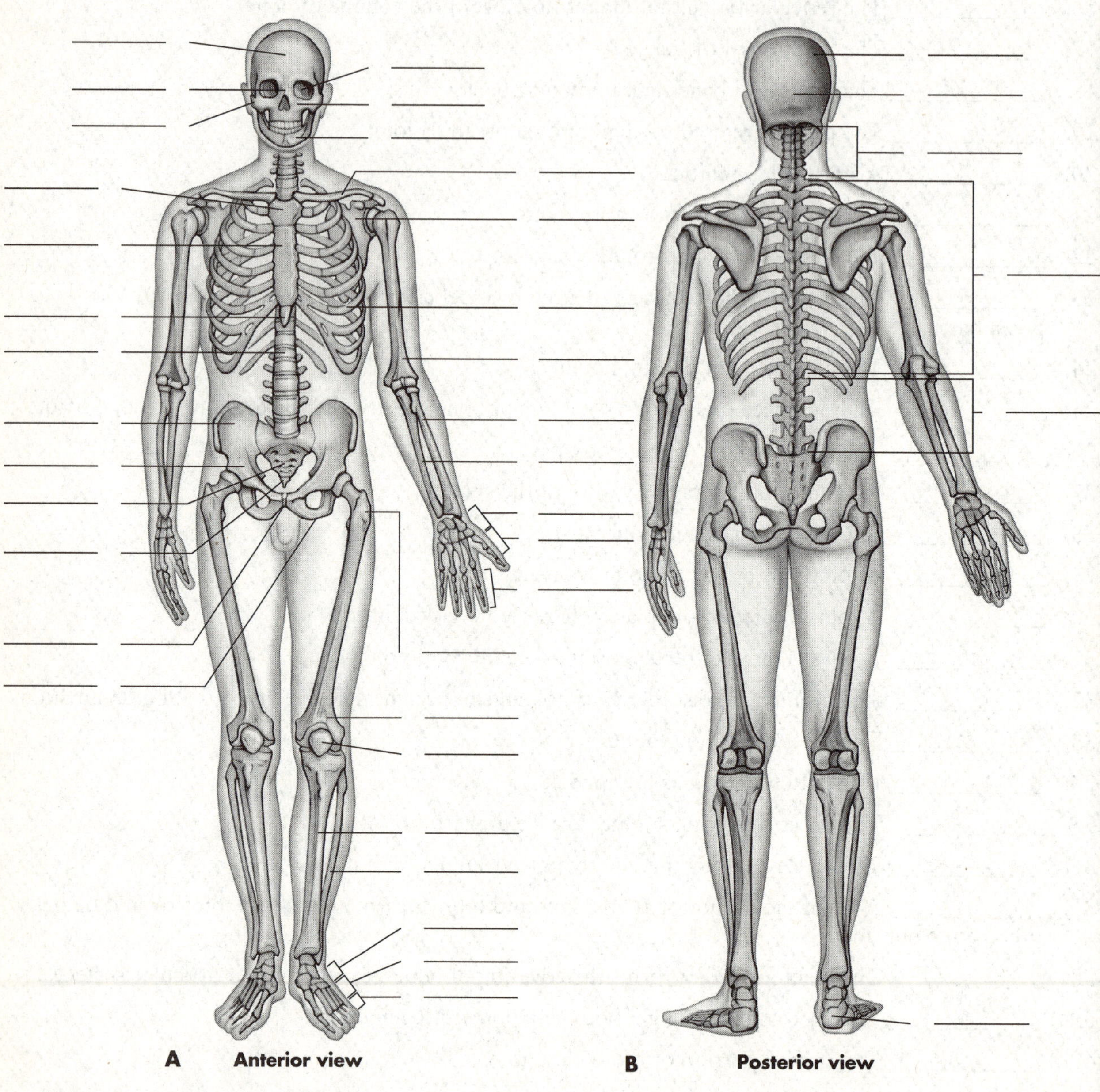

2. Label the types of fractures found in this image.

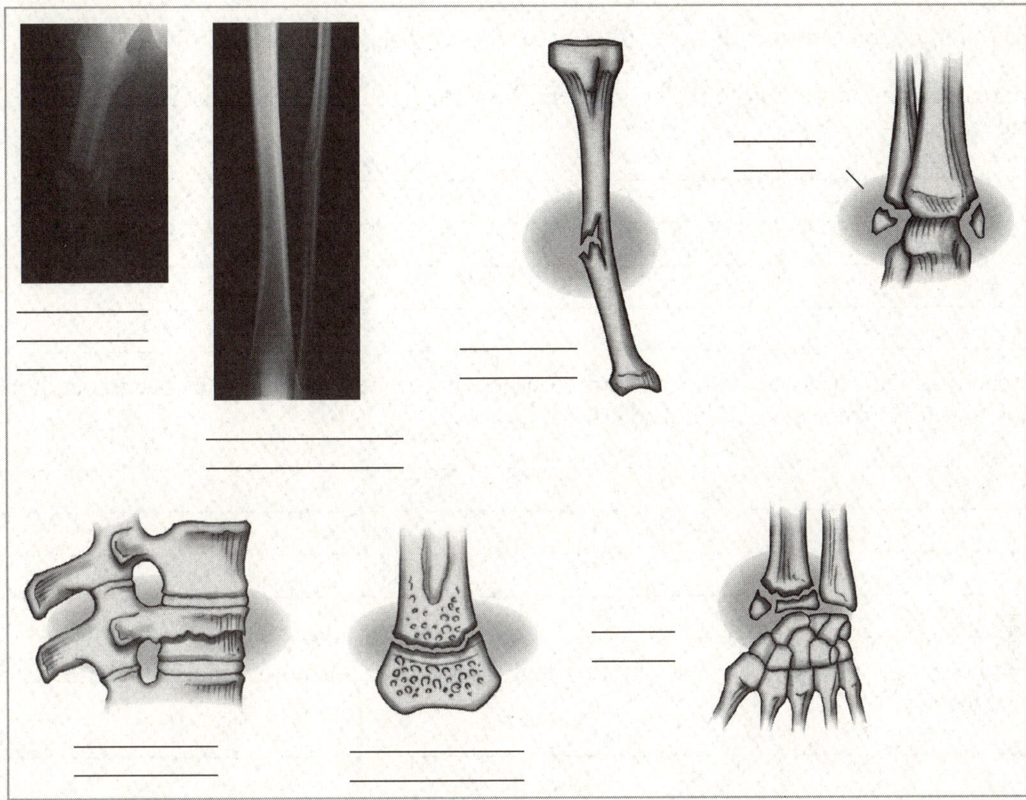

LEARNING ACTIVITY: TRUE/FALSE

Indicate whether the following statements are true or false by placing a T or an F on the line that precedes each statement.

_______ 1. The bones of the human skeleton have seven main functions.

_______ 2. Women build bone until about age 30 and then begin to lose about 1% of their bone mass annually.

_______ 3. Babies are born with more cartilage and bones than adults.

_______ 4. Older adult bones heal faster than in children.

_______ 5. The axial skeleton consists of both the upper and lower extremities, as well as the clavicles and the scapula, which form the pectoral girdle.

_______ 6. Many times, a scoliatic spine appears to have an S or C shape.

_______ 7. The most telling symptom of kyphosis is the rounded back.

_______ 8. Arthritis can occur at any age; however, it most commonly develops in young adults.

_______ 9. Colles's fractures occur in the ankle and affect both bones of the lower leg (the tibia and the fibula).

_______ 10. In a compound fracture, bone is shattered into a multitude of bony fragments.

CRITICAL THINKING

Answer the following questions to the best of your ability. Utilize the textbook as a reference.

1. If a patient has an injury to the skeletal system, how might the medical assistant be able to assist the patient?

2. How can the medical assistant stay current with new information that may be occurring in medicine? Why is staying current in one's field so critical?

3. When obtaining a medical history from a patient, why is it important to check the patient's past medical history?

RESEARCH ACTIVITY

Utilize Internet search engines to research the following topics and write a brief description of what you find. It is important to utilize reputable websites.

1. Using the Internet as a research source, conduct further research on two conditions/diseases of the skeletal system. These conditions can be ones that are found in the textbook or others that you may be interested in learning more about. Conduct your research with the idea of learning more about the conditions/diseases than what is found in the textbook. Write an essay on what you learned, including how the disease presents itself, the possible cause of the condition, the treatment, and any new technology that may be available in the future to address the condition/disease. Be sure to cite your resources.

Chapter 24

The Muscular System

CHAPTER OUTLINE

General review of the chapter:

Functions of Muscle
Types of Muscle Tissue
Energy Production for Muscle
Structure of Skeletal Muscles
Major Skeletal Muscles
Common Disorders Associated with the Muscular System

STUDENT STUDY GUIDE

Use the following guide to assist in your learning of the concepts from the chapter.

I. The Muscular System

1. Muscle Characteristics

   A. Contains bundles of parallel muscle tissue ________.
   B. Muscles ________ when a message is sent from the ________ via nerves.
   C. The human body has more than ________ muscles.
   D. Muscles make up more than ________ of body weight.

2. The Functions of the Muscular System

   i. ______________________________
   ii. ______________________________
   iii. ______________________________
   iv. ______________________________

3. Skeletal Muscles

   A. Attached to __________ bones.
   B. Wrapped in layers of __________ tissue.
   C. Stimulated by _________ neurons.

4. Smooth Muscles

   A. Found in tissue in the walls of __________ organs.
   B. Responsible for the movement of __________ organs.

5. Adenosine Triphosphate (ATP)

   A. The type of chemical energy needed for __________ or repeated muscular __________.
   B. Can be produced by either __________ or __________ means.

6. The Effects of Oxygen Debt
   A. Occurs when skeletal muscles are used for more than _________ or _________ minutes.
   B. Lack of oxygen intake reduces the body's ability to produce energy _________, causing _________ production.
   C. The body can only utilize this energy for about _________ seconds, depending on the individual, before severe fatigue sets in, making it very difficult to recover.
   D. Oxygen "owed" to body is the debt and can only be recovered by _________ respiration, which allows more oxygen into the _________ to reach the _________.

II. The Pathology of the Muscular System

1. Atrophy
   A. Lipoatrophy is atrophy of the _________ _________.
   B. The signs and symptoms of atrophy include the apparent _________ of a muscle group and extreme _________ and _________ associated with atrophic muscle groups.
   C. Treatment includes _________ exercises of the immobilized muscle.

2. Fibromyalgia
   A. More common in _________ than _________.
   B. The signs and symptoms include mild to severe _________ pain and _________.
   C. _________ _________ syndrome is a common symptom.

3. Criteria for Determining Fibromyalgia
   A. The American College of _________ identified specific criteria.
   B. Must show _________ to _________ trigger or tender points to be considered for this diagnosis, as well as a history of widespread pain lasting at least _________ months.

4. Treatment for Fibromyalgia
   A. Geared toward improving the quality of _________ and reducing _________.
   B. Common medications used in treatment include the following:
      i. ______________________________
      ii. ______________________________
      iii. ______________________________
      iv. ______________________________
      v. ______________________________

5. Ganglion Cyst
   A. More common in _________ than _________.
   B. The signs and symptoms include masses occurring typically on the _________, _________, and _________.
   C. _________ swelling can occur.

6. Treatment for a Ganglion Cyst
   i. ______________________________
   ii. ______________________________
   iii. ______________________________

7. Lyme Disease
   A. Carried by _________ and transmitted through a bite of an infected _________.
   B. The signs and symptoms include the following:
      i. ______________________________
      ii. ______________________________
      iii. ______________________________
      iv. ______________________________

8. The Prevention of and Treatment for Lyme Disease
   A. Prevention includes the following:
      i. ______________________________
      ii. ______________________________
      iii. ______________________________
   B. Treatment includes the use of _________, _________, or _________.

9. Muscular Dystrophy
   A. There are _____ major forms of muscular dystrophy.
   B. The signs and symptoms include _________, _________, and _________.

10. Treatment for Muscular Dystrophy
   A. _________ _________ to prevent contraction
   B. _________ for support
   C. Corrective _________ surgery
   D. The Emery-Dreifuss and myotonic forms may necessitate a _________ because of the cardiac problems associated with these forms

11. Rotator Cuff Tears
   A. Common in _________ muscles/tendons.
   B. Caused by many years of _________ of these muscles/tendons.
   C. Also caused by one single _________ injury.

12. Treatment for Rotator Cuff Tears
   i. ______________________________
   ii. ______________________________
   iii. ______________________________
   iv. ______________________________
   v. ______________________________
   vi. ______________________________

13. Shin Splints
   A. Usually caused by _________ or _________ conditioning of the leg muscles.
   B. Found in persons with _________ feet or _________ arches.
   C. The signs and symptoms include the following:
      i. ______________________________
      ii. ______________________________
      iii. ______________________________

14. Treatment for Shin Splints
   i. ______________________________
   ii. ______________________________
   iii. ______________________________
   iv. ______________________________

15. Sprains
   A. Very common in _________.
   B. Often occurs in the _________ of major joints.
   C. The signs and symptoms include the following:
      i. ______________________________
      ii. ______________________________
      iii. ______________________________
      iv. ______________________________

16. Strains
    A. A chronic strain occurs from _________ and _________ movement.
    B. An acute strain can occur from _________ lifting of a heavy object.
    C. The signs and symptoms include the following:
        i. ______________________________
        ii. ______________________________
        iii. ______________________________
        iv. ______________________________
        v. ______________________________
        vi. ______________________________
        vii. ______________________________
17. The Signs, Symptoms, and Treatment for Tendonitis
    A. The signs and symptoms include pain and _________ in the affected area.
    B. Treatment involves physical therapy, including _________ to increase range of motion.
18. Tetanus
    A. Tetanus is an often fatal, _________ disease.
    B. Caused by _________ bacterium.
    C. The signs and symptoms include the following:
        i. ______________________________
        ii. ______________________________
        iii. ______________________________
        iv. ______________________________
        v. ______________________________

KEY TERMINOLOGY REVIEW

Match the selected key terms to their definitions below.

a. Antagonist
b. Aponeurosis
c. Aspiration
d. Atrophy
e. Cardiac muscle
f. Contracture
g. Endomysium
h. Epimysium
i. Fascia
j. Fascicles
k. Fibromyalgia
l. Ganglion cyst
m. Insertion
n. Ligament
o. Lyme disease
p. Muscular dystrophy
q. Myasthenia gravis
r. Origin
s. Orthoses
t. Oxygen debt
u. Perimysium
v. Prime mover (agonist)
w. Skeletal muscle
x. Smooth muscle
y. Sprain
z. Strain
aa. Striated
bb. Synergist
cc. Tendon
dd. Tendonitis
ee. Tetanus
ff. Tonicity

1. ____________ A muscle that counteracts, or opposes, the action of another muscle.

2. ____________ A condition in which shortened muscles around joints cause abnormal and sometimes painful positioning of the joints.

3. ____________ Connective tissue that connects bones or connects cartilage to a joint.

4. ____________ The amount of oxygen "owed" to the body that is needed to recover.

5. ____________ A chronic autoimmune neuromuscular disease characterized by varying degrees of weakness of the skeletal or voluntary muscles of the body.

6. ____________ A benign saclike swelling or cyst.

7. ____________ Inflammation of the tendon.

8. ____________ One of a group of genetic diseases characterized by progressive weakness and degeneration of the skeletal or voluntary muscles that control movement.

9. ____________ Consists of a group of fibers held together by connective tissue.

10. ____________ A fibrous sheath that holds connective tissue together.

11. ____________ A wide, thin, sheetlike tendon made up of fibrous connective tissue that typically attaches muscles to other muscles.

12. ____________ Orthopedic appliances used for support.

13. ____________ An injury to either a muscle or a tendon.

14. ____________ The body's ability to maintain posture through a continual partial contraction of skeletal muscles.

15. ____________ The band of connective tissue found at each end of a muscle that attaches the muscle to a bone.

16. ____________ The sections of a muscle.

17. ____________ An injury to a ligament.

18. ____________ Responsible for dividing a muscle into sections.

19. ____________ The loss of muscle mass and strength that occurs with the disuse of muscles over a long period of time.

20. ____________ A disorder in which musculoskeletal pain and fatigue are present.

21. ____________ Caused by the *Borrelia burgdorferi* bacterium.

22. ____________ The covering of connective tissue that surrounds the individual muscle cell.

23. ____________ Composed of elongated, spindle-shaped cells.

24. ____________ The attachment to the bone that is more fixed or still.

25. ____________ A muscle that acts with another muscle, most often a prime mover, to produce movement.

26. ____________ Thin fascia that covers muscles.

27. ____________ Removal of fluid by suction.

28. ____________ The attachment point on the bone that moves.

29. ____________ Striped in appearance.

30. ____________ A muscle that is the primary actor in a given movement.

31. ____________ Has a single central nucleus and is found in the heart.

32. ____________ An often fatal, infectious disease caused by the bacterium *Clostridium tetani*.

APPLIED PRACTICE

1. Label the muscles found on the images of the anterior and posterior views of the muscular system.

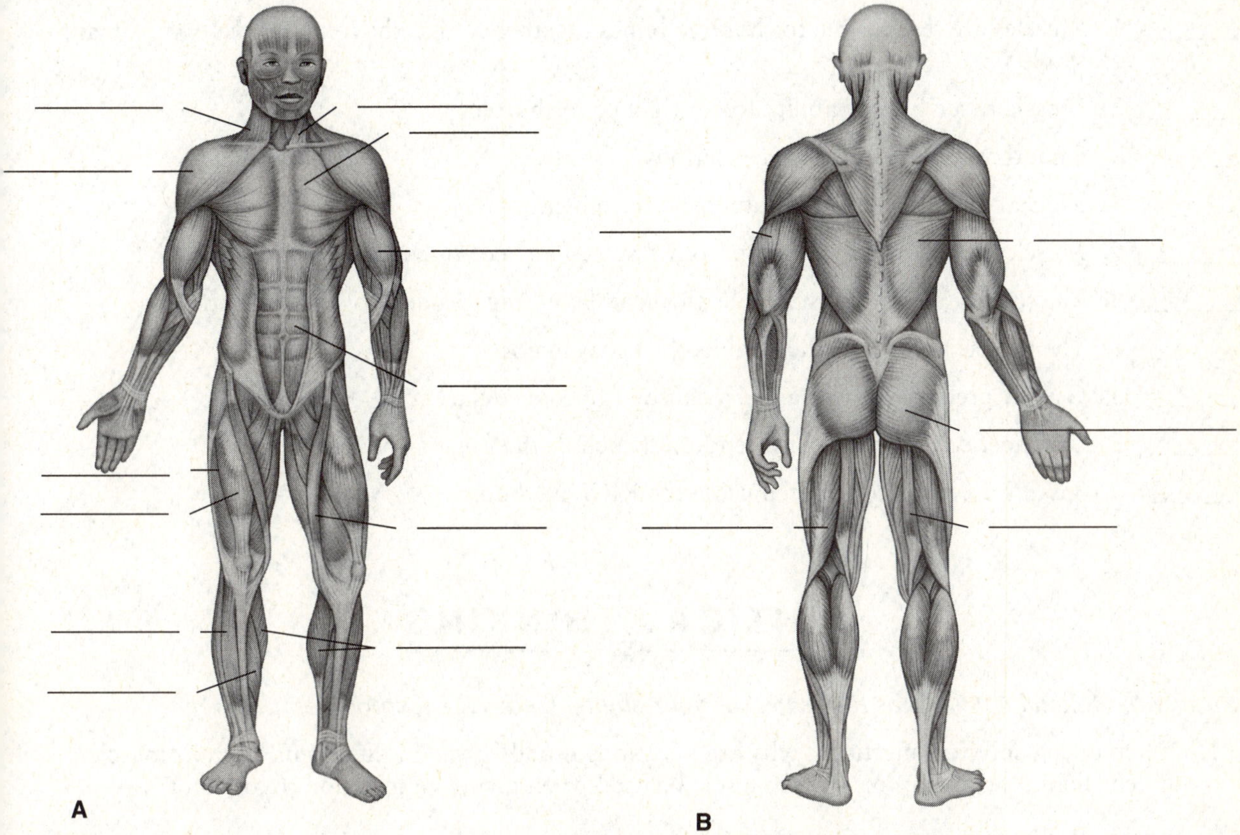

A

B

2. Label the muscles of the head, neck, and face found in this image.

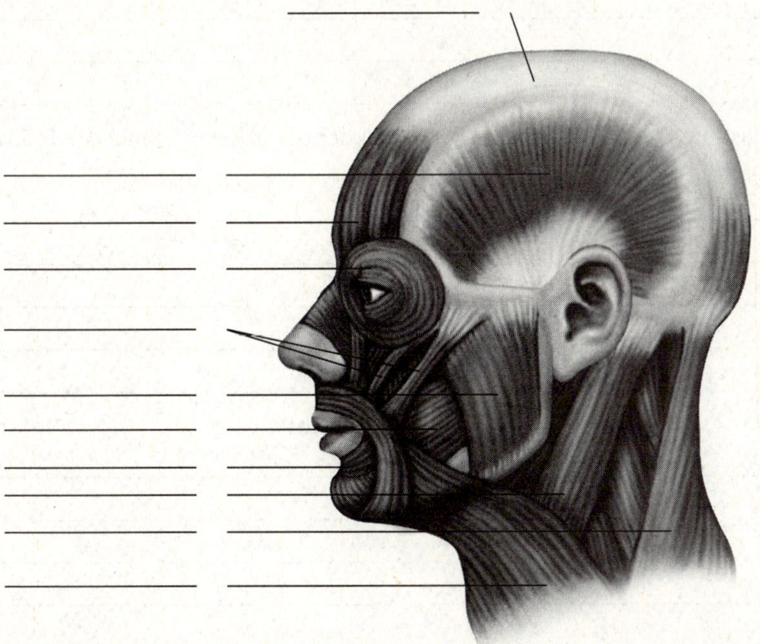

LEARNING ACTIVITY: TRUE/FALSE

Indicate whether the following statements are true or false by placing a T or an F on the line that precedes each statement.

_______ 1. Muscles are responsible for holding bones together so that the joints of the body remain stable.

_______ 2. Muscle tissue has the ability to contract or to shorten.

_______ 3. Smooth muscle cells contain striations.

_______ 4. Skeletal muscle controls involuntary movement.

_______ 5. Muscle fatigue usually develops as a result of an accumulation of lactic acid.

_______ 6. The splenius capitis muscle pulls the head from side to side and to the chest.

_______ 7. The muscle that flexes the thigh is the psoas major.

_______ 8. Genetic predisposition may be a cause of fibromyalgia.

_______ 9. The most common areas for tendonitis include the fingers and toes.

_______ 10. Sprains are generally treated using the RICE method.

CRITICAL THINKING

Answer the following questions to the best of your ability. Utilize the textbook as a reference.

1. When giving children injections, why are injections usually given in the vastus lateralis muscle? When should the gluteus maximus muscle be used when giving an injection to an adult?

____

____

____

____

____

2. As a medical assistant, what should you do if a patient is upset or concerned about his or her health?

____

____

____

____

____

3. How does regular exercise help older adults stay healthy?

____

____

____

____

____

RESEARCH ACTIVITY

Utilize Internet search engines to research the following topics and write a brief description of what you find. It is important to utilize reputable websites.

1. Using the Internet as a research source, conduct further research on two conditions/diseases of the muscular system. These conditions can be ones that are found in the textbook or others that you may be interested in learning more about. Conduct your research with the idea of learning more about the conditions/diseases than what is presented in the textbook. Write an essay on what you learned, including how the disease presents itself, the possible cause of the condition, the treatment, and any new technology that may be available in the future to address the condition/disease. Be sure to cite your resources.

Chapter 25
The Nervous System

CHAPTER OUTLINE

General review of the chapter:

Structure and Functions of the Nervous System
Neurons
Nerve Fibers, Nerves, and Tracts
Nerve Impulses and Synapses
Central Nervous System
Peripheral Nervous System
Common Disorders Associated with the Nervous System

STUDENT STUDY GUIDE

Use the following guide to assist in your learning of the concepts from the chapter.

I. An Overview of the Central Nervous System

1. The Nervous System
   A. Acts to correlate both __________ and __________ factors that affect our bodies by gathering, storing, and deciphering both external and internal information.
   B. Decides how to __________ and __________ in an appropriate manner in order to satisfy certain needs.
   C. Of these needs, the most important is __________.
2. Types of Neurons: Motor Neurons
   A. Usually have several __________ and only one __________.
   B. Axons may be several feet long and reach from the __________, __________ to the area that is to be activated.
   C. Dendrites resemble __________ __________ and are unsheathed.

3. Motor Neurons: On the following image, indicate the location of the axon, dendrite, and myelin sheath.

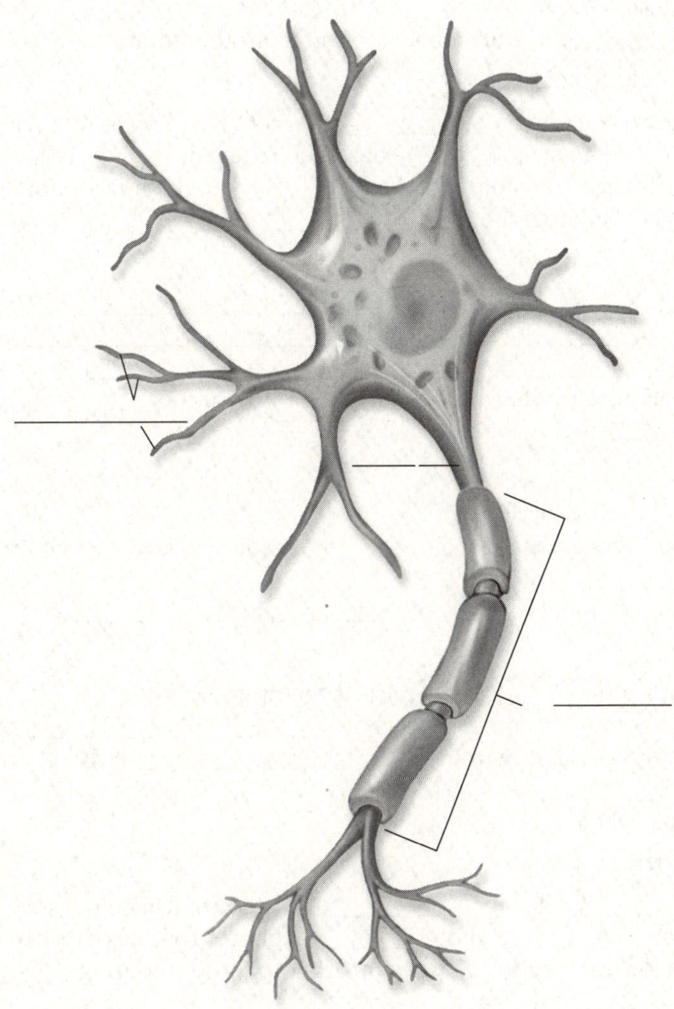

4. Sensory Neurons
   A. They lack true __________, are sheathed, and more closely resemble __________.
   B. Transmit impulses directly to the __________ __________ __________.
5. Nerve Fibers
   A. Single, elongated process, usually an axon or __________ process from a __________ neuron.
   B. Nerve fibers in the peripheral nervous system (PNS) are wrapped in __________.
   C. Nerve fibers in the central nervous system (CNS) do not contain __________ __________, and thus damage to the CNS is permanent, whereas damage to a __________ nerve can be reversed.
6. Myelinated Sheaths
   A. Myelin is a thick __________ substance.
   B. Myelin sheaths have both an inner sheath of __________ and an outer sheath, or __________, composed of Schwann cells.
   C. __________ __________ are needed for the process of regenerating a damaged nerve fiber.

7. Tracts
   A. All nerve fibers that are housed within the nerve tract must have the same __________, __________, and __________.
   B. The spinal cord contains __________ tracts that are __________, which ascend to the brain, and __________ tracts that descend from the brain.
8. Nerve Impulses and Synapses
   A. Each receptor has its own __________ at which it will react to a stimulus, and each will only respond when its __________ has been reached.
   B. The impulse is then transmitted via a __________, which is a knoblike branch ending.
   C. The process is similar to the __________ __________.
9. An Overview of the Brain
   i. ______________________________
   ii. ______________________________
   iii. ______________________________
   iv. The three membranes that encompass the brain are the __________, the __________, and the __________.
10. The Brain
    A. Manages all bodily functions and __________.
    B. Functions and movement are __________ by specific areas of the brain.
    C. Generates __________.
    D. Is the basis for rational thought, __________, and __________.
11. The Cerebrum
    A. The cerebrum is the __________ part of the brain.
    B. Controls higher thought processes such as __________ __________, reasoning, and judgment.
    C. The cerebrum is divided by the __________ __________ into left and right halves called __________ __________.
    D. Each hemisphere has __________ __________.
12. The Cerebral Cortex
    A. Houses __________ of the __________ in the entire nervous system.
    B. Composed of __________ and __________ matter that lies directly below it.
    C. Responsible for interpreting sensory information and initiating __________ __________.
    D. Stores __________ and creates __________.
13. The Diencephalon
    A. Literally means the __________ portion of the brain.
    B. Made up of the __________ and the __________.
14. The Thalamus
    A. The thalamus is two large masses of __________cell bodies connected by a third mass.
    B. Serves as a relay center for all sensory impulses, with the exception of __________.
15. The Hypothalamus
    A. Lies beneath the __________.
    B. Primarily regulates the __________ nervous activity associated with behavior and emotional expression.
    C. Responsible for a variety of __________ functions that occur throughout the body.
16. The Brainstem
    A. Resembles a __________.
    B. Contains the __________, the __________, and the __________.
    C. These structures relay important information to the cerebrum, including __________, __________, and other sensory data.

17. The Midbrain

    A. Located just below the __________ and above the __________.
    B. Associated with __________ __________ and the tracking movements of the eyes.
    C. The lower two segments are associated with the sense of __________.

18. The Pons

    A. A broad band of white matter anterior to the __________ that is between the midbrain and the __________ __________.
    B. Contains __________ __________ linking the cerebellum and medulla oblongata to higher cortical areas.
    C. Plays a vital role in __________ and __________ motor control.

19. The Medulla Oblongata

    A. Connects the __________ and the rest of the brain to the spinal cord.
    B. The nerve centers in this area are vital to the body's __________ because they exert control of the circulation of blood by regulating both the __________ and arterial blood pressure.
    C. Different areas of the medulla oblongata are also responsible for involuntary bodily functions, including __________, __________, __________, __________, and __________.

20. The Cerebellum

    A. Located in the back of the skull below the cerebrum and behind the pons and the __________ __________.
    B. The cerebellum is the __________ largest portion of the brain.
    C. The surface has a large __________ of gray cell bodies and white matter on its interior.
    D. Coordinates voluntary and involuntary __________ of movement.
    E. Adjusts muscles to automatically maintain __________.

21. A Review of the Brain: Label the parts of the brain as found on the image.

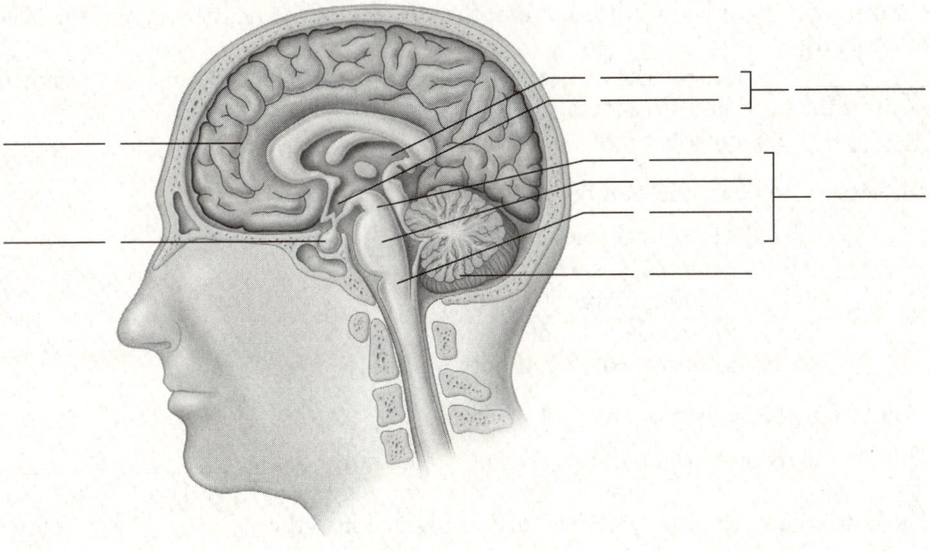

22. The Spinal Cord

    A. Connects the brain with the __________ nerves.
    B. Consists of gray matter (cell bodies) in the __________ __________.
    C. Consists of white matter (__________ __________) in the outer layer.
    D. Like the brain, it is surrounded by __________ fluid.
    E. Impulses are transmitted through the spinal cord along __________.
    F. The spinal cord is encased in the __________ __________.

G. The four divisions of the spinal cord are __________, __________, __________, and __________.

H. The levels of the spinal column are numbered (e.g., cervical level 5 is noted as __________).

I. Spinal nerves exit through __________ (openings) in the vertebrae.

23. Cerebrospinal Fluid

A. Circulates around the brain and spinal cord in the __________ space.
B. Provides __________ and __________ for the brain and spinal cord.
C. Contains nourishment and __________.
D. Produced in the __________ __________ of the ventricles of the brain.

24. Cranial Nerves and Their Functions: Name the nerves that provide each function listed.

A. __________: Provides the sense of smell.
B. __________: Provides vision.
C. __________: Conducts motor impulses to four of the six external muscles of the eye and to the muscle that raises the eyelid.
D. __________: Conducts motor impulses to control the superior oblique muscle of the eyeball.
E. __________: Provides sensory input from the face, nose, mouth, forehead, and top of the head; motor fibers to the muscles of the jaw (chewing).
F. __________: Conducts motor impulses to the lateral rectus muscle of the eyeball.
G. __________: Controls the muscles of the face and scalp, the lachrymal glands of the eye and the submandibular and sublingual salivary glands, and input from the tongue for the sense of taste.
H. __________: Provides input for hearing and equilibrium.
I. __________: Provides a general sense of taste, regulates swallowing, and controls the secretion of saliva.
J. __________: Controls the muscles of the pharynx, larynx, thoracic, and abdominal organs; swallowing; voice production; the slowing of the heartbeat; and the acceleration of peristalsis.
K. __________: Controls the trapezius and sternocleidomastoid muscles, permitting movement of the head and shoulders.
L. __________: Controls tongue movement.

25. Spinal Nerves: Indicate the number of each.

A. ________ pair(s) of cervical spinal nerves
B. ________ pair(s) of thoracic spinal nerves
C. ________ pair(s) of lumbar spinal nerves
D. ________ pair(s) of sacral spinal nerves
E. ________ pair(s) of coccygeal spinal nerves

26. The Autonomic Nervous System

A. The final division of the nervous system occurs in the __________ __________ __________.
B. The autonomic nervous system is further divided into the __________ and __________ nervous systems.

27. The Sympathetic Division

A. Branches from the __________ thoracic and the first three __________ spinal nerves form the first part of the sympathetic division of the ANS.
B. The cell bodies of these nerve fibers are located in the __________ __________ of the spinal cord.
C. The axons of the nerve cells leave the spinal nerves and enter almost immediately into masses of nerve cell bodies, which are called __________ __________.

D. Spinal nerves that synapse with the __________ __________ tend to produce widespread __________ when activated.
E. This occurrence is thought to prepare the body for __________ or __________.
F. During fight or flight, a person experiences increased alertness in conjunction with an increase in __________ __________and other bodily functions.
G. At this point, the somatic nervous system stimulates the __________ __________ to release __________, the hormone that causes the familiar adrenaline rush.

28. The Parasympathetic Division
A. Long fibers that branch from __________ __________ III, VII, IX, and X in conjunction with the long fibers of __________ __________ II, III, and IV form the first stage of the parasympathetic division.
B. Cranial nerve fibers extend via the __________ nerve to ganglia serving the thoracic, abdominal, and pelvic viscera.
C. The fibers of the sacral spinal nerves form the __________ nerve, which branches to synapse with small ganglia near or within the organs to be innervated.
D. The cell bodies of these ganglia serve the __________ __________, __________, __________, and __________ __________.
E. The parasympathetic division works to conserve energy and innervate the digestive system; thus, its function earned the nickname "__________."
F. Instead of the adrenaline rush that is felt with the somatic nervous system, a __________ in metabolism and bodily function occurs.

II. The Pathology of the Nervous System

1. Alzheimer's Disease
A. __________ history often plays a role in the development of this disease, along with __________ and __________.
B. Onset is most frequent in the later stages of life, generally ages __________ to __________.

2. Signs and Symptoms of Alzheimer's Disease
A. Mild __________ of recent events is the first symptom.
B. The ability to think and rationalize __________.
C. Thought processes are __________.
D. __________ may become difficult to understand.
E. __________ and __________ skills dissipate.
F. __________ patterns change during the later stages.
G. Patients (may) become __________, __________, aggressive, or __________.
H. Eventually, patients are unable to __________, __________, or __________ for themselves.

3. Treatment for Alzheimer's Disease
A. Medications may __________ the progression of the disease in the __________ stages.
B. Patients must continue to take medication throughout their life to avoid __________.

4. Amyotrophic Lateral Sclerosis
A. Breaks down the __________ that are responsible for __________.
B. The disease is also known as motor __________ disease.

5. Signs and Symptoms of Amyotrophic Lateral Sclerosis
A. Loss of control of __________ muscle movement, including that of the arms, legs, and trunk.
B. __________ muscle movement, such as that associated with the __________ of the heart and the smooth muscle of the internal organs, is not generally affected.
C. Depending on the form of ALS, the loss of __________ __________ (dementia) or sensory symptoms may occur.

6. Bell's Palsy

   A. Generally not a serious condition, but does affect the __________ of the face.
   B. Caused by damage to a __________ __________; a facial nerve runs beneath each ear to the muscles on that side of the face.
   C. Also known as __________ palsy.
   D. Named after Dr. Charles Bell, who first documented the disorder in __________.

7. Signs, Symptoms, and Treatment of Bell's Palsy

   Signs and symptoms include the following:

   A. __________ __________ of the face.
   B. Facial __________ and lack of expression on the afflicted side.

   Treatment includes the following:

   A. __________ at the onset ensures good recovery.
   B. Without treatment, it may resolve on its own in a few __________ or __________.

8. Disk Disorders

   A. Disk disorders include painful deterioration of the disks that support the __________ __________.
   B. Signs and symptoms include the following:
      i. ______________________________
      ii. ______________________________
      iii. ______________________________
      iv. ______________________________

9. Treatment for Disk Disorders

   i. ______________________________
   ii. ______________________________
   iii. ______________________________
   iv. ______________________________
   v. ______________________________

10. Encephalitis

   A. Often caused by a __________.
   B. Primarily affects __________ and the __________.

11. Epilepsy and Seizures

   A. The cause of epilepsy is __________.
   B. Epilepsy is often the result of another condition, such as a __________ __________, __________, __________ __________, or __________ __________.
   C. Seizures affect about _____ of the population.

12. Types of Headaches

   i. ______________________________
   ii. ______________________________
   iii. ______________________________
   iv. ______________________________

13. Huntington's Chorea

   A. Huntington's chorea is a hereditary degenerative disorder of the cerebral and __________ __________.
   B. Also referred to as __________ __________.
   C. Generally, onset begins during the mid to late __________; sometimes occurs in juveniles.

14. Signs and Symptoms of Huntington's Chorea

i. ______________________________
ii. ______________________________
iii. ______________________________
iv. ______________________________
v. ______________________________
vi. ______________________________

15. Treatment for Huntington's Chorea

A. __________ and __________ are used to regulate pain, spasms, and seizures.
B. Death occurs within __________ years of diagnosis.

16. Hydrocephalus

A. Commonly occurs in __________.
B. Characterized by an excessive amount of CSF __________ in the brain, causing the brain to __________ against the skull.
C. Without proper treatment, this condition can result in __________ __________.

17. Signs and Symptoms of Hydrocephalus

i. ______________________________
ii. ______________________________
iii. ______________________________
iv. ______________________________

18. Signs and Symptoms of Meningitis

i. ______________________________
ii. ______________________________
iii. ______________________________
iv. ______________________________
v. ______________________________

19. Treatment for Meningitis

i. ______________________________
ii. ______________________________
iii. ______________________________
iv. ______________________________
v. ______________________________
vi. ______________________________

20. Multiple Sclerosis

A. MS is a chronic, debilitating autoimmune disease that affects the __________ and the __________ __________.
B. There is no known ______.
C. The body directs the __________ and white blood cells to attack the __________ __________ surrounding the nerves in the brain and the spinal cord.
D. __________ and injury to the sheath and nerves result; __________ is possible.
E. Transmission of nerve impulses are impeded, making __________, __________, or __________ difficult.

21. Signs and Symptoms of Multiple Sclerosis

i. ______________________________
ii. ______________________________
iii. ______________________________
iv. ______________________________
v. ______________________________
vi. ______________________________

vii. ______________________________
viii. ______________________________
ix. ______________________________
x. ______________________________

22. Neuralgia

A. __________ __________, __________ (including surgery), __________, and __________ may all lead to neuralgia.

B. The signs and symptoms of neuralgia include the following:

i. ______________________________
ii. ______________________________

23. Treatment for Neuralgia

A. Rest, stretching, and __________
B. Aspirin, __________, or ibuprofen
C. Narcotic pain killers, __________ __________, and anesthetic agents administered via __________ injection
D. Surgical procedures to decrease __________

24. Parkinson's Disease

A. Parkinson's disease is a __________ disorder.
B. Caused by the __________ of nerve cells in the parts of the brain that control __________.
C. Because of degeneration, there is a shortage of the neurotransmitter __________, causing the __________ impairment that characterizes the disease.
D. Causes __________, __________ changes, __________, __________ disturbances, __________ impairment, and __________difficulties.
E. __________ over time.

25. Signs and Symptoms of Parkinson's Disease

i. ______________________________
ii. ______________________________
iii. ______________________________
iv. ______________________________
v. ______________________________
vi. ______________________________

26. Treatment for Parkinson's Disease

A. Administration of __________.
B. __________ must eventually be discontinued because of __________ __________.
C. __________ intervention helps minimize involuntary movement.

27. Signs and Symptoms of Sciatica

A. Sharp pain from the __________ __________, down the back of the __________.
B. Pain may be worse during periods of __________, as well as at __________.
C. Increased pain when the __________ changes.

28. Treatment for Sciatica

i. ______________________________
ii. ______________________________
iii. ______________________________
iv. ______________________________
v. ______________________________
vi. ______________________________

29. Spina Bifida

A. Spina bifida is the most frequently __________, permanently __________, and devastating of all birth defects.
B. Affects approximately 1 out of every __________ newborns in the United States.
C. More children have spina bifida than __________ __________, __________ __________, and __________ __________ combined.
D. The spine fails to __________ properly during the first month of pregnancy.
E. All nerve damage is __________.

30. Forms of Spina Bifida

i. ____________________
ii. ____________________
iii. ____________________
iv. ____________________

31. Signs and Symptoms of Spina Bifida: Closed Neural Tube

A. Defects are __________.
B. Some individuals show no __________.
C. Others have __________, causing __________ and __________ dysfunction.

32. Signs and Symptoms of Spina Bifida: Meningocele

A. The __________ protrude from the spinal opening.
B. There may be no __________.
C. Symptoms are similar to those of __________ neural tube defects.

33. Signs and Symptoms of Spina Bifida: Myelomeningocele

A. Myelomeningocele is the most __________ form.
B. The entire spinal cord is __________.
C. __________ may be partial or complete below the area of the __________.

34. Treatment for Spina Bifida

A. Some children may need __________ intervention as they grow and develop.
B. __________ forms may not require any __________.
C. Surgery __________ has been tried; however, complications can be great for both the mother and the fetus.

35. Treatment for the Complications of Paralysis

A. Treatment is aimed at reducing __________.
B. __________ therapy may be helpful in hemiplegic patients with complications due to stroke.

36. Complications Associated with Paralysis

i. ____________________
ii. ____________________
iii. ____________________
iv. ____________________

37. Strokes

A. Strokes are the __________ leading cause of death in the United States.
B. The __________ __________ dies when the blood supply to the brain is decreased by __________ or __________.
C. Brain cells can die when the __________ supply is interrupted for more than a few minutes.
D. __________ is important in the diagnosis and treatment of strokes.

38. Signs and Symptoms of a Stroke

i. ____________________
ii. ____________________

iii. ____
iv. ____
v. ____
vi. ____

39. Treatment for a Stroke

A. __________ intervention is vital.
B. Stabilize condition by either __________ blood clots or stopping the __________.
C. __________ may be necessary.
D. Administer medications to control __________ of the brain and __________ __________.
E. Medications and treatments are given after the incident to __________ the chance of __________.

40. Transient Ischemic Attacks

A. TIAs are frequently precursors of __________.
B. __________ can last anywhere from a few seconds to hours.

41. Signs and Symptoms of Transient Ischemic Attacks

i. ____
ii. ____
iii. ____

42. Treatment for Transient Ischemic Attacks

i. ____
ii. ____

43. Methods for Reducing the Risk of Future Transient Ischemic Attacks

i. ____
ii. ____
iii. ____
iv. ____
v. ____

44. Types of Trauma to the Brain

A. Subdural __________ cause pressure in the brain that must be relieved by __________.
B. A __________ is an injury caused by abrupt jarring of, or a blow to, the head.
C. A __________ is bruising of the brain.
D. Skull fractures known as __________ can cause brain injury.

45. Signs and Symptoms of Brain Trauma

i. ____
ii. ____
iii. ____
iv. ____
v. ____
vi. ____
vii. ____

46. Treatment for Brain Trauma

A. __________ therapy
B. Medications to suppress seizures, such as ______________ and ____________.

KEY TERMINOLOGY REVIEW

Match the vocabulary term to the correct definition below.

a. Afferent
b. Alzheimer's disease
c. Amyotrophic lateral sclerosis (ALS)
d. Autonomic nervous system (ANS)
e. Bell's palsy
f. Central nervous system (CNS)
g. Cerebrospinal fluid (CSF)
h. Concussion
i. Contusion
j. Corpus callosum
k. Efferent nerves
l. Encephalitis
m. Epilepsy
n. Fissure
o. Hemiplegia
p. Interneurons
q. Meninges
r. Meningitis
s. Motor neurons
t. Multiple sclerosis (MS)
u. Neurons
v. Neuralgia
w. Neurilemma
x. Paraplegia
y. Parkinson's disease
z. Peripheral nervous system (PNS)
aa. Quadriplegia
bb. Sciatica
cc. Seizure
dd. Sensory neurons
ee. Sheaths
ff. Somatic nervous system (SNS)
gg. Spina bifida
hh. Stroke
ii. Sulcus
jj. Tract

1. ____________ Inflammation of the brain.
2. ____________ Weakness or paralysis of the muscles that control expression on one side of the face.
3. ____________ An outer sheath of myelin.
4. ____________ Membranes that encompass the brain.
5. ____________ Refers to a pain that runs along the sciatic nerve.
6. ____________ Often considered to be the "blood" of the nervous system.
7. ____________ Made up of nerves that connect the CNS to the other parts of the body.
8. ____________ A chronic, potentially debilitating disease that affects the brain and spinal cord; there is no known cure.
9. ____________ Also known as Lou Gehrig's disease.
10. ____________ Nerves where the impulse is transmitted from the neural cell body to stimulate the target muscle or organ.
11. ____________ Transmit sensory information through a peripheral process.
12. ____________ Bruising of the brain.
13. ____________ Occurs when abnormal and often intense bursts of electrical activity are produced within the brain.
14. ____________ Responsible for controlling involuntary bodily functions.
15. ____________ A deep groove in the brain.
16. ____________ Typically presents as a tremor of a limb, especially when the body is at rest.
17. ____________ Often referred to as associative neurons because they are located entirely within the CNS.
18. ____________ Nerves that conduct impulses to the CNS.
19. ____________ Refers to paralysis from approximately the shoulders down.

20. ____________ A shallow groove.
21. ____________ Term used for general nerve pain.
22. ____________ A disorder associated with misfiring or interference.
23. ____________ Stimulates the adrenal gland to release epinephrine.
24. ____________ A group of nerve fibers within the CNS.
25. ____________ Receives impulses from the entire body, requiring it to process information and respond with appropriate actions.
26. ____________ Control most of the body's functions as they cause muscles to contract, glands to secrete, and organs to function properly.
27. ____________ Formed by accessory cells.
28. ____________ An infection of the meninges that surround and protect the brain and spinal cord.
29. ____________ Refers to paralysis from approximately the waist down.
30. ____________ Known in medicine as a cerebrovascular incident.
31. ____________ An injury caused by abrupt jarring of, or a blow to, the head that may result in a loss of consciousness.
32. ____________ Nervous system tissue that is made up of specialized nerve cells.
33. ____________ Stimulates the adrenal gland to release epinephrine.
34. ____________ Occurs when paralysis affects one side of the body.
35. ____________ A progressive degenerative disease that attacks the brain and its cognitive functioning.
36. ____________ The largest nerve tract that joins the right and left hemispheres of the brain.

APPLIED PRACTICE

Read the scenarios below and answer the questions that follow.

Scenario 1

A 20-year-old female patient presents to your office with the following symptoms: Headache ×3 days, temperature of 103.2°F, dizziness, and blurred vision. She said that since she woke up this morning she has not been able to move her head. In her medical chart, you make a note that "the patient states 'My neck is so stiff, I can't bend it.' Her head appears bent forward toward her chest."

1. What would you suspect the diagnosis might be based on her symptoms? *(Medical assistants never make a diagnosis; this is a question about your knowledge of the signs and symptoms of various conditions.)*

   ____

Scenario 2

A 59-year-old male patient presents to your office with observable right-side facial drooping, specifically near the mouth. The patient states that he "woke up this way" and he "can't feel anything on the entire right side of my face."

1. What would you suspect the diagnosis might be on the basis of his symptoms? *(Medical assistants never make a diagnosis; this is a question about your knowledge of the signs and symptoms of various conditions.)*

   ____

2. What is the treatment for this condition?

   ____

Scenario 3

As an administrative medical assistant, one of your duties is transcribing for the neurologists in the office where you work. Dr. Preston dictated notes on a patient whom he saw in the emergency room last night. He dictates "17-year-old male patient presents to the ER with suspected countercoup injury of the head with a 4-inch laceration on the right temporal region of his skull. Due to the extent of the contusion, the patient will remain hospitalized for observation for 48 hours."

1. What is the difference between a concussion and a contusion?

____

____

LEARNING ACTIVITY: MULTIPLE CHOICE

Circle the correct answer to each of the questions below.

1. Which of the following applies to a cerebrovascular accident?
   a. It is the third leading cause of death in the United States.
   b. It is caused by a virus.
   c. Brain tissue dies when the blood supply to a part of the brain is decreased.
   d. All of the above

2. Which of the following are signs and symptoms of encephalitis?
   a. Headache
   b. Stiff neck and back
   c. Drowsiness
   d. All of the above

3. Sciatica ______________________________.
   a. usually causes very intense pain
   b. is caused by inflammation due to a pinched root
   c. usually occurs on one side of the body
   d. All of the above

4. Which of the following diseases has a cause that is unknown?
   a. ALS
   b. TIA
   c. Trigeminal neuralgia
   d. Multiple sclerosis

5. The corpus callosum ______________________________.
   a. controls most of the body's functions
   b. joins the right and left hemispheres of the brain
   c. is divided into grey and white matter
   d. All of the above

6. Which of the following make up the central nervous system?
   a. Nerves
   b. Cells
   c. Brain and spinal cord
   d. All of the above

7. Which of the following applies to epidural and subdural hematomas?
   a. They develop when the head receives a blow.
   b. They are typically seen in the elderly.
   c. They are a bruising of the brain.
   d. None of the above

8. Which of the following are associated with epilepsy?
   a. Often occurs after a head or neck injury has healed.
   b. The cause is unknown.
   c. It is a weakness or paralysis of the muscles that control expression on one side of the face.
   d. It is an inflammation of the brain caused by a virus.

9. Which of the following is not associated with meningitis?
   a. It is similar to encephalitis.
   b. It may be caused by a virus or bacteria.
   c. It has a high death rate if untreated.
   d. It is an autoimmune disease.

10. Motor neurons are ______________________________.
   a. greatly affected in ALS
   b. considered afferent nerves
   c. housed within the nerve tract
   d. structurally like a stem

CRITICAL THINKING

Answer the following questions to the best of your ability. Utilize the textbook as a reference.

1. A patient, a 57-year-old female named Katie Gilpatrick, has come into the office and is exhibiting signs of high stress. How can the medical assistant help relieve the patient's stress?

   ____
   ____
   ____
   ____

2. A fellow health care worker comes to work and states that she cannot do very much because she has "a migraine." She was out late last night at a party and states that the headache is not because she had some drinks. She hopes that you will help her through the day by taking care of some of her patients. She is incorrect in diagnosing herself with a migraine because it is a specific type of headache, and she has not been diagnosed with migraines by a physician. Explain why it is unlikely that someone with a true migraine would be able to come to work and function even at a slow pace.

   ____
   ____
   ____
   ____

3. Why is it important to be aware of the laws in your state regarding driving and neurological disorders?

RESEARCH ACTIVITY

Utilize Internet search engines to research the following topics and write a brief description of what you find. It is important to utilize reputable websites.

1. Visit The Parkinson's Disease Foundation at www.pdf.org. Click on the "News and Events" tab on the top of the page, then select "Science News". Choose an article of interest and provide a summary of the information discussed within the article. Discuss what interested you most about the article that you selected.

CHAPTER 26
The Special Senses

CHAPTER OUTLINE

General review of the chapter:

The Eye and the Sense of Vision
Common Refractive Disorders
Disorders Related to Structural Irregularities of the Eye
Infectious Eye Disorders
Age-Related Eye Disorders
Other Eye Disorders
The Ear and the Sense of Hearing
Hearing Loss
Common Disorders Associated with the Outer Ear
Common Disorders Associated with the Middle Ear
Common Disorders Associated with the Inner Ear
The Senses of Taste and Smell
The Sense of Touch

STUDENT STUDY GUIDE

Use the following guide to assist in your learning of the concepts from the chapter.

I. The Eye and the Sense of Vision

1. An Overview of the Eye and the Sense of Vision
   A. The eye is a __________, __________organ composed of specialized structures that work together to facilitate vision.
   B. Light rays pass through the __________, __________, __________, and vitreous humor to the retina where they stimulate sensory receptors.
   C. Nerves in the eye control the amount of __________ entering the eye through the __________, the focusing of the light by the lens on the __________, and the transmission of the resulting images to the __________.
   D. The eye is made up of the eyeball and its internal structures, which perform the complex process of translating __________ into __________, and external structures that support and protect the eyeballs.

2. The Iris
   A. The iris is part of the __________ layer.
   B. Contains the __________, or eye color.
   C. Has a __________ in the center, called the __________, which controls the amount of light entering the eye.

3. The Innermost Layer of the Eye
   A. Contains the __________ cells in the retina called __________ and __________ that translate light rays into nerve impulses that are transmitted to the brain.
   B. The fovea centralis retinae contains only __________.
   C. The optic nerve enters at the __________ disk and carries this information from the eye to the brain.
   D. A reflexive process called ______________ adjusts the eye's optical powers to maintain a clear image at various distances.
4. Eyelids, or Palpebrae
   A. Eyelids close over the eyeballs, protecting them from __________ __________, __________ __________, and __________.
   B. They also keep the eyes moist by preventing __________ from evaporating.
   C. __________ in the margins protect the eye from foreign matter.
   D. The superior and inferior __________ meet at the __________ at each corner of the eye.
5. The Lacrimal Apparatus
   A. The lacrimal gland secretes __________ through ducts on the surface of the __________ of the __________ lid.
   B. __________cleanse the eyes and keep them moist.
   C. At the inner corner of each eye are two ducts, the __________ __________, which collect and drain the tears in the lacrimal __________.
6. Extrinsic Eye Muscles
   A. Six short extrinsic eye muscles connect the eyeball to the __________ __________.
   B. Muscles provide the eyeball with support and __________ movement.
   C. Four of these muscles, the __________ muscles, are straight; two are oblique, or slanted.
7. The Characteristics of Refractive Disorders of the Eye
   A. Refractive disorders are the most __________ disorders of the eye.
   B. Characterized by the __________ of the eye to __________ correctly.
   C. Caused by factors such as __________ and changes in the __________ of the eyeball and the various eye muscles.
8. Astigmatism
   A. Caused by irregularities in the __________ of the __________ and __________ that cause light to focus on the retina but spread out over an area.
   B. Signs and symptoms include __________ near or distance vision.
   C. Treatment involves the use of __________ lenses or surgery to reshape the __________.
9. Myopia
   A. Also known as __________.
   B. The lens focuses the light in front of the __________.
10. Hyperopia
    A. Also known as __________.
    B. The lens focuses light behind the __________.
    C. __________ objects are seen more clearly than objects that are __________.
11. Presbyopia
    A. Characterized by a loss of __________ in the lens, usually as a result of __________.
    B. Signs and symptoms include difficulty in focusing on __________ objects.
12. Strabismus
    A. Also called ________ eyes or ________ eyes.
    B. Signs and symptoms include poor ________ ________ and diplopia, or ________ vision.

C. Treatment for strabismus
   i. ______________________________
   ii. ______________________________
   iii. ______________________________
   iv. ______________________________

13. Blepharoptosis
   A. Usually a __________ condition that occurs when the muscles of the eyelid are not strong enough to __________ it.
   B. Signs and symptoms include abnormal __________ of one or both __________.
   C. __________ is the only treatment option.

14. Exophthalmos
   A. Usually caused by __________ or __________ disease.
   B. Unilateral exophthalmos may be caused by an __________ __________.
   C. Signs and symptoms include __________ __________ of one or both eyeballs.

15. Blepharitis
   A. Inflammation of the __________ of the __________.
   B. Signs and symptoms include redness, __________, and swelling of the eyelids.
   C. Treatment includes warm __________ and __________ antibiotic therapy.

16. Conjunctivitis
   A. Conjunctivitis is an __________ of the conjunctiva.
   B. Commonly known as __________.
   C. Causes of conjunctivitis
      i. ______________________________
      ii. ______________________________
      iii. ______________________________
      iv. ______________________________
      v. ______________________________

17. Hordeolums
   A. Caused by __________, generally *Staphylococcus*.
   B. May accompany blocked or infected eyelid __________ or __________ eyelids.
   C. Contaminated __________ that touch the eye area may cause the infection.
   D. Painful hordeolums can occur __________ the eyelids.
   E. Signs and symptoms of hordeolums
      i. ______________________________
      ii. ______________________________
      iii. ______________________________
      iv. ______________________________
   F. Treatment includes a warm, wet __________ applied to the area that may help to relieve the pain.

18. Cataracts
   A. Cataracts are a clouding or __________ of the __________ that prevents light from entering.
   B. The cause is unclear, but there may be a correlation between the formation of cataracts and __________, __________, and excessive exposure to __________.
   C. Signs and symptoms of cataracts
      i. ______________________________
      ii. ______________________________
      iii. ______________________________
   D. Treatment for cataracts
      i. ______________________________
      ii. ______________________________

19. Dry Macular Degeneration
    A. Dry macular degeneration is the deterioration of the macula, the __________ portion of the __________.
    B. Small yellow deposits called __________ form under the macula, causing it to thin and dry out, leading to a loss of __________vision.
    C. This form has a __________ progression than does the wet type; however, it sometimes turns into the wet type.
20. Wet Macular Degeneration
    A. __________ new blood vessels grow under the __________ and the macula.
    B. These blood vessels may then __________ and leak fluid, which causes the macula to __________ or lift up, impairing or destroying the central vision.
    C. Vision loss may be __________and __________.
21. Nyctalopia
    A. The inability to see well in __________ light.
    B. Occurs in patients with __________ __________ and __________.
    C. May be due to a vitamin __________ deficiency.
    D. Can be provoked by __________ __________ .
22. Amblyopia
    A. Also called __________.
    B. This disorder, seen in __________, occurs when the muscles are weaker in one eye than in the other.
    C. Patients with more severe amblyopia may suffer from various vision-related disorders, such as __________ __________ __________.
    D. For treatment, a __________ may be worn over the stronger eye to strengthen the muscles of the weaker eye.
23. Corneal Abrasion
    A. Results from __________, __________, or both.
    B. Can be very __________.
    C. The patient will be very sensitive to __________ and will have difficulty opening the affected eye.
    D. Treatment may include mild __________ and resting the eye.
24. Diplopia
    A. Also called __________ __________.
    B. Frequently follows __________ to the eye or head.
    C. Can be caused by a disease of any of the following structures:
        i. ____
        ii. ____
        iii. ____
        iv. ____
        v. ____
        vi. ____
25. Glaucoma
    A. Characterized by __________ pressure in the eye brought on by an excessive amount of __________ humor.
    B. If left untreated, the __________ can lead to damage of the __________ __________ and, eventually, blindness.
    C. Types of glaucoma include ________________ and ________________.
    D. Glaucoma has no symptoms, so it must be diagnosed by ______________ ______________ in a doctor's office.

E. Treatment includes eye drops to lower __________ __________, as well as possible __________ or conventional surgery.

26. Nystagmus or Nystaxis

A. Characterized by __________, __________, __________ eye movements.
B. May be __________ or acquired.
C. Usually results in some __________ of vision.
D. Signs and symptoms include __________ eye movements that may be __________, __________, or even __________.

27. Retinopathy

A. Patients with __________ are prone to diabetic retinopathy.
B. This nerve damage is a result of __________ __________ and can lead to permanent blindness.

28. Photophobia

A. Also known as __________ to light.
B. Sometimes caused by __________, __________, __________, or inflammation of the eyes.

II. The Senses of Hearing, Taste, and Smell

1. The Three Main Divisions of the Ear

i. ______________________________
ii. ______________________________
iii. ______________________________

2. The Structure and Function of the External Ear

A. The pinna, or auricle, funnels sound waves through the __________ __________ to the __________ membrane.
B. The auditory canal, or auditory meatus, is S-shaped and secretes __________, or __________.
C. The tympanic membrane, or eardrum, separates the __________ ear from the __________ ear.

3. The Structure and Function of the Middle Ear

A. The middle ear is a tiny cavity in the __________ bone of the skull.
B. Contains three small bones: the __________ (hammer), the __________ (anvil), and the __________ (stirrup).
C. The function of the middle ear
i. Transmits __________ __________.
ii. __________ air pressure on both sides of the tympanic membrane.
iii. Protects the ear from __________ __________ .
iv. Sound vibrations are transmitted by __________ from the tympanic membrane to the __________ __________ and into the inner ear.

4. The Structure and Function of the Inner Ear

A. The inner ear is a bony labyrinth in the temporal bone that is made up of the __________, the __________, and __________ semicircular canals.
B. The bony and membranous labyrinths are separated by __________.
C. Tiny _____ cells function as receptors for hearing and balance.
D. The cochlea resembles a __________ __________.
E. The cochlear duct runs between the __________ and __________ chambers.

5. The Two Most Common Types of Hearing Disorders

A. Conductive
i. Temporary hearing loss; sound is not conducted efficiently through the __________ __________ to the __________ and __________ __________.
ii. __________ __________ can be corrected.

B. Sensorineural
   i. Permanent hearing loss is caused by damaged __________ or __________ __________ from the inner ear to the brain.
   ii. __________ __________ cannot be corrected.

6. Impacted Cerumen
   A. Cerumen is produced by the __________ __________ as lubrication.
   B. Impacted cerumen obstructs the __________ __________.
   C. Affects __________ adults.
   D. Exacerbated by the use of a ____________ swab.
   E. Signs and symptoms include blocked or ______________ hearing, a ____________ feeling in the ear, and ____________.
   F. Treatment includes softening the ____________, then flushing with a __________.
   G. If left untreated, impacted cerumen leads to __________.

7. Ruptured Tympanic Membrane
   A. Caused by __________ or __________ air pressure on both sides of the membrane.
   B. Signs and symptoms of a ruptured tympanic membrane
      i. ____
      ii. ____
   C. Treatment for a ruptured tympanic membrane
      i. ____
      ii. ____
      iii. ____

8. Otitis Media
   A. __________ __________(swimmer's ear) is an inflammation of the outer ear.
   B. __________ __________ is an inflammation of the middle ear.
   C. Signs and Symptoms of otitis media
      i. ____
      ii. ____
      iii. ____
      iv. ____
      v. ____
   D. Treatment for otitis media
      i. Eliminating the cause of the __________.
      ii. Oral __________ and decongestants
      iii. __________ __________ every 1 to 2 days

9. Otosclerosis
   A. Otosclerosis is a __________ condition
   B. The tissue surrounding the staples grows __________.
   C. Prevents __________ from transmitting sound vibrations.
   D. Signs and symptoms include hearing loss in one or both ears, __________, and __________.
   E. Treatment includes the use of a ____________ or surgery.

10. Tinnitus
   A. Causes of tinnitus
      i. ____
      ii. ____
      iii. ____
      iv. ____
      v. ____
   B. Signs and symptoms include __________ or __________ in one or both ears.
   C. Some relief is provided by the use of __________ __________, __________, and medications such as __________ and antidepressants.

11. Ménière's Disease

A. Caused by changes in ______ volume in the ______ ear.

B. Signs and symptoms of Ménière's disease

i. ______
ii. ______
iii. ______
iv. ______
v. ______
vi. ______
vii. ______
viii. ______
ix. ______

C. Treatment for Ménière's disease

i. ______
ii. ______
iii. ______
iv. ______
v. ______

12. Presbycusis

A. Caused by loud noises, __________, __________, or the side effects of medications.

B. Occurs in both ears and affects __________ and __________ tones.

C. Treatment typically involves the use of a __________ __________.

13. How the Senses of Taste and Smell Function Together

A. __________ cells respond to the changes in the chemical concentrations that activate the smell __________.

B. Receptors send information to the brain via __________ __________.

C. __________ move from the nose to the mouth region, stimulating the __________ __________.

14. The Four Types of Taste Cells

i. ______
ii. ______
iii. ______
iv. ______

15. The Sense of Touch

A. The sense of touch is the oldest, most __________ sense.

B. It is the first sense that humans experience in the __________ and the last one lost before __________.

C. Found over the __________ body.

D. Originates in the __________.

E. Nerve endings in the __________, called receptors, transmit __________ to the brain via the spinal cord.

F. More nerve endings equal more __________.

KEY TERMINOLOGY REVIEW

Match the vocabulary term to the correct definition below.

a. Accommodation

b. Aqueous humor

c. Canthus

d. Choroid

e. Ciliary body
f. Cones
g. Conjunctiva
h. Cornea
i. Diabetic retinopathy
j. Ciplopia
k. Ectropion
l. Entropion
m. Fundus
n. Hearing loss
o. Hordeolums
p. Hypertensive retinopathy
q. Insufflation
r. Labyrinth
s. Lacrimal sac
t. Macula lutea
u. Nasolacrimal duct
v. Orbit
w. Ossicles
x. Palpebral fissure
y. Papilledema
z. Pupil
aa. Refraction problems
bb. Focea centralis retinae
cc. Retina
dd. Retinal detachment
ee. Rods
ff. Sclera
gg. Vertigo
hh. Vitreous chamber
ii. Vitreous humor

1. ______________ Provides nutrients to the cornea, lens, and other tissues.
2. ______________ Located in the middle of the macula lutea, a yellow spot on the back of the eye.
3. ______________ Empties into the nasal cavity.
4. ______________ Can be divided into two main conditions: Conductive (temporary) and Sensorineural (permanent).
5. ______________ The posterior, or back, section of the eyeball cavity located behind the lens.
6. ______________ Also known as sties, which are very common and frequently contagious.
7. ______________ Lines the sclera and absorbs extra light entering the eye.
8. ______________ The floor of the tympanic cavity.
9. ______________ A reflexive process that adjusts the eye's optical powers to maintain a clear image at various distances.
10. ______________ Responsible for holding and moving the lens.
11. ______________ Causes nerve damage as a result of hypertension and can lead to permanent blindness.
12. ______________ A maze of bones inside the inner ear.
13. ______________ They are sensitive to bright light and are used to see color.
14. ______________ Controls the amount of light entering the eye.
15. ______________ A form of severe dizziness.
16. ______________ The inability to focus correctly, it occurs because light rays change direction when they pass through the eye.
17. ______________ A yellow spot on the back of the eye.
18. ______________ A mucous membrane that lines the underside of the eyelids and the anterior part of the eyeball.
19. ______________ An inflammation at the optic nerve, usually caused by a tumor, which increases pressure in the eye.
20. ______________ Frequently referred to as the "window" of the eye because it allows light to enter.

21. ______________ Occurs when the retina has separated from the underlying choroid layer.
22. ______________ The introduction of gas, vapor, or powder into a cavity every 1 to 2 days.
23. ______________ The white part of the eye.
24. ______________ A very thick fluid in the vitreous chamber.
25. ______________ A disease of the retina and a condition that patients with diabetes tend to have.
26. ______________ The photosensitive cells in the retina.
27. ______________ It empties into the nasolacrimal duct, which empties into the nasal cavity.
28. ______________ Also known as double vision.
29. ______________ The innermost layer of the eye.
30. ______________ An abnormal condition in which the lower eyelid everts, or turns outward.
31. ______________ The outer and inner corners of the eye where the superior and inferior palpebrae meet.
32. ______________ The opening between the eyelids that allows light to enter.
33. ______________ The cavity in the skull that houses the eyeball.
34. ______________ A condition where the eyelid inverts, or folds inward.
35. ______________ The name of the three small bones found in the middle ear.

APPLIED PRACTICE

Read the scenario below and answer the questions that follow.

1. On the image provided, label the parts of the eyeball and its anatomical structures.

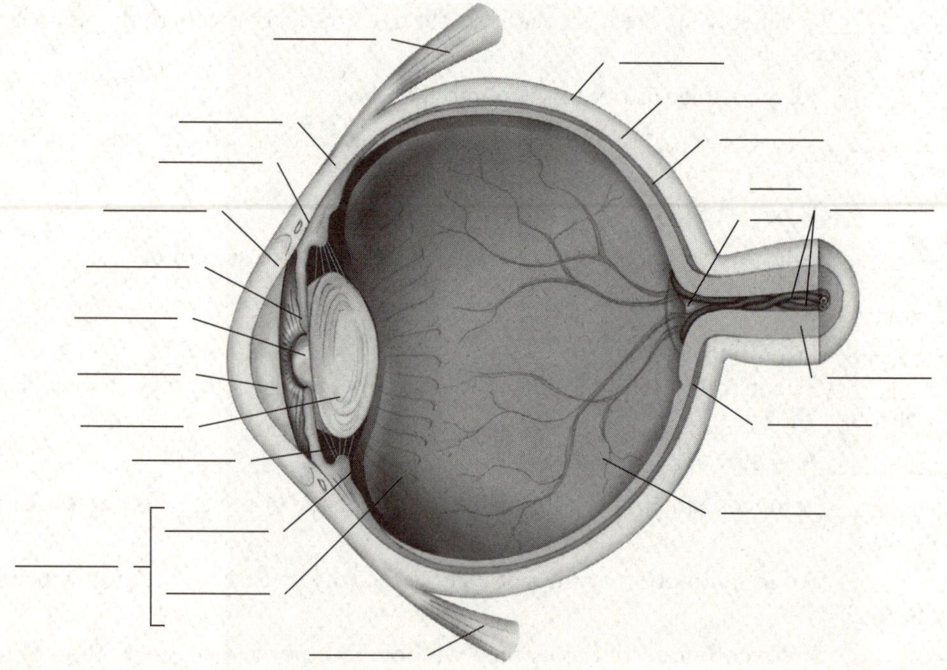

2. On the image provided, label the parts of the ear and its anatomical structures.

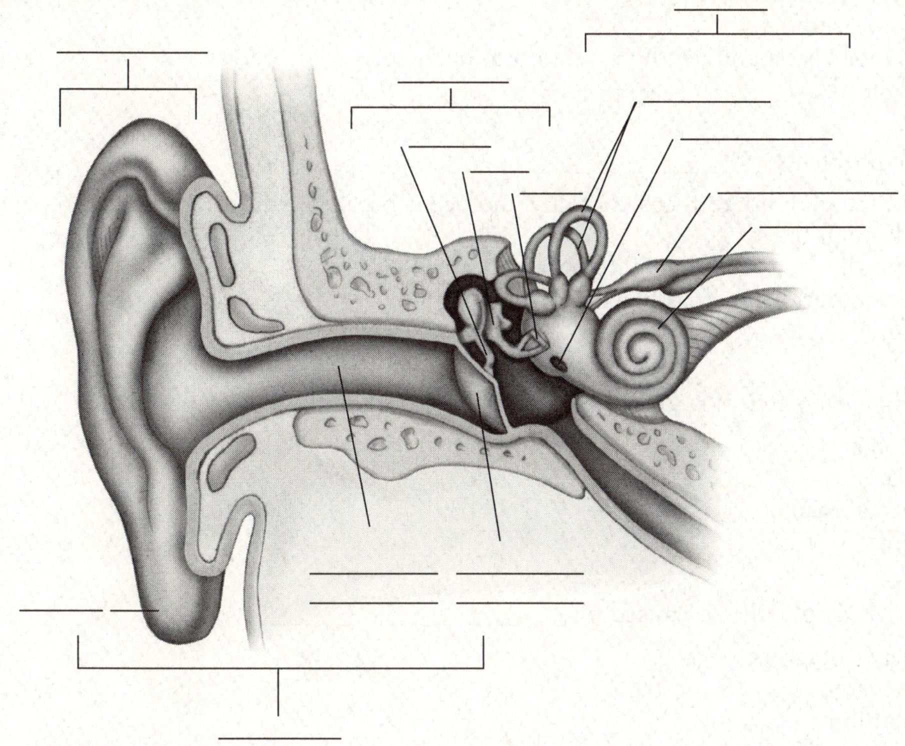

LEARNING ACTIVITY: MULTIPLE CHOICE

Circle the correct answer for each of the following questions.

1. Which of the following may develop due to maternal infections during the first 5 or 6 weeks of pregnancy?
   a. Strabismus
   b. Sensorineural deafness
   c. Congenital ear problems
   d. All of the above

2. How can intraocular pressure be reduced?
   a. Eyedrops
   b. Oral medications
   c. Surgery
   d. All of the above

3. Labyrinthitis is also known as ______________________.
   a. Otosclerosis
   b. Otitis media
   c. Nyctalopia
   d. Presbycusis

4. The developing infant ______________________.
   a. has poor visual acuity
   b. is often farsighted
   c. lacks color vision and depth perception at birth
   d. All of the above

5. Refraction problems ______________________.
   a. involve the inability to focus correctly and occur because light rays change direction when they pass through the eye
   b. are typically seen more in children then in the elderly
   c. include conditions such as blepharoptosis
   d. All of the above

6. The use of an eye patch is recommended for which of the following conditions?
   a. Glaucoma
   b. Nystagmus
   c. Corneal abrasion
   d. Diplopia

7. Hypertensive retinopathy is caused by ______________________.
   a. a variety of factors
   b. hypertension
   c. hypotension
   d. diabetes

8. Recurrent ear infections may be treated with ______________________.
   a. myringotomy
   b. keratotomy
   c. osteotomy
   d. None of the above

9. Taste and smells are most acute ______________________.
   a. at birth
   b. by the toddler stage
   c. in young adults
   d. None of the above

10. The eyes continue to grow and mature ______________________.
    a. throughout one's life
    b. until adulthood
    c. until the eighth or ninth year of life
    d. None of the above

CRITICAL THINKING

Answer the following questions to the best of your ability. Utilize the textbook as a reference.

1. When dealing with patients who have visual difficulties, why should you understand the rules for driving in your state?

2. If the physician is running behind schedule and patients must wait, what should you do?

RESEARCH ACTIVITY

Utilize Internet search engines to research the following topics and write a brief description of what you find. It is important to utilize reputable websites.

1. Visit different websites that deal with speech and hearing loss. What information can you find to help families with speech and hearing deficiencies? What websites did you find most useful? Could these websites be beneficial to staff members of an EENT (eye, ear, nose, and throat) practice? If so, why?

CHAPTER 27
The Circulatory System

CHAPTER OUTLINE

General review of the chapter:

Overview of the Circulatory System
The Heart
Blood Vessels
Blood Pressure
Pulmonary and Systemic Circulation
Blood
Blood Types
The Lymphatic System
Common Disorders Associated with the Circulatory System

STUDENT STUDY GUIDE

Use the following guide to assist in your learning of the concepts from the chapter.

I. An Overview of the Circulatory System

1. The Heart
   A. Responsible for ____________ the blood thorough the blood ____________ throughout the body.
   B. Provides ___________ blood to and removes ___________ from the cells of the body.
   C. Made up of __________ muscle ____________.
   D. Beats an average of ___________ to ___________ beats per minute or about ___________ times a day.
   E. Located in the ________________, in the center of the chest cavity.
   F. Located toward the __________ side of the ____________.
   G. The tip of the heart at the lower edge is called the ___________.
   H. The ____________ is located directly in front of the heart.
2. The Blood Vessels
   A. Responsible for carrying the blood through the ______________ to get _____________ and release ___________________.
   B. Carries the ___________ blood to all the ___________ of the body.
3. The Blood
   A. Carries the ____________ and waste products through the ______________.
   B. A major waste product is ____________________.
4. The Lymphatic System
   1. Responsible for ____________ substances to and from the ________________ system.
   2. It is also a part of the _____________ system.

5. The Chambers of the Heart
   A. Divided into ______________ chambers.
   B. The ______________ are the receiving chambers of the heart.
   C. The ________________ are the pumping chambers.
6. Heart Valves
   A. Act as restraining gates to control the direction of _________________.
   B. Situated at the entrances and exits to the _____________.
   C. When properly functioning, allow blood to flow only in the _____________ direction by blocking it from _____________ to the previous _____________.
7. The Tricuspid Valve
   A. The tricuspid valve is an ________________ valve.
   B. The prefix tri-, meaning _________, indicates that this valve has _________ leaflets or _________.
8. The Pulmonary Valve
   A. The pulmonary valve is also called the ______________ valve.
   B. Located between the right ____________ and the pulmonary artery.
9. The Mitral Valve
   A. The mitral valve is also called the ___________ valve.
   B. Has _________ cusps.
   C. Blood flows through the _______________ valve to the left ventricle.
10. The Valves of the Heart (Label the location of each valve of the heart.)

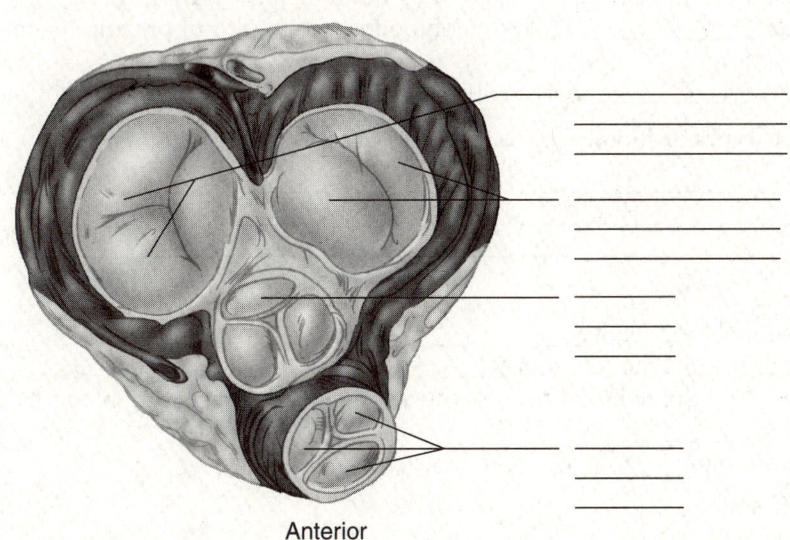

11. The Great Vessels of the Heart (Explain what each vessel does.)
   A. The aorta ____.
   B. The pulmonary arteries ________________________________.
   C. The pulmonary veins __________________________________.
   D. The inferior and superior vena cava _____________________.

12. The Normal Flow of Blood Through the Heart
    A. ______________ blood from all of the tissues, except the lungs, enters a relaxed right ______________ via two large veins called the ______________ and the ______________.
    B. The right ______________ contracts and blood flows through the ______________ valve into the relaxed right ____________.
    C. The right ______________ then contracts and blood is pumped through the pulmonary valve into the ______________ artery, which carries the blood to the lungs.
    D. The left __________ receives blood that has been oxygenated by the lungs. This blood enters the relaxed left __________________ from the four ________________ veins.
    E. The left ______________ contracts and blood flows through the ______________ valve into the relaxed left ______________.
    F. When the left ______________ contracts, the blood is pumped through the aortic valve and into the aorta, the ______________ artery in the body.
    G. The ______________ carries blood to all parts of the body, except the lungs.

13. The Conduction System of the Heart
    A. The _______________ _______________ system controls the heart rate.
    B. Special tissue conducts ______________ impulses that ______________ different chambers to ______________ in the correct order.

14. The Phases of the Cardiac Cycle
    A. Phase 1: ______________________
    B. Phase 2: ______________________
    C. Phase 3: ______________________

15. Blood Pressure
    A. A measurement of the force exerted by blood against the walls of a ____________.
    B. During _______________ systole, blood is under a lot of pressure from ______________ contraction.
    C. During ___________ diastole, blood is not being ___________ from the heart.

16. The Three Types of Blood Vessels (List and explain each type.)
    i. ____
    ii. ____
    iii. ____

17. Veins
    A. Transport blood from _____________ tissues to the heart.
    B. Have thin walls that contain ____________.
    C. __________ force blood to flow toward the heart, preventing blood from _________ in the lower ____________.
    D. Veins are more ____________ than arteries.

18. Korotkoff Sounds
    A. The sounds heard as the ___________ wall __________ when the blood pressure cuff compresses.
    B. Classified according to ___________ different phases

19. Average Normal Blood Pressure Readings
    A. Newborn: ____________
    B. 6–9 years: ____________
    C. 10–15 years: ____________
    D. 16 years to adulthood: ____________
    E. Adult: ____________

20. Physiological Factors Affecting Blood Pressure
    i. ______________________________
    ii. ______________________________
    iii. ______________________________
    iv. ______________________________

21. Pulmonary Circulation
    A. The route that blood takes from the ____________ to the ____________ and then back to the ____________.
    B. The function of pulmonary circulation is to ____________ the blood.

22. The Physiology of the Lymphatic System
    A. Collects excess ________ fluid throughout the body and returns it to the ________ system, purifying it as it passes through the system.
    B. Assists the ___________ system in __________ substances throughout the body.
    C. Defends against the invasion of ____________.

23. Lymphatic Vessels
    A. Form a network of ____________ throughout the body.
    B. Serve as one-way pipes conducting ____________ from the ____________ toward the ____________ cavity.
    C. These vessels begin as very small ____________ ____________ in the tissues.
    D. Excessive tissue fluid enters these __________ to begin the trip back to the __________ system.
    E. ____________ merge into large lymph vessels that have ____________ along their length.
    F. Lymph vessels finally drain into one of two large lymph ____________.

24. Lymph Nodes
    A. Lymph nodes are small organs composed of ____________ tissue that are located along the route of the ___________ vessels.
    B. The functions of the lymph nodes
       i. ______________________________
       ii. ______________________________
       iii. ______________________________

25. Tonsils
    A. Tonsils are lymphatic tissue located on each side of the ____________.
    B. There are three sets of tonsils
       i. ______________________________
       ii. ______________________________
       iii. ______________________________
    C. Act as ________ to protect the body.

26. The Spleen
    A. Located in the ____________ of the abdomen.
    B. Consists of lymphatic tissue that is highly infiltrated with ________ ___________.

27. The Thymus Gland
    A. Located in the upper portion of the ____________.
    B. Essential for the proper development of the ____________ system.
    C. Assists the body with the ____________ function and the development of ___________.

II. The Composition and Function of Blood

1. The Blood
    A. The average adult has about _______ liters of blood.
    B. Circulates through the body in the vessels of the _____________ system.
    C. Blood is a mixture of _________ with _________.

2. The Functions of Blood
   i. ____________________
   ii. ____________________
   iii. ____________________
3. Erythrocytes
   A. Erythrocytes are ____________ blood cells.
   B. There are ____________ erythrocytes per cubic millimeter of ____________.
   C. The life span of an erythrocytes is ____________ days.
4. Leukocytes
   A. Leukocytes are ____________ blood cells
   B. Provide protection against ____________.
   C. There are __________ leukocytes per cubic millimeter of ____________.
5. Neutrophils
   A. Neutrophils are the most common ____________.
   B. Categorized as ____________.
   C. Develop in the ____________ marrow.
6. Eosinophils
   A. Eosinophils are one of the least common ____________.
   B. Categorized as ____________.
   C. Develop in the ____________ marrow.
   D. Engulf and destroy ____________ cells.
   E. Release ____________ chemicals that kill ____________ that invade the body.
7. Basophils
   A. Categorized as ____________.
   B. The nucleus of a basophil has ____________ lobes.
   C. Release ____________ at the site of tissue damage.
8. Lymphocytes
   A. Categorized as ____________ because the granules in their cytoplasm are nearly invisible.
   B. Begin their development in the ____________ marrow.
   C. Lymphocytes are present in the blood and in the ____________ nodes, ____________ tissues, and the organs of the ____________ system.
9. Monocytes
   A. Monocytes are ____________ that engulf and destroy all types of invading microorganisms, cancerous cells, dead leukocytes, and cellular debris.
   B. Found in the ____________ and in the ____________ nodes of the ____________ system.
10. Thrombocytes (Platelets)
   A. Different from other blood cells because they are only _______ ____________.
   B. Active in the ____________ process.
   C. Begin their development in the red marrow as stem cells, which then become ____________.
   D. Thrombocytes are the smallest of all the elements of the ____________.
   E. They are not ____________ cells.
   F. They are critical in ____________, or hemostasis.
   G. Leads to the formation of ____________, which converts fibrinogen to fibrin.
11. Blood Types (List the four blood types.)
   i. ____________________
   ii. ____________________
   iii. ____________________
   iv. ____________________

12. Universal Donor
    A. Because type __________ blood has neither marker __________ nor __________, it will not react with __________ or __________ antibodies.
    B. In an emergency, type __________ blood may be given to a person with any of the other blood types.
    C. A person with type __________ blood has no __________ against the other blood types and, therefore, in an emergency, can receive any type of blood.

13. The Rh Factor
    A. A person with the Rh factor in his or her red blood cells is said to be ______________.
    B. Since this person has the Rh factor, he or she will not make ______________ antibodies.
    C. A person without the Rh factor is Rh ______________ and will produce ______________ antibodies.

III. The Pathology of the Circulatory System

1. Anemia
    A. Anemia is a condition characterized by abnormally ______________ numbers of healthy ______________ blood cells circulating in the body.
    B. Often considered to be the most common dysfunction of the ______________ blood cells.
    C. Affects about ______________ Americans.

2. Common Signs and Symptoms of Anemia
    i. ______________________________
    ii. ______________________________
    iii. ______________________________
    iv. ______________________________
    v. ______________________________
    vi. ______________________________
    vii. ______________________________
    viii. ______________________________
    ix. ______________________________
    x. ______________________________

3. Causes of Anemia
    A. ______________ production of healthy red cells by the bone marrow.
    B. ______________ erythrocyte destruction.
    C. ______________ and ______________ deficiencies in the diet that can also slow down the production of ______________.

4. Iron Deficiency Anemia
    A. Occurs when there is not enough ______________ in the body.
    B. Iron deficiency anemia is the most ______________ type of anemia.
    C. Symptoms include ______________, ______________, ______________, and ______________.

5. Vitamin Deficiency Anemia
    A. Vitamin B12 is essential for normal ______________ production. Some people have difficulty absorbing B12, resulting in a vitamin B12 deficiency, a condition known as ______________ anemia.

6. Hemolytic Anemia
    A. Occurs when there are not enough ______________ blood cells in the blood.
    B. Caused by a ______________ destruction of red blood cells with which the bone marrow cannot keep up.

7. Sickle Cell Anemia
   A. The abnormal ___________ shape and sharp edges of this sickled ___________ are very different from the smooth, rounded contours of a normal erythrocyte.
   B. Repeated sickling causes these fragile ___________ to have a shortened life span, resulting in ___________.
8. Aplastic Anemia
   A. Occurs when the body stops producing enough ___________ blood cells.
   B. Aplastic anemia is a rare and ___________ condition.
   C. Treatment includes ___________, ___________, and a ___________.
9. Aneurysm
   A. An aneurysm is an abnormal ___________ or ___________ of a portion of an ___________, related to a weakness in the vessel wall.
   B. Can be congential or ___________.
   C. High blood pressure and ___________ disease may contribute to the formation of certain types of aneurysms.
10. Treatment for Aneurysms
    A. Surgical intervention may be required to repair the __________ and prevent __________.
    B. Some patients may also be candidates for __________ placement within the affected vessel.
11. Arrhythmias
    A. An arrhythmia is an __________ heartbeat caused by a disturbance of the normal __________ activity of the heart.
    B. Can be __________________, especially when they significantly impact the pumping function of the blood.
12. Causes of Arrhythmias
    i. ______________________________
    ii. ______________________________
    iii. ______________________________
    iv. ______________________________
13. Signs and Symptoms of Arrhythmias
    i. ______________________________
    ii. ______________________________
    iii. ______________________________
    iv. ______________________________
    v. ______________________________
    vi. ______________________________
    vii. ______________________________
14. Treatment for Arrhythmias
    i. ______________________________
    ii. ______________________________
    iii. ______________________________
15. Arteriosclerosis
    A. Often referred to as ______________________________.
    B. Arteriosclerosis is the thickening and loss of ______________ of the ______________.
    C. Causative factors include the following:
       i. ______________________________
       ii. ______________________________
       iii. ______________________________
       iv. ______________________________

16. Symptoms of and Treatment for Arteriosclerosis
    A. Symptoms include:
        i. ______________________________
        ii. ______________________________
        iii. ______________________________
    B. Treatment includes relieving the ______________ and ______________.

17. Atherosclerosis
    A. Narrowing and ______________ of the vessel ______________ of the ______________.
    B. Caused by a buildup of ______________ material and ______________ within the vessel.

18. Cardiogenic Shock
    A. Cardiogenic shock is the collapse of the ______________ system.
    B. Characterized by ______________ and fluid shifting away from the heart.
    C. Shock leads to inefficient ______________ function.

19. Symptoms of and Treatment for Cardiogenic Shock
    A. Symptoms of cardiogenic shock
        i. ______________________________
        ii. ______________________________
        iii. ______________________________
        iv. ______________________________
    B. Treatment for cardiogenic shock
        i. ______________________________
        ii. ______________________________
        iii. ______________________________
        iv. ______________________________

20. Cardiomyopathy
    A. Cardiomyopathy is a disease of the ___________, or heart muscle, resulting in ___________ dysfunction.
    B. Thought to be ___________ and idiopathic.

21. Symptoms of and Treatment for Cardiomyopathy
    A. Signs and symptoms include an enlarged ___________.
    B. Treatment for cardiomyopathy
        i. ______________________________
        ii. ______________________________
        iii. ______________________________

22. Endocarditis
    A. Endocarditis is an inflammation of the ___________ of the heart, including the heart ___________.
    B. Most commonly caused by a ______________ infection.
    C. Frequently affects patients with existing abnormal conditions of the heart ___________.

23. Symptoms of and Treatment for Endocarditis
    A. Symptoms of endocarditis
        i. ______________________________
        ii. ______________________________
        iii. ______________________________
        iv. ______________________________
        v. ______________________________
    B. Treatment generally consists of ___________.

24. Myocarditis

A. Myocarditis is an inflammation of the ____________ layer of the heart.
B. The most common cause is a ____________ infection.

25. Symptoms of and Treatment for Myocarditis

A. Symptoms of myocarditis
   i. ____________
   ii. ____________
   iii. ____________
   iv. ____________
   v. ____________
   vi. ____________
B. The best treatment is the ____________ of the inflammation, bed rest, and a ____________ diet.

26. Pericarditis

A. Pericarditis is an inflammation of the ____________.
B. Most commonly seen as a complication of a ____________ or ____________ infection.

27. Symptoms of and Treatment for Pericarditis

A. Symptoms of pericarditis
   i. ____________
   ii. ____________
   iii. ____________
   iv. ____________
B. Treatment for pericarditis
   i. ____________
   ii. ____________
   iii. ____________

28. Cerebrovascular Accident

A. Occurs when the blood flow to the brain stops, allowing brain cells to ____________.
B. The two types of stroke are ____________ and ____________.

29. Symptoms of a Cerebrovascular Accident

i. ____________
ii. ____________
iii. ____________
iv. ____________
v. ____________

30. Causes of Congestive Heart Failure

i. ____________
ii. ____________
iii. ____________
iv. ____________
v. ____________
vi. ____________
vii. ____________

31. Signs and Symptoms of Congestive Heart Failure

i. ____________
ii. ____________
iii. ____________

32. Treatment for Congestive Heart Failure

i. ______
ii. ______
iii. ______
iv. ______

33. Cor Pulmonale

A. Also known as ______ heart disease.
B. Causes the ______ ventricle to ______.
C. A symptom of cor pulmonale is ______, or an ______ heart.

34. Coronary Heart Disease

A. Also called ______ disease.
B. A ______ of the blood vessels that supply blood and oxygen to the heart muscle.

35. Factors that Increase the Risk of Coronary Heart Disease

i. ______
ii. ______
iii. ______
iv. ______
v. ______
vi. ______
vii. ______
viii. ______

36. Symptoms of and Treatment for Coronary Heart Disease

A. Symptoms of coronary heart disease
   i. ______
   ii. ______
   iii. ______
B. Treatment includes ______ and ______.

37. Myocardial Infarction

A. Affects more than ______ people each year.
B. Occurs when the blood supply to a part of the ______ is severely reduced or stopped.

38. Treatment for Myocardial Infarction

i. ______
ii. ______
iii. ______
iv. ______

39. Leukemia

A. Malignant cancer of the ______ and ______.
B. Involves the uncontrolled growth of ______ cells.
C. Can be acute or ______.

40. Symptoms of Leukemia

i. ______
ii. ______
iii. ______
iv. ______
v. ______
vi. ______
vii. ______
viii. ______

ix. ____
x. ____
xi. ____

41. Treatment for Leukemia

A. ____________ is used to kill leukemia cells with strong anticancer drugs.
B. ____________ therapy is used to kill cancer cells by exposure to high-energy ____________.
C. ____________ transplant

42. Mitral Stenosis

A. Caused by insufficient closing of the ____________.
B. Leads to ____________, or a ____________ backward.
C. May cause a ____________.
D. Treatment includes ____________ to strengthen heart function.

43. Varicose Veins

A. Enlarged walls that are ____________ and ____________ above the surface of the skin.
B. Caused when the ____________ in the veins ____________.
C. Affect ____________ out of ____________ people in the United States.

44. Prevention of Varicose Veins

i. ____
ii. ____
iii. ____
iv. ____
v. ____
vi. ____

45. Symptom Relief of Varicose Veins

i. ____
ii. ____
iii. ____
iv. ____
v. ____

KEY TERMINOLOGY REVIEW

Without using your textbook, write a sentence using the selected vocabulary terms in the correct context.

1. ***Auscultation***

____

____

2. ***Bruit***

____

____

3. ***Bradycardia***

____

____

4. ***Carditis***

____

____

5. *Carotid artery*

6. *Cyanosis*

7. *Cor pulmonale*

8. *Dyspnea*

9. *Hemophilia*

10. *Hypoxia*

11. *Inferior vena cava*

12. *Ischemia*

13. *Occlusion*

14. *Petechiae*

15. *Purkinje fibers*

16. *Sinoatrial node*

17. *Sphyagomanometer*

18. *Superior vena cava*

____

____

19. *Thoracocenesis*

____

____

20. *Thrombophlebitis*

____

____

APPLIED PRACTICE

1. List the primary pulse points of the body.

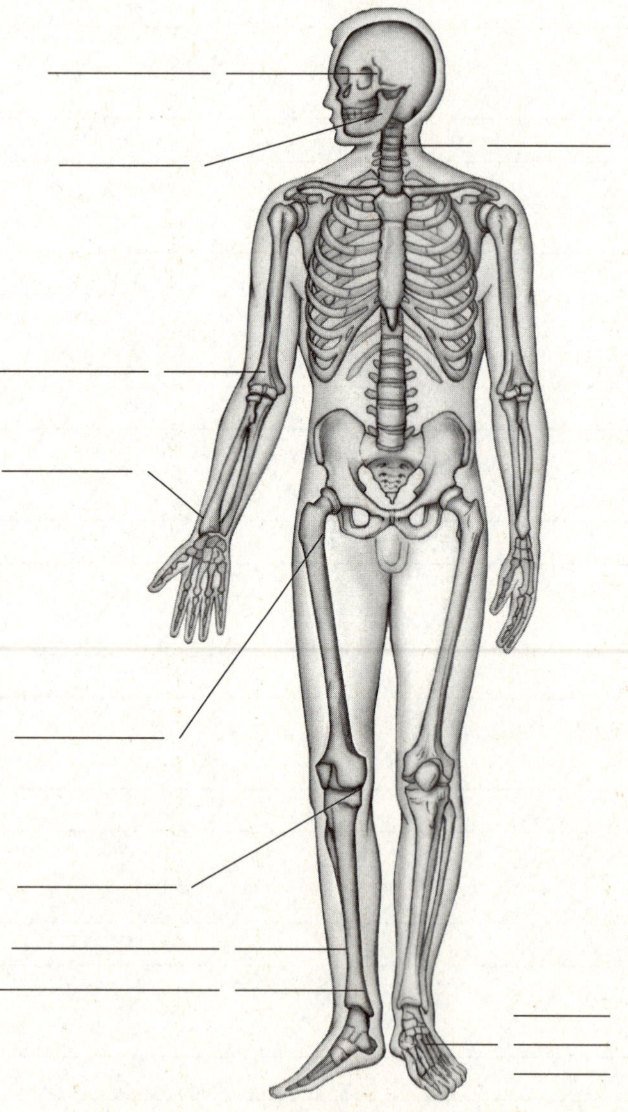

2. Provide the names of the ducts and nodes of the lymphatic system.

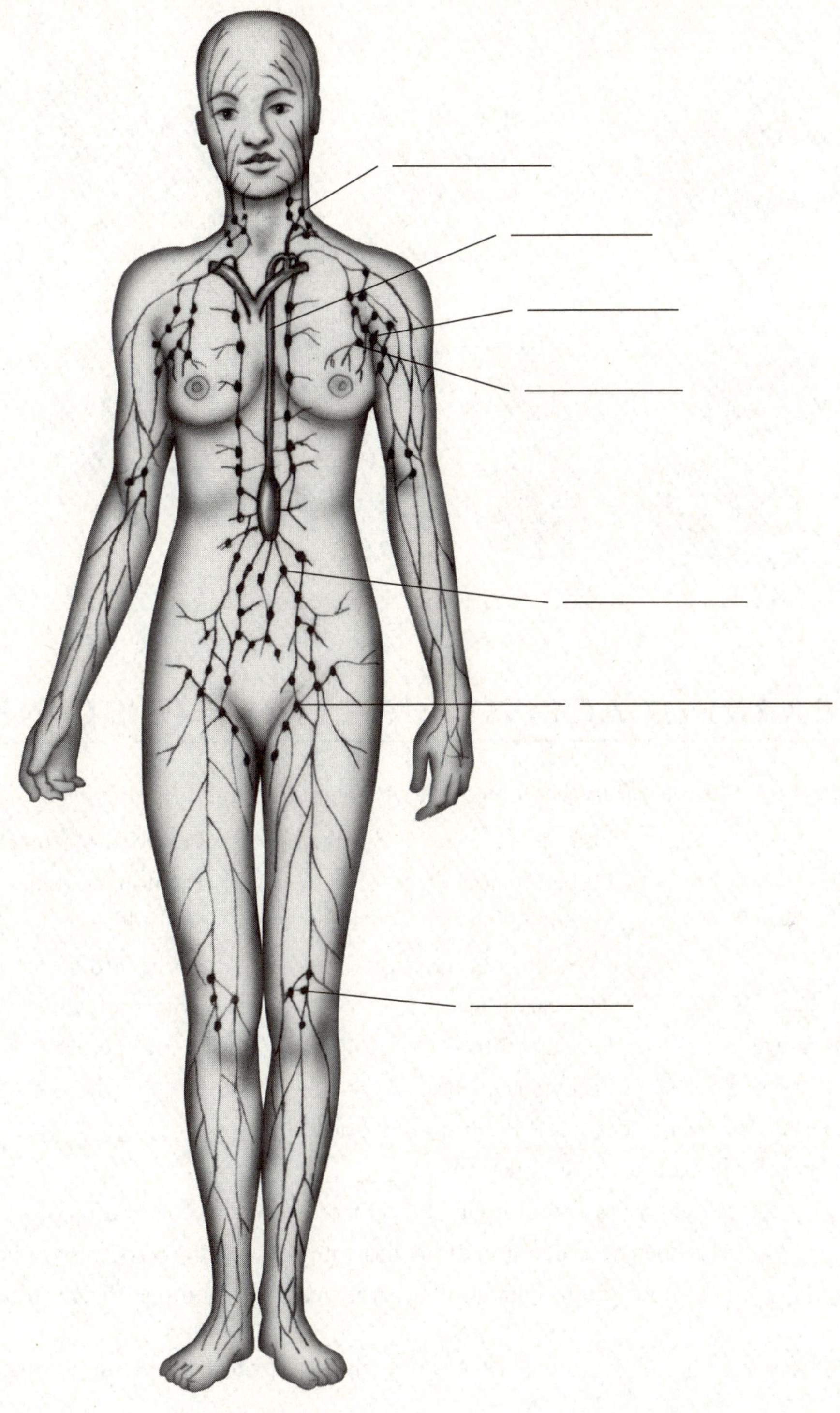

3. Provide the name of each formed element of blood.

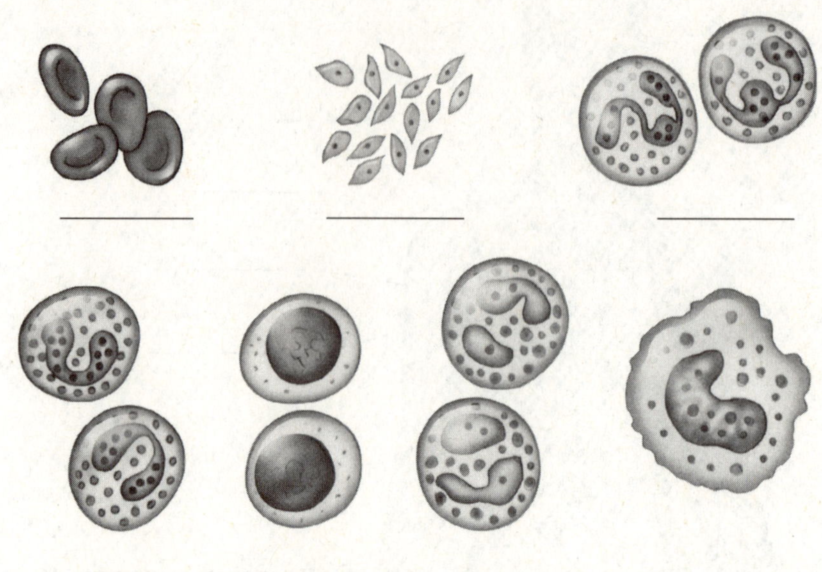

LEARNING ACTIVITY: FILL IN THE BLANK

Using words from the list below, fill in the blanks to complete the following statements.

Agglutination	Flutter	Pulmonary artery
Aneurysm	Hypertension	Pulmonary vein
Buffers	Hypotension	Septum
Cardic arrest	Myocardial infarction	Tachycardia
Cardic tamponade	Myocardium	Tricuspid valve
Congestive heart failure	Pericardium	Venipuncture
Fibrillation	Prehypertension	

1. A systolic pressure of greater than 120 is considered borderline ________________.
2. The middle layer, or heart muscle, is called the ________________.
3. ________________ is the process of removing blood from the veins for examination.
4. ________________ is defined as congestion of the heart muscle and the restriction of heart movement.
5. ________________ is a condition in which the heart is unable to pump sufficient blood to the other organs.
6. Symptoms of a ________________ include a squeezing pain or heavy pressure in the middle of the chest.
7. When the electrical system has problems, ________________ can occur.
8. The AV bundle extends from the AV node into the intraventricular ________________.
9. The ________________ is the outer lining of the heart.
10. ________________ occurs when an antigen on the surface of red blood cells binds to antibodies in the plasma.

11. On its return from the lungs, oxygenated blood enters the left atrium via the ________________.
12. When an occlusion leads to the heart stopping, it is known as ________________.
13. Blood pressure ranging from 120/80 to 139/89 is a symptom of ________________.
14. The blood contains ________________, which are mechanisms within the blood that balance the pH level.
15. ________________ is an abnormally fast heartbeat of more than 100 beats per minute.
16. ________________ is an abnormal condition in which a person's blood pressure is much lower than usual.
17. After going through the ________________, the blood enters the right ventricle.
18. Common locations for an ________________ include the aorta, brain, leg, and intestine.
19. Blood leaves the right ventricle through the pulmonary valve to go to the lungs, via the ________________.
20. If the heart trembles, it is known as ________________.

CRITICAL THINKING

Answer the following questions to the best of your ability. Utilize the textbook as a reference.

1. You are working at the front desk and looking out at the patients who have been waiting for their appointments. One man appears to be holding his left hand in front of his chest, he seems to be SOB, and his face looks sweaty or clammy. What is your first thought about this patient? Describe what the danger signs are to you even though the patient has not come up to the desk to voice a complaint about how he is feeling. What might you ask the patient and how would you handle this situation?

____

____

____

____

____

2. You are performing an EKG. As it is printing, you notice that there is a normal waveform and complex, but the number of beats per minute is more than 100. What do you think the problem could be? Speculate on what the doctor might diagnose.

____

____

____

3. When providing care to a patient, how can you help to ensure that their privacy is protected?

RESEARCH ACTIVITY

Utilize Internet search engines to research the following topics and write a brief description of what you find. It is important to utilize reputable websites.

1. Visit www.americanheart.org and navigate through the website. Pay particular attention to the link entitled "For Healthcare Professionals". Explain what information you think is most useful in this section and why.

CHAPTER 28
The Immune System

CHAPTER OUTLINE

General review of the chapter:

Anatomy of the Immune System
The Immune System and the Body's Defenses
Common Disorders Associated with the Immune System

STUDENT STUDY GUIDE

Use the following guide to assist in your learning of the concepts from the chapter.

I. The Immune System

1. The Composition of the Immune System
   i. ______________________________
   ii. ______________________________
   iii. ______________________________
   iv. ______________________________
   v. ______________________________
2. The Structures Central to the Immune System
   A. Central lymphoid tissue is composed of __________ __________.
   B. Peripheral lymphoid tissue consists of the __________ __________, __________, and __________________ lymphoid tissue.
3. The Immune System
   A. Operates __________ the body.
   B. The structures are part of the __________ system, which is a subsystem of the __________ system.
   C. The primary function of the lymphatic system is to defend the body against invasion by pathogens such as __________, __________, and __________.
   D. Through the immune response, the __________, __________, and __________ work together to attack organisms and substances that invade body systems and cause disease.
   E. __________, or white blood cells (WBCs), combine to seek out and destroy harmful organisms.
   F. ________________ medications and __________ can suppress the immune system.
4. The Bone Marrow
   A. Comprises the __________ __________ tissue.
   B. Contains __________ cells that create all of the cells that make up the tissues and structures of the immune system.

C. Produces __________ __________ cells, __________ __________ cells, and platelets, along with _____ cells and natural killer cells.

5. The Location and Purpose of the Thymus Gland

   A. Comprises the __________ __________ tissue.
   B. Located posterior to the __________, in the anterior __________.
   C. Manufactures infection-fighting _____ cells and helps distinguish normal _____ cells from those that attack the body's own tissues.

6. The Compartments of the Thymus Gland

   A. Consist of an outer __________ and an internal __________.
   B. __________ lymphoid cells enter the cortex, reproduce, and mature; they then move to the medulla where they reenter the ____________.

7. The Peripheral Lymphatic System

   A. Consists of the __________ __________, __________, and other lymphoid tissue.
   B. Lymphatic __________, lymphatic __________, and lymphatic __________ are part of the peripheral lymphatic system.

8. Lymph Nodes

   A. Take many different __________ and __________.
   B. Most are __________ __________ and are about 1 inch long.
   C. They are covered with a __________, __________ capsule.
   D. The node is subdivided into different compartments by ________________ ________________ .

9. B Lymphocytes

   A. The __________ __________ are the primary locations where B lymphocytes reproduce prolifically.
   B. Responsible for the production of circulating __________.
   C. Each unique type of B cell produces only one type of __________.
   D. When an __________ enters the body, these B lymphocytes rapidly undergo __________ and divide.

10. The Spleen

   A. Located in the __________ of the abdomen.
   B. Consists of lymphatic tissue that is highly __________ by blood vessels.
   C. The spleen's blood vessels are lined with __________, which swallow and digest debris in the blood such as worn-out red blood cells and __________.

11. Tonsils

   A. Located in the depressions of the mucous membranes of the __________ and the __________.
   B. The function of the tonsils is to __________ __________ and aid in the __________ of white blood cells.

12. Phagocytes

   A. Phagocytes are a type of white blood cell that attacks the __________ __________.
   B. A number of different cells are considered to be phagocytes, but the most common are __________, which primarily fight bacteria.

13. Lymphocytes

   A. A type of white blood cell that allows the body to __________ and __________ previous invading organisms.
   B. Originates in the __________ __________ and either stays there and matures into B cells or moves to the __________ __________, where they mature into T cells.

14. B and T Lymphocytes
    A. B lymphocytes and T lymphocytes have __________ __________ within the immune system.
    B. B lymphocytes seek out invading __________ and send __________ to attach onto them.
    C. T cells __________ the organisms that the B lymphocytes have __________.
15. Antibodies
    A. Immunoglobulins are __________ that function as antibodies.
    B. The terms antibody and __________ are often used interchangeably.
    C. Antibodies are found in __________, __________ __________, and many secretions.
    D. Structurally, antibodies are globulins, which means that they are __________ and __________ by plasma cells derived from the B cells of the immune system.
16. The B Cells of the Immune System
    A. Activated upon __________ to their specific antigen and ________________ into plasma cells.
    B. Although antibodies can recognize an antigen and lock onto it, they are not capable of __________ it; that is the job of the _____ cells.
17. T Cells
    A. T cells are a part of the system that destroys antigens which have been tagged by antibodies or cells that have been infected or __________ __________.
    B. Assist other cells, such as __________.
    C. Antibodies can __________ toxins produced by different organisms.
    D. Antibodies can activate a group of proteins called __________, which are also part of the immune system.
18. Innate Immunity
    A. Everyone is born with innate, or __________, immunity.
    B. Provided, in part, by the external barriers of the body, including the __________ and __________ __________ that line the __________, __________, and ____________ tract.
    C. If this outer defensive wall is broken, such as by a cut in the skin, __________ __________ __________ on the skin attack any invading microorganisms.
19. Active Immunity
    A. Active immunity is __________.
    B. The individual has lifelong ***protection*** against the disease.

II. The Pathology of the Immune System
1. Allergies
    A. An __________ is any substance capable of causing an allergic reaction.
    B. Most allergic reactions are a result of an immune system that responds to a __________ __________.
    C. When a harmless substance such as pollen is encountered by a person who is allergic to that substance, the immune system may react dramatically by producing __________ that attack the allergen.
2. Anaphylaxis
    A. Sometimes occurs after a __________ or __________ is introduced into the patient.
    B. During anaphylaxis, __________ of the neck can cause breathing to be impeded, which can lead to __________ and death.
3. Signs and Symptoms of Allergies
    i. ____
    ii. ____

iii. ______________________________

iv. ______________________________

v. ______________________________

vi. ______________________________

vii. ______________________________

4. Treatments for Allergies

   A. __________ or __________ help combat allergy symptoms.
   B. Reactions to certain __________ __________ may be treated by the use of air filters and dehumidifiers.
   C. Alternative treatment includes __________ and __________ treatment.
   D. In severe cases, optimal treatment may be identified only through __________ __________ __________ and desensitization.
   E. If anaphylaxis occurs, it is important for the physician to immediately order medications (such as __________) that will stop the process.

5. Cancer

   A. A group of many related diseases that all pertain to __________.
   B. Cancer cells are unlike normal cells, which grow and, through __________, divide. Normal cells "know" when to stop growing.

6. Cancer Cells

   A. Do not __________ or __________ like normal cells; they grow and spread very rapidly.
   B. Cancer cells continue to __________ and __________ erratically and do not die.
   C. They are not well __________, nor do they work on behalf of the body.
   D. They also make use of the body's resources at the expense of __________ cells.
   E. Usually, cancer cells clump together to form __________.
   F. A __________ tumor can destroy the __________ cells around it, damaging the body's healthy tissue.
   G. Sometimes cancer cells break away from the __________ __________ and travel to other areas of the body, where they keep growing, and form new tumors; this process is called __________.

7. Signs and Symptoms of Cancer

   i. ______________________________

   ii. ______________________________

   iii. ______________________________

   iv. ______________________________

   v. ______________________________

   vi. ______________________________

8. Treatment for Cancer

   A. __________, __________, __________, or a combination of all three
   B. The choice of treatment generally depends on the __________ of cancer and the __________ to which the cancer has spread within the body.

9. Surgery

   A. Surgery is the __________ form of cancer treatment.
   B. _____ out of every _____ persons with cancer may require surgery to remove it.
   C. During surgery, some __________ cells or tissue may also be removed to ensure that all of the cancer is removed.

10. Chemotherapy

   A. Medicines, which are sometimes taken in pill form but are more often given __________
   B. Usually given over a number of __________ or __________.

C. Often, a permanent IV catheter, called a ____________, is placed under the skin into one of the larger blood vessels of the __________ __________.

11. Radiation Therapy

A. Uses high-energy waves, such as __________, to damage and destroy cancer cells.
B. Causes tumors to __________ and, in some cases, __________ completely.
C. Radiation therapy is one of the most __________ treatments for cancer.

12. Immunotherapy

A. Immunotherapy is the most __________ form of cancer therapy.
B. It is a technique that involves creating __________ __________ __________ that are "programmed" to specifically target cancer cells.
C. Empowers the body's own __________ __________ to target only cancer cells, rather than also destroying healthy cells.

13. Possible Causes of Chronic Fatigue Syndrome

i. ____________________
ii. ____________________
iii. ____________________
iv. ____________________
v. ____________________

14. Signs and Symptoms of Chronic Fatigue Syndrome

i. ____________________
ii. ____________________
iii. ____________________

15. Treatment for Chronic Fatigue Syndrome

A. Generally begins with a thorough evaluation of the patient's __________ __________ history.
B. Both the _______ and ________ of sleep are important.
C. Educating the patient, with emphasis on becoming an __________ __________ in the treatment regimen. is extremely important in the treatment of CFS.

16. Infectious Mononucleosis

A. Characterized by an increase in white blood cells that are ____________, that is, containing a ________ ________.
B. Often develops in young adults between the ages of _____ and _____.
C. Commonly referred to as ________________.
D. The _________ period for mononucleosis is generally between 4 and 8 weeks.

17. Signs and Symptoms of Mononucleosis

i. ____________________
ii. ____________________
iii. ____________________
iv. ____________________

18. Treatment for Mononucleosis

A. Getting plenty of ______.
B. Gargling with __________ or using _______________ to soothe the throat.
C. Taking _____________ and _____________ medications to reduce fever and relieve sore throat and headache.

19. Types of Lymphedema

A. Primary lymphedema can be ________ and has several stages.
B. Secondary lymphedema is generally caused by an ____________ of or __________ to the lymph system that interrupts the normal lymphatic flow.

20. Causes of Primary Lymphedema
    i. ______________________________
    ii. ______________________________
    iii. ______________________________

21. Causes of Secondary Lymphedema
    i. ______________________________
    ii. ______________________________
    iii. ______________________________

22. Treatment for Lymphedema
    A. ______________________ (CDT) and ______________________ (MDT)
    B. CDT is used primarily in the treatment of lymphedema and ______________________.
    C. Other treatments for lymphedema
        i. ______________________________
        ii. ______________________________
        iii. ______________________________
        iv. ______________________________
        v. ______________________________

23. Rheumatoid Arthritis
    A. One out of every ______ persons suffers from chronic rheumatoid arthritis.
    B. Individuals with a family history of rheumatoid arthritis are ______ times more likely to develop the disease.
    C. Occurs when the body's immune defenses attack tissue in the ________, leading to pain and degeneration of the ____________________.
    D. The disease and its treatment also increase __________; patients often have a shorter life expectancy than their healthy peers.

24. Signs and Symptoms of and Treatment for Rheumatoid Arthritis
    A. Signs and symptoms include pain and ___________ in the joints.
    B. Treatment is based on medication regimens and educating the patient on how to ______________________.
    C. Drugs are used to _______ and _______ the symptoms, and help the patient to function at a more productive level.

25. Systemic Lupus Erythematosus
    A. Called a __________ disorder because its effects may appear in many parts of the body.
    B. Ninety percent of patients with SLE are women, who are generally diagnosed before ___________.
    C. There is a ______________ as well; the risk of developing SLE rises if a close family member has it.
    D. It is a chronic, lifelong condition with periods of ___________ and __________.

26. Possible Signs and Symptoms of Systemic Lupus Erythematosus
    A. _________ and ______ in the joints.
    B. General _________, _________, _________, and _________.
    C. _________ (discoid) lesions that are raised and scaly.
    D. _________, or inflamed blood vessels, characterized by red marks in any area of the body.

E. Sometimes, ________________ appear, especially on the leg, where they may develop into _________.

F. In some people, the tips of the fingers and toes may develop ____________________.

27. Treatment of Systemic Lupus Erythematosus

A. Usually aimed at reducing the immune response using drugs such as ____________.
B. The course of the disease for a given individual is difficult to predict, but with immediate treatment, most patients can expect to have a __________________.

KEY TERMINOLOGY REVIEW

Match the vocabulary term to the correct definition below.

a. Acquired active immunity
b. Active immunity
c. Adenoids
d. Allergy
e. Anaphylaxis
f. Antibodies
g. Antigen
h. Artificially acquired active immunity
i. Autoimmune diseases
j. B lymphocytes
k. Chemotherapy
l. Chronic fatigue syndrome (CFS)
m. Complement
n. Cortex
o. Germinal centers
p. Immune response
q. immune system
r. Immunosuppressants
s. Infectious mononucleosis
t. Lymphedema
u. Medulla
v. Metastasis
w. Natural immunity
x. Neutrophils
y. Oncogenes
z. Passive immunity
aa. Radiation therapy
bb. Rheumatoid arthritis (RA)
cc. Systemic lupus erythematosus (SLE)
dd. T lymphocytes
ee. Trabeculae
ff. Vaccine

1. ______________ Medications that suppress the immune system.
2. ______________ Has no single known cause, although some authorities believe that it is a condition shared by many different underlying diseases rather than a separate disorder.
3. ______________ Contains fragments of a disease organism or small amounts of a weakened disease organism.
4. ______________ Occurs when the person is exposed to a live pathogen, develops the disease, and becomes immune as a result of the primary immune response.
5. ______________ The process wherein cancer cells break away from the original tumor and travel to other areas.
6. ______________ The cells responsible for the production of circulating antibodies, which are specialized proteins that lock onto specific antigens.
7. ______________ An extreme, often life-threatening, response to an antigen.

8. _______________ Uses high-energy waves, such as X-rays, to damage and destroy cancer cells.

9. _______________ An inherited immunity to certain diseases.

10. _______________ Inward-pointing compartments that make up part of the lymph nodes.

11. _______________ Induced by a vaccine, which is a substance that contains the antigen and that stimulates a primary response against the antigen without causing symptoms of the disease.

12. _______________ One set of three that make up the tonsils.

13. _______________ A viral infection caused by the Epstein-Barr virus (EBV).

14. _______________ Cells that circulate through the lymph nodes, the bloodstream, and the lymphatic ducts to seek out any infection.

15. _______________ A hypersensitivity to a normally harmless substance.

16. _______________ Along with the medulla, it is one of two basic parts of the lymph nodes.

17. _______________ Consists of tissues, organs, and physiological processes that identify abnormal cells, foreign substances, and foreign tissues, and defends against substances that might be harmful to the body.

18. _______________ An autoimmune disorder wherein people produce abnormal antibodies in their blood that target tissues within their own body instead of foreign infectious agents.

19. _______________ The most common type of phagocytes, these attack an invading organism.

20. _______________ The primary locations where B lymphocytes reproduce prolifically.

21. _______________ The production of immunity by infection or with a vaccine.

22. _______________ An example of a chronic autoimmune disease.

23. _______________ A group of proteins activated by antibodies that assist in destroying bacteria, viruses, or infected cells.

24. _______________ "Borrowed" from another source; lasts for only a short time.

25. _______________ A foreign substance that invades the body.

26. _______________ The response in the body that creates autoimmune diseases, in which the body attacks itself.

27. _______________ A treatment where anticancer drugs are used to treat the cancerous growth or tumor.

28. _______________ The genes controlling cell growth and multiplication.

29. _______________ A condition that results from a damaged or dysfunctional lymphatic system.

30. _______________ Along with the cortex, it is one of two basic parts of the lymph node.

31. _______________ They are specialized proteins that lock onto specific antigens.

32. _______________ Occurs when the cells, tissues, and organs that make up the immune system work together to attack organisms and substances that invade body systems and cause disease.

APPLIED PRACTICE

1. Label the components of the lymphatic system.

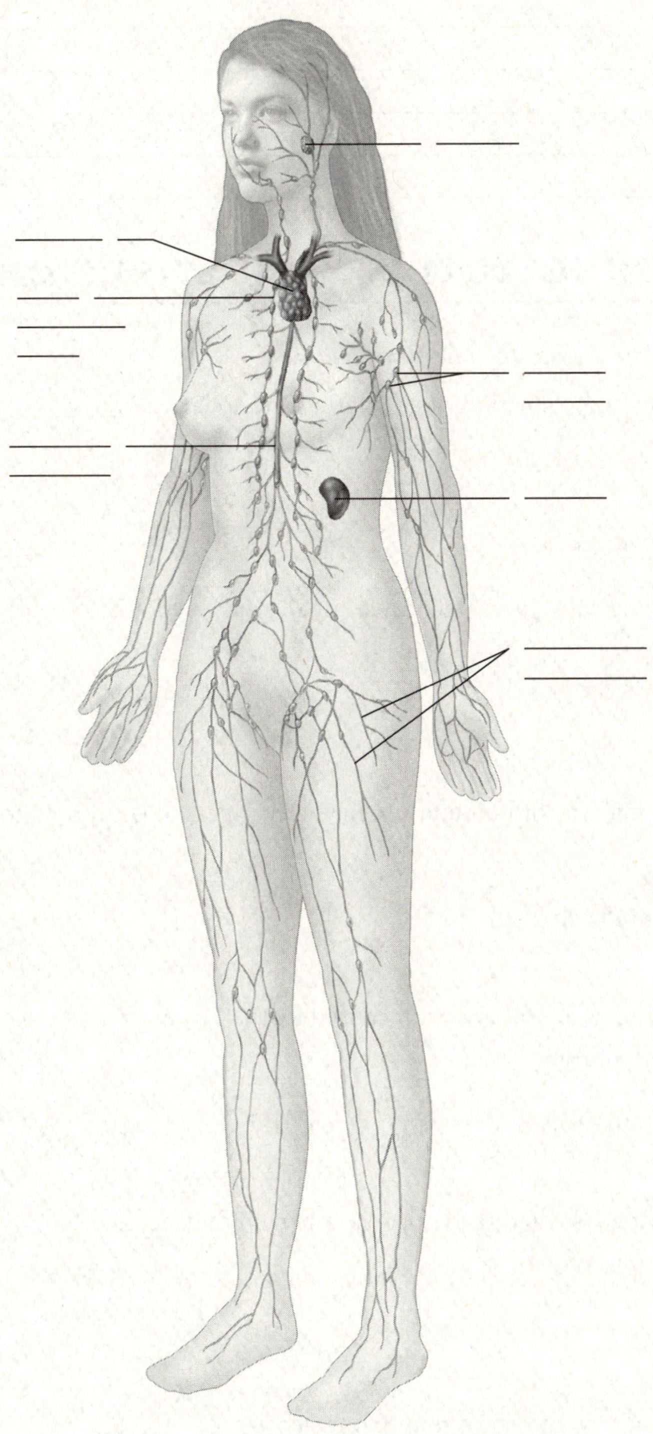

2. A patient has just been diagnosed with several allergies. It is her first visit and you are providing patient education and various instructions. How would you explain (in layman's terms) antigens and allergens to the patient?

____

____

____

____

____

____

LEARNING ACTIVITY: MULTIPLE CHOICE

Circle the correct answer to each of the questions below.

1. The cells responsible for production of circulating antibodies are ____________________.
   a. T cells
   b. B cells
   c. A cells
   d. None of the above

2. Which of the following substances may cause an allergic reaction?
   a. Dust
   b. Mold
   c. Pollen
   d. All of the above

3. Which of the following type of immunity occur when a person is exposed to a live pathogen.
   a. Active
   b. Acquired active
   c. Artificially acquired active
   d. Natural

4. Which of the following is a viral infection caused by the Epstein-Barr virus?
   a. Chronic fatigue syndrome
   b. Lymphedema
   c. Infectious mononucleosis
   d. Systemic lupus erythematosus

5. Which of the following risk factors predispose a person to cancer?
   a. Suppressed immune system
   b. Exposure to radiation
   c. Viruses
   d. All of the above

6. Which statement is false with regard to mononucleosis?
   a. It is caused by a herpes virus.
   b. It is much more severe in young children.
   c. It is characterized by an increase in white blood cells.
   d. It is often spread through saliva.

7. Which of the following allow the body to remember and recognize previous invading organisms?
   a. Lymphocytes
   b. Neutrophils
   c. Phagocytes
   d. Leukocytes

8. When an antigen is detected, several types of cells work together to recognize and respond to it. These cells trigger the lymphocytes to produce antibodies. This process is known as ________________.
   a. active immunity
   b. acquired active immunity
   c. humoral immunity
   d. None of the above

9. The thymus gland enlarges during ______________.
   a. birth
   b. childhood
   c. puberty
   d. None of the above

10. Which of the following contains stem cells that create all the cells that make up the tissues and structures of the immune system?
    a. Bone marrow
    b. Liver
    c. Thymus gland
    d. Lymph nodes

CRITICAL THINKING

Answer the following questions to the best of your ability. Utilize the textbook as a reference.

1. Why do the frequency and severity of infections and incidence of autoimmune disease generally increase in elderly persons?

   ____

   ____

   ____

   ____

2. While at work, why should medical assistants not wear strong-smelling perfumes or aftershave lotions?

   ____

   ____

   ____

   ____

RESEARCH ACTIVITY

Utilize Internet search engines to research the following topics and write a brief description of what you find. It is important to utilize reputable websites.

1. Research an autoimmune disease that is of interest to you. Identify the signs and symptoms of the disease, how a diagnosis is made, and treatment options. Also, research support groups, societies, or foundations for that disease. Write an essay on your findings and be sure to cite the websites where you found your information.

Chapter 29
The Respiratory System

CHAPTER OUTLINE

General review of the chapter:

Overview of the Respiratory System
Organs of the Respiratory System
Mechanism of Breathing
Respiratory Volumes and Capacities
Common Disorders Associated with the Respiratory System

STUDENT STUDY GUIDE

Use the following guide to assist in your learning of the concepts from the chapter.

I. The Respiratory System

1. The Process of Breathing
   A. When we breathe, we inhale __________ and exhale ________________.
   B. Respiration is achieved through the __________, ______________, ______________, ___________, and ______________.
   C. Oxygen enters the respiratory system through the __________ and the __________.
2. The Path Taken by Oxygen During Breathing (List the path that oxygen takes during breathing.)
   i. Oxygen passes through the ________.
   ii. And through the ________, where speech sounds are produced.
   iii. Through the lungs and the bronchioles that connect to tiny sacs, the ________
   iv. After the gas exchange, it then diffuses through the ________ into the ________ ________.
   v. The waste-rich blood from the veins releases _______ _______ into the _______.
   vi. The ________ helps pump air into and carbon dioxide out of the _______.
   vii. Upon ________, carbon dioxide follows the reverse of the path taken by oxygen flowing into the lungs.
3. The Functions of the Nose
   A. __________ and moistens inhaled air.
   B. Warms the ______.
   C. Assists with _________.
4. The Internal Structure of the Nose
   A. The septum is a ________ structure.
   B. The septum is lined with ________ membrane.
   C. The conchae connects the ________ tube, the ________, and the ________ duct.
   D. The palatine bone of the skull makes up the ________ palate and separates the nose from the ________.

5. The Pharynx
   A. The pharynx is a ____________________ tube that is about _____ inches long.
   B. Contains the ____________.
   C. Consists of three parts: the ________________, the ________________, and the ________________.

6. The Larynx (The "Voice Box")
   A. The epiglottic cartilage, also called the __________________, closes over the ____________ during swallowing to keep food out of the ____________.
   B. The cricoid cartilage serves as a landmark for performing a ______________________ when the airway is obstructed.

7. The Trachea
   A. The trachea is a cartilaginous tube about ____ inch wide and ______ inches long that extends between the _________ and the main _________.
   B. The interior of the trachea is lined with ________ _____________ and __________ that trap foreign matter.
   C. The most important function of the trachea is to serve as an __________ ____________ through which air reaches the lungs.
   D. The epiglottis is a flap of __________ that covers the trachea when swallowing occurs to prevent food from entering the trachea.

8. The Main Branches of the Trachea
   A. The main branches of the trachea that extend into the lungs are called the ____________.
   B. The right bronchus is the __________, ___________ branch located along the ________ side of the heart.
   C. The left bronchus is __________ and more ____________.
   D. After entering the lungs at the hilum, the __________ subdivide into the ____________ tree, which continues to branch out into smaller and smaller branches called _______________.

9. Alveoli
   A. The alveoli are small air _____ at the terminal end of the _______________.
   B. They _________ and __________ with inhalation and exhalation.
   C. They are surrounded by a network of _______________ for gas exchange.

10. The Structure of the Lungs
    A. The lungs contain ___________, ____________, and ____________.
    B. The lungs are spongy, __________, and highly ____________.

11. The Functions of the Lungs
    i. ____
    ii. ____
    iii. ____

12. External Respiration (List and explain the elements of external respiration.)
    i. ____
    ii. ____
    iii. ____

13. The Action of the Diaphragm
    A. ___________ and moves downward.
    B. Causes a ___________ in pressure, or __________ thoracic pressure, within the chest cavity.
    C. Air enters the lungs to __________ the pressure during ____________.

14. Intercostal Muscles
    A. External intercostal muscles assist ______________, raise the ______ ______, and enlarge the __________ cavity.

B. Internal intercostal muscles assist ____________, reduce the size of the __________ cavity, and force air from the __________.

15. Respiratory Volume and Capacity

A. ______________ function tests are used to measure lung _________ and ______________.

B. Such tests are used in human ____________ testing.

16. Types of Lung Volume (Explain each type.)

A. Tidal volume: ______________________________

B. Inspiratory reserve volume: ______________________________

C. Expiratory reserve volume: ______________________________

D. Residual volume: ______________________________

17. Types of Lung Capacity (Explain each type.)

A. Inspiratory capacity: ______________________________

B. Vital capacity: ______________________________

C. Functional residual capacity: ______________________________

D. Total lung capacity: ______________________________

18. Other Respiratory Measurements (Explain each type.)

A. Respiratory rate: ______________________________

B. Minute ventilation: ______________________________

C. Dead space: ______________________________

D. Alveolar ventilation: ______________________________

II. The Pathology of the Respiratory System

1. Asthma

A. Asthma is a chronic ____________ disease of the ____________.

B. Causes of asthma

i. Irritations that cause ________ and

ii. Affect the _______ and/or _________ _____,

iii. Resulting in _______, which adds to the irritation.

C. Treatment includes an ____________ for acute episodes and long-term ____________ for the prevention of episodes.

2. Chronic Obstructive Pulmonary Disease (COPD)

A. COPD is a combination of related diseases—chronic __________ and ________________.

B. ____________ is a major cause.

C. Air and other __________ may increase risk.

D. A diagnosis is made through ____________ and ____________.

E. Signs and symptoms of chronic obstructive pulmonary disease

i. ______________________________

ii. ______________________________

iii. ______________________________

iv. ______________________________

F. Treatment for chronic obstructive pulmonary disease

i. ______________________________

ii. ______________________________

iii. ______________________________

iv. ______________________________

3. Bronchitis

A. Bronchitis is a respiratory disease in which the _________ ________ in the _________ passages become ________.

B. As the irritated __________ swells and grows thicker, it narrows or shuts off the tiny airways to the ________.

4. Signs and Symptoms of Acute Bronchitis
   i. ____________________
   ii. ____________________
   iii. ____________________
   iv. ____________________
   v. ____________________
   vi. ____________________

5. Signs and Symptoms of Chronic Bronchitis
   A. A persistent cough that produces __________, white, or __________ phlegm.
   B. Sometimes ____________ and breathlessness.
   C. The symptoms of chronic bronchitis are worsened by ______ ______________.

6. Treatment for Acute Bronchitis
   A. Conventional treatment for acute bronchitis
      i. ____________________
      ii. ____________________
      iii. ____________________
      iv. ____________________

7. Emphysema
   A. Emphysema is a long-term, ____________ lung disease in which the _________ that support the physical shape and function of the _______ are destroyed.
   B. Deterioration is _________ and may go unnoticed.
   C. ____________ smoking is by far the most common cause.

8. Risk Factors for Emphysema
   i. ____________________
   ii. ____________________
   iii. ____________________
   iv. ____________________
   v. ____________________
   vi. ____________________

9. Signs and Symptoms of Emphysema
   i. ____________________
   ii. ____________________
   iii. ____________________

10. Treatment for Emphysema
   i. ____________________
   ii. ____________________
   iii. ____________________
   iv. ____________________
   v. ____________________

11. The Common Cold
   A. A common cold is an inflammation of the _____________ respiratory tract.
   B. Many cold viruses are highly _______________.
   C. The common cold can be spread by ________.

12. Signs and Symptoms of the Common Cold
   i. ____________________
   ii. ____________________

iii. ______________________
iv. ______________________
v. ______________________
vi. ______________________
vii. ______________________
viii. ______________________
ix. ______________________
x. ______________________
xi. ______________________

13. Treatment for the Common Cold
    A. Antibiotics are __________ against cold viruses.
    B. Over-the-counter cold preparations do not cure a common cold or __________ its duration.
    C. For fever, sore throat, and headache, mild _______ __________ may be helpful.
    D. For a runny nose and nasal congestion, ________________ or ________________ may be useful.

14. Measures for Slowing the Spread of the Common Cold
    i. ______________________
    ii. ______________________
    iii. ______________________
    iv. ______________________

15. Hay Fever
    A. Hay fever is also called _________ ___________ ___________ or pollinosis.
    B. It is a seasonal allergy in which the __________ ___________ of the nose and eyes become ___________.
    C. About _____ million Americans experience hay fever symptoms each month.

16. Hay Fever
    A. Symptoms of hay fever
        i. ______________________
        ii. ______________________
        iii. ______________________
        iv. ______________________
        v. ______________________
        vi. ______________________
    B. Treatment for hay fever
        i. ______________________
        ii. ______________________
        iii. ______________________

17. Influenza
    A. Influenza is an illness caused by ______________ that infect the respiratory tract.
    B. It is often more serious than the __________ __________.
    C. Most people who get the flu recover completely in ____ to ____ weeks.

18. Signs and Symptoms of Influenza
    i. ______________________
    ii. ______________________
    iii. ______________________
    iv. ______________________
    v. ______________________

19. The Flu Vaccine
    A. The flu vaccine is the best defense against ____________________.

B. The flu vaccine should be received by ___________________, the _______________, those who are __________________, and _______________.

20. Lung Cancer

A. Lung cancer is the leading cause of _________ deaths in both women and men in the United States and throughout the world.

B. ___________ percent of the cases occur in __________ and former ___________.

C. Other causes are ___________, ____________________, and __________ exposure.

21. Treatment for Lung Cancer

i. ______________________________

ii. ______________________________

iii. ______________________________

22. Pleurisy

A. Pleurisy is an _____________ of the __________ that surrounds and protects the lungs.

B. Causes of pleurisy

i. ______________________________

ii. ______________________________

iii. ______________________________

iv. ______________________________

C. Symptoms of pleurisy

i. ______________________________

ii. ______________________________

iii. ______________________________

iv. ______________________________

v. ______________________________

D. Treatment includes _________________ drugs and _________ medicine.

23. Pneumonia

A. Pneumonia is an inflammation of the lung or lungs caused by __________, _________, ____________, or ___________________.

B. ________________ *pneumoniae* is the most common bacteria.

C. Symptoms of pneumonia

i. ______________________________

ii. ______________________________

iii. ______________________________

D. Treatment for pneumonia

i. ______________________________

ii. ______________________________

iii. ______________________________

24. Legionnaire's Disease

A. Legionnaire's disease is a type of __________________.

B. Usually affects ____________ or __________________ persons.

C. Caused by the ____________ germ, which is spread throughout ____________.

25. Pneumothorax

A. Occurs when air enters the chest _________ of the lungs.

B. Occurs most frequently when the lung has been _________ through trauma.

C. Signs and symptoms are _____________, _________________, _________________, and ______________.

D. Treatment must be given quickly to prevent ______________ of the heart and lungs.

26. Pulmonary Edema

A. Pulmonary edema is a condition in which _______ accumulates in the lungs.

B. Can be a __________ condition, or it can develop suddenly and quickly become life threatening.
C. Most cases are caused by a failure of the heart's ________ chamber, the left ________, to pump adequately.
D. Symptoms include shortness of breath with ___________, respiratory distress after ________, ___________ breathing, and coughing.
E. Treatment must be __________ to reduce the amount of fluid.

27. Pulmonary Embolism
   A. A pulmonary embolism is a ______ clot that travels to the ___________.
   B. The result is a __________ infarct.
   C. Causes include extended periods of ___________, surgery or ____________, obesity, and ________ disease.
   D. Symptoms of a pulmonary embolism
      i. ____________________
      ii. ____________________
      iii. ____________________
      iv. ____________________
      v. ____________________
      vi. ____________________
   E. Treatment includes medications to eliminate the _____ or thin the blood and ______ the blood pressure.

28. Sinusitis
   A. Sinusitis is an infection of the ___________ of the sinuses.
   B. Infection occurs because of lack of ___________.
   C. Usually caused by a _______ infection, a ______, or a ___________ infection.
   D. Symptoms include ______ and __________ in the facial area and green or ________ nasal discharge.
   E. Treatment includes __________, moist heat for _________, and prevention of sinus _____.

29. Tuberculosis
   A. Caused by the _________________ tuberculosis complex of bacteria.
   B. Individuals become infected by inhaling __________ from an infected person.
   C. Symptoms of tuberculosis
      i. ____________________
      ii. ____________________
      iii. ____________________
      iv. ____________________
      v. ____________________
      vi. ____________________
      vii. ____________________

KEY TERMINOLOGY REVIEW

Use the key terms found at the beginning of the chapter to complete the sentences below.

Apnea	Cyanosis	Nares
Arterial blood gases	Dyspnea	Orthopnea
Asphyxia	Expiration	Pleura
Bronchodilators	Hemoptysis	Sinuses
Carbon dioxide	Hilum	Tonsils
Cilia	Inspiration	Visceral pleura

1. ________________ is a compound of carbon and oxygen.
2. Three pairs of ________ reside in the pharynx.
3. The external entrances of the nose are called the __________.
4. The absence of breathing for more than 19 seconds is termed ________.
5. Difficulty breathing is known as ____________.
6. The bases of the lungs are called _________.
7. __________ are hairlike projections.
8. _____________ is another term for suffocation.
9. The ____________ covers the outer surface of the lungs and the inside of the thoracic cavity.
10. The symptom of coughing up blood, which can occur with tuberculosis, is known as ___________.
11. If a patient has trouble breathing unless a certain position is maintained (such as with the head elevated), it is termed ______________.
12. ______________________ are measured by drawing blood out of the arteries.
13. ________________ occurs as a result of lack of oxygen in the tissues.
14. ________________ open the bronchial passages.
15. ________________, also defined as inhalation, involves a precise sequence of events.
16. ________________ are hollow spaces, or cavities, located around the eyes, cheeks, and nose.
17. The pleural space separates two layers of the pleura—the parietal pleura and the ________________.
18. Quiet exhalation, or ____________, is ordinarily a passive process.

APPLIED PRACTICE

1. Label the sections of the nasal cavity and the pharynx.

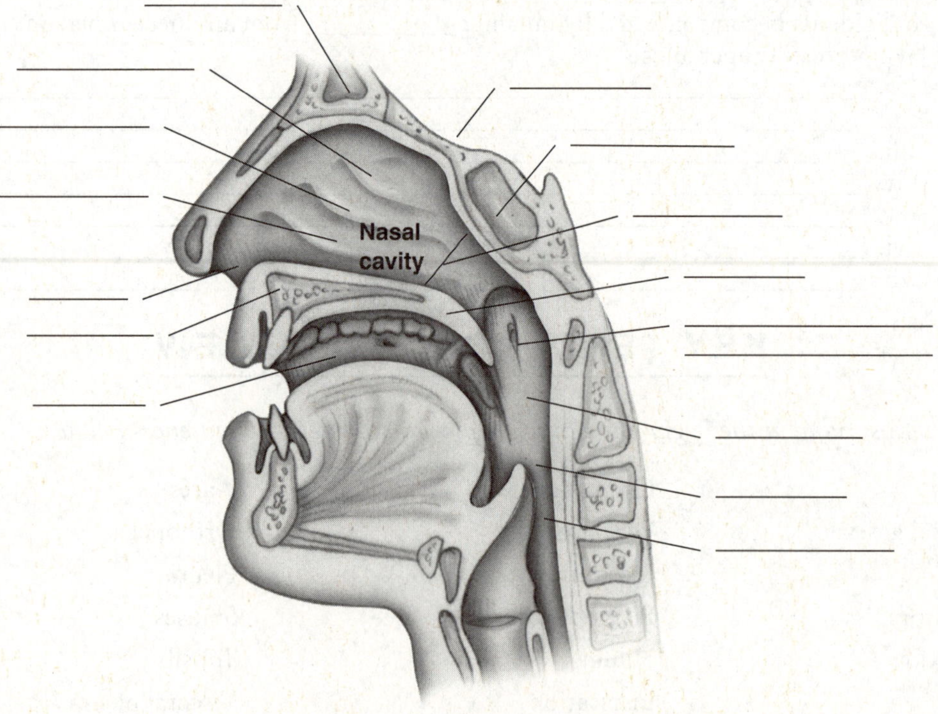

2. When working with children who have asthma, why should you be aware of the medication requirements of the school districts in your area?

LEARNING ACTIVITY: TRUE/FALSE

Indicate whether the following statements are true or false by placing a T or an F on the line that precedes each statement.

_______ 1. The upper respiratory tract includes the larynx, the trachea, the bronchioles, and the lungs.

_______ 2. The nose is part of the apparatus of respiration and voice.

_______ 3. The pharynx consists of two parts: the nasopharynx and the oropharynx.

_______ 4. The tonsils are part of the immune system and help with infection control.

_______ 5. The thyroid cartilage, or Adam's apple, is the smallest of the cartilage structures.

_______ 6. When the vocal cords are long and relaxed, high sounds are produced.

_______ 7. The respiratory rates in older adults may lower as the cumulative effects of pollution, smoking, and disease wear on the integrity of the tissues.

_______ 8. At birth, the lungs are pinkish in color, but as adulthood approaches they turn a dark slate-gray.

_______ 9. The right lung has three lobes, but the left lung only has two.

_______ 10. Asthma is related to the same process that causes allergic reactions.

CRITICAL THINKING

Answer the following questions to the best of your ability. Utilize the textbook as a reference.

1. You have a patient with obstructive lung disease who wants to know why he has a hard time breathing. This person has a form of COPD that does not allow him to exhale very much. Explain briefly here, as if explaining to the patient, why he feels so short of breath.

____

____

____

____

2. SARS (severe acute respiratory syndrome) was spread from China to North America by infected persons traveling by airplane. How can we control the entry of microbes into a country? What should China have done to prevent the spread of the disease within and outside of China? Should the Chinese government have shared information about SARS with the world immediately in case it spread?

____

____

____

____

RESEARCH ACTIVITY

Utilize Internet search engines to research the following topics and write a brief description of what you find. It is important to utilize reputable websites.

1. Visit www.lungusa.org. What information do you think will be most useful with regard to patient education? What is "hidden" asthma and what age group does it commonly effect? How can this information be useful to patients?

CHAPTER 30
The Digestive System

CHAPTER OUTLINE

General review of the chapter:

Organs of the Digestive System
Common Disorders Associated with the Digestive System

STUDENT STUDY GUIDE

Use the following guide to assist in your learning of the concepts from the chapter.

I. The Digestive System

1. The Digestive System

   A. The digestive system __________ food, __________ food, and __________ waste products.
   B. The three main functions are ___________, ____________, and ___________.

2. The Tongue

   A. The tongue is a ___________ muscle covered with a __________ membrane.
   B. The three areas of the tongue
      i. ____
      ii. ____
      iii. ____
   C. Papillae and taste buds are located on the ________ of the tongue.

3. The Teeth (List the types of teeth.)

   i. ____
   ii. ____
   iii. ____
   iv. ____

4. The Structure of the Tooth

   A. The ________ is the portion embedded in the top of the gum between the crown and the root.
   B. The ________ is the portion embedded in the gums.
   C. The _________ covers the exposed part of the crown.

5. The Anatomy of the Tooth—From the Crown to the Root

   A. __________ is the calcified, mostly mineral tissue that forms the bulk of the tooth.
   B. ____________ ___________ are the fibers that anchor teeth to bony sockets in the maxillary bone and the mandible.
   C. The____________ is the protective layer on the dentin that anchors the periodontal ligament.

6. The Pharynx

   A. The pharynx is the beginning of the _______________.
   B. It also opens to the _______________.

7. The Esophagus
   A. Carries food to the ____________.
   B. It is about ____________ inches long.
   C. Wave-like muscular contractions, called ____________, move food to the ____________.
8. The Stomach
   A. Can hold ___________ to ___________ liters.
   B. Secretes ___________ that aid in digestion.
   C. Processes food into a ____________ state.
   D. Prepares food for further ___________ and ___________ in the small intestine.
9. The Sphincters of the Stomach
   A. The sphincters of the stomach are muscular __________.
   B. Allow the flow of food in a __________ direction.
   C. The stomach has __________ sphincters.
   D. The lower esophageal sphincter is found between the __________ and the top of the stomach.
   E. The pyloric sphincter is between the __________ and the __________.
10. The Stomach's Role in Digestion
    i. ____________________
    ii. ____________________
    iii. ____________________
    iv. ____________________
11. The Small Intestine
    A. The small intestine is a tube about _________ feet long, _________ inch in diameter.
    B. Attaches to the _________ at the _________ sphincter.
    C. Ends at the _________ orifice at the beginning of the large intestine.
12. The Sections of the Small Intestine (List the three sections.)
    i. ____________________
    ii. ____________________
    iii. ____________________
13. The Large Intestine
    A. The large intestine begins at the ___________ orifice.
    B. The large intestine is about ___________ feet long.
    C. The functions of the large intestine
       i. ____________________
       ii. ____________________
       iii. ____________________
14. The Sections of the Large Intestine (List the four sections.)
    i. ____________________
    ii. ____________________
    iii. ____________________
    iv. ____________________
15. The Salivary Glands (List the three pairs.)
    i. ____________________
    ii. ____________________
    iii. ____________________
16. The Liver
    A. Stores _______ and several vitamins.
    B. The products of the liver include _______, _______, _______, _______, and _______.

17. The Pancreas

A. The pancreas is about ______ to ______ inches long.
B. Produces ____________ enzymes.
C. Serves the ____________ function.
D. It is part of two body systems: ____________ and ______________.
E. Its function is to secret the hormone ____________.

II. The Pathology of the Digestive System

1. Appendicitis

A. Appendicitis is an ____________ of the appendix.
B. Symptoms include acute pain on the __________ point of the abdomen.
C. Treatment is ____________ _____________ of the appendix.

2. Cirrhosis

A. Cirrhosis is damage to the liver caused by ____________.
B. Chronic ______________ of the liver prevents normal liver function.
C. Symptoms of cirrhosis

i. ____
ii. ____
iii. ____
iv. ____
v. ____
vi. ____
vii. ____
viii. ____
ix. ____

3. Treatment for Cirrhosis

i. ____
ii. ____
iii. ____
iv. ____
v. ____

4. Colitis

A. Colitis is an inflammation of the __________ intestine.
B. Symptoms of colitis

i. ____
ii. ____
iii. ____
iv. ____
v. ____

5. Colorectal Cancer

A. Begins as __________ polyps.
B. Treatment includes _________________, _______________, and _____________.

6. Constipation

A. Causes of constipation

i. ____
ii. ____
iii. ____
iv. ____

B. Treatment for constipation
    i. ______________________________
    ii. ______________________________
    iii. ______________________________
    iv. ______________________________

7. Crohn's Disease

    A. Crohn's disease is a chronic ______________ of the ______________.
    B. Common symptoms include ________________, ______________, and ______________.

8. Diverticulosis

    A. Diverticulosis is outpouching in the ______________ intestinal wall.
    B. There is a higher incidence in the ______________.
    C. Can be prevented with a _______ ________ diet.

9. Diverticulitis

    A. Diverticulitis is an inflammation of the diverticulum in the walls of the ____________.
    B. Symptoms of diverticulitis
        i. ______________________________
        ii. ______________________________
        iii. ______________________________
        iv. ______________________________
        v. ______________________________
        vi. ______________________________
        vii. ______________________________

10. Gastroesophageal Reflux Disease (GERD)

    A. GERD is a backflow of the _________ juices into the ______________.
    B. The lower ____________ sphincter does not close.
    C. Symptoms of gastroesophageal reflux disease
        i. ______________________________
        ii. ______________________________
        iii. ______________________________
        iv. ______________________________
        v. ______________________________
        vi. ______________________________
    D. Complications of gastroesophageal reflux disease
        i. ______________________________
        ii. ______________________________
        iii. ______________________________
        iv. ______________________________
        v. ______________________________
        vi. ______________________________

11. Hemorrhoids

    A. Hemorrhoids are dilated veins in the walls of the ____________.
    B. Symptoms include __________ with elimination.
    C. Treatment involves _________ changes, topical medication, and _________ (if severe).

12. Hiatal Hernia

    A. The upper stomach protrudes into the chest through the ____________ hiatus.
    B. Causes of a hiatal hernia
        i. ______________________________
        ii. ______________________________
        iii. ______________________________
        iv. ______________________________

v. ____________________
vi. ____________________
vii. ____________________
viii. ____________________

C. Symptoms of a hiatal hernia
i. ____________________
ii. ____________________
iii. ____________________
iv. ____________________
v. ____________________
vi. ____________________

13. Inguinal Hernia
A. The intestine pushes through the __________ wall in ________ area.
B. Causes include __________ in the abdominal wall; heavy lifting; and __________ as a result of coughing, laughing, or bending.
C. Symptoms include a bulge in the abdomen when ________, ________, or __________.
D. The only treatment is __________.

14. Irritable Bowel Syndrome (IBS)
A. IBS is a common __________ condition.
B. Causes include ________.
C. Treatment includes ________ modifications, medications, and __________.
D. Symptoms of IBS
i. ____________________
ii. ____________________
iii. ____________________
iv. ____________________
v. ____________________
vi. ____________________
vii. ____________________

15. Oral Cancer
A. Risk factors include age, ______, smoking, the use of ______ ______, and ______ exposure.
B. Symptoms of oral cancer
i. ____________________
ii. ____________________
iii. ____________________
iv. ____________________
v. ____________________

C. Treatment for oral cancer includes __________, __________, and __________.

16. Pancreatic Cancer
A. The most common type is ______________ of the pancreas.
B. Symptoms of pancreatic cancer
i. ____________________
ii. ____________________
iii. ____________________
iv. ____________________
v. ____________________
vi. ____________________

C. Treatment includes ____________________, __________, and __________.

17. Peptic Ulcer Disease (PUD)
A. PUD is characterized by a lesion in the lining of the ________, ________, or ________.
B. ________ ulcers are common.

C. Can be aggravated by ___________ infection.
D. Symptoms of PUD
i. ______________________________
ii. ______________________________
iii. ______________________________
iv. ______________________________

18. Treatment for Peptic Ulcer Disease
i. ______________________________
ii. ______________________________
iii. ______________________________
iv. ______________________________
v. ______________________________

19. Pyloric Stenosis
A. Pyloric stenosis is a condition where the ___________ sphincter ________ and thickens.
B. Symptoms include ____________________, ______________, and ____________.
C. Treatment for pyloric stenosis is _____________.

KEY TERMINOLOGY REVIEW

Match the selected key terms to their definitions below.

a. Cholelithiasis
b. Colorectal cancer
c. Diverticulitis
d. Diverticulosis
e. Esophagus
f. Gallbladder
g. Hemorrhoid
h. Hernia
i. Large intestine
j. Liver
k. Mastication
l. Pancreas
m. Pancreatic cancer
n. Peptic ulcer disease (PUD)
o. Pharynx
p. Pyloric stenosis
q. Small intestine
r. Stomach

1. ______________ A hollow, sac-like organ.
2. ______________ May be secondary to colitis.
3. ______________ The formation or presence of stones or calculi in the gallbladder or common bile duct.
4. ______________ Lies posterior to the mouth.
5. ______________ Caused by an imbalance in stomach acids.
6. ______________ Begins at the ileocecal orifice.
7. ______________ May be the result of stool in the diverticulum.
8. ______________ An abnormal protrusion of an organ or part of an organ through the wall of the body cavity that contains it.
9. ______________ The organ that is posterior to the stomach.
10. ______________ The tube leading from the pharynx to the stomach.
11. ______________ Occurs in infants, usually before 5 months of age.
12. ______________ The largest glandular organ.
13. ______________ Associated with constipation or chronic diarrhea.
14. ______________ Another word for chewing.

15. _______________ The green membranous sac below the liver.
16. _______________ Caused by pressure on and a weakening of the intestinal wall.
17. _______________ A condition that typically develops in the exocrine glands.
18. _______________ Attaches to the stomach at the pyloric spincter.

APPLIED PRACTICE

1. Label each part of the digestive system.

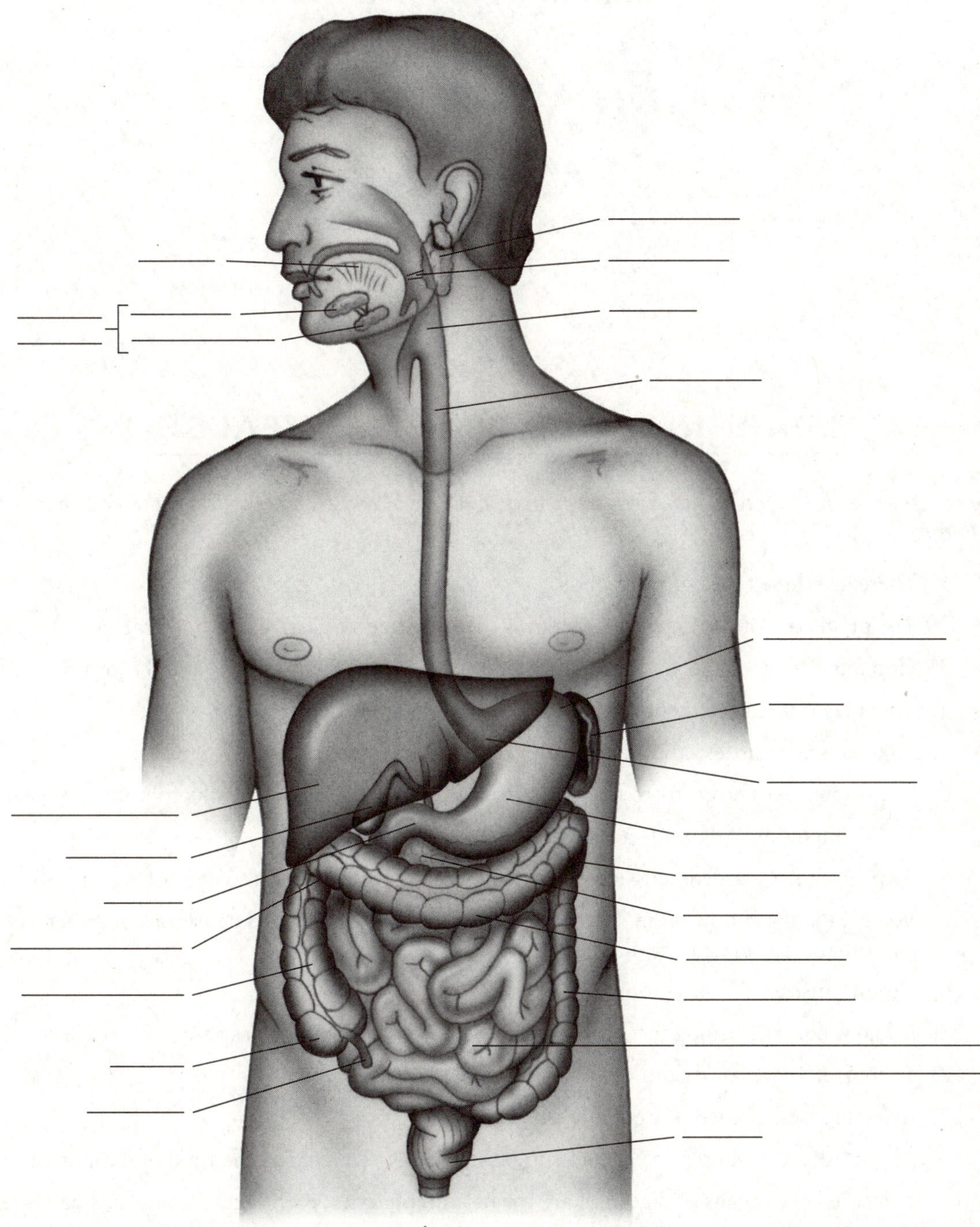

2. Label each part of the oral cavity.

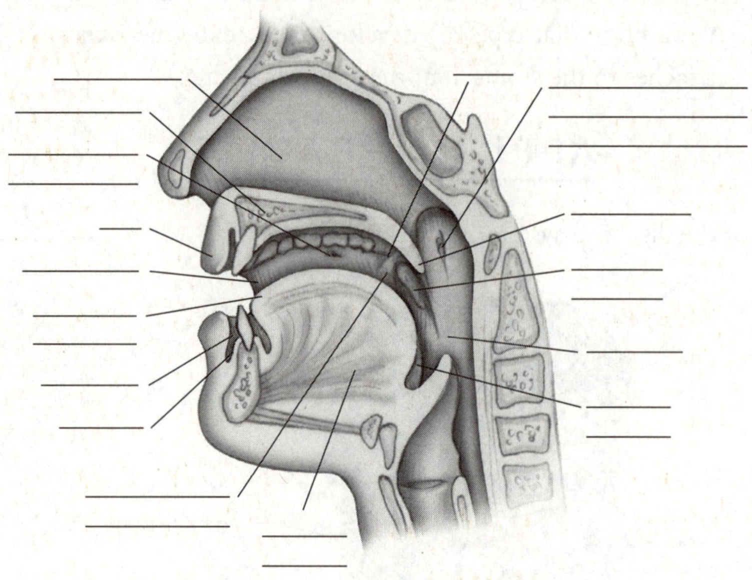

LEARNING ACTIVITY: TRUE/FALSE

Indicate whether the following statements are true or false by placing a T or an F on the line that precedes each statement.

_______ 1. There are three types of taste buds.

_______ 2. The main part of the digestive system is the digestive or gastrointestinal tract.

_______ 3. Humans have two sets of teeth: 25 deciduous teeth (the baby teeth) and 35 permanent teeth.

_______ 4. The incisor teeth are the largest teeth in the permanent set.

_______ 5. Enamel is the hardest and most compact part of the tooth.

_______ 6. Deciduous teeth erupt from the gums from the age of about 7 months to about 2½ years.

_______ 7. The submandibular glands are located below the tongue.

_______ 8. Anyone can get appendicitis, but it occurs most often between the ages of 10 and 30.

_______ 9. Volvulus is the condition in which the bowel twists on itself and causes an obstruction that is painful and requires immediate surgery.

_______ 10. Crohn's disease is contagious.

_______ 11. A hiatal hernia is thought to contribute to the weakening of this sphincter muscle.

_______ 12. There is no cure for irritable bowel syndrome.

_______ 13. Age increases the risk of oral cancer.

_______ 14. About 50% of pancreatic cancers can be surgically removed at the time of diagnosis.

_______ 15. The accessory organs of digestion are the mouth, pharynx, esophagus, stomach, small intestine, large intestine, and rectum.

CRITICAL THINKING

Answer the following questions to the best of your ability. Utilize the textbook as a reference.

1. Mr. McNeill is experiencing constipation and has called in for advice on how to deal with this. Try to recall what you have read in this chapter of your textbook and use your common sense to list a few things that may help. After you have done that, check the book and review the items that you may not have remembered.

2. Some digestive disorders, such as stomach ulcers, IBS, and GERD, may be associated with a person's lifestyle. As a member of the health care profession, what is your role when assisting in the care of these patients? What should you avoid doing when providing care?

RESEARCH ACTIVITY

Utilize Internet search engines to research the following topics and write a brief description of what you find. It is important to utilize reputable websites.

1. As a medical assistant, it will be your responsibility to instruct patients on how to prepare for certain types of diagnostic tests, such as a colonoscopy, endoscopy, or sigmoidoscopy. Select a condition from your textook, research the types of tests performed for diagnosis, select one of the tests, and research the instructions that would be provided to patients. Write a short essay explaining the condition, the procedure, and the preparatory instructions that patients should be given prior to the procedure. Cite your Internet sources.

CHAPTER 31
The Urinary System

CHAPTER OUTLINE

General review of the chapter:

Organs of the Urinary System
Urine
Common Disorders Associated with the Urinary System

STUDENT STUDY GUIDE

Use the following guide to assist in your learning of the concepts from the chapter.

I. The Urinary System

1. Urine
   A. Urine is the waste product produced by the __________.
   B. Contains mostly water, as well as __________ and __________ compounds.
   C. Drains from the __________, through the __________, to the __________.
2. The Structure of the Kidneys
   A. Located at the __________ region of the abdominal cavity between the __________ thoracic and __________ lumbar vertebrae.
   B. The kidneys are encased in three capsules for protection: the __________, the __________, and the __________.
3. The Nephron
   A. Each kidney contains more than 1 __________ nephrons.
   B. A nephron consists of a __________ capsule and a renal __________.
4. Ureters
   A. Ureters are composed of three layers
      i. ______________________________
      ii. ______________________________
      iii. ______________________________
   B. They are about ______ to ______ inches long and less than ______ inch in diameter.
5. The Urinary Bladder
   A. The urinary bladder consists of four layers
      i. ______________________________
      ii. ______________________________
      iii. ______________________________
      iv. ______________________________
   B. Stretches to hold ________.
   C. The urge to urinate typically occurs when an adult bladder holds ______ to ______ mL of urine.
   D. The bladder empties through the _________ and the _________ meatus.

6. The Urethra
   A. In males, the urethra is approximately ______ cm long and transports urine and _________.
   B. The male urethra has three sections: the ____________, the ____________, and the ____________.
   C. In females, the urethra is approximately ______ cm long and transports only urine.
   D. The external opening of the female urethra is situated between the ________ and the opening of the __________.
7. Facts About Urine
   A. Consists of ___________, ______________, and ______________.
   B. An adult passes about ______ to ______ mL of urine daily.
   C. Characteristics of normal urine
      i. ____
      ii. ____
      iii. ____
      iv. ____

II. The Pathology of the Urinary System

1. Cystitis
   A. Caused by a ________________ infection of the __________ tract.
   B. Most prevalent in ____________ active women, ages ______ to ______, because of anatomical configuration.
   C. Symptoms include ___________ and ___________________________ urination.
   D. Treatment includes _____________ and ______________.
2. Interstitial Cystitis
   A. Interstitial cystitis is an inflammation of the __________________.
   B. Affects mostly ______________.
   C. Its cause is ________________.
   D. It is not responsive to _____________.
3. Glomerulonephritis
   A. Can lead to ________ failure.
   B. Causes include _____________, ________________, ______________________, and _____________________________.
   C. Symptoms glomerulonephritis
      i. ____
      ii. ____
      iii. ____
      iv. ____
      v. ____
      vi. ____
   D. Treatment includes __________, __________, __________, and __________.
4. Incontinence
   A. Commonly seen in women who have had _________________.
   B. Types of incontinence include _________________, ____________, __________________, and ___________________.
   C. Treatment includes _______________, _______________, _________________, and _________________________.
5. Kidney Stones, or Renal Calculi
   A. Kidney stones are harmless in the ___________.
   B. They become problematic when passed into the __________.
   C. Symptoms include _______________, _____________________, and ___________________.

D. Treatment includes ______________ and ________________.
E. Prevention includes controlling the ________________ and ________________.

6. Polycystic Kidney Disease (PKD)
   A. Symptoms of PKD
      i. ________________
      ii. ________________
      iii. ________________
      iv. ________________
      v. ________________
      vi. ________________
   B. ___________ focuses on the symptoms and their complications.
7. Pyelonephritis
   A. Causes of pyelonephritis
      i. ________________
      ii. ________________
      iii. ________________
      iv. ________________
   B. Symptoms of pyelonephritis
      i. ________________
      ii. ________________
      iii. ________________
      iv. ________________
      v. ________________
   C. Treatment is typically the use of ____________.
   D. If left untreated, __________ and possible kidney ___________ may occur.
8. Types of Dialysis (List and briefly explain the two types.)
   i. ________________
   ii. ________________

KEY TERMINOLOGY REVIEW

Without using any material from your textbook, write a sentence using the selected vocabulary terms in the correct context.

1. *ascites*

____

____

2. *cystitis*

____

____

3. *dialysis*

____

____

4. *dysuria*

____

____

5. *enuresis*

6. *hilum*

7. *lithotripsy*

8. *micturition*

9. *nephrons*

10. *renal calculi*

11. *renal pelvis*

12. *urinary meatus*

APPLIED PRACTICE

Using the information found in the chapter, answer the questions following the scenario below.

Scenario

Mr. Bai Feng, born 8-13-66, presents to the office today with a fever of 99.7°F, noticeable beads of sweat on his brow, and complaints of right-sided pain in his lower back. He states, "I am in so much pain I can't stand up straight and I feel like I always have to urinate." A urine specimen is obtained for urinalysis and shows positive for blood in the urine, as well as other abnormalities. His urine specimen is sent to the laboratory for further testing.

1. Based on his urinalysis and symptoms, what would be a likely diagnosis? (Keep in mind that a medical assistant never diagnoses a patient; this is your opinion based on information found in the textbook.)

2. Draw a picture of the urinary system (kidneys, ureters, urinary bladder, and urethra). Circle the area of the urinary system that is likely to be the causative factor for Mr. Feng's pain.

LEARNING ACTIVITY

Match the vocabulary term to the correct definition below.

a. Acute renal failure
b. Chronic renal failure
c. Cortex
d. Frequency
e. Glomerulonephritis
f. Incontinence
g. Interstitial cystitis
h. Kidney stones
i. Kidneys
j. Medulla
k. Polycystic kidney disease (PKD)
l. Pyelonephritis
m. Ureters
n. Urethra
o. Urinary bladder
p. Void

1. _______________ Caused by deposits of mineral salts in the kidney.
2. _______________ The outer layer of a kidney.
3. _______________ A muscular sac in the pelvic cavity that serves as a reservoir for urine.
4. _______________ A kidney disease that hampers the kidneys' ability to remove waste and excess fluids.
5. _______________ The involuntary and unpredictable flow of urine.
6. _______________ The middle portion of the kidney.
7. _______________ Two muscular tubes that carries the newly formed urine from each kidney down to the bladder.
8. _______________ The need to void often.
9. _______________ An infection of the kidney and renal pelvis.
10. _______________ A musculomembranous tube extending from the bladder to the urinary meatus.

11. ____________ Occurs when something causes a change in the filtering function of the kidneys.
12. ____________ A pair of bean-shaped organs located at the back of the abdominal cavity.
13. ____________ A painful inflammation of the bladder wall.
14. ____________ To urinate.
15. ____________ A disorder in which clusters of cysts develop primarily within the kidneys.
16. ____________ A gradual and progressive loss of kidney function.

CRITICAL THINKING

Answer the following questions to the best of your ability. Utilize the textbook as a reference.

1. Why are the elderly more susceptible to becoming dehydrated?

____

____

____

____

____

2. When discussing urinary issues with patients, what cultural considerations should be given?

____

____

____

____

____

____

____

____

____

____

____

____

RESEARCH ACTIVITY

Utilize Internet search engines to research the following topics and write a brief description of what you find. It is important to utilize reputable websites.

1. Visit www.kidney.org. As you navigate through the site, what information do you find that would be helpful for a patient who is in need of a kidney transplant? What information is available for healthcare technicians? How could this website be beneficial for a urology/nephrology office?

____

____

____

CHAPTER 32
The Endocrine System

CHAPTER OUTLINE

General review of the chapter:

- Function of the Endocrine System
- Pituitary Gland
- Pineal Gland
- Thyroid Gland
- Parathyroid Glands
- Pancreas
- Adrenal Glands
- Ovaries
- Testes
- Placenta
- Gastrointestinal Mucosa
- Thymus Gland
- Common Disorders Associated with the Endocrine System

STUDENT STUDY GUIDE

Use the following guide to assist in your learning of the concepts from the chapter.

I. The Endocrine System

1. Types of Glands
   - A. Exocrine glands secrete __________ to an _________ surface, but do not circulate into the ______________.
   - B. Endocrine glands secrete __________ that __________ within the body.
2. The Functions of the Endocrine System
   - i. ______________________________
   - ii. ______________________________
   - iii. ______________________________
   - iv. ______________________________
   - v. ______________________________
3. The Connection Between the Nervous and Endocrine Systems
   - A. The nervous system works closely with the ____________ system.
   - B. The nervous system helps maintain ______________.
   - C. The _______________, located in the brain, is the link between the two systems.
4. The Pituitary Gland
   - A. Regulates all of the other ___________ in the _________ system.
   - B. Located near the ___________ of the ___________.

C. Attached to the ____________ by the ____________ stalk.
D. The pituitary gland has two lobes: the ________________ and the ________________.

5. Anterior Lobe Hormones (List each hormone.)
   i. ______________________________
   ii. ______________________________
   iii. ______________________________
   iv. ______________________________
   v. ______________________________
   vi. ______________________________
   vii. ______________________________

6. The Hormones and the Functions of the Posterior Lobe of the Pituitary Gland (List the functions of each hormone.)

   A. Antidiuretic hormone (ADH)
      i. ______________________________
      ii. ______________________________
      iii. ______________________________
      iv. ______________________________
   B. Oxytocin
      i. ______________________________
      ii. ______________________________

7. The Pineal Gland

   A. Located at the ____________ end of the ________________.
   B. Secretes __________ and ____________.

8. The Thyroid Gland

   A. Located anterior to the __________, just below the __________ cartilage.
   B. The thyroid gland is approximately _____ cm long and _____ cm wide.
   C. Weighs _____ grams.
   D. Secretes _______ hormones.

9. The Parathyroid Glands

   A. Located around the ________ and lower aspect of the thyroid gland.
   B. Each gland is _____ mm in diameter.
   C. Each gland weighs _____ grams.
   D. Secretes parathyroid _________.

10. Parathyroid Hormone (PTH)

   A. The functions of PTH
      i. ______________________________
      ii. ______________________________

11. The Pancreas

   A. Contains small clusters of cells called the __________________ that secrete hormones.
   B. __________ types of cells make up the islets of Langerhans.

12. Pancreas Cells (List each cell and briefly explain its function.)
   i. ______________________________
   ii. ______________________________
   iii. ______________________________

13. The Adrenal Gland

   A. The adrenal gland is ____________ in shape.
   B. The adrenal __________ is the outer portion of the gland.
   C. The adrenal __________ is the inner portion of the gland.

14. The Adrenal Cortex (List the three types of hormones manufactured by the adrenal cortex.)
    i. ______
    ii. ______
    iii. ______
15. The Adrenal Medulla
    A. The adrenal medulla is the ______ portion of the ______ glands.
    B. Synthesizes, ______, and stores ______.
16. Primary Catecholamines (List the functions of each hormone.)
    A. Dopamine
        i. ______
        ii. ______
        iii. ______
    B. Epinephrine
        i. ______
    C. Norepinephrine
        i. ______
        ii. ______
        iii. ______
        iv. ______
        v. ______

II. The Pathology of the Endocrine System
1. Acromegaly
    A. Commonly affects ______ adults.
    B. The most serious health consequences of acromegaly
        i. ______
        ii. ______
        iii. ______
        iv. ______
    C. Commonly characterized by abnormal growth of the ______ and ______.
2. Signs and Symptoms of Acromegaly
    i. ______
    ii. ______
    iii. ______
    iv. ______
    v. ______
    vi. ______
    vii. ______
    viii. ______
    ix. ______
    x. ______
    xi. ______
    xii. ______
    xiii. ______
    xiv. ______
    xv. ______
    xvi. ______
3. Treatment for Acromegaly
    A. Reduce ______ production to ______ levels.
    B. Surgical removal of the ______.

C. __________ therapy.
D. __________ therapy of the pituitary gland.

4. Addison's Disease

A. Addison's disease is an ____________ disease in which the body attacks itself.
B. May be caused by _________ of the adrenal glands, cancer, or _____________ into the glands.
C. It is a rare condition that occurs in _____ in _________ Americans.
D. Diagnosed by _______ and ________ tests that measure _______________ hormone levels.

5. Signs and Symptoms of Addison's Disease

i. ____
ii. ____
iii. ____
iv. ____
v. ____
vi. ____
vii. ____
viii. ____
ix. ____
x. ____
xi. ____
xii. ____

6. Treatment for Addison's Disease

A. Replace the ______________ hormones and prescribe sodium _____________.
B. Administer intramuscular ________________ injections.

7. Cushing's Syndrome

A. Possibly caused by a _______________.
B. Treatment includes ___________ and ____________.

8. Signs and Symptoms of Cushing's Disease

i. ____
ii. ____
iii. ____
iv. ____
v. ____
vi. ____

9. Diabetes Mellitus

A. Diabetes mellitus is a silent disease that may not be detected until it is at an _____ stage.
B. Approximately _____ million people have been diagnosed with diabetes, but an estimated _____ million are undiagnosed.

10. Juvenile Diabetes

A. Typically diagnosed in ________ who cannot produce sufficient quantities, if any, of ________.
B. Patients are dependent on __________ injections for the rest of their lives.

11. Type 2 Diabetes

A. Type 2 diabetes is the most _____________ form of the disease.
B. Results from ________ resistance combined with a relative ________ deficiency.
C. There is a very strong correlation between _________ and type 2 diabetes.

12. Signs and Symptoms of Diabetes

A. _______________ (frequent urination)
B. _______________ (excessive thirst)
C. _______________ (excessive hunger)

13. Treatment for Diabetes

A. Type 1 diabetes can usually be treated only by ______________ the __________.
B. Type 2 diabetes is treated with ______, __________, and oral ___________ medications.
C. May be preventable with modest lifestyle changes, including a healthy ______, __________, and ________ management.

14. Achondroplasia

A. Achondroplasia is the most common type of ___________, occurring in 1 in 25,000 children.
B. Abnormal ___________ growth is usually diagnosed at birth.
C. Development of motor skills may be ________, but intellectual development is normal.

15. The Physical Characteristics of Achondroplasia

i. ______________________________
ii. ______________________________
iii. ______________________________
iv. ______________________________
v. ______________________________
vi. ______________________________
vii. ______________________________
viii. ______________________________

16. Treatment for Achondroplasia

A. In addition to social and family support, treatment focuses on the ____________ and ______________ of medical complications.
B. ____________ may be performed to relieve pressure on the ________ system.
C. Dental and _________ work may be necessary to correct _____________ and preserve dental health.

17. Signs and Symptoms of and Treatment for Gigantism

A. Signs and symptoms of gigantism
   i. ______________________________
   ii. ______________________________
   iii. ______________________________
B. Treatment includes ___________ therapy and _________ removal of the tumor.

18. Signs and Symptoms of Hyperthyroidism

i. ______________________________
ii. ______________________________
iii. ______________________________
iv. ______________________________
v. ______________________________
vi. ______________________________
vii. ______________________________
viii. ______________________________
ix. ______________________________
x. ______________________________
xi. ______________________________

19. Treatment for Hyperthyroidism

A. ____________ medications
B. Radioactive _________ to destroy the thyroid
C. ___________

20. Hypothyroidism

   A. Since it develops slowly, only about half of the _____ million cases in the United States are diagnosed early.

   B. Untreated, it can lead to other conditions. Constant stimulation causes the release of _________ hormones, which can cause the _________ gland to _________.

   C. Untreated hypothyroidism is associated with a higher risk of ___________ disease because of the high levels of _______________ _____________ (LDL).

   D. Other complications include __________, _________________, and _________________.

21. Other Disorders Related to the Endocrine System (List and briefly explain each.)

   i. ____

   ii. ____

   iii. ____

   iv. ____

   v. ____

   vi. ____

   vii. ____

   viii. ____

   ix. ____

   x. ____

   xi. ____

   xii. ____

   xiii. ____

   xiv. ____

   xv. ____

   xvi. ____

   xvii. ____

KEY TERMINOLOGY REVIEW

Match the vocabulary term to the correct definition below.

a. Acromegaly
b. Addison's disease
c. Adrenal glands
d. Cardiomegaly
e. Cushing's disease
f. Diabetes mellitus

g. Dwarfism
h. Exophthalmos
i. Gestational diabetes
j. Gigantism
k. Goiter
l. Grave's disease
m. Hashimoto's thyroiditis
n. Hyperthyroidism
o. Hypothyroidism
p. Insulin-dependent diabetes mellitus
q. Islets of Langerhans
r. Lipolysis
s. Myxedema
t. Non–insulin-dependent diabetes mellitus
u. parathyroid glands
v. pineal gland
w. pituitary gland
x. thymus gland
y. thyroid gland

1. ____________ Called "The Master Gland".
2. ____________ A possible symptom of hypothyroidism, in which the eyeballs protrude beyond their normal protective orbit when the tissues behind them swell.
3. ____________ Juvenile diabetes; also known as type 1 diabetes.
4. ____________ When the cortex of the adrenal gland is damaged, decreasing the production of adrenocortical hormones.
5. ____________ Produce parathormone.
6. ____________ The destruction of fats promoted by growth hormone (GH).
7. ____________ A rare disorder caused by the hypersecretion of cortisol.
8. ____________ Small clusters of cells within the pancreas.
9. ____________ Results from excessive secretion of growth hormone (GH) during childhood, before the closure of the bone growth plates.
10. ____________ Pregnancy-related diabetes.
11. ____________ An enlarged heart.
12. ____________ The most common form of hyperthyroidism.
13. ____________ This condition, along with cretinism and Hashimoto's disease, can result from hyposecretion of calcitonin and its companion hormones, T3 and T4.
14. ____________ Characterized by elevated thyroid hormone levels.
15. ____________ A hormonal disorder that results from the overproduction of growth hormone (GH) by the pituitary gland.
16. ____________ Also known as Type 2 diabetes, or adult-onset diabetes.
17. ____________ Condition where the body is unable to produce enough insulin to properly control blood sugar levels.
18. ____________ Releases melatonin.
19. ____________ An autoimmune inflammation of the thyroid.
20. ____________ When the thyroid produces inadequate amounts of thyroid hormones.
21. ____________ Achondroplasia is the most common type of this abnormal skeletal growth condition, which occurs in children.
22. ____________ Releases thymosin and thymopoietin.
23. ____________ This gland secrets thyroxine, tri-iodothyronine, and calcitonin.
24. ____________ The most common cause is Hashimoto's thyroiditis, an autoimmune inflammation of the thyroid.
25. ____________ Located on top of each kidney.

APPLIED PRACTICE

Follow the directions as instructed with each question below.

1. Using the information from the following patient chart, correctly identify the possible endocrine gland disorder based on the patient's signs and symptoms.

> Mikovich, Anya, 10-26-1982
> 4/02/20XX, 3:45 P.M.
> Wt: 134 lbs T: 98.6° F P: 104 bpm, bounding
> BP: 118/78
> cc: Pt presents to office complaining of restlessness, heart palpitations, tremors, sweating. She states, "I am unable to relax and have been sweating a lot recently. I always feel hot." She is displaying exophthalmos and has lost 6 lbs since her last visit 3 months ago, though she claims she hasn't been trying to lose weight.
>
> Adam Bello, RMA

2. Label the primary gland of the endocrine system as seen on the image provided.

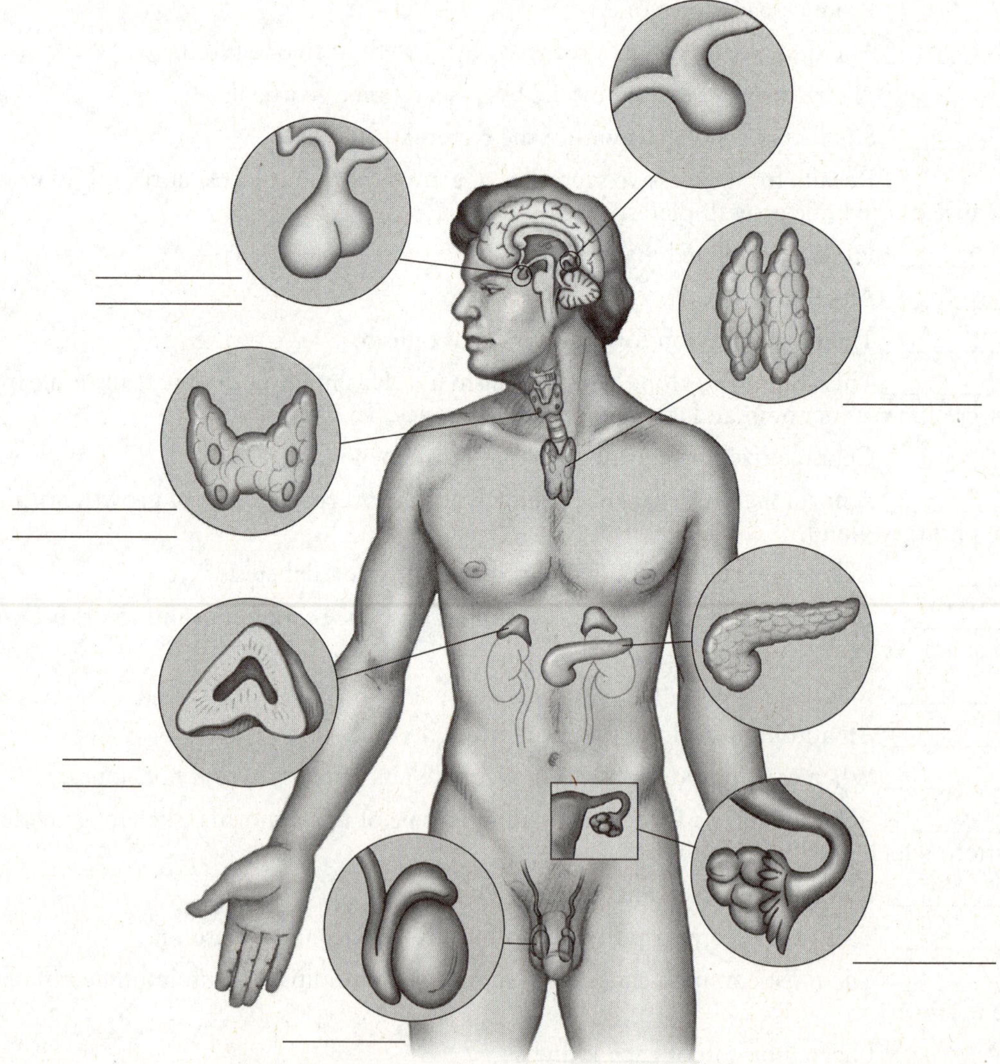

LEARNING ACTIVITY: TRUE/FALSE

Indicate whether the following statements are true or false by placing a T or an F on the line that precedes each statement.

_______ 1. The nerve cells in the hypothalamus control the pituitary gland by producing chemicals that either suppress or stimulate hormone secretion from the pituitary gland.

_______ 2. Depression is commonly associated with disorders related to the hormone serotonin.

_______ 3. Diabetes mellitus is very rare in children.

_______ 4. A myxedema coma can be triggered by sedatives, infection, or other stress.

_______ 5. Insulin and glucagon are secreted by the pancreas.

_______ 6. Hyposecretion of the adrenal cortex results in dwarfism.

_______ 7. Progesterone is a steroid hormone.

_______ 8. Copulation can occur without testosterone.

_______ 9. The thymus is part of the endocrine gland.

_______ 10. Von Rechlinghausen's disease results in degeneration of the bones due to excessive production of parathyroid hormone.

CRITICAL THINKING

Answer the following questions to the best of your ability. Utilize the textbook as a resource.

1. A pregnant patient who is overdue for going into labor may need a hormone to help stimulate the process of uterine contractions. What hormone may be given? What endocrine gland would produce this hormone naturally? What else does this hormone stimulate?

____

____

____

____

2. Why is it important to understand your state laws regarding individuals with diabetes who drive school buses and other forms of public transportation?

____

____

____

____

RESEARCH ACTIVITY

Utilize Internet search engines to research the following topics and write a brief description of what you find. It is important to utilize reputable websites.

1. Visit www.diabetes.org. Research information as to how diabetes plays an ethnic and cross-cultural role. What facts do you find most surprising regarding this topic? How prevalent is diabetes within your ethnic race or culture?

____

____

CHAPTER 33

The Reproductive System

CHAPTER OUTLINE

General review of the chapter:

The Female Reproductive System
The Menstrual Cycle
The Male Reproductive System
Common Disorders Associated with the Female Reproductive System
Common Disorders Associated with the Male Reproductive System

STUDENT STUDY GUIDE

Use the following guide to assist in your learning of the concepts from the chapter.

I. The Female Reproductive System

1. The Uterus
   A. The uterus is a hollow, _______-shaped organ.
   B. Located in the anterior ________ cavity between the ________ and the symphysis _______, above the bladder and in front of the ________.
   C. The functions of the uterus
      i. ______________________________
      ii. ______________________________
      iii. ______________________________
2. Layers of the Uterine Wall
   i. ______________________________
   ii. ______________________________
   iii. ______________________________
3. Fallopian Tubes
   A. The fallopian tubes are also called the ________ tubes or the ____________.
   B. Functions include moving ________ from the ___________ to the uterus.
   C. The three layers of the fallopian tubes
      i. ______________________________
      ii. ______________________________
      iii. ______________________________
4. Features of the Fallopian Tubes
   i. ______________________________
   ii. ______________________________
   iii. ______________________________
   iv. ______________________________
   v. ______________________________

5. Ovaries
   A. Located on both sides of the ____________.
   B. Attached to the __________ by the __________ ligament.
   C. Controlled by the hormones from the __________ gland.
   D. The microscopic structure includes the ______ (the outer layer) and the __________.
6. The Vagina
   A. The vagina is a _______________ tube.
   B. Extends from the _______ cervix to the ___________.
   C. Located between the ___________ and the __________.
7. The Five Organs of the Vulva That Make Up the External Female Genitalia
   i. ______________________________
   ii. ______________________________
   iii. ______________________________
   iv. ______________________________
   v. ______________________________
8. Breasts
   A. Breasts are also called __________ glands.
   B. Composed of compound __________ structures consisting of _____ to _____ glandular tissue lobes separated by the septa of the connecting tissue.
   C. The __________ is the dark, pigmented circular area of skin found on each breast.
   D. The _________ is the elevated area in the center of the __________.
9. Prolactin
   A. Prolactin is the _________________ produced by the anterior lobe of the pituitary gland.
   B. Stimulates the ____________ glands to produce __________.
10. An Overview of the Menstrual Cycle
   A. The menstrual cycle is normally _____ days.
   B. It has _____ phases.
   C. The occurrence of _______________ ends the menstrual cycle.

II. The Pathology of the Female Reproductive System
   1. Disorders of the Female Reproductive System (Briefly explain each of the following disorders.)
      A. Abruptio placentae: ______________________________
      B. Amenorrhea: ______________________________
      C. Breech presentation: ______________________________
      D. Cervical polyps: ______________________________
      E. Condyloma: ______________________________
      F. Cystocele: ______________________________
      G. Ectopic pregnancy: ______________________________
   2. Cancers of the Female Reproductive System (List the three types and briefly explain each.)
      i. ______________________________
      ii. ______________________________
      iii. ______________________________
   3. Types of Ovarian Cancer (List the three types and briefly explain each.)
      i. ______________________________
      ii. ______________________________
      iii. ______________________________
   4. Signs and Symptoms of Early Stage Ovarian Cancer
      i. ______________________________
      ii. ______________________________

iii. ______________________________
iv. ______________________________
v. ______________________________
vi. ______________________________
vii. ______________________________
viii. ______________________________
ix. ______________________________
x. ______________________________
xi. ______________________________
xii. ______________________________
xiii. ______________________________
xiv. ______________________________

5. Signs and Symptoms of Advanced Ovarian Cancer

i. ______________________________
ii. ______________________________
iii. ______________________________
iv. ______________________________
v. ______________________________
vi. ______________________________

6. Treatment for Ovarian Cancer

A. Treatment is based on the type, __________, and _________ of the cancer.
B. Can include __________, __________ therapy, ___________, and _________ therapies.
C. ____________ therapies, such as traditional Chinese medicines or special diets, are sometimes used.

7. Uterine Cancer (Endometrial Cancer)

A. Generally develops in the _________ tissues of the __________.
B. If detected and _________ early, treatment is usually very successful.

8. Factors That Can Increase the Risk of Uterine Cancer

i. ______________________________
ii. ______________________________
iii. ______________________________
iv. ______________________________
v. ______________________________
vi. ______________________________

9. Signs and Symptoms of Uterine Cancer

i. ______________________________
ii. ______________________________
iii. ______________________________
iv. ______________________________
v. ______________________________
vi. ______________________________
vii. ______________________________
viii. ______________________________

10. Uterine Fibroids

A. Uterine fibroids are ________ growths or tumors.
B. They are made up of ______ cells and other tissues that grow within the wall of the _______.
C. Can occur as a ________ growth or as a _________ of ___________.
D. Common in women of _______________ age.
E. ________________ women are the most susceptible of all racial groups.
F. There is a higher risk of fibroids among women who are ____________.

11. Signs and Symptoms of Uterine Fibroids
    i. ____________________
    ii. ____________________
    iii. ____________________
    iv. ____________________
    v. ____________________
    vi. ____________________
    vii. ____________________
12. Treatment for Uterine Fibroids
    A. ____________ medications for mild symptoms
    B. ____________ hormone agonists to decrease the size of the fibroids
    C. ____________ agents may stop or slow the growth of fibroids.
13. Pelvic Inflammatory Disease (PID)
    A. PID is an infection of the upper ________ area.
    B. Caused by disease-carrying ____________.
    C. Can affect the ________, ovaries, and ________ tubes.
    D. If untreated, can cause ________.
14. Signs and Symptoms of and Treatment for Pelvic Inflammatory Disease
    A. Signs and symptoms of PID
        i. ____________________
        ii. ____________________
        iii. ____________________
        iv. ____________________
        v. ____________________
        vi. ____________________
    B. Treatment for PID involves treating the underlying ____________.
15. Ovarian Cysts
    A. Ovarian cysts are ______ filled with ______ or a semisolid material that develops on or within the ovary.
    B. Functional cysts are relatively common and usually disappear within ______ days without treatment.
16. Signs and Symptoms of Ovarian Cysts
    A. A constant, dull ________ pain
    B. Abdominal ________ or ________
17. Treatment for Ovarian Cysts
    A. Oral ____________ may be prescribed.
    B. If larger than ______ cm or persisting for longer than ______ weeks, the cyst may require surgical removal.
18. Preeclampsia
    A. Preeclampsia is ________ during pregnancy.
    B. If untreated, can result in true ________.
    C. Symptoms of preeclampsia
        i. ____________________
        ii. ____________________
        iii. ____________________
        iv. ____________________
19. Premenstrual Syndrome (PMS)
    A. PMS is also called ____________ ____________ disorder.
    B. Estimated to affect ______% of women who menstruate.

C. Only _____ to _____% of menstruating women are severely impaired by PMS.
D. It is believed that PMS is associated with the amount of ___________ produced.

20. Signs and Symptoms of Premenstrual Syndrome
   i. ______________________________
   ii. ______________________________
   iii. ______________________________
   iv. ______________________________
   v. ______________________________
   vi. ______________________________
   vii. ______________________________
   viii. ______________________________
   ix. ______________________________
   x. ______________________________
   xi. ______________________________
   xii. ______________________________
   xiii. ______________________________
   xiv. ______________________________
   xv. ______________________________
   xvi. ______________________________

21. Treatment for Premenstrual Syndrome
   i. ______________________________
   ii. ______________________________
   iii. ______________________________
   iv. ______________________________
   v. ______________________________
   vi. ______________________________

22. Disorders of the Female Reproductive System (Briefly explain each.)
   A. Prolapsed uterus: ______________________________
   B. Rh factor: ______________________________
   C. Salpingitis: ______________________________
   D. Spontaneous abortion: ______________________________
   E. Toxic shock syndrome: ______________________________

23. Breast Cancer
   A. Affects women primarily and about _____% of men.
   B. ________ percent of breast cancers develop in the tiny ______ that extend from the _________ of the mammary glands to the nipple.
   C. Cancer may also develop in the ____________.
   D. The most serious cancers are _________ cancers, which spread from their origin into other tissues.

24. Risk Factors for Breast Cancer
   A. ___________ history
   B. Women who begin ________________ at an early age or experience a late menopause

25. Signs and Symptoms of Breast Cancer
   A. A ___________ in the breast, under the arm, or above the collarbone
   B. _______ discharge
   C. Nipple __________

26. Factors to Be Considered When Treating Breast Cancer
   i. ______________________________
   ii. ______________________________

iii. ____________________
iv. ____________________
v. ____________________

27. Surgical Treatment for Breast Cancer (List the four types of surgery.)

i. ____________________
ii. ____________________
iii. ____________________
iv. ____________________

28. Cervicitis

A. Cervicitis is an inflammation of the __________.
B. Symptoms include ________ or ____________ vaginal discharge; frequent and __________ urination; pain during ____________; and ____________ bleeding after intercourse, between menstrual periods, or after menopause.

29. Treatment for Cervicitis

A. ________________ are used to treat an underlying ____________ infection.
B. If the infection is ________, such as genital herpes, an _____________ medication is given.
C. The person's sexual partner may also be treated to prevent ______________.

30. Dysmenorrhea

A. Signs and symptoms include dull or throbbing pain, usually centered in the __________ abdomen and radiating toward the ________ back or ___________.
B. Some women may also experience nausea and vomiting, ___________, irritability, _________, or dizziness.

31. Treatment for Dysmenorrhea

A. Controlled by treating the ____________ disorder.
B. ____________________________________, such as acetaminophen and ibuprofen, are used to relieve pain.
C. Aromatherapy and __________ are helpful for some women.

32. Endometriosis

A. Occurs when _____________ tissue is found __________ the uterus.
B. One theory as to the cause of endometriosis is that, during menstruation, some of the ____________ tissue backs up through the ____________ tubes into the abdomen.

33. Signs and Symptoms of Endometriosis

i. ____________________
ii. ____________________
iii. ____________________
iv. ____________________
v. ____________________
vi. ____________________
vii. ____________________
viii. ____________________

34. Treatment for Endometriosis

A. Early diagnosis and treatment may limit ______ growth and help prevent __________.
B. Pregnancy, ______________, and other hormones appear to delay the onset of endometriosis.
C. Treatment with medication focuses on treating the ___________.
D. __________ is generally reserved for women with severe endometriosis.

35. Fibrocystic Breast Disease

A. Fibrocystic breast disease involves common, _________ changes in the tissues of the breast.
B. It is common in __________ breasts.

C. The condition usually subsides with ___________.
D. Estimated to affect more than _____% of all women.

36. Signs and Symptoms of Fibrocystic Breast Disease
i. ______
ii. ______
iii. ______
iv. ______
v. ______

37. Treatment for Fibrocystic Breast Disease
i. ______
ii. ______
iii. ______
iv. ______
v. ______

38. Sexually Transmitted Infections (STIs)
A. Transmitted via the exchange of ________, ________, and other bodily fluids, or by direct contact with the affected areas of people with STIs.
B. STIs are also called ___________ diseases.

39. The Most Common Sexually Transmitted Infections in the United States
i. ______
ii. ______
iii. ______
iv. ______
v. ______
vi. ______

40. Reducing the Risk of Contracting a Sexually Transmitted Infection
i. ______
ii. ______
iii. ______

41. Sexually Transmitted Infections (List and briefly explain each.)
i. Acquired immune deficiency syndrome (AIDS): ______
ii. Candidiasis: ______
iii. Chancroid: ______
iv. Chlamydial infection: ______
v. Genital herpes: ______
vi. Genital warts: ______
vii. Gonorrhea: ______
viii. Hepatitis: ______
ix. Syphilis: ______
x. Trichomoniasis: ______

42. Vaginitis
A. An inflammation of the vagina that can result in discharge, _________, or ________.
B. The most common cause is a change in the normal balance of vaginal _______ or an ______.
C. Reduced ___________ levels after menopause are another contributing factor.
D. The most common types of vaginitis
i. ______
ii. ______
iii. ______
iv. ______

III. The Male Reproductive System

1. The Scrotum
   A. The scrotum is a pouch-like structure behind the _________.
   B. It is suspended from the __________ region.
   C. It is divided into _____ sacs by a septum.
2. The Penis
   A. Composed of _____________ tissue covered by skin.
   B. The size and shape of the penis vary; the average erect penis is about _____ to _____ cm in length.
   C. Covered with a loose fold of skin called the __________, or __________.
3. The Epididymis
   A. The epididymis is a coiled tube lying on the posterior aspect of the __________.
   B. It is between _____ and _____ feet in length.
   C. It is coiled into a space that is less than _____ cm in length and ends at the ________ __________.
   D. Its function is to serve as the storage site for maturing __________.
4. The Ductus Deferens
   A. The ductus deferens is a slim, muscular tube about _____ cm in length that is continuous with the ___________.
   B. It is the excretory duct of the _________.
   C. Extends from a point adjacent to the ______ and enters the abdomen at the ______ canal.
5. The Two Seminal Vesicles
   A. The vesicles are connected by a narrow ______ to the _____________.
   B. Form the _____________ duct.
   C. Produce an __________ fluid that becomes part of the seminal fluid, or semen.
6. The Prostate Gland
   A. Lies behind the _______ bladder.
   B. Wraps around the first _____ cm of the urethra.
   C. It is about _____ cm wide.
   D. Secretes an __________ fluid that aids in maintaining the viability of the ____________.
7. The Male Urethra
   A. The male urethra is approximately _____ cm long.
   B. It is divided into three sections: ___________, ___________, and _____________.
   C. Extends from the bladder to the ________ orifice at the end of the __________.

IV. The Pathology of the Male Reproductive System

1. Disorders of the Male Reproductive System (Briefly explain each.)
   A. Anorchism: ______________________________
   B. Aspermia: ______________________________
   C. Azoospermia: ______________________________
   D. Carcinoma of the testes: ______________________________
   E. Cryptorchidism: ______________________________
   F. Phimosis: ______________________________
   G. Prostatitis: ______________________________
   H. Varicocele: ______________________________
2. Benign Prostatic Hyperplasia (BPH)
   A. BPH is also known as ______________________________.
   B. May occur in men _____ years of age and older.
   C. By age _____, four out of five men have an enlarged ____________.

3. Signs and Symptoms of Benign Prostatic Hyperplasia
   i. ____________________
   ii. ____________________
   iii. ____________________
   iv. ____________________
   v. ____________________
   vi. ____________________
   vii. ____________________
   viii. ____________________
4. Treatment for Benign Prostatic Hyperplasia
   i. ____________________
   ii. ____________________
   iii. ____________________
   iv. ____________________
5. Epididymitis
   A. Epididymitis is an inflammation or __________ of the epididymis.
   B. The most severe pain and swelling are usually associated with the ________ form.
   C. Symptoms may last for more than _____ weeks after treatment begins.
   D. Can occur anytime after the onset of puberty, but is most common between the ages of _____ and _____.
6. Risk Factors for Epididymitis
   A. Infection of the ________, __________, __________, or _________ _________
   B. A narrowing of the __________
   C. Use of a __________ catheter
7. Causes of Epididymitis
   A. Can be caused by the same organisms that cause some ____ or as a result of ______ surgery.
   B. Generally caused by _____-generating __________ associated with infections in other parts of the body.
   C. Can also be caused by an injury to or ___________ of the scrotum.
8. Signs and Symptoms of Epididymitis
   A. Sudden redness and swelling of the ___________
   B. The affected __________ is hard and sore.
   C. Enlarged _________ nodes in the groin that may cause scrotal pain
9. Treatment for Epididymitis
   A. Because it can cause __________, ___________ therapy must be initiated as soon as symptoms appear.
   B. Patients are advised to wear _________ ___________ when they resume normal activities.
10. Erectile Dysfunction
    A. Erectile dysfunction is the inability to achieve or __________ an _________.
    B. Is not an ___________ part of aging.
    C. Occurs when not enough blood is supplied to the ___________.
11. Risk Factors for Erectile Dysfunction
    i. ____________________
    ii. ____________________
    iii. ____________________
    iv. ____________________
    v. ____________________
    vi. ____________________
    vii. ____________________

viii. ____________________
ix. ____________________
x. ____________________
xi. ____________________
xii. ____________________
xiii. ____________________
xiv. ____________________
xv. ____________________

12. Treatment for Erectile Dysfunction
    i. ____________________
    ii. ____________________
    iii. ____________________
    iv. ____________________
    v. ____________________

13. Hydrocele
    A. Hydrocele is a painless buildup of __________ fluid around one or both __________ that causes swelling in the __________ or groin area.
    B. Can be __________ or acquired.

14. Signs and Symptoms of Hydrocele
    A. The scrotum may have a __________ tinge.
    B. The swelling is __________, may be soft or firm, and cannot be reduced by changing its position or gently pushing it up.
    C. The swelling may change in __________.

15. Prostate Cancer
    A. Prostate cancer is a __________ tumor that grows in the __________ gland.
    B. It is the second leading cause of cancer __________ in men.
    C. By age 50, ______ in ______ American men has some __________ cells in the prostate gland.
    D. The average age of diagnosis is ______.

16. Risk Factors for Prostate Cancer
    i. ____________________
    ii. ____________________
    iii. ____________________
    iv. ____________________
    v. ____________________

17. Signs and Symptoms of Prostate Cancer
    i. ____________________
    ii. ____________________
    iii. ____________________
    iv. ____________________
    v. ____________________
    vi. ____________________
    vii. ____________________
    viii. ____________________
    ix. ____________________

18. Treatment for Prostate Cancer
    i. ____________________
    ii. ____________________
    iii. ____________________
    iv. ____________________
    v. ____________________

vi. ____________________

vii. ____________________

viii. ____________________

KEY TERMINOLOGY REVIEW

Match the vocabulary term to the correct definition below.

a. Breast cancer
b. Bulbourethral glands
c. Cervicitis
d. Epididymitis
e. Episiotomy
f. Erectile dysfunction
g. Fallopian tubes
h. Fibrocystic breast disease
i. Myomectomy
j. Ovaries
k. Ovulation
l. Ovum
m. Prostate cancer
n. Prostate gland
o. Salpingo-oophorectomy
p. Sexually transmitted infections
q. Spermatozoa
r. Urethra
s. Uterine cancer
t. Uterus

1. ____________ Most cases are caused by a sexually transmitted infection such as gonorrhea and chlamydia.
2. ____________ A type of surgery performed for uterine fibroids.
3. ____________ Contains six sets of ligaments.
4. ____________ A term for more than 20 different infections.
5. ____________ Move the egg from the ovary to the uterus.
6. ____________ The process where a Graafian follicle ruptures on the ovarian cortex and an ovum is released into the pelvic cavity and into one of the fallopian tubes.
7. ____________ The most common cause of pain in the scrotum.
8. ____________ Extends from the bladder to the urethral orifice at the end of the penis.
9. ____________ Composed of glandular, connective, and muscular tissue.
10. ____________ Second leading cause of death by cancer in women (second only to lung cancer).
11. ____________ The most common cancer among American men.
12. ____________ Procedure that is performed to prevent tearing of the perineum during delivery.
13. ____________ Also called adenocarcinoma.
14. ____________ Produced by the testes.
15. ____________ Located inferior to the prostate and on either side of the urethra.
16. ____________ An egg or reproductive cell.
17. ____________ Also referred to as mammary dysplasia.
18. ____________ Removal of the ovaries and the fallopian tubes.
19. ____________ Their function is to produce estrogen and progesterone.
20. ____________ A symptom of prostate cancer.

APPLIED PRACTICE

1. Label the uterus, ovaries, and associated structures.

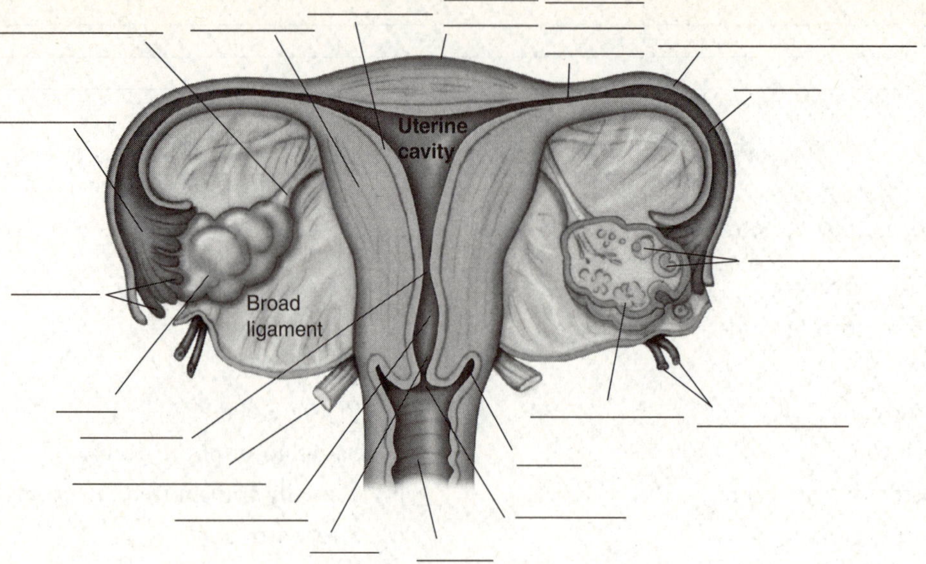

2. Label the structures of the male reproductive system.

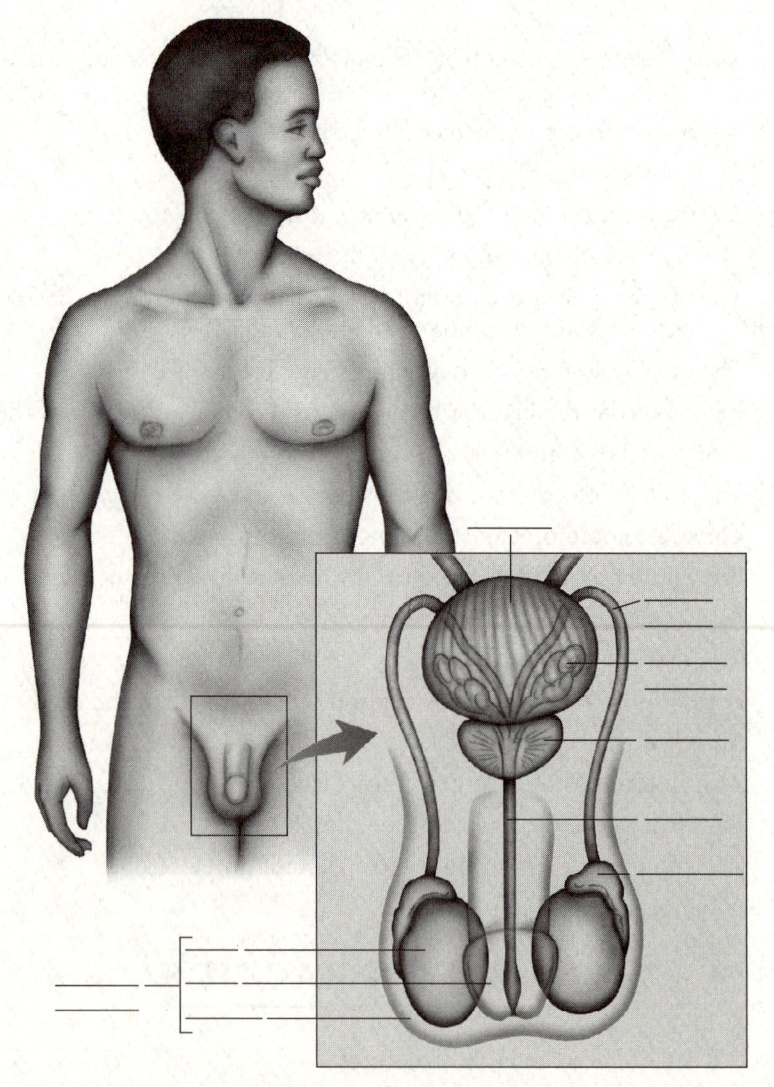

LEARNING ACTIVITY: FILL IN THE BLANK

Using words from the list below, fill in the blanks to complete the following statements.

Benign prostatic hyperplasia	Ovarian cysts
Cervical cancer	Pelvic inflammatory disease (PID)
Circumcision	Perineum
Dysmenorrhea	Premenstrual syndrome (PMS)
Endometriosis	Scrotum
Hydrocele	Testes
Hysterectomy	Urethritis
Menarche	Uterine fibroids
Ovarian cancer	Vaginitis

1. Phimosis is typically treated by performing a ____________________.
2. Anorchism is a congenital absence of one or both _________.
3. ___________occurs at the age of puberty.
4. The main symptom of a _________ is a swollen scrotum or groin area.
5. The ______________ is between the vulva and the anus.
6. ____________________ is an enlargement of the prostate gland.
7. Symptoms of epididymitis include chills, fever, and acute ____________.
8. To test for __________, a pap test is typically performed.
9. A genitourinary infection caused by a parasite that is usually asymptomatic (without symptoms) in both males and females; can produce itching and/or burning and a foul-smelling discharge and result in ___________ in women.
10. Typically, by the time ____________ is diagnosed, the cancer is usually at an advanced stage.
11. ______________ is defined as the symptoms that develop just prior to the onset of a menstrual period.
12. ______________ are not disease related and typically disappear on their own.
13. Epididymitis is characterized by sudden redness and swelling of the __________.
14. ___________ is described as painful cramping associated with menstruation.
15. A ______________ involves the removal of the uterus.
16. ________________ is the most common and serious complication of STIs among women.
17. Although the cause of _____________ is unknown, one theory suggests that delayed childbearing increases the risk.
18. _____________ usually, but not always, shrink or disappear after menopause.

CRITICAL THINKING

Answer the following questions to the best of your ability. Utilize the textbook as a reference.

1. A patient asks you if you think that her infant son should be circumcised. What do you do?

____

____

2. How can you ensure a patient's privacy when you are calling to talk with them by phone?

RESEARCH ACTIVITY

Utilize Internet search engines to research the following topics and write a brief description of what you find. It is important to utilize reputable websites.

1. Visit www.cdc.gov. As you navigate through the site, what information would be helpful to provide a patient who has a sexually transmitted disease?

CHAPTER 34
Infection Control

CHAPTER OUTLINE

General review of the chapter:

History of Asepsis
Microorganisms
The Infection Control System
Universal Precautions
Implementing OSHA Guidelines
Hepatitis
HIV and AIDS
Multidrug-Resistant Organisms
Bioterrorism

STUDENT STUDY GUIDE

Use the following guide to assist in your learning of the concepts from the chapter.

I. Infection Control

1. Microorganisms: A Definition

   A. Microorganisms, also called ___________, are living organisms that can be seen only with a ___________.

   B. Microorganisms include __________, __________, ________, and __________.

2. The Scientific Fields of the Study of Microorganisms (List and briefly explain each.)

   i. ______________________________
   ii. ______________________________
   iii. ______________________________
   iv. ______________________________

3. The Stages of the Infection Process (Explain each stage.)

   A. Invasion: ______________________________
   B. Multiplication: ______________________________
   C. Incubation period: ______________________________
   D. Prodromal period: ______________________________
   E. Acute period: ______________________________
   F. Recovery period: ______________________________

4. Preventing the Spread of Infection

   A. Prevent the spread of __________________ microorganisms.
   B. __________________ the microorganisms.

5. The Body's Barriers to Infection (List the four barriers that the body provides against infection.)

   i. ______________________________
   ii. ______________________________

iii. ______________________________
iv. ______________________________

6. Genetic and Acquired Immunity
   A. Genetic immunity does not involve ________________.
   B. Acquired immunity may be achieved through active or ________________ means.
7. Natural Active and Artificial Active Immunity
   A. Natural active immunity develops as a result of having recovered from a ______________
   B. Artificial active immunity is the result of receiving a ________________ containing an inactivated or attenuated organism.
8. Types of Acquired Immunity
   A. Active acquired natural immunity is achieved by having the ________, which results in the production of ________________ and "memory cells" that respond if the antigen reappears.
   B. Active acquired artificial immunity is achieved by administering a ________ that stimulate the production of ________________ and "memory cells" to prevent that disease from occurring.
   C. Passive acquired natural immunity is achieved by receiving someone else's ______________ such as from the mother to the fetus through the placenta or through breast milk.
   D. Temporary protection for passive acquired artificial immunity is achieved from ________________.
9. Cardinal Signs of Inflammation
   i. ______________________________
   ii. ______________________________
   iii. ______________________________
   iv. ______________________________
10. The Centers for Disease Control and Prevention's (CDC's) Two-tiered Precautionary System
   A. Universal precautions apply to ________ patients and assume that all ______________ fluids and ________________ are infected with ________________.
   B. Standard precautions apply to ________ patients regardless of medical condition or the ris of spreading ________________.
   C. Transmission-based precautions apply to patients who are suspected of carrying ________________ diseases or who are known to be ________________.

II. Universal Precautions and Aseptic Techniques
1. The Requirements of Bloodborne Pathogen Standards
   A. Employees must follow ________________ precautions to impede contact with ________________ material.
   B. Employees must consider all ________________ fluids contagious if unable to differentiat among ________________ fluids.
2. Following the Standard Precautions
   A. Medical professionals should change gloves between ________________ or if gloves are ________________.
   B. Medical professionals should wash their hands ________ or when ________________.
   C. Medical professionals should avoid direct ________________ resuscitation.
   D. Medical professionals should use ________________ waste containers for contaminated material.
3. Hand Sanitizing and Hygiene
   A. Hand sanitizing is one of the best means of reducing the spread of ________________ in a health care facility and at home.

B. Hand hygiene recommendations include not wearing ________________ fingernails.
C. Natural fingernails should be kept short (less than ________ inch long).

4. The CDC's Guidelines for Respiratory Hygiene/Cough Etiquette

A. Signs are to be posted to remind people to cover their ________________ and ________________ when coughing and to dispose of tissues properly.
B. Perform ________________ hygiene after contact with respiratory secretions.
C. Provide at least ________________ feet of space around persons with respiratory infections whenever possible.

5. The CDC's Safe Injection Practices

A. Use ________________ technique.
B. No ________________ vials should be kept in the immediate treatment area.
C. Do not use bags or bottles of intravenous (IV) solutions among ________________ patients.

6. Airborne Precautions

A. Used for patients who are known to be infected with ________________ that are transmitted via ________ droplet ________________.
B. Often involve patient ________________ in a private room if hospitalized, as well as the use of a ________________ and ________________ by all health care personnel who come in contact with the patient.
C. The transport of the patient should be as ________________ as possible, with the patient wearing a ________________ during transport.
D. All reusable patient care equipment should be ________________ and ________________ before use on another patient.

7. Droplet Precautions

A. Used for patients suspected of being infected with ________________ spread by ________________ during sneezing, coughing, and talking.
B. A ________________ should be worn if a caregiver is within ________ feet of an infected patient.
C. ________________ and gloves are worn if there is a chance of coming in contact with the blood or bodily fluids of suspected patients.
D. All reusable equipment should be ________________ and ________________.

8. Contact Precautions

A. Used when infections are difficult to treat and the likelihood of ________ transmission among patients and health care providers is high.
B. Precautions include isolating ________ and wearing ________________ and gloves.
C. If there is a chance of coming in contact with bodily fluids, a ______________ and eyewear should be worn.

9. Latex Sensitivity

A. Before touching a patient while wearing latex gloves, ask the patient if there is a history of latex ________________.
B. High-risk patients, such as those with congenital defects and indwelling ________________, must always be assessed for latex ________________.
C. Patients with allergies to ________________, chestnuts, kiwi, and ________ may have cross sensitivity to latex.

10. The Occupational Safety and Health Administration's Goals and Guidelines

A. Aim to minimize exposure to hepatitis __________ and HIV.
B. Programs include ______________ determination, method of compliance, and ______________ evaluation.

11. Items That Employers Should Have Available to Ensure Worker Safety
    i. ____________
    ii. ____________
    iii. ____________
    iv. ____________
    v. ____________
    vi. ____________

12. Disposing of Infectious Waste (List the guidelines for disposal.)
    i. ____________
    ii. ____________
    iii. ____________
    iv. ____________
    v. ____________
    vi. ____________
    vii. ____________
    viii. ____________
    ix. ____________

13. Physical and Chemical Barriers
    A. Used to maintain ____________ control.
    B. Prevent ____________ infections and hospital/medical facility-acquired infections.
    C. Barrier is achieved when medical and ____________ asepsis are maintained.

14. Medical Asepsis
    A. Medical asepsis is the elimination of ____________ that have left the body.
    B. Surgical asepsis is the practice of creating and maintaining a ____________ environment in which ____________ are destroyed before they enter the body.

15. Practicing Medical Asepsis Hygiene Habits
    i. ____________
    ii. ____________
    iii. ____________
    iv. ____________
    v. ____________
    vi. ____________

16. Medical Asepsis in the Facility
    A. Practices in addition to personal hygiene and equipment cleanliness
        i. Keep examination rooms ____________.
        ii. ____________ trash cans.
        iii. Replace ____________ containers appropriately.
        iv. Look for insect ____________.
        v. Separate well patients from ____________ patients in seating areas.

17. Steps for Proper Hand Hygiene
    i. ____________
    ii. ____________
    iii. ____________
    iv. ____________
    v. ____________
    vi. ____________
    vii. ____________
    viii. ____________
    ix. ____________
    x. ____________

18. Alcohol-Based Hand Sanitizers
    A. Hand sanitizers were recently approved by the _______________.
    B. Unless the hands are visibly _________________ or the professional has used the restroom or _________________, the use of hand sanitizers is an alternative to using soap and water.
    C. Approximately ________ to ________ mL of solution should be placed in the palm and vigorously worked into the hands and wrists for ________ to ________ seconds.

19. Personal Protective Equipment
    A. Worn in order to accomplish the following
        i. ______________________________
        ii. ______________________________
        iii. ______________________________

20. Procedures for Applying Gloves
    i. ______________________________
    ii. ______________________________
    iii. ______________________________
    iv. ______________________________
    v. ______________________________

21. Procedures for Removing Gloves
    i. ______________________________
    ii. ______________________________
    iii. ______________________________
    iv. ______________________________
    v. ______________________________

22. Steps for Performing Isolation Techniques
    i. ______________________________
    ii. ______________________________
    iii. ______________________________
    iv. ______________________________
    v. ______________________________
    vi. ______________________________
    vii. ______________________________
    viii. ______________________________
    ix. ______________________________
    x. ______________________________

23. Steps for Removing Barrier Protection
    i. ______________________________
    ii. ______________________________
    iii. ______________________________
    iv. ______________________________
    v. ______________________________
    vi. ______________________________
    vii. ______________________________
    viii. ______________________________

III. Surgical Asepsis

1. Surgical Asepsis: Sanitizing Instruments
    A. Prevents pathogens from _______________ or _______________ pathogens.
    B. Should be used for instruments that only touch the _______________ surface.

2. Sanitizing Equipment and Supplies (List the equipment and the supplies used.)

   i. ______________________________
   ii. ______________________________
   iii. ______________________________
   iv. ______________________________
   v. ______________________________
   vi. ______________________________
   vii. ______________________________

3. Disinfecting Instruments (Explain the use of each of the following methods.)

   A. Alcohol: ______________________________
   B. Chlorine: ______________________________
   C. Formaldehyde: ______________________________
   D. Hydrogen peroxide: ______________________________
   E. Glutaraldehyde: ______________________________

4. Sterilizing Instruments

   A. Any ____________ that touch wounds or internal body ____________ must be sterilized.
   B. Sterile gloves must be worn when touching ____________ equipment.
   C. The process of putting on sterile or nonsterile gloves is called ____________.

5. The Autoclave

   A. Autoclaves are used for ____________.
   B. Autoclaves cause ____________ to explode, thus killing them.
   C. Types of autoclaves
      i. ______________________________
      ii. ______________________________
      iii. ______________________________
      iv. ______________________________

6. Cleaning an Autoclave

   A. An autoclave should be ____________ before each use.
   B. If detergent is used, the autoclave should be ________ thoroughly before use.
   C. The air exhaust valve must be ____________ and free of lint before use.

7. Wrapping Instruments and Materials

   A. Wrappings must be ____________ and strong.
   B. Types of wrappings
      i. ______________________________
      ii. ______________________________
      iii. ______________________________
      iv. ______________________________
   C. The wrapping generally has ____________ layers.
   D. The hinges of instruments should be in an ____________ position, the tubing should be free of kinks, and ____________ should be unassembled.

8. Autoclave Indicator Tapes

   A. Indicator tapes are placed in the ____________.
   B. The lines on the tape change color during the process to indicate that the appropriate ____________ has been reached.

9. Autoclave Sterilization Pouches and Bags

   A. The instrument must be ____________ and ____________.
   B. The pouch must not rupture during ____________.
   C. The pouch must have ____________ indicators inside and outside.

10. Autoclave Trays
    A. Used only for those instruments that will be used ____________.
    B. Trays are ____________.
    C. A ____________ is usually placed under instruments to absorb moisture.
    D. The lid should be placed on the tray ____________ after sterilization.
11. Handling Individual Packs
    A. Items should be wrapped in ____________ packs.
    B. When individual packs are opened, the contents must be removed without introducing ____________.
    C. Solutions should be ____________ separately.
12. Time and Pressure Requirements
    A. Always follow the ____________ requirements.
    B. Items will not be sterilized if the time or ____________ is changed.
13. Drying Autoclaved Goods
    A. Improperly dried items can lead to ____________ growth.
    B. Procedures for drying goods
       i. Open the autoclave door ____________ inch before the drying cycle.
       ii. Run the drying cycle per the ____________ instructions.
14. Sterilization Indicators
    A. Used to indicate ____________.
    B. The appearance of dots or a change in ____________ indicates that proper sterility has been achieved.
15. The Shelf Life of Autoclaved Packages
    A. The oldest items should always be used ____________.
    B. Items are considered sterile for ________ to ________ days.
    C. The shelf life is ________ month(s), but depends on how the item was wrapped.

IV. Hepatitis, AIDS, and Bioterrorism
1. Hepatitis A (HAV)
    A. Transmitted when ____________ waste contaminates the food or water supply.
    B. The incubation period is ________ to ________ days.
2. Symptoms of Hepatitis A
    i. ________________________________
    ii. ________________________________
    iii. ________________________________
    iv. ________________________________
    v. ________________________________
    vi. ________________________________
    vii. ________________________________
3. Hepatitis B (HBV)
    A. Transmitted through ____________ fluids.
    B. HBV is a potentially fatal disease that can be passed from one drug user to another when sharing a ____________ needle.
    C. Infection with HBV ____________ the risk of contracting HIV and HAV.
    D. The incubation period for this liver infection is ________ to ________ days, with a rapid onset of symptoms.
4. Symptoms of and Treatment for Hepatitis B
    A. About ________% of infected persons have no signs or symptoms.
    B. Treatment for all forms of hepatitis is a ____________ diet and rest for several weeks.

5. Hepatitis B Vaccine

   A. Routine vaccines are recommended from birth to age ________.
   B. Vaccination is recommended for ______________ groups.
   C. Any personnel with a high risk of contact with ______________ and bodily fluids should be encouraged to receive the vaccine.
   D. If an employee decides not to get vaccinated, a ______________ must be signed and placed in the employee's file.

6. Types of Hepatitis B Vaccine

   A. Types include ______________ and ______________.
   B. Vaccines are administered in ______________ doses.

7. Cautions About Receiving the Vaccine

   A. Persons who are sensitive to ______________ or any of the other components found in the vaccine should not receive it.
   B. ______________ mothers or persons with ______________ disease should be cautious about receiving the vaccine.

8. Hepatitis C

   A. Hepatitis C is the most ______________ form of new cases each year.
   B. The symptoms are similar to hepatitis ________.
   C. The treatment of choice is ______________ and ______________.

9. Hepatitis D

   A. Transmitted through the use of ______________ drugs and/or ______________ contact.
   B. The symptoms are ______________ severe than for the other types.
   C. Often seen in conjunction with ______________ and ______________ cases.

10. The Hepatitis E and G Viruses

   A. Hepatitis E is the result of exposure to food contaminated with human ______________.
   B. It is a major infectious disease in developing countries because of poor ______________ conditions.
   C. This form of hepatitis is ______________ in the United States.
   D. Recently, hepatitis G has been isolated as a ______________ infection.

11. HIV and AIDS

   A. There are more than ________ million persons living with HIV in the United States.
   B. The virus was first identified in the United States in ______________.
   C. Worldwide, more than ________ million people are infected with HIV.

12. Survival Characteristics of the Human Immunodeficiency Virus

   A. HIV cannot survive on ______________ objects.
   B. HIV can survive in bodily ______________.

13. AIDS-Related Complex (ARC)

   A. ARC develops before ______________ and is milder.
   B. Symptoms of ARC
      i. ______________________________
      ii. ______________________________
      iii. ______________________________
      iv. ______________________________
      v. ______________________________
      vi. ______________________________
      vii. ______________________________
      viii. ______________________________

14. Developing AIDS
    A. It can take ________ years or more for HIV infection to advance to AIDS.
    B. A person who becomes infected with HIV develops ____________________.
    C. A person may experience swollen ________________________ glands for a number of years.
    D. After the immune system is severely compromised, ________________ can occur.
    E. The final stage of HIV infection is ________________________.
15. Other HIV-related Conditions (List four opportunistic infections that can occur as a result of a suppressed immune system.)
    i. ____________________
    ii. ____________________
    iii. ____________________
    iv. ____________________
16. Risk Factors for AIDS (List persons who are at highest risk for contracting HIV.)
    i. ____________________
    ii. ____________________
    iii. ____________________
    iv. ____________________
    v. ____________________
17. Symptoms of AIDS
    i. ____________________
    ii. ____________________
    iii. ____________________
    iv. ____________________
    v. ____________________
    vi. ____________________
    vii. ____________________
    viii. ____________________
    ix. ____________________
    x. ____________________
    xi. ____________________
    xii. ____________________
18. Caring for a Person with AIDS
    A. Procedures for protecting the caregiver
        i. ____________________
        ii. ____________________
        iii. ____________________
        iv. ____________________
    B. Procedures for protecting the patient
        i. ____________________
        ii. ____________________
        iii. ____________________
19. Multidrug-Resistant Organisms (MDROs)
    A. MDROs are bacteria and other __________ that have developed a resistance to __________ drugs.
    B. Examples of MDROs
        i. ____________________
        ii. ____________________
        iii. ____________________
        iv. ____________________

v. ______________________________
vi. ______________________________

20. Risk Factors for Acquiring MDROs
    i. ______________________________
    ii. ______________________________
    iii. ______________________________
    iv. ______________________________
    v. ______________________________

21. Symptoms of Staph Infection
    i. ______________________________
    ii. ______________________________
    iii. ______________________________
    iv. ______________________________

22. Bioterrorism
    A. Bioterrorism is the deliberate release of ___________, __________, or other agents that can cause illness and death in humans, animals, or plants.
    B. Biological agents can be spread through the __________, __________, or __________.

23. Category A Agents or Toxins (List six examples.)
    i. ______________________________
    ii. ______________________________
    iii. ______________________________
    iv. ______________________________
    v. ______________________________
    vi. ______________________________

KEY TERMINOLOGY REVIEW

Use the key terms found at the beginning of the chapter to finish the sentences below. Key terms may be more than one word in length.

1. ______________ bacteria require an oxygen supply to live.
2. ______________ kills all microorganisms, both pathogenic and nonpathogenic.
3. Microorganisms normally found on the skin may enter the body through a ______________ and may cause infections.
4. The body has a natural protective mechanism called ______________.
5. Microorganisms that are normally found on the skin and in the urinary, gastrointestinal, and respiratory tracts are known as ______________.
6. ______________ is the state of being free from germs, infection, and any form of microbial life.
7. During the process of inflammation, phagocytes engulf, digest, and destroy ______________.
8. ______________ bacteria can survive without oxygen.
9. The principles of asepsis are applied in the hospital setting to prevent the spread of ______________.
10. ______________ destroys most or all pathogens on inanimate objects with the use of chemicals such as iodine, chlorine, alcohol, and phenol.
11. The pathogen present in the ______________ is the beginning of the chain of infection.
12. MRSA is highly resistant to ______________.
13. Leukocytes actively fight pathogenic microorganisms with the process of ______________.

14. ______________ such as *Staphylococcus* (staph), *Streptococcus* (strep), and malaria can cause disease.

15. The gastrointestinal tract, containing hydrochloric acid (HCl), causes a ______________ action that destroys disease-producing bacteria.

APPLIED PRACTICE

Follow the directions as instructed with each question below.

1. Identify the links of the cycle of infection, as well as the incubation and prodromal periods.

> **Scenario**
>
> Shandra Graham, CMA (AAMA), did not know that she was infected with the flu virus when she went to work at Peachtree Medical Center. She forgot to wash her hands after she had coughed just prior to assisting her patient, Adam Kenney, into the examination room. While she was checking Mr. Kenney's blood pressure, Shandra sneezed and, unfortunately, was unable to cover her mouth.
>
> Two days later, Mr. Kenney developed some muscle aches that he had attributed to his exercise regimen. By day 5 after his office visit, Mr. Kenney had a high fever, chills, and intense muscular aches.

a. Who, in this scenario, represents the reservoir host within the cycle of infection?

____

b. What is the means of exit of the infectious pathogen?

____

c. What is the means of transmission of the pathogen?

____

d. Who is the susceptible host?

____

e. What is the incubation period for the reservoir host?

____

____

____

f. What is the prodromal period for the person who became infected?

____

____

____

2. Using what you have learned from the chapter, arrange the following steps in order to reflect the process of sanitization, disinfection, and sterilization of instruments. Read through all of the steps carefully. When you find what you think is the first step, write its corresponding letter in the space provided for step one. Continue this process until you have assigned the final step.

a. Completely immerse instruments in a container of disinfectant, cover, and let soak for the recommended length of time.
b. With hinges open, allow instruments to air dry on a cotton towel.
c. Remove instruments from the disinfectant, rinse thoroughly, and dry with paper towels.
d. Place contaminated instruments in an empty basin, cover the basin, and transport to the cleaning area.
e. Load the autoclave.

f. Read MSDS for disinfectant and check the expiration date.
g. Place disinfected instruments in the center of dry wrapping paper.
h. Fold wrapping paper as directed and apply sterilization indicator tape.
i. Place instruments in a neutral low-suds detergent.
j. Remove the instruments to a clean container using sterile transfer forceps.
k. Check the distilled water level in the autoclave reservoir, and add distilled water as necessary.
l. Use a soft brush on all serrated and smooth edges, grooves, and open hinges; cleaning one instrument at a time.
m. Turn on the autoclave.
n. Put on disposable gloves and then utility gloves before handling the disinfectant.

Step 1: ___________
Step 2: ___________
Step 3: ___________
Step 4: ___________
Step 5: ___________
Step 6: ___________
Step 7: ___________
Step 8: ___________
Step 9: ___________
Step 10: ___________
Step 11: ___________
Step 12: ___________
Step 13: ___________
Step 14: ___________

LEARNING ACTIVITY: MULTIPLE CHOICE

Circle the correct answer to each of the questions below.

1. Since ________________, the United States has been screening all blood for HIV antibodies.
   a. 1980
   b. 1990
   c. 1978
   d. 1985
2. The initial signs of HIV infection may include ______________.
   a. symptoms of an opportunistic infection
   b. flulike symptoms such as fever, sore throat, swollen glands, and muscle aches
   c. symptoms of Kaposi's sarcoma
   d. no symptoms in the primary stage
3. Waterless hand sanitizers kill ________% of common microorganisms in 15 seconds.
   a. 90
   b. 95
   c. 99.9
   d. 100
4. The ordinary hygiene habits of everyday life are a form of ______________________.
   a. medical asepsis
   b. surgical asepsis
   c. bloodborne asepsis
   d. None of the above

5. The CDC Special Pathogens Branch and the CDC National Center for Preparedness, Detection, and Control of Infectious Diseases (NCPDCID) ________________________________.
   a. monitor outbreaks of the category illnesses
   b. have goals that include developing rapid diagnostic tests
   c. offer assistance in control and prevention during outbreaks
   d. All of the above

6. Sodium hypochlorite is actually ____________.
   a. alcohol
   b. salt with chloride
   c. household bleach
   d. None of the above

7. The personal protective equipment you will wear for various tasks is determined by ___________.
   a. actual or anticipated exposure to microorganisms
   b. actual or anticipated exposure to blood and bodily fluids and OPIM
   c. actual or anticipated exposure to nosocomial infections
   d. actual or anticipated exposure to hepatitis B or HIV/AIDS

8. An exposure control program must be implemented in each facility and must include the following ________________________________.
   a. exposure determination
   b. method of compliance
   c. postexposure evaluation
   d. All of the above

9. The hepatitis B vaccine has been available since __________.
   a. 1965
   b. 1974
   c. 1982
   d. 2000

10. By which of the following means can the AIDS virus enter the body?
   a. Vaginal, anal, or oral intercourse with a person who has the virus
   b. Receiving an organ transplant from a donor who has the virus
   c. Receiving artificial insemination with the sperm of a man who has the virus
   d. All of the above

CRITICAL THINKING

Answer the following questions to the best of your ability. Utilize the textbook as a reference.

1. What is the main premise of Standard and Universal Precautions and the Bloodborne Pathogen Standard? What impact on patient discrimination do you think this has had?

   ____

   ____

   ____

   ____

2. You are working on preparing the sterile field and go to the autoclave for the paper-wrapped packs of instruments that you ran earlier that day. The tape on the outside of the packs has the darkened stripes so you know that the outside of the pack has been sterilized. The physician is behind schedule and irritated about that. There are no extra instruments for this particular procedure, which is why you

planned ahead and autoclaved them earlier. You open all of the packs and transfer the contents to the sterile tray and put the sterile cover over it. As you clean up the empty paper and packages, you notice that the sterilization indicator from the inside of the packs had not changed color. What would you do? Say nothing and assume that the tape on the outside indicated that the entire package had been sterilized? Tell the doctor that it will take another 40 minutes to re-autoclave the items and get them ready for the procedure? Say nothing because you fear the physician's anger or even losing your job?

RESEARCH ACTIVITY

Utilize Internet search engines to research the following topics and write a brief description of what you find. It is important to utilize reputable websites.

1. Research the website for the Occupational Safety and Health Administration, www.osha.gov.
   What information can be found for health care facilities? List some facts found within the website.

CHAPTER 35
Vital Signs

CHAPTER OUTLINE

General review of the chapter:

Interviewing the Patient
Correct Documentation
Measuring Weight and Height
Vital Signs
Temperature
Pulse
Respiration
Blood Pressure
Pain
Body Fat Measurement

STUDENT STUDY GUIDE

Use the following guide to assist in your learning of the concepts from the chapter.

I. Documentation of Patient Information

1. Reasons for Maintaining the Patient's Medical Record
   i. ______________________________
   ii. ______________________________
   iii. ______________________________
   iv. ______________________________
   v. ______________________________
   vi. ______________________________
   vii. ______________________________
2. Contents of the Patient's Medical Record
   i. ______________________________
   ii. ______________________________
   iii. ______________________________
   iv. ______________________________
   v. ______________________________
   vi. ______________________________
   vii. ______________________________
   viii. ______________________________
   ix. ______________________________
3. Types of Diagnosis (Explain each of the following types.)
   A. Final or medical diagnosis: ______________________________
   B. Clinical diagnosis or working diagnosis: ______________________________
   C. Differential diagnosis: ______________________________

4. Steps for Gathering Information to Ensure Proper Charting
   A. Before a patient has a physical examination or is seen by the physician, a __________ __________ must be obtained.
   B. The initial patient interview is conducted by the medical assistant and the information gathered becomes part of the __________ __________ __________.
   C. After the initial data have been gathered, the patient's __________ __________, __________, and __________ are measured.
   D. The physician then examines the patient and __________ the information obtained.
5. The Initial Patient Interview
   A. Performed to obtain information on the patient's __________ and __________ __________ and treatments.
   B. It is important to ensure the patient's __________ during the interview.
6. Considerations When Interviewing a Patient
   A. Review the __________ __________ before the interview.
   B. Ask the patient's __________ to interview him or her.
   C. Use an "__________" comment to put the patient at ease.
   D. Provide __________ during the interview.
   E. Be aware of __________ and __________ cues.
   F. Avoid making __________ responses.
   G. Avoid providing medical __________.
   H. Treat __________ topics with respect.
   I. Document according to __________ __________.
7. Charting Guidelines
   i. __________
   ii. __________
   iii. __________
   iv. __________
   v. __________
   vi. __________
   vii. __________
   viii. __________
   ix. __________
   x. __________
   xi. __________
   xii. __________
   xiii. __________
8. The Six Cs of Charting
   A. C __________ own words must be used exactly and be in quotes.
   B. C __________ must be used when recording information.
   C. C __________ is essential.
   D. C __________ of entries saves time and chart space.
   E. C __________ order of information is critical.
   F. C __________ of patient information is mandatory.
9. Weighing a Patient
   A. Frequent weight monitoring is particularly important for certain patients (List patients who would benefit from such monitoring.)
      i. __________
      ii. __________
      iii. __________
      iv. __________

10. Obtaining a Patient's Weight
    A. Typically done with clothing __________.
    B. Shoes should be __________.
    C. Patients who cannot stand may be weighed on a __________ or a __________.
11. Measuring a Patient's Height
    A. Measured __________ shoes.
    B. Heel, buttocks, and the back of the head should be touching the measuring __________ or bar.
    C. Convert inches and feet to __________ by multiplying by 2.5.
    D. Convert from centimeters to __________ by dividing by 2.5.

II. Temperature

1. Vital Signs (List what is considered to be a vital sign.)
    i. ______________________________
    ii. ______________________________
    iii. ______________________________
    iv. ______________________________
    v. ______________________________
2. Factors That Affect Body Temperature
    i. ______________________________
    ii. ______________________________
    iii. ______________________________
    iv. ______________________________
    v. ______________________________
    vi. ______________________________
    vii. ______________________________
    viii. ______________________________
    ix. ______________________________
    x. ______________________________
3. Fever
    A. A fever is also known as __________.
    B. A fever is a temperature that is above __________ (38°C).
    C. Indicates that the body is producing greater __________ than what is being __________.
    D. Indicates that the body is __________.
    E. __________ or __________ develops if the body temperature exceeds 105.8°F (41°C).
    F. A temperature above __________ (43°C) is typically fatal.
4. Common Types of Fevers
    i. ______________________________
    ii. ______________________________
    iii. ______________________________
    iv. ______________________________
5. Signs of a Fever
    i. ______________________________
    ii. ______________________________
    iii. ______________________________
    iv. ______________________________
    v. ______________________________
6. Hypothermia
    A. Hypothermia is indicated by a temperature that is below __________ (36°C).
    B. A temperature below __________ (34°C) is typically fatal.

C. Clinical signs of hypothermia

i. ___

ii. ___

iii. ___

iv. ___

7. Sites for Measuring Body Temperature (Explain why each site might be selected.)

A. Oral: ___

B. Rectal: ___

C. Axillary: ___

D. Tympanic (aural): ___

8. Normal Temperature Values

A. Oral: ___

B. Rectal: ___

C. Axillary: ___

D. Ear (aural): ___

E. Temporal artery: ___

9. Considerations When Taking an Oral Temperature

A. Make sure that the patient closes his or her mouth ___ around the thermometer.

B. Some facilities do not require the use of the degree symbol (°) when documenting this measurement.

C. The thermometer is inserted under the tongue on either side of the ___ ___.

D. For an accurate measurement, the patient must be advised not to ___ during the procedure.

E. Oral temperature should only be measured if ___ minutes have elapsed since the patient has taken fluids or smoked.

10. Considerations When Taking an Axillary Temperature

A. Axillary temperatures register ___ (0.6°C) lower than oral temperatures.

B. The axillary method is the least ___ of the temperature measurements, but it is recommended for small children or patients who have had ___ surgery.

C. This method is affected by ___; therefore, the underarm area should be ___ in order to obtain an accurate reading.

11. Considerations When Taking an Aural Temperature

A. This method uses the ___ ___ area at the end of the external auditory canal.

B. Tympanic thermometers are able to detect ___ waves in the ear canal and calculate body temperature from this data.

12. Considerations When Taking a Temporal Artery Temperature

A. This method is a new, noninvasive procedure involving a device that measures the temperature over the temporal artery located close to the skin surface on the ___ and the ___ area.

B. When the probe/scanner is passed over the surface of the forehead toward the temple, it can read the peak ___ temperature.

13. Types of Thermometers

i. ___

ii. ___

iii. ___

iv. ___

14. Steps for Measuring a Rectal Temperature

A. If the patient is a child, explain the procedure to both the ___ and the ___.

B. Instruct the patient to lie on his or her left side with the top leg bent (this is called the __________ position).
C. Place a small amount of __________ on a tissue and dip the probe into the __________.
D. With one hand, raise the upper __________ to expose the anus, or anal opening.
E. With the other hand, gently insert the lubricated thermometer _____ inch into the anal canal.
F. Hold the thermometer in place until the __________ is signaled, and then withdraw the thermometer.
G. Dispose of the __________ __________ in a biohazard waste container.
H. Wipe the anus from __________to __________ to remove excess lubricant.

15. Steps for Accurately Using the Tympanic Thermometer
A. Remove the thermometer from its base. The display will read "__________".
B. Attach the __________ __________ cover to the earpiece.
C. With one hand, gently pull __________ on the patient's __________ ear if the patient is an adult or pull back and __________ if the patient is an infant or a child who is 3 years of age or younger.
D. Gently insert the plastic covered tip of the probe into the __________ __________.
E. Press the __________ __________, which activates the thermometer.
F. Observe the temperature reading in the __________ __________.

16. Steps for Accurately Obtaining an Axillary Temperature
A. Ask the patient to expose the __________.
B. Using a tissue, pat the area dry of __________.
C. Place the covered probe into the __________ __________.
D. When the thermometer __________, remove the thermometer and discard the probe cover in a waste container.

17. Steps for Using a Chemical Disposable Thermometer
A. Identify the patient, explain the procedure, and __________ the patient's __________.
B. Place the thermometer strip on the patient's __________.
C. Read the correct temperature by reading the __________ __________.
D. The reading is taken by noting the __________ reading among the dots that changed color.
E. The strip is kept in place for about __________ seconds and is read by the color change on the strip.

18. Steps for Using a Temporal Artery Thermometer
A. Identify the patient, explain the procedure, and __________ the patient's __________ aside.
B. Place the probe __________ on the center of the forehead and depress the __________ __________.
C. Keep the button depressed and slowly slide the probe on the __________ across the __________ to the hairline.
D. Lift the probe from the forehead and place it on the _________ just behind the __________.
E. Release the __________ and read the temperature.

III. Pulse and Respiration

1. The Pulse
A. The pulse is the number of times that the heart __________ per __________ (bpm).
B. A wave of blood is created each time the __________ __________ of the heart contracts.
C. Each pulse beat is one __________ __________, or one heartbeat.
D. A normal heartbeat is about __________ times per minute.
E. Increased __________ results in a faster pulse rate.

2. Factors That Influence the Pulse Rate

    i. ____________________
    ii. ____________________
    iii. ____________________
    iv. ____________________
    v. ____________________
    vi. ____________________
    vii. ____________________
    viii. ____________________
    ix. ____________________

3. Average Pulse Rates by Age

    A. Less than 1 year: __________ bpm
    B. 2–6 years: __________ bpm
    C. 6–10 years: __________ bpm
    D. 11–16 years: __________ bpm
    E. Adult: __________ bpm
    F. Older adult: __________ bpm

4. Characteristics of the Pulse

    i. ____________________
    ii. ____________________
    iii. ____________________
    iv. ____________________

5. Rate and Volume of the Pulse

    A. The __________ describes the number of pulse beats per minute.
    B. The __________ refers to the strength of the pulse.
    C. The volume is influenced by the __________ of the heartbeat, the __________ of the arterial walls, and __________.
    D. A variance in the __________ of the pulse may indicate heart disease.

6. Rhythm

    A. Refers to the __________, or __________, of the beats.
    B. Normally, the intervals between each heartbeat are of the same __________.
    C. A pulse with an irregular rhythm is known as a __________, or __________.
    D. It is not considered abnormal if the heart occasionally __________ a beat. This is referred to as an __________ pulse.

7. Common Pulse Sites

    i. ____________________
    ii. ____________________
    iii. ____________________
    iv. ____________________
    v. ____________________
    vi. ____________________
    vii. ____________________
    viii. ____________________
    ix. ____________________

8. Steps for Measuring a Radial Pulse Rate

    A. Explain the procedure to the patient and ask the patient about any recent __________ __________ or __________.
    B. Place your fingertips on the __________ __________ on the thumb side of the wrist.
    C. Check the __________ of the pulse.

D. Start counting the pulse beats when the second hand on your watch is at ____, ____, ____, or ____.
E. Count the pulse for __________ __________ __________.
F. Immediately write down the number of __________ __________ per __________.

9. Steps for Taking an Apical-Radial Pulse
   A. The first person places the ear pieces of the stethoscope in his or her ears, with the opening in the __________ facing __________.
   B. Locate the __________ of the patient's heart by palpating to the left __________ __________ space at the __________ line.
   C. The second person locates the __________ __________ on the thumb side of the wrist 1 inch below the base of the thumb.
   D. The first person places the __________ __________ of the stethoscope at the __________ of the heart.
   E. When the __________ __________ is heard, a nod is made to the second person and counting begins. Ideally, the count should begin when the __________ __________ of a watch is at the 3, 6, 9, or 12.
   F. Count for __________ __________ minute.
   G. Record the rate and quality of the heartbeat. Include both ________ and ________ rates, using the designation AP.
   H. Calculate the pulse deficit by ________ the radial pulse rate from the ________ pulse rate.

10. Respiration
    A. Respiration is the exchange of __________ and __________ __________.
    B. It consists of one __________ and one __________.
    C. Each __________ and __________ of a patient's chest equals one respiration.
    D. Taken typically at the same time as a __________.

11. The Characteristics of Respiration
    i. ______________________________
    ii. ______________________________
    iii. ______________________________
    iv. ______________________________

12. Respiratory Rate Ranges by Age Group
    A. Newborn: __________
    B. 1 year old: __________
    C. 2–10 years: __________
    D. 11–18 years: __________
    E. Adult: __________

13. Circumstances That Alter Respiration
    i. ______________________________
    ii. ______________________________
    iii. ______________________________
    iv. ______________________________
    v. ______________________________
    vi. ______________________________
    vii. ______________________________
    viii. ______________________________
    ix. ______________________________
    x. ______________________________

14. Terms for Describing Breathing Sounds
    i. ______________________________
    ii. ______________________________

iii. ____________________
iv. ____________________
v. ____________________
vi. ____________________
vii. ____________________

IV. Blood Pressure

1. Symptoms of Hypertension and Hypotension
   A. Symptoms of Hypertension
      i. ____________________
      ii. ____________________
      iii. ____________________
   B. Symptoms of Hypotension
      i. ____________________
      ii. ____________________
2. Blood Pressure Readings (Briefly explain each.)
   A. Systolic pressure: ____________________
   B. Diastolic pressure: ____________________
   C. Pulse pressure: ____________________
3. The Five Phases of the Korotkoff Sounds
   A. The first __________ sound is heard.
   B. The sound becomes __________.
   C. The sound becomes less __________ and develops a __________ sound.
   D. The sound begins to __________.
   E. The sound __________.
4. Blood Pressure Guidelines (List what the readings would be for each of the following.)
   A. Hypertension: __________ or above
   B. Prehypertension: __________ to __________
   C. Normal: __________ or below
   D. Optimal: __________ or below
5. Average Normal Blood Pressure Readings
   A. Newborn: __________
   B. 6–9 years: __________
   C. 10–15 years: __________
   D. 16 years to adulthood: __________
   E. Adulthood: __________
6. Physiological Factors Affecting Blood Pressure
   i. ____________________
   ii. ____________________
   iii. ____________________
   iv. ____________________
7. Other Factors Affecting Blood Pressure
   i. ____________________
   ii. ____________________
   iii. ____________________
   iv. ____________________
   v. ____________________
   vi. ____________________
   vii. ____________________
   viii. ____________________

ix. ____________________

x. ____________________

8. Other Terms Related to Abnormal Readings

A. Benign: __________-__________ of elevated blood pressure without symptoms.
B. Essential: Primary __________ of unknown cause. May be __________ determined.
C. Secondary: Elevated blood pressure associated with other conditions such as __________ disease, __________, __________, and obesity.
D. Malignant: Rapidly developing elevated blood pressure that may become __________ if not treated immediately.
E. Renal: Elevated blood pressure as a result of __________ disease.
F. Orthostatic: A __________ __________ in blood pressure that occurs when a patient rapidly moves from a lying to a standing position.
G. Postural: A temporary fall in blood pressure from __________ __________ for extended periods of time.

9. Conditions That Require Blood Pressure to Be Monitored Regularly

i. ____________________
ii. ____________________
iii. ____________________
iv. ____________________
v. ____________________
vi. ____________________
vii. ____________________
viii. ____________________
ix. ____________________
x. ____________________
xi. ____________________
xii. ____________________

10. Equipment for Measuring Blood Pressure

i. ____________________
ii. ____________________

11. The Components of the Stethoscope

i. ____________________
ii. ____________________
iii. ____________________
iv. ____________________
v. ____________________
vi. ____________________
vii. ____________________

12. Causes of Errors in Blood Pressure Readings

A. Equipment: The cuff is the __________ __________, or air leaks around the __________ or __________.
B. Procedure: The patient's arm is __________ __________, or the medical assistant is too far from the __________ to accurately read the gauge.
C. Patient: The patient's arm is __________ __________ to obtain an accurate reading.

V. Pain

1. Pain—The Fifth Vital Sign

A. Pain is highly __________ and personal.
B. It is important to document a __________ of the pain.
C. It is important to observe the __________ signs of pain when talking with the patient.

D. Use of a __________ pain measurement scale can be useful.
E. Assessment is necessary to establish a __________ plan.

2. Characteristics of Pain (Briefly explain each type.)
   A. Acute pain: ____________________
   B. Chronic pain: ____________________
   C. Radiating pain: ____________________
   D. Referred pain: ____________________
   E. Intractable pain: ____________________
   F. Phantom pain: ____________________
3. Other Terms Used to Describe Pain
   i. ____________________
   ii. ____________________
   iii. ____________________
   iv. ____________________
   v. ____________________

VI. Body Fat Measurement

1. Steps for Using Calipers to Measure Skin-Fold Fat
   A. Grasp the __________ in the __________ __________ with your thumb and index finger.
   B. Place the calipers over the __________ and __________.
   C. Grasp the __________ __________ beneath the shoulder blade and obtain the caliper reading and record it.
   D. Determine the __________ __________ of body fat, using a table provided by the manufacturer.
2. Steps for Accurately Calculating the Body Mass Index
   A. Insert the patient's __________ and __________ into the formula; use __________ and __________ or kilograms and meters according to facility policy.
   B. Formula BMI = ____________________

KEY TERMINOLOGY REVIEW

Without using your textbook, write a sentence using the selected key terms in the correct context.

1. *Afebrile:*
   ____
   ____
2. *Apical:*
   ____
   ____
3. *Asymptomatic:*
   ____
   ____
4. *Basal metabolism:*
   ____
   ____

5. *Baseline:*

6. *Cyanosis:*

7. *Dysrhythmia:*

8. *Febrile:*

9. *Frenulum linguae:*

10. *Hypertension (HTN):*

11. *Hyperthermia:*

12. *Hyperventilation:*

13. *Hypoventilation:*

14. *Manometer:*

15. *Metabolism:*

16. *Palpatory method:*

17. *Phantom pain:*

18. *Pulse deficit:*

19. *Radiating pain:*

20. *Referred pain:*

21. *Subjective symptom:*

22. *Syncope:*

23. *Tachycardia:*

24. *Thready pulse:*

APPLIED PRACTICE

Follow the directions as instructed with each question below.

1. A patient, who has a normal baseline temperature of 98.6°F has had the following average body temperatures over the past 5 days: **Day 1: 101.2°F, Day 2: 100.1°F, Day 3: 98.6°F, Day 4: 99.0°F, Day 5: 101.3°F.** How would you describe this fever? Explain your answer.

2. Your patient is a 43-year-old female. Her blood pressure is 157/92. What is the patient's pulse pressure? Is the pulse pressure normal? Explain your answer.

3. You are preparing a new patient for a physical examination. Because the patient has recently moved from a European country, he would like the medical assistant to tell him his body temperature in Celsius rather than Fahrenheit. When obtaining his temperature, the thermometer reads 99.0°F. How does this convert to Celsius? What is the conversion formula?

LEARNING ACTIVITY: FILL IN THE BLANK

Using words from the list below, fill in the blanks to complete the following statements.

Note: Some terms are used in more than one statement.

Anthropometric	Heat waves	Rhythm
Anthropometry	Korotkoff sounds	Sphygmomanometer
Apnea	Movement	Symptom
Arterial	Orthostatic hypotension	Tachypnea
Blood pressure	Pulse	Tympanic membrane thermometer
Bradypnea	Rate	Volume
Core	Rectal	Walls
Eupnea	Respirations	

1. Oral and ________________ temperatures measure the body's ________________ temperature.
2. ________________ are counted by watching, listening, or feeling the ________________ of inspiration and expiration on the patient's back, stomach, or chest.
3. The three aspects to note when taking a pulse are ________________, ________________, and ________________.
4. The ________________ ________________ are the sounds actually heard as the ________________ wall distends during the compression of the blood pressure cuff.
5. ________________ ________________ refers to the lowered ________________ ________________ that occurs when a patient moves from lying down to an erect position.
6. The ________________ is the instrument used for measuring the pressure that the blood exerts against the ________________ of the artery.
7. The ________________ ________________ ________________ or aural thermometer is so named because it is able to detect ________________ ________________ within the ear canal and near the eardrum.
8. A respiratory rate of below 12 (called ______________) or above 40 (called ______________) in an adult should be considered a serious symptom.
9. ________________ means the absence of breathing for longer than 19 seconds, and ________________ means normal breathing.
10. Weight and height are ______________ measurements since they relate to ______________, the science of size, proportion, weight, and height.

CRITICAL THINKING

Answer the following questions to the best of your ability. Utilize the textbook as a reference.

1. Why might you take vitals while a patient is receiving a treatment?

____

____

____

____

2. If a patient walks in without an appointment and presents as extremely short of breath (SOB) and appears weak, do you think that you should spend the time doing weight, height,

and all of the vitals before alerting the doctor of the patient's immediate condition? Explain your answer.

RESEARCH ACTIVITY

Utilize Internet search engines to research the following topics and write a brief description of what you find. It is important to utilize reputable websites.

1. Choose a health condition related to a vital sign (e.g., hypertension, obesity, etc.). Research informational websites related to your chosen condition. What type of information is included in the informational websites? How can this information be useful for patients?

CHAPTER 36
Assisting with Physical Examinations

CHAPTER OUTLINE

General review of the chapter:

Preparing the Examination Room
Patient History
Equipment and Supplies Used for Physical Examinations
Examination Methods Used by the Physician
Adult Examination
Assisting the Physician with a Physical Examination
Sequence of Examination Procedures

STUDENT STUDY GUIDE

Use the following guide to assist in your learning of the concepts from the chapter.

I. Preparing the Examination Room and Examination Methods

1. The Medical Assistant's Role in the Patient's Physical Exam

   i. ______________________________
   ii. ______________________________
   iii. ______________________________
   iv. ______________________________
   v. ______________________________
   vi. ______________________________
   vii. ______________________________
   viii. ______________________________
   ix. ______________________________
   x. ______________________________

2. Cleaning the Examination Room

   A. Place the used gown in the __________ receptacle or waste container.
   B. Clean the examination table, allow it to dry, and __________ it with fresh paper.
   C. Clean and __________ used equipment.
   D. Disinfect all surfaces with __________.
   E. Close all biohazard containers, __________, and remove if full.
   F. Ensure that the room is clean and clutter and __________ free.

3. Features of the Examination Room (List the items typically found in an examination room.)

   i. ______________________________
   ii. ______________________________
   iii. ______________________________

iv. ____
v. ____
vi. ____
vii. ____
viii. ____

4. Examination Room Safety Issues (List the safety considerations for the examination room.)

i. ____
ii. ____
iii. ____
iv. ____
v. ____
vi. ____
vii. ____
viii. ____
ix. ____

5. Preparing the Examination Room

A. Prepare __________ and __________ for the physician.
B. Ensure that the equipment is not within the __________ of the patient.
C. Position the __________ __________ to provide the correct __________ for the physician.
D. Ensure that the examination light is positioned so that it does not __________ __________.
E. Use proper __________ __________ when assisting with patient care.

6. Ensuring Patient Comfort and Privacy

A. Keep the thermostat around __________ to __________ °F.
B. Provide __________ and __________, as needed, to keep the patient warm.
C. Ensure that the examination room is __________ -__________ to decrease odors.
D. Clearly explain how to put on the __________ __________.
E. Inform the patient where to place his or her __________.
F. Leave the room when the patient is __________, unless assistance is required.
G. Knock and receive __________ when reentering the examination room.

7. Information Provided on the Patient Registration Form

i. ____
ii. ____
iii. ____
iv. ____
v. ____
vi. ____
vii. ____
viii. ____
ix. ____
x. ____
xi. ____

8. The Purpose of the Patient's History

A. Assists the physician in assessing the patient's __________ __________ __________.
B. Helps determine a __________ of the patient's present problem or __________.

9. Contents of the Medical History

i. ____
ii. ____
iii. ____
iv. ____

v. ____________________

vi. ____________________

10. The Chief Complaint

A. The chief complaint is referred to as the __________ __________.
B. Usually consists of one or two __________.
C. Symptoms are either __________ or __________.
D. __________ symptoms, such as vertigo or pain, are felt by the patient but are not apparent to an observer and cannot be __________.
E. __________ symptoms, such as a rash or fever, are felt by the patient, are apparent to an observer, and can be __________.
F. Symptoms are usually documented using the patient's own __________.

11. Steps for Interviewing a Patient and Preparing for an Examination

A. __________ the patient, greet the patient warmly, and __________ yourself.
B. Provide a __________ area in which to conduct the interview.
C. Ask the patient to fill in the __________ information on the patient data form.
D. Record the chief complaint in the patient's __________ __________ as appropriate.
E. Ask the patient other __________ -__________ questions to gather more information about the chief complaint to record under present illness.
F. Use __________ skills during interview.
G. Ask the patient about __________. Record allergies in __________ ink as required by office policy.
H. If the patient states that he or she does not have any allergies, record in __________ __________ according to office policy.
I. Correct any errors by drawing __________ __________ through the error; then date and __________ the correction.
J. Ask the patient to provide a __________ specimen, if required, or ask the patient to empty his or her bladder.
K. Explain what __________ the patient should remove, where the opening of the examination gown should be, and where the patient should sit and wait.

12. The Present Illness (PI)

A. Provides a more complete, expansive description of the __________ __________.
B. Must contain a detailed description of the symptom(s), including the __________, __________, and __________ of each.
C. Each __________ should be documented as to its relationship to the __________ __________.

13. Obtaining a Past Medical History

A. Includes all __________ and __________ __________ that the patient has experienced in the past.
B. The dates of __________ __________, __________, __________, and __________ __________, including over-the-counter drugs, are noted whenever possible.

14. Information Included on a Complete Medical History

i. ____________________

ii. ____________________

iii. ____________________

iv. ____________________

v. ____________________

vi. ____________________

vii. ____________________

viii. ____________________

ix. ____________________

15. The Family Medical History
   A. A family medical history is a record of the health problems of the patient's __________ relatives.
   B. Information on __________ relatives should include __________ __________, __________ __________ __________, and __________ __________ __________, as well as the age at which the individual died.

16. Information Contained in the Patient's Personal History
   i. ____________________
   ii. ____________________
   iii. ____________________
   iv. ____________________
   v. ____________________
   vi. ____________________
   vii. ____________________

17. Steps for Documenting a Chief Complaint
   A. Review briefly the patient's __________ __________ before greeting the patient.
   B. Ask __________-__________ questions to gather information about why the patient is being seen today.
   C. Maintain eye __________ and actively __________ to the patient's responses.
   D. Ask the patient to rate pain on a scale of __________ to __________.
   E. Document the __________ __________ and __________ __________ correctly on the correct form in the patient's own words.
   F. Thank the patient and explain that the __________ will be in shortly to examine him or her.
   G. Make sure that the patient is __________ before you leave the room.

18. The Inspection Method of Physical Examination
   A. Accomplished by visually examining the __________ surface of the body.
   B. Notes are made regarding any unusual __________, __________, __________, __________, or symmetry of the areas being inspected.

19. The Palpation Method of Physical Examination
   A. Performed by using the __________ to feel the skin and accessible underlying __________.
   B. Used to determine any unusual __________, __________, __________, or texture.
   C. Oftentimes, abnormalities and __________ and __________ in the abdomen can be discovered through palpation.

20. The Percussion Method of Physical Examination
   A. To use this method, two fingers of one hand are placed on the patient's __________ and then struck with the __________ and __________ __________ of the other hand.
   B. The physician uses his or her fingers to percuss the chest wall and abdomen by gentle __________ or __________, which produces sounds or vibrations.
   C. An alteration in the standard, expected sound or vibration aids in determining the presence of __________ or __________ in a cavity.

21. The Auscultation Method of Physical Examination
   A. Using this method, the physician listens to __________ that are found within the body.
   B. These sounds must be differentiated from __________ body sounds by the physician.
   C. The auscultation method can also be performed by placing the __________ directly over the body surface.

22. The Mensuration Method of Physical Examination
   A. Special tools are used to measure the __________ or specific __________.
   B. To determine a patient's __________, a scale is used.

C. A __________ is used to measure the range of motion of a joint.
D. __________ are used to determine the amount of body fat.

23. The Manipulation Method of Physical Examination
   A. This method is the passive assessment of the __________ of a joint.
   B. When a physician is using this examination method, he or she may __________ the joint for __________ and warmth.

II. Preparing the Examination Room and Examination Methods

1. The Role of the Medical Assistant in Assisting with a Physical Examination
   A. Positions and __________ the patient.
   B. Hands instruments, __________, and supplies to the physician.
   C. Documents and __________ specimens.
   D. Acts as a __________ to the behavior of the physician and the patient.
   E. Carries out __________ plans.
   F. Schedules __________ tests.
2. Draping the Patient
   A. Used to protect the patient's __________ and provide some warmth.
   B. Drape must not obstruct the __________ view or interfere with the area being examined.
   C. Sterile drapes are used during __________ procedures.
3. The Role of the Medical Assistant in Positioning the Patient
   A. Provides the patient with clear __________ on what position to assume.
   B. Ensures the patient's __________.
4. Nine Standard Positions for Examinations and Procedures
   i. ____________________
   ii. ____________________
   iii. ____________________
   iv. ____________________
   v. ____________________
   vi. ____________________
   vii. ____________________
   viii. ____________________
   ix. ____________________
5. The Supine Position
   A. The supine position is also known as the __________ __________ position.
   B. The patient lies flat on his or her back, with hands at the __________.
   C. Be sure that the patient's feet are supported by __________ the table.
   D. This is the position used to examine anything on the anterior or __________ surface of the body.
   E. Drape the patient from the __________ down to over the feet.
   F. This position may not be comfortable for patients who are short of breath or have __________ __________ problems.
   G. Placing a __________ under the patient's head and under the knees may make him or her more comfortable.
6. The Dorsal Recumbent Position
   A. The patient is lying flat on his or her back with knees __________ and feet __________ on the table.
   B. This position relieves strain on the __________ __________ and relaxes the __________ muscles.

C. Used to inspect the __________; __________; __________; and __________, __________ or perineal areas.
D. Can be used for __________ exams of the vagina and rectum.
E. Patients with __________ __________ may find this position uncomfortable.

7. The Lithotomy Position

A. Similar to the __________ __________ position except that the patient's feet are placed in stirrups attached to the side of the table.
B. After the feet are in place in the stirrups, the patient is instructed to __________ __________ until the buttocks are positioned at the edge of the table.
C. Patients with severe __________ or those who are severely __________ or in late-term pregnancy may find this position impossible.

8. The Fowler's Position

A. In this position, the head of the table is raised to a __________-degree angle.
B. This position is useful for examinations of the __________, __________, or __________ body.
C. The drape should be placed over the patient's __________, covering the __________.

9. The Semi-Fowler's Position

A. This position is similar to the Fowler's position, but the head of the table is at a __________ degree angle instead of 90 degrees.
B. Used for __________-__________ examinations, patients with breathing difficulties, or patients suffering from general malaise.
C. The Fowler's or semi-Fowler's positions are more comfortable for patients who have __________ __________ injuries or __________ difficulties.

10. The Prone Position

A. Requires the patient to lie face down, flat on his or her stomach, or the __________ surface of the body, with the head turned to the __________ and arms either __________ the body or __________ under the head.
B. It is the opposite of the __________ position.
C. The drape should cover the patient from the __________ back to over the feet.
D. Used for __________ exams and certain types of surgery.
E. Unsuitable for patients with __________ problems, women in __________-__________ pregnancies, or the __________.

11. The Sims', or Lateral, Position

A. Requires the patient to lie on the __________ side with the right leg sharply bent upward and the left leg slightly bent.
B. The patient's weight is mainly on the __________ area.
C. The right arm is __________ next to the __________ for support.
D. Used for rectal exams, rectal __________, __________, and __________ and pelvic exams.

12. The Knee–Chest Position

A. The patient lies in the __________ position and then pulls the knees up to a __________ position with the thighs at a 90-degree angle to the table and the __________ in the air.
B. The head is turned to one side and the arms may be placed __________ __________ __________ or on either side of the head for comfort and support.
C. Most patients need assistance to assume this position correctly and should never be left __________ in this position at any time.
D. Used for __________ exams, __________, and rectal and vaginal exams.

E. The drape should be placed from the __________ __________ at an angle covering the __________ area.
F. A __________ drape, which is a drape with a precut opening in the appropriate area, may be used.
G. Many physicians have __________ tables available for this type of exam.

13. The Trendelenburg Position
    A. This position is not normally used in a physician's office except in cases of __________ or low blood pressure.
    B. The patient lies in the __________ position and the end of the table is raised to about a __________-degree angle with the patient's legs bent at the knees over the end of the table.
    C. Used for __________ surgeries.

14. The Proctological (Jackknife) Position
    A. Used for proctological examinations conducted with a __________.
    B. This position is similar to the __________-__________ position, but with a greater bend at the hips.
    C. The patient will lie face down with the __________ at the __________ of the table.

KEY TERMINOLOGY REVIEW

Write a sentence using the selected key terms in the correct context.

1. *amplify:*

____

____

2. *bimanual:*

____

____

3. *chief complaint (CC):*

____

____

4. *goniometer:*

____

____

5. *inspection:*

____

____

6. *laryngeal mirror:*

____

____

7. *manipulation:*

____

____

8. ***mensuration:***

9. ***objective symptom:***

10. ***ophthalmoscope:***

11. ***palpation:***

12. ***present illness (PI):***

13. ***reflex hammer:***

14. ***review of systems (ROS):***

15. ***subjective symptom:***

16. ***tongue depressor:***

17. ***turgor:***

18. ***vaginal speculum:***

APPLIED PRACTICE

Follow the directions as instructed with each question below.

1. Next to each of the supplies shown below, name the supply and state its purpose.

Supplies	Purpose

2. Provide the name of the position for each of the pictures provided below.

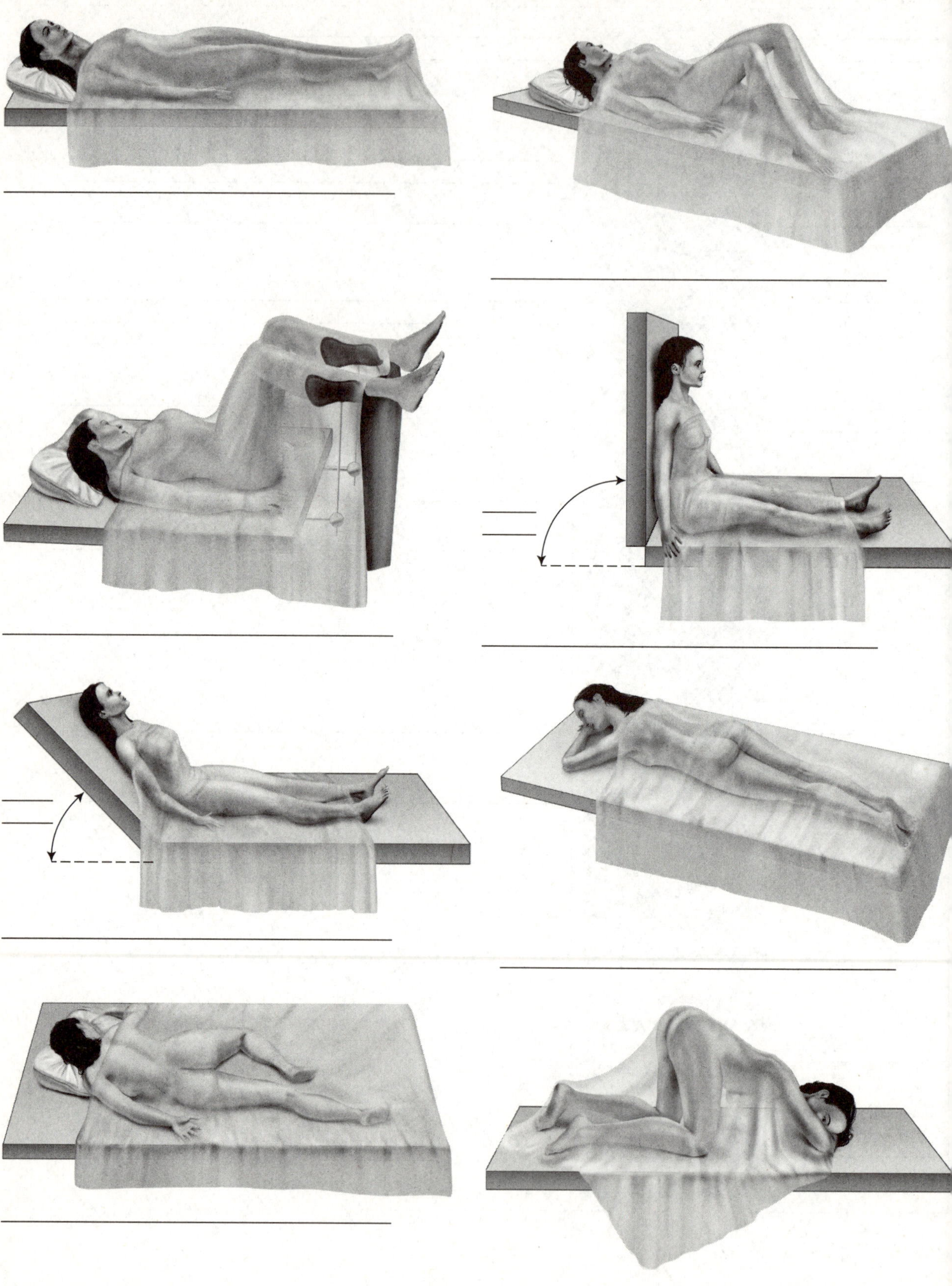

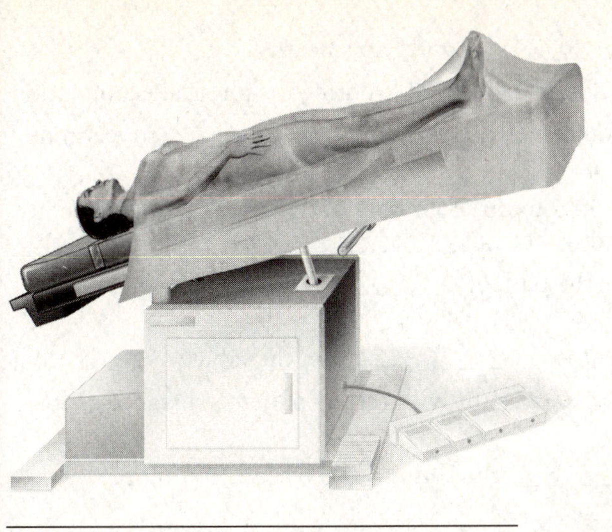

____

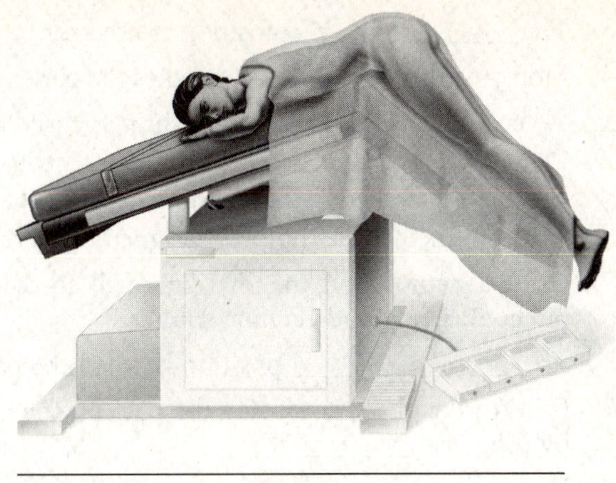

____

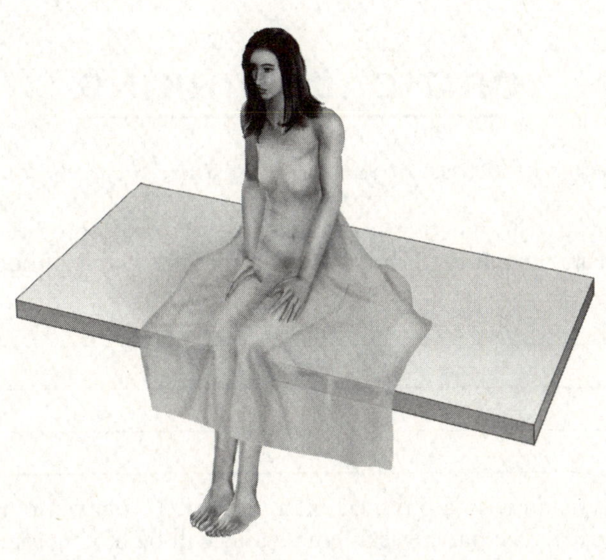

____

LEARNING ACTIVITY: FILL IN THE BLANK

Using words from the list below, fill in the blanks to complete the following statements. Note: Some terms are used in more than one statement.

Auscultate	Pelvic exams	Tuning fork
Bladder	Percussion	Tympanic membrane
Bowel sounds	Rate	Underlying body parts
Depth	Rhythm	
Fowler's	Sitting erect	
Frequency	Snellen chart	
Lithotomy	Speculum	

1. Using a stethoscope the physician will ________________ the patient's breathing sounds, noting the ________________, ________________, pitch, ________________, and location.
2. ________________ is the process of using the fingertips to tap the body lightly but sharply in order to assess the position and size of the ________________.

3. The ______________ position is used for ______________ and Pap smears.
4. Emptying the ___________ makes the patient feel more comfortable during the physical examination.
5. When using an otoscope, the light is focused through the disposable ______________ to examine the outer ear, then the ______________ (eardrum).
6. A ______________ is a metal instrument that comes in different sizes and has two prongs extending from the handle that are designed to vibrate at a specific ______________.
7. Using a stethoscope, the physician will auscultate the patient's ______________ for frequency, pitch, gurgling, and clicking sounds.
8. The ______________ position is when the patient is ______________ on the table.
9. Prior to the physician seeing the patient, the medical assistant will test the patient's distance vision by using a ______________.
10. Using a stethoscope, the physician will ______________ the sounds of the heart, noting the ______________, rhythm, pitch, and quality.

CRITICAL THINKING

Answer the following questions to the best of your ability. Utilize the textbook as a reference.

1. During a patient's clinical visit, whether for a physical examination or another reason, the medical assistant visually inspects the patient. Think of what may be visible about the patient that the MA may note.

____

____

____

____

2. You are assisting a physician with a physical examination. You have prepared all of the supplies and have any equipment ready. The patient is a female and will be having a pelvic exam along with the physical examination. Although the physician does not need you to assist him, you are expected to be present with the doctor anyway. State why the MA would be present in this situation. Would the same be true if the patient were a male? Would the same be true if the doctor was a female and the patient were a male?

____

____

____

____

____

RESEARCH ACTIVITY

Utilize Internet search engines to research the following topics and write a brief description of what you find. It is important to utilize reputable websites.

1. It is very important to be aware of the cultural norms of the patients seen in the medical office. Cultural norms can affect a patient's approach to having a physical examination. Select a culture.

Research this culture online or by interviewing individuals whom you know from this culture. Discover the cultural differences and/or barriers that may affect the success of performing a physical examination on a patient.

CHAPTER 37

Assisting with Medical Specialties

CHAPTER OUTLINE

General review of the chapter:

The Role of the Medical Assistant
Allergy
Dermatology
Cardiovascular System
Endocrinology
Gastrointestinal System
Lymphatic System
Musculoskeletal System
Nervous System

STUDENT STUDY GUIDE

Use the following guide to assist in your learning of the concepts from the chapter.

I. Diagnosing and Testing Allergies and Skin Disorders

1. Allergic Reactions
   A. May be localized, such as a mosquito bite, or ________, such as asthma or anaphylactic shock.
   B. Respiratory symptoms include wheezing, __________, coughing, and nasal __________.
2. Allergic Condition: Asthma
   A. Condition seen most frequently in ___________ in which wheezing, coughing, and ___________ are the major symptoms.
   B. Asthmatic attacks may be caused by ____________ inhaled in the air and ingested in food and drugs.
   C. Treatment is _____________ and the control of the __________ factors.
3. Allergic Condition: Contact Dermatitis
   A. Involves ____________ and _____________ of the skin.
   B. Treatment consists of topical and ___________ medications.
4. Symptoms of a Severe Allergic Reaction
   i. ______________________________
   ii. ______________________________
   iii. ______________________________
   iv. ______________________________
   v. ______________________________
   vi. ______________________________
   vii. ______________________________
   viii. ______________________________

5. Scratch or Skin Testing
   A. Used to determine the specific substances that cause an __________ reaction in the patient.
   B. If a __________ forms within __________ minutes after placing an allergen on the skin, an allergy is indicated.
   C. The patient should be advised to remain in the physician's office for at least __________ minutes after testing has been completed.
6. Intradermal Allergy Test
   A. Performed by injecting _____ to _____ mL of an allergen extract into the anterior surface of the forearm.
   B. Several tests (_____ to _____) can be performed on each arm.
   C. The test is considered to be more accurate than a ________ test.
7. Patch Tests
   A. Consists of placing a small amount of the __________ onto the ________ forearm and then covering it with a plastic wrap.
   B. Several patch tests can be performed at the same time and these are read after the patches have remained in place for _____ to _____ hours.
   C. The test is used to detect the ________ agents in contact dermatitis.
8. Radioallergosorbent Test (RAST)
   A. Measures blood levels of ____________ to particular antigens.
   B. The test is expensive, but it is more sensitive and useful for patients who have __________ problems.
9. Skin Lesions
   A. Skin lesions can occur whenever the normal surface of the skin is invaded or ___________.
   B. A skin lesion is not always a sign of ________.
10. Cellulitis
    A. Cellulitis is an ______________ of the cellular or _________ tissue caused by either _________ or _____________ infection of a cut or lesion.
    B. Treatment includes ________ and application of _________ compresses.
11. Psoriasis
    A. Psoriasis is a chronic inflammatory condition consisting of discrete _______ or _______ lesions covered with ________ scaling.
    B. It is not contagious and is thought to be an ___________ disease.
12. Acne Vulgaris
    A. Acne vulgaris is an inflammatory disease of the ____________ glands and hair follicles that results in __________ and ___________.
    B. Treatment includes systemic and ____________ antibiotics.
13. Scleroderma
    A. Scleroderma is a chronic, progressive ____________ disease that affects the blood __________ and ___________ tissue of the skin and other organs.
    B. Integumentary symptoms include hardening of the skin, pallor, edema, and fixating of skin to ____________ tissues.
14. Neoplasms
    A. Neoplasms are biopsied by surgically removing a small amount of ________ for testing.
    B. Benign growths may grow in size but are usually ____________.
    C. Malignant growths are ________ and tend to take over surrounding tissues.

15. Types of Benign Neoplasms (Briefly explain each type.)
    A. Dermatofibroma: ______
    B. Hemangioma: ______
    C. Keloid: ______
    D. Keratosis: ______
    E. Leukoplakia: ______
    F. Lipoma: ______
    G. Nevus: ______
16. Types of Malignant (Cancerous) Neoplasms (Briefly explain each type.)
    A. Basal cell carcinoma: ______
    B. Kaposi's sarcoma: ______
    C. Malignant melanoma: ______
    D. Squamous cell carcinoma: ______
17. Diagnostic Tests and Procedures to Treat Integumentary System Disorders (Briefly explain each type.)
    A. Adipectomy: ______
    B. Chemobrasion: ______
    C. Cryosurgery: ______
    D. Curettage: ______
    E. Dermabrasion: ______
    F. Dermoplasty: ______
    G. Electrocautery: ______
    H. Exfoliative cytology: ______
    I. Frozen section: ______
    J. Fungal scrapings: ______
    K. Lipectomy: ______
    L. Marsupialization: ______
    M. Plication: ______
    N. Rhytidectomy: ______
    O. Sweat test: ______
    P. Tzanck test: ______
18. Steps for Obtaining a Wound Culture (List each step in this procedure.)
    i. ______
    ii. ______
    iii. ______
    iv. ______
    v. ______
    vi. ______
    vii. ______
    viii. ______
    ix. ______
    x. ______
    xi. ______
    xii. ______
    xiii. ______

II. Examinations and Diagnostic Procedures

1. Precipitating the Causes of Cardiovascular Disease
    i. ______
    ii. ______

iii. ______________________________
iv. ______________________________

2. The Most Common Symptoms of Cardiovascular Disease
   i. ______________________________
   ii. ______________________________
   iii. ______________________________
   iv. ______________________________
   v. ______________________________

3. Angiography
   A. X-rays are taken after the injection of an ________ material into a blood _______.
   B. Can be performed on the _______ as an __________ angiogram.

4. Arterial Blood Gases
   A. Measurement of the amount of _______, ________ ________, and ________ in the blood.
   B. Provide a valuable evaluation of cardiac failure, hemorrhage, and __________ failure.

5. The Artificial Pacemaker
   A. Controls the beating of the heart through a series of __________ electrical impulses.
   B. An external pacemaker has the ___________ on the outside of the body.

6. Cardiac Catheterization
   A. Cardiac catheterization is a diagnostic procedure to detect _______________.
   B. Collects cardiac blood samples and determines the ____________________ within the cardiac area.

7. Cardiac Enzymes
   A. Cardiac enzymes are complex ___________ that are capable of inducing chemical changes within the body.
   B. Taken by blood sample to determine the severity of ________ disease or damage.

8. Diagnostic Tests for Cardiovascular Conditions (Briefly explain each type.)
   A. Cardiolysis: ______________________________
   B. Cardiorrhaphy: ______________________________
   C. Cardioversion: ______________________________
   D. Commissurotomy: ______________________________
   E. Doppler ultrasonography: ______________________________
   F. Electrocardiography: ______________________________
   G. Embolectomy: ______________________________
   H. Lipoproteins: ______________________________
   I. Percutaneous balloon valvuloplasty: ______________________________
   J. Percutaneous transluminal coronary angioplasty:
   ____
   K. Phleborrhaphy: ______________________________
   L. Prothrombin time: ______________________________
   M. Stress test: ______________________________
   N. Venography: ______________________________

9. Coronary Artery Disease (CAD)
   A. CAD usually results from ________________________.
   B. If enough of the heart muscle is denied an oxygen-rich blood supply, a _______________, or heart attack, may occur.

10. Congestive Heart Failure (CHF)
    A. CHF may result from _______________.
    B. Symptoms occur because the heart muscle becomes ___________ and is less able to pump blood to the rest of the body.

11. Factors That Reduce the Risk of Heart Disease
    i. ____________________
    ii. ____________________
    iii. ____________________
    iv. ____________________
    v. ____________________
    vi. ____________________
    vii. ____________________

12. Dysrhythmia
    A. Dysrhythmia is an abnormality of the ________ or ________ of the heartbeat.
    B. Caused by a disturbance of the _________ system in the heart.

13. The Glands of the Endocrine System (List and explain both types.)
    i. ____________________
    ii. ____________________

14. Diabetes Mellitus
    A. Diabetes mellitus is one of the most common ____________ imbalances.
    B. Characterized by ____________________ (too much sugar in the blood).

15. Types of Diabetes Mellitus (Explain both types.)
    A. Type 1: ____________________
    B. Type 2: ____________________

16. Procedures and Diagnostic Tests for the Endocrine System (Briefly explain each.)
    A. Blood serum test: ____________________
    B. Fasting blood sugar: ____________________
    C. Glucose Tolerance Test (GTT): ____________________
    D. Parathryroidectomy: ____________________
    E. 17-hydroxycorticosteroids (17-OHCS): ____________________
    F. 17-ketosteroids (17-KS): ____________________
    G. Protein blood iodine test (PBI): ____________________
    H. Radioactive iodine uptake test (RAIU): ____________________
    I. Radioimmune assay test (RIA): ____________________
    J. Serum glucose test: ____________________
    K. Thymectomy: ____________________
    L. Thyroid echogram: ____________________
    M. Thyroparathyroidectomy: ____________________
    N. Total calcium: ____________________

17. Procedures and Diagnostic Tests for the Digestive System (Briefly explain each.)
    A. Air contrast barium enema: ____________________
    B. Anastomosis: ____________________
    C. Cholecystectomy: ____________________
    D. Cholecystogram: ____________________
    E. Choledocholithotomy: ____________________
    F. Choledocholithotrispy: ____________________

G. Colostomy: ____
H. Endoscopic retrograde cholangiopancreatography (ERCP):
____
I. Esophagram: ____
J. Esophagogastrostomy: ____
K. Fistulectomy: ____
L. Gastrectomy: ____
M. Gastrointestinal endoscopy: ____
N. Gastric lavage: ____
O. Glossectomy: ____
P. Hepatic lobotomy: ____
Q. Ileostomy: ____
R. Intravenous cholangiogram: ____
S. Jejunostomy: ____
T. Proctoplasty: ____
U. Vagotomy: ____

18. Gastroesophageal Reflux Disease (GERD)

A. GERD is one of the most common ______________ disorders.
B. It is also known as ___________ or ______________.

19. Treatment for Gastroesophageal Reflux Disease

A. Eating small meals ____________ times a day.
B. Eating at least ___________ to ____________ hours before bedtime.
C. Moderating coffee and ____________ intake.

20. Diverticular Disease

A. Diverticula are the small ____________ found mainly in the ___________ part of the colon or _____________ intestine.
B. A diverticulum is a _____________ of the inner lining of the _________ wall through the muscular layers of _____________.
C. Diverticulitis is an _________________ of one or more __________, causing severe pain, muscle spasms, nausea, and fever.

21. Sigmoidoscopy

A. A sigmoidoscopy is also called a ____________ or _______________ examination.
B. It is an examination of the _____________ of the sigmoid colon for diagnostic purposes.

22. Assisting During a Sigmoidoscopy

A. For this procedure, the patient may be placed in the ________ position or on a _________ examination table.
B. The patient should be given detailed instructions on how to empty his or her ___________ prior to the procedure.
C. The patient should sign a consent form for both the ____________ and any ____________ taken.

23. Colonoscopy

A. Performed in an office or as a hospital outpatient procedure because an __________ sedative is administered prior to the procedure.
B. Allows the physician to examine more of the ___________ intestine than is done in the sigmoidoscopy.
C. The American Cancer Society recommends that all individuals over the age of ___________ have a colonoscopy.

24. Steps for Administering a Disposable Enema

i. ____________________

ii. ____________________

iii. ____________________

iv. ____________________

v. ____________________

vi. ____________________

vii. ____________________

viii. ____________________

ix. ____________________

x. ____________________

xi. ____________________

25. Testing for Occult Blood

A. Instruct the patient to follow the guidelines for preparation as listed by the ______________ of the test kit.

B. Guidelines should be observed for __________ days prior to collecting specimens and should continue until all __________ samples have been obtained.

26. The Lymphatic System

A. Contains the __________ glands, ducts, nodes, tonsils, __________ gland, and spleen.

B. It is the basis of the body's defense, or __________, system.

C. The system protects the body against the invasion of foreign ____________.

D. Works in conjunction with the ____________ system to purify the blood and drain fluids throughout the body.

27. Immunity

A. Immunity is the body's ability to defend itself against ____________ organisms and toxic substances.

B. It is either natural or ____________.

28. Procedures and Diagnostic Tests for the Lymphatic System (Briefly explain each.)

A. Bone marrow aspiration: ____________________

B. ELISA: ____________________

C. Lymphadenectomy: ____________________

D. Lymphangiogram: ____________________

E. Splenopexy: ____________________

F. Western blot: ____________________

29. Musculoskeletal System Specialists

A. ____________ treat the body by realigning the skeletal system to promote healing.

B. ____________ see patients with join inflammations and treat patients with autoimmune disorders.

C. ____________ use manual adjustment of the spine to promote healing and maintain homeostasis.

30. Procedures and Diagnostic Tests for the Musculoskeletal System (Briefly explain each.)

A. Aldolase: ____________________

B. Antinuclear antibody (ANA): ____________________

C. Anterior cruciate ligament (ACL) reconstruction:

____

D. Arthrocentesis: ____________________

E. Arthrodesis: ____________________

F. Arthrography: ______________________
G. Arthroplasty: ______________________
H. Arthrotomy: ______________________
I. Creatine phosphokinase (CPK):
____
J. C-Reactive Protein (CRP): ______________________
K. Electromyography: ______________________
L. Fasciectomy: ______________________
M. Goniometry: ______________________
N. Lactic dehydrogenase (LDH):
____
O. Laminectomy: ______________________
P. Menisectomy: ______________________
Q. Myelography: ______________________
R. Phosphorus (P) blood test: ______________________
S. Photon absorptiometry: ______________________
T. Reduction: ______________________
U. Serum glutamic oxaloacetic transaminase (SGOT):
____
V. Serum glutamic pyruvic transaminase (SGPT):
____
W. Serum rheumatoid factor (RF):
____
X. Thermography: ______________________

31. Physicians Specializing in the Nervous System
A. A ____________ specializes in treating and diagnosing conditions of the nervous system.
B. A ____________ performs surgical procedures on the nervous system because of disease or trauma.
C. A ____________ treats mental and neurological conditions that affect behavior.

32. Neurological Tests and Procedures (Briefly explain each.)
A. Babinski's sign: ______________________
B. Carotid endarterectomy: ______________________
C. Cerebral angiogram: ______________________
D. Cordectomy: ______________________
E. Craniotomy: ______________________
F. Electromyogram: ______________________
G. Laminectomy: ______________________
H. Pneumoencephalography: ______________________
I. Positron emission tomography (PET):
____
J. Romberg's sign: ______________________
K. Sympathectomy: ______________________
L. Trephination: ______________________
M. Vagotomy: ______________________

33. Cerebral Vascular Accident (CVA)
A. A CVA is also known as a ____________.
B. Risk factors for CVA
i. ______________________
ii. ______________________
iii. ______________________

iv. ______________________________
v. ______________________________
vi. ______________________________
vii. ______________________________

34. Symptoms of a cerebral vascular accident

i. ______________________________
ii. ______________________________
iii. ______________________________
iv. ______________________________
v. ______________________________
vi. ______________________________
vii. ______________________________

35. Dementia

A. Dementia is a condition that results in the progressive loss of ____________ and intellectual ability.
B. Can occur at any age and is not a normal result of ____________.
C. Approximately half of all dementia patients suffer from ____________ disease.

KEY TERMINOLOGY REVIEW

Use the key terms found at the beginning of the chapter to finish the sentences below. Key terms may b more than one word in length.

1. Asthmatic attacks may be caused by ____________ inhaled from the air or ingested in food or drugs.
2. ____________ is defined as excessive thirst.
3. The allergic interaction of an antigen and an antibody causes the release of ____________, which is the substance that produces the signs and symptoms of allergies.
4. ____________ or hidden blood in feces may be an indication of bleeding in the gastrointestinal tract.
5. ____________ are formed in reaction to the scratch testing of allergens.
6. Intracranial pressure may be evaluated by testing for the ____________.
7. As the coronary arteries narrow, the blood flow to the heart muscle is lessened and ____________ may occur.
8. An ____________ is a granular white cell that captures invading microorganisms and antibody–antigen reactions through phagocytosis.
9. ____________ is the branch of medicine dealing with malignant neoplasms or tumors.
10. The medical term for excessive sweating is ____________.

APPLIED PRACTICE

Follow the directions as instructed with each question below.

1. Identify each of the following skin lesions.

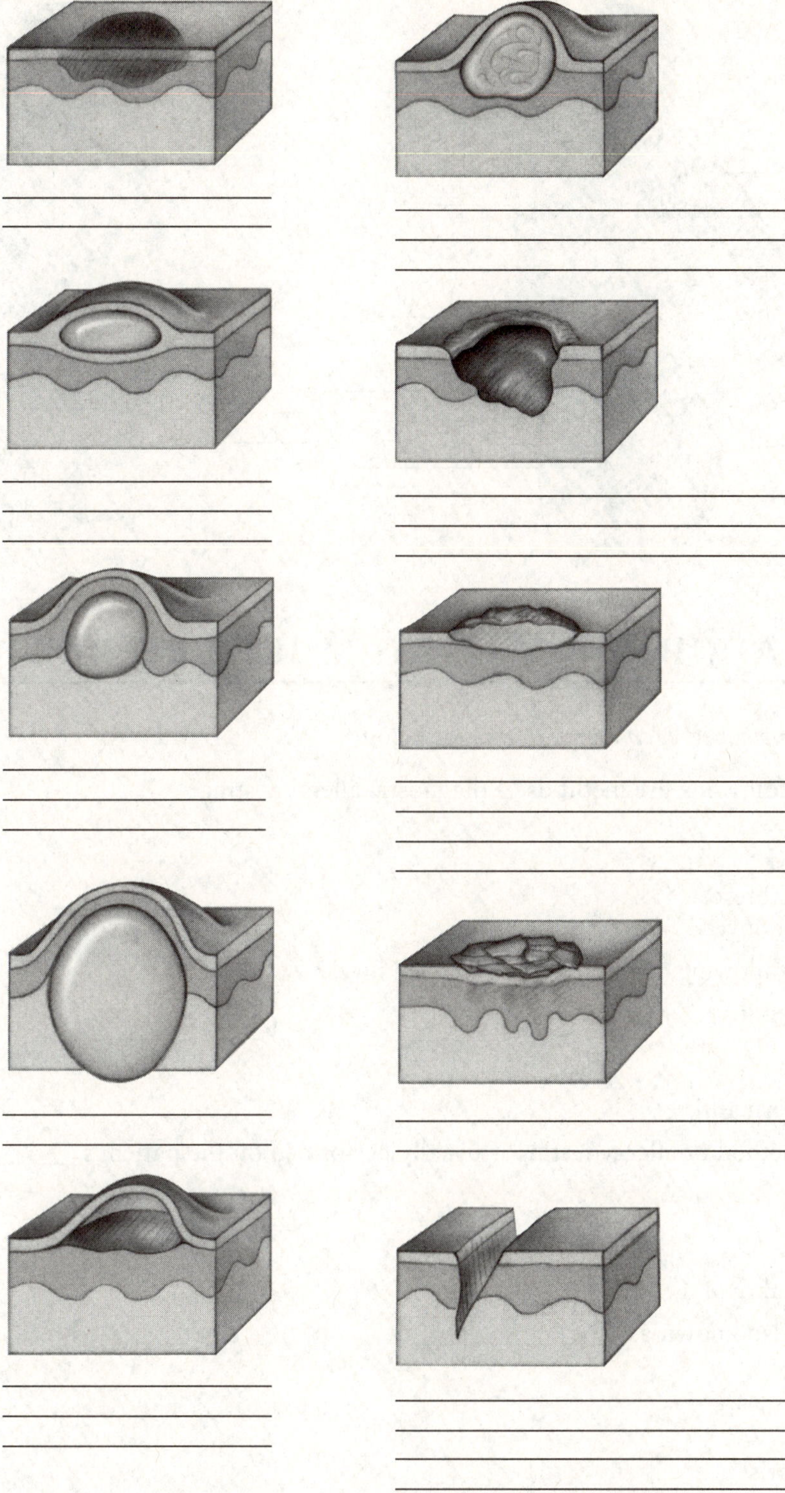

2. Using the drawings below, name each of the sites where referred abdominal pain can occur.

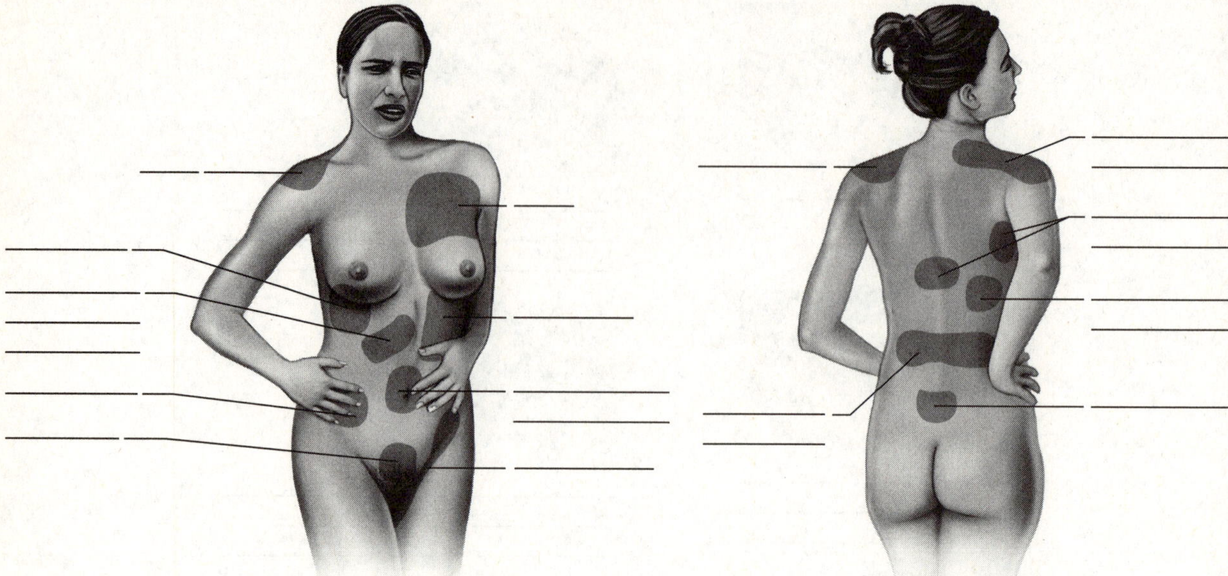

LEARNING ACTIVITY: MULTIPLE CHOICE

Circle the correct answer to each of the questions below.

1. Which of the following are methods of diagnostic allergy testing?
   a. RAST Test
   b. Scratch test
   c. Intradermal test
   d. All of the above
2. Which of the following conditions is also called hives?
   a. Allergic rhinitis
   b. Eczema
   c. Urticaria
   d. Contact dermatitis
3. The scratch method of allergy testing is usually performed on the patient's ______________.
   a. Back
   b. Leg
   c. Foot
   d. All of the above
4. Bedsores are also known as ______________.
   a. erysipelas
   b. decubitus ulcers
   c. psoriasis
   d. acne vulgaris
5. Which of the following is a type of cancer therapy?
   a. Chemotherapy
   b. Cryotherapy
   c. Radiotherapy
   d. All of the above

6. Using the results of diagnostic tests such as bone and liver scans and other information gathered from the physical examination to determine the size, depth, and degree of spread of the initial tumor is called ______________________.
   a. staging a tumor
   b. grading a tumor
   c. biopsying a tumor
   d. All of the above
7. Dermatofibroma is defined as a(n) ______________________.
   a. benign tumor of dilated vessels
   b. fibrous tumor of the skin
   c. epithelial tumor of the basal cell layer of the epidermis
   d. epidermal cancer
8. Cardiolysis is the surgical procedure ______________________________________.
   a. to separate adhesions, which involves a resectioning of the ribs and sternum
   b. that uses a balloon inside a vessel to alter the structure of the vessel by dilating it
   c. to remove an aneurysm
   d. done to change the size of an opening
9. For very high-risk patients, the new goal is to have an LDL ______________________.
   a. under 130 mg/dL
   b. below 100 mg/dL
   c. below 93 mg/dL
   d. None of the above
10. Hormones are regulated by ______________________.
    a. the nervous system
    b. endocrine control
    c. a feedback system
    d. All of the above

CRITICAL THINKING

Answer the following questions to the best of your ability. Utilize the textbook as a reference.

1. Read the following case study. How would you respond?

   Benito Salvatore, a 65-year-old business executive, is scheduled to have a sigmoidoscopy with Dr. Bahjat. When David Slate, RMA, escorts him to the procedure room, Mr. Salvatore confides that he is extremely nervous and is concerned that he did not prepare well enough for the sigmoidoscopy.

   ____

   ____

   ____

   ____

2. What would you do if a patient refused to participate in a teaching session regarding their condition and treatment?

   ____

   ____

   ____

   ____

RESEARCH ACTIVITY

Utilize Internet search engines to research the following topics and write a brief description of what you find. It is important to utilize reputable websites.

1. Select one or two of the procedures/diagnostic tests discussed in the chapter. Research the procedure/diagnostic test on the Internet. Why may the test be performed, how is the test performed, and what are the outcomes that are expected from the test? Write an essay on your findings. Be sure to cite your sources.

CHAPTER 38
Assisting with Reproductive and Urinary Specialties

CHAPTER OUTLINE

General review of the chapter:

Reproductive System
Female Reproductive System
Male Reproductive System
Sexually Transmitted Infections (STIs)
Urinary System

STUDENT STUDY GUIDE

Use the following guide to assist in your learning of the concepts from the chapter.

I. Assisting with Specialty Examinations of the Female Reproductive System

1. Examination of the Female Reproductive Organs
   i. ______________________________
   ii. ______________________________
   iii. ______________________________
   iv. ______________________________
2. The Importance of the Clinical Breast Examination (CBE)
   A. Over a lifetime, __________ in __________ women will develop breast cancer.
   B. __________, __________ __________ __________ (CBE), __________ __________ __________ (BSE) and MRIs are tools for early detection.
   C. Women who are at a greater risk of developing breast cancer should have an __________ and a __________every year.
3. Steps for the Breast Examination
   A. The patient lies in the __________ position.
   B. The patient is typically asked to place her hand behind her __________ on the side that is being examined first.
   C. This position allows the physician to examine the __________ nodes under the __________.
   D. The physician __________ the breast using his or her fingertips in a __________ manner around all of the breast tissue to search for lumps, tenderness, or inflammation.
   E. In addition, any __________ or __________ of the skin around the breast and nipple is noted.
   F. The nipples are checked for __________, __________, or discharge.
4. The Health Benefits of Breast Self-Examination (BSE)
   A. The overall goal should be for the patient to be __________with her own breasts and to report any __________ immediately to her physician.

B. The physician may advise the patient to perform BSE every __________, usually __________ week after the menstrual period ends.
C. Women who have reached __________ should examine their breasts on the same day each month.

5. Correct Application of Fingertips for a Breast Self-Examination in the Shower

A. Raise the right __________.
B. Use the left hand to examine the __________ __________.
C. Then raise the left arm and use the right hand to examine the __________ __________.
D. Using flat __________, check breast tissue and __________ tissue, gently feeling for any lump or thickening.

6. Correct Application of Fingertips for a Breast Self-Examination in Front of a Mirror

A. Inspect the breasts for any __________ in shape while the arms are at the side of the body.
B. Look for __________, __________, or __________ of the skin; lumps; or changes in the __________, such as inversion.
C. Gently squeeze both nipples and look for ______________________.
D. Raise the arms __________ and look for size, shape, and __________ changes in each breast.
E. With palms resting on __________, flex chest muscles, looking for any obvious differences in the breasts.

7. Correct Application of Fingertips for a Breast Self-Examination Lying Down

A. To examine the right breast, place a __________ or folded towel behind the right shoulder and place the right hand __________ the head.
B. Using the hand with fingers flat, gently press the breast tissue, using small __________ motions starting at the __________ __________ of the breast at the 12 o'clock position and spiraling toward the __________.
C. Gently squeeze the nipple of each breast between the thumb and index finger, noting any __________ or __________.

8. Recommendations from the American Cancer Society for Breast Examinations

A. A baseline mammogram should be done at age __________.
B. Women older than age __________ should have a yearly breast examination by a physician and a mammogram every 1 to 2 years.
C. Women older than age __________ should have a yearly breast examination by a physician and a yearly mammogram.

9. Instructions for a Patient Prior to a Pap Test

A. Avoid sexual intercourse for at least ________ hours before the examination.
B. She should not schedule a Pap test during a time when she may have her __________.
C. Schedule the Pap test for at least __________ days after the last day of menstruation.

10. The Pelvic Examination

A. Begins with an examination of the external genitalia for __________, __________, or __________.
B. Next, the vaginal __________ is inserted into the vagina to inspect the vagina and cervix for __________, __________, __________, or discharge.
C. Vaginal specula may be either __________, and need to be sanitized and sterilized after each use, or disposable, and meant for one use only.

11. The Importance of the Pap Smear

i. ____
ii. ____
iii. ____

12. Human Papilloma Viruses (HPVs)

    A. Responsible for the majority of __________ cancer cases and for genital warts.
    B. Women who become sexually active at an early age, as well as those who have had __________ __________, are at higher risk of infection from HPV.
    C. A new vaccine, __________, prevents infection.
    D. __________ of cervical cancers and __________ of genital warts will not be prevented by these vaccines.

13. The Older "Dry" Method of Pap Smear Collection

    A. Separate slides are made by the __________.
    B. The medical assistant labels the slides C, V, and E (__________, __________, and __________ canal) based on the source of the cells.
    C. The MA then sprays them with a __________ spray to preserve the cells.

14. The Newer, More Accurate "Liquid" Method of Pap Smear Collection

    A. Requires the __________ to be collected in a manner similar to that used in the dry method.
    B. The plastic vaginal __________ or __________ that is used is swirled in a liquid __________ medium in order to suspend and preserve the sample.

15. Prenatal Care and Postnatal Care

    A. __________ __________ is provided to pregnant women before delivery, including a series of visits and specific tests to promote the health of both the mother and the fetus.
    B. __________ __________ covers the time from the delivery of the infant through the mother's __________-week __________ follow-up appointment.

16. The First Trimester of Pregnancy

    A. Includes the period of time from __________ of the embryo in the uterus through the __________ week.
    B. The period in which the embryo is most __________ to substances that may cause birth defects.
    C. After the __________week, the embryo is referred to as a __________.

17. The Second Trimester of Pregnancy

    A. Begins at the end of the __________ week and continues to the end of the __________ month.
    B. It is the stage at which the refinement of all the __________ takes place.
    C. Fetal movement, also called __________, may be felt.

18. The Third Trimester of Pregnancy

    A. The period from the end of the __________ month to birth is marked by an increase in the *size* and __________of the fetus.
    B. During this stage, the fetus usually assumes a __________-__________ position.
    C. It is said to have reached the age of __________ (able to sustain life on its own) at 7 months.

19. Elements of the First Prenatal Visit (List the procedures that are typically performed and ordered during this visit.)

    i. ____
    ii. ____
    iii. ____
    iv. ____
    v. ____
    vi. ____

20. The Contents of the Prenatal History

i. ______________________________
ii. ______________________________
iii. ______________________________
iv. ______________________________
v. ______________________________
vi. ______________________________

21. The Contents of the Past Obstetrical History

A. __________, or the number of times that the patient has been pregnant (not necessarily delivered)
B. __________, or births after 20 weeks of gestation, regardless of whether the infant was born alive or dead
C. The number of __________ or the number of fetuses that did not reach the age of viability

22. Information Requested for the Present Pregnancy History

i. ______________________________
ii. ______________________________
iii. ______________________________
iv. ______________________________
v. ______________________________

23. Follow-Up Prenatal Visits

A. Every __________weeks through the __________ week
B. Return every __________ weeks up to the __________ week, and then every week until delivery.
C. During a prenatal visit, the physician will typically do the following
   i. ______________________________
   ii. ______________________________
   iii. ______________________________
   iv. ______________________________
   v. ______________________________

24. The Medical Assistant's Role During Follow-Up Visits

i. ______________________________
ii. ______________________________
iii. ______________________________
iv. ______________________________
v. ______________________________
vi. ______________________________
vii. ______________________________

25. Amniocentesis

A. Amniocentesis is the puncturing of the __________ __________ using a needle and syringe for the purpose of withdrawing __________ fluid for testing.
B. Can assist in determining fetal __________, __________, and __________ disorders.

26. Procedures and Diagnostic Tests for the Female Reproductive System (Briefly explain each type.)

A. Chorionic villus sampling (CVS): ______________________________
B. Colposcopy: ______________________________
C. Conization: ______________________________
D. Culdoscopy: ______________________________
E. Human chorionic gonadotropin (HCG): ______________________________
F. Hysterosalpingography: ______________________________

G. Hysteroscopy: ____
H. Kegel exercises: ____
I. Laparotomy: ____
J. Laparoscopy: ____
K. Oophorectomy: ____
L. Panhysterectomy: ____
M. Panhysterosalpingo-oophorectomy: ____
N. Pelvimetry: ____
O. Salpingo-oophorectomy: ____

27. Screening Tests Performed During Pregnancy

A. The __________-__________ (AFP) test is a blood test taken between the 15th and 18th week of pregnancy to detect __________ __________ defects.
B. The __________ __________ __________ is a special ultrasound test of the fetus to screen for the risk of Down syndrome and other birth defects.

28. Amniocentesis

A. Performed between the __________ and __________ week of gestation.
B. Involves using a fine needle to take a sample of __________ __________ from the sac around the fetus.
C. Fluid containing __________ __________ is cultured, grown in a laboratory, and screened to detect __________ defects such as Down syndrome.
D. Used to assess fetal __________, __________, and __________.
E. Recommended for women older than __________ and those who have a family history of genetic defects.

29. Glucose Tolerance Test

A. Performed to test for gestational __________.
B. Performed between the __________ and __________ week of pregnancy.
C. After fasting, the patient is given a specific dosage of __________ and blood is taken 1 hour later.
D. An elevated test result requires an additional, more comprehensive 3-hour __________ __________ test.
E. A diet that is low in __________, moderate in carbohydrates, and high in __________, as well as regular exercise, is recommended.

30. Group B *Streptococcus*

A. Commonly found in the __________ and __________ tract; normally does not cause illness.
B. A vaginal culture at __________ to __________ weeks is recommended.
C. One to __________ percent of infants may be infected, and the infection may be life threatening.
D. A patient who tests positive will be treated with __________ during labor to prevent fetal infection.

31. Ultrasound

A. Used to determine the __________, __________ __________, __________ of the fetus, and obvious birth defects.
B. Generally performed at __________ to __________ weeks, and is generally painless.

32. The Process of Birth

A. The first stage of labor varies in length and ends with __________ __________ (widening of the cervix) and __________ (thinning of the cervical walls).
B. Stage two, the pushing stage, occurs from the period of complete __________ and __________ through the birth of the fetus.
C. Stage three is the period from the birth of the fetus to the __________ of the __________.

33. Possible Complications During Birth
   A. __________ __________ is a complication in which the placenta develops in the lower portion of the uterus, blocking the opening of the cervix.
   B. __________ __________is a complication that occurs when the placenta tears away from the uterine wall, resulting in hemorrhaging and fetal distress.
   C. Hypertension during pregnancy, or __________ __________, occurs in roughly 10% of pregnancies.
   D. __________ is when protein in the urine and edema occur.
34. Postpartum Visit
   A. Should be scheduled approximately __________ weeks after delivery.
   B. Provides time to evaluate the overall __________ __________ of the patient and provide contraceptive information if desired.
   C. The postpartum visit includes the following
      i. ______________________________
      ii. ______________________________
      iii. ______________________________
      iv. ______________________________
35. Methods of Contraception
   A. Barrier contraceptive methods include use of male and female __________, __________, shields, __________, sponges, and __________ caps.
   B. Hormonal methods use hormones to change the levels of female hormones in the body to prevent __________ or __________ of the fertilized ovum.
   C. An intrauterine device (IUD) is a small device with __________ that is placed in the uterus by the physician.
   D. Natural family planning is also known as the __________ __________ or, most recently, fertility-awareness-based birth control, a method in which intercourse is avoided around the time of ovulation.
   E. __________ __________ involves the withdrawal of the male's penis before ejaculation in the vagina.

II. Assisting with Specialty Examinations of the Male Reproductive System
   1. Circumcision
      A. Circumcision is surgical removal of the end of the __________, or __________, of the penis.
      B. The primary reason for this procedure is ease of __________.
      C. Circumcision is also a __________ practiced in some religions.
   2. Procedures and Diagnostic Tests for the Male Reproductive System (Briefly explain each type.)
      A. Castration: ______________________________
      B. Epididymectomy: ______________________________
      C. Erickson Sperm Separation: ______________________________
      D. Fluorescent treponemal antibody absorption: ______________________________
      E. Orchidopexy: ______________________________
      F. Orchiectomy: ______________________________
      G. Prostatectomy: ______________________________
      H. Testosterone toxicology: ______________________________
      I. Transurethral resection of the prostate (TURP): ______________________________
      J. Venereal disease research laboratory (VDRL): ______________________________
   3. Steps for Instructing a Male Patient to Perform a Testicular Exam
      A. __________ the patient and introduce yourself.
      B. Explain to the patient that he or she should perform the examination in the __________ or right after a warm shower, which causes the __________ __________ to relax.

C. Using the testicular model or illustration, explain that he should place his middle and index fingers underneath the __________ and thumb on top and use a gentle motion to roll the __________ between the fingers.
D. Indicate on the model or illustration the location of the __________, a soft tubular cord behind the testis that stores and carries sperm.

4. Vasectomy

A. Involves cutting the __________ __________ and tying off the ends to prevent sperm from being transported out of the testes.
B. After a vasectomy, the man still achieves an __________ and ejaculates, but without the presence of __________.
C. Another birth control method should be used for _____–_____ weeks afterward or until a sample taken after the vasectomy confirms the absence of sperm.
D. In some cases, the procedure is __________, but a vasectomy should be considered a __________ form of birth control.

5. Sexually Transmitted Infectionss (STIs)

A. Transmitted by sexual contact from __________ to person or __________ to child.
B. Caused by __________.
C. Generally treated successfully with __________.
D. Viral STDs, such as __________, __________ __________ , __________, and __________, are incurable.

6. Symptoms of a Sexually Transmitted Infection

i. ____
ii. ____
iii. ____
iv. ____

7. Bacterial Vaginosis (BV)

A. BV is the most common __________ __________ in women of childbearing age.
B. Certain behaviors increase the risk of infection, such as __________ __________ and douching.
C. Symptoms include a thin __________ or __________ discharge with an unpleasant fishy odor.
D. Increases susceptibility to other __________.
E. Treatment is important for __________ women.

8. Chlamydia Infections

A. Caused by the bacterium __________ __________.
B. In males, it is characterized by __________ and __________.
C. May lead to __________ __________ __________ in women.
D. Infected females have an increased risk of __________ pregnancy and sterility.
E. Infants born to infected mothers may develop __________ or __________.
F. Can be successfully treated with __________ or __________.

9. Genital Human Papilloma Virus Infection

A. __________ __________, or __________, are found in clusters on the external sexual organs of both males and females, and internally in the female in the vagina and cervix and in the anus and rectum of the male.
B. Can be discovered in the female by a __________ __________, although the patient may not have visible signs of warts.
C. Genital warts increase a female's risk of developing __________ __________.

10. Genital Herpes

A. Genital herpes is caused by __________ __________ __________ __________ (HSV-1) and type 2 (HSV-2).

B. There is no known cure for herpes, but __________ may lessen the duration of symptoms.
C. __________ are usually self-limiting, but may reoccur during stressful situations.

11. Gonorrhea

A. Gonorrhea is an STD that is caused by the organism __________ __________, a bacterium that grows well under warm, moist conditions.
B. Can grow in the __________, __________ __________, and uterus in the female.
C. Can grow in the __________, __________, __________, and __________ of both males and females.
D. In the male, gonorrhea is characterized by __________ __________, clear at first, and then becoming thick and milky, burning, itching, and producing pain upon urination.
E. Females are often __________, and then they develop a yellowish-green discharge.
F. Other symptoms include __________ __________, __________ __________, anal discharge, and fever.

12. Treatment for Gonorrhea

A. Large doses of __________ or __________ with follow-up examinations.
B. If left untreated, gonorrhea can cause __________ in males and females.
C. Gonorrhea can be diagnosed by __________ and __________ __________.
D. Many people who have gonorrhea also have __________ and must be treated for both.

13. Human Immunodeficiency Virus (HIV)

A. Causes __________ __________ __________ (AIDS), the final stage of HIV infection.
B. It is a very delicate virus that cannot survive __________ of the body.
C. It is not spread by casual contact or day-to-day activities such as __________ __________, __________, or sitting on toilet seats.

14. Methods of Transmission of Human Immunodeficiency Virus

A. __________, __________, or anal sex with someone who is infected.
B. Sharing __________ or __________ with someone who is infected.
C. Being exposed as a __________ or infant to HIV before or during birth or breastfeeding.
D. Coming in contact with __________ that is infected.

15. Preventing the Transmission of Human Immunodeficiency Virus

i. ______________________________
ii. ______________________________
iii. ______________________________
iv. ______________________________
v. ______________________________
vi. ______________________________
vii. ______________________________

16. Lymphogranuloma Venereum (LGV)

A. LGV is an STD that is caused by three strains of the bacterium __________ __________.
B. It is difficult to diagnose because the symptoms are __________ to that of other conditions.
C. Can be mistaken for __________ STDs like syphilis and genital herpes.
D. Untreated, LGV may cause __________ obstruction and __________ (massive swelling of the scrotum).

17. Pelvic Inflammatory Disease (PID)

A. PID is the term used to describe inflammation of the vagina, cervix, uterus, and __________ __________ in the female.
B. If left untreated, __________ __________ may develop in the fallopian tube, which then blocks the movement of the ovum in the tubes.
C. If the tubes are completely blocked, __________ cannot reach the ovum to cause fertilization.

D. If partially blocked, a fertilized ovum may begin to grow in the __________ __________ instead of in the uterus.
E. Diagnosed by __________ __________ and an ultrasound of the abdomen.
F. Can result in __________ __________, __________, and even death if untreated.
G. __________ can cure PID.
H. Treatment does not correct any damage already done to the __________ organs.

18. Syphilis

A. Syphilis is an STD that is caused by the bacterium __________ __________.
B. Spread by direct person-to-person contact with a __________ __________, or sore.
C. Sores may occur on the genitals, anus, __________, __________, and __________.
D. May be transmitted to a newborn by an infected mother, resulting in __________ or developmental delays or death after birth.
E. A primary chancre occurs in about __________ weeks or up to __________ months after exposure.
F. Secondary-stage signs are a __________ on the palms of the hands, the soles of the feet, and elsewhere on the body, along with fever, swollen glands, __________ __________, and fatigue.
G. The latent stages occur __________ to __________ years after the first two stages have disappeared.
H. The disease will damage the brain, heart, liver, and other internal organs, causing __________, __________, blindness, and death.
I. Diagnosed by __________-__________ microscopic examination of chancre material or by blood tests for the presence of syphilis antibodies (RPR, VDRL).
J. During the primary stage, a single, large dose of __________ may cure the patient.

19. Trichomoniasis

A. Trichomoniasis is a protozoal infection caused by the organism __________ __________, resulting in an infection of the lower genitourinary tract.
B. Causes a white or yellow, __________ __________ discharge with a foul odor in females.
C. The male is usually __________, except for __________ itching.
D. A diagnosis is made by obtaining a sample of vaginal __________ and preparing a slide with normal saline solution.
E. Treatment for both males and females is a course of the antibiotic __________ or __________ taken orally.

20. Symptoms of Urinary Tract Disorders

A. Increased urine production is seen in __________.
B. Frequent urination is seen in __________ __________ infections.
C. Swelling and weight gain are seen in __________ __________ __________ (CHF) and renal dysfunction.
D. Decreased urinary output is seen in urinary __________.

21. Procedures and Diagnostic Tests for the Urinary System (Briefly describe each.)

A. Creatinine clearance: ____
B. Cystography: ____
C. Cystoscopy: ____
D. Extracorporeal shockwave lithotripsy (ESWL): ____
E. Excretory urography: ____
F. Hemodialysis: ____
G. Intravenous pyelogram (IVP): ____
H. Kidney, ureters, bladder (KUB): ____
I. Meatotomy: ____
J. Peritoneal dialysis: ____
K. Retrograde pyelogram: ____

L. Sound: ________________________________
M. Urography: ________________________________
N. Ultrasonography of the kidneys: ________________________________

22. Benign Prostate Hyperplasia (BPH)

A. As the __________enlarges, it presses on the urethra and causes restriction of the flow of urine.
B. Restricted urinary flow can result in __________ __________, interruption of the __________ __________, and difficulty starting to urinate.

23. Prostate Cancer

A. Prostate cancer is a slow-growing __________ tumor of the prostate gland.
B. May spread to the adjacent __________ __________ and male reproductive organs, as well as to the lymph nodes and bones.
C. It is the __________ most common form of cancer in men, with one in eight males affected.
D. Its cause is unknown, but age, heredity, and a __________-__________ diet increase the risk of developing it.

24. Symptoms of Prostate Cancer

i. ________________________________
ii. ________________________________
iii. ________________________________
iv. ________________________________
v. ________________________________

25. Screening for Prostate Cancer

A. Prostate-specific antigen (PSA) __________ __________and a __________ rectal examination
B. The PSA test checks for a __________ released by the prostate.
C. If levels are elevated, then a __________ of prostate tissue is done, usually in the office.
D. If the results are positive for cancer cells, then a __________ __________ is done to detect possible spread of the disease.
E. PSA results of under __________ are considered to be normal.

26. Treatment for Prostate Cancer

i. ________________________________
ii. ________________________________
iii. ________________________________
iv. ________________________________
v. ________________________________

27. Acute and Chronic Renal Failure

A. Kidney failure is the inability of the kidneys to adequately __________ __________ waste products from the blood.
B. Acute kidney failure has a rapid onset of a few days to a few __________.
C. Causes of acute kidney failure
   i. ________________________________
   ii. ________________________________
   iii. ________________________________

28. Symptoms of Acute Renal Failure

i. ________________________________
ii. ________________________________
iii. ________________________________
iv. ________________________________
v. ________________________________
vi. ________________________________

29. Diagnosing Acute Renal Failure (List the types of tests and diagnostic procedures used.)
   i. ______________________________
   ii. ______________________________
   iii. ______________________________
   iv. ______________________________
   v. ______________________________
30. Chronic Renal Failure
   A. Chronic renal failure is a slow __________, decline in kidney function over a period of months to several years.
   B. Acute kidney failure can become chronic if, after treatment, the kidneys do not __________ recover.
   C. Any condition that can cause acute renal failure can cause __________ __________ failure.
31. Common Causes of Chronic Renal Failure
   i. ______________________________
   ii. ______________________________
   iii. ______________________________
   iv. ______________________________
   v. ______________________________
32. Symptoms of Chronic Renal Failure
   A. Patient may experience mild symptoms, including __________ and elevated __________ __________ nitrogen.
   B. As the condition progresses, __________, lack of __________ __________, anemia, loss of appetite, and shortness of breath affect the patient's quality of life.
33. Diagnosing Chronic Renal Failure
   A. Diagnosis is based on patient __________, __________, and blood tests for the levels of __________ and blood urea nitrogen.
   B. Chronic renal failure is __________ if not treated.
   C. Survival for patients with end-stage renal disease is a ________ ________.
34. Treatment for Chronic Renal Failure
   A. Various medications to adjust __________ __________, regulate __________ __________, and counteract anemia.
   B. Restriction of __________ and __________ in the diet.
   C. When these treatments are no longer effective, kidney __________ or __________ are the alternatives.
   D. Most patients with advanced kidney failure die within __________ to __________ years even with dialysis.

KEY TERMINOLOGY REVIEW

Write a sentence using the selected key terms in the correct context.

1. *amenorrhea*

____

____

2. *carcinoma in situ*

____

____

3. *chancre*

4. *chorionic villus sampling (CVS)*

5. *dysplasia*

6. *eclampsia*

7. *ectopic pregnancy*

8. *endometrium*

9. *fundus*

10. *gonads*

11. *gravida*

12. *human papilloma viruses (HPVs)*

13. *lochia*

14. *menarche*

15. *nocturia*

16. *oxytocin*

17. *para*

18. *parturition*

19. *placenta abruptio*

20. *placenta previa*

21. *preeclampsia*

22. *puerperium*

23. *quickening*

APPLIED PRACTICE

Follow the directions as instructed with each question below.

1. Sometimes patients are not ready either physically or emotionally to fully understand their medical diagnosis. The medical assistant must be able to clearly explain, in simple language, any terms that are confusing to the patient. The medical assistant must utilize many teaching methods to facilitate the patient's comprehension of his or her diagnosis and treatment plan. List three teaching methods that the medical assistant can utilize to help the patient.

2. Many states mandate that suspicions of abuse be reported. How would you go about reporting any suspicion you may have?

LEARNING ACTIVITY: FILL IN THE BLANK

Using your text as necessary, fill in the blanks to the following questions.

1. ACS suggests that women in their twenties and thirties have a ________ as part of a periodic regular health exam by a health professional every 3 years.
2. Females develop breast cancer 100 times more frequently than males, probably due to the effects of ___________.
3. Prior to the patient scheduling a Pap test, the medical assistant should advise her not to douche for _____–_____ hours before the examination.
4. The pelvic examination begins with an examination of the ________________.
5. Women who become sexually active at an early age, as well as those who have multiple partners, are at ___________ risk of infection from HPV.
6. The Pap smear is ______% accurate in detecting cervical carcinoma.
7. The third trimester is the period from the end of the _______ month to birth.
8. The normal FHT is _____–_____ beats per minute.
9. Condoms have an effectiveness rate of about ______%.
10. Women are fertile for about ______ years of their adult lives.
11. An alternative birth control method should be used for _____–_____ weeks after a vasectomy or until a sample confirms the absence of sperm.
12. The symptoms of gonorrhea do not appear in females until _____ months after exposure.
13. ______________ has no known cause and is the most common vaginal infection in women of childbearing age.
14. Untreated, gonorrhea can cause ___________ in both males and females and can spread to the blood or joints.
15. Benign prostate hyperplasia (BPH) is an enlargement of the prostate gland that may occur after age ______.

CRITICAL THINKING

Answer the following questions to the best of your ability. Utilize the textbook as a reference.

1. Imagine the following scenario: You are a female. You have completed your externship and have been hired by a urology clinic for your first full-time medical assistant position. You are directed by the physician to instruct a patient in how to perform a testicular self-exam. You are suddenly nervous about doing this with a real patient even though you have practiced this in your medical assisting program with other students. Describe in one or two paragraphs how you would feel and what you would do or tell yourself to bolster your own comfort and confidence.

2. A patient, 18-year-old Maria Riojas, has come in with a chief complaint of bleeding between her periods. This will be her third GYN visit since menarche, and she is still quite apprehensive about the examination and getting undressed. She says that she hopes that the doctor won't have to do a pelvic examination today; she just wants a stronger or different birth control pill. Her friend told her that she has breakthrough bleeding because she is on the wrong pill. What would you say to the patient?

3. A patient comes in with her husband, and she asks that he be allowed to come into the examination room with her. When you ask her to disrobe, she looks hesitant, then looks at her husband and doesn't move to take the gown and drape. What do you anticipate is happening? What should you do?

4. A patient who is 6 months pregnant calls in saying that she has been bleeding a little (just spotting) all morning and wanted to let the doctor know. She wants an appointment for Thursday and today is Monday. What would you say?

RESEARCH ACTIVITY

Utilize Internet search engines to research the following topics and write a brief description of what you find. It is important to utilize reputable websites.

1. Select one procedure and diagnostic test for the female reproductive system and one procedure and diagnostic test for the male reproductive system. Conduct research on each using online resources and/or your school or local library. Write a paragraph on what you learned about each procedure/diagnostic test, including why the test is done, how the test is done, and what type of treatment might be available if the test result is positive. Be sure to cite your sources.

CHAPTER 39

Assisting with Eye and Ear Care

CHAPTER OUTLINE

General review of the chapter:

The Study of the Eye
Assessing Visual Acuity
Irrigation of the Eye
Instillation of Eye Medication
Patient Safety Guidelines
Changes in the Aging Eye
Assisting the Visually Impaired Patient
The Study of the Ear
Hearing Acuity
Hearing Assessment
Assisting the Hearing-Impaired Patient
Examination of the Nose and Throat

STUDENT STUDY GUIDE

Use the following guide to assist in your learning of the concepts from the chapter.

I. The Study of the Eye

1. The Ophthalmologist
   A. Performs eye ___________ and eye ___________.
   B. Prescribes medications, _________________, and contact lenses.
2. The Doctor of Optometry (OD)
   A. Also referred to as an _______________.
   B. Performs eye examinations, prescribes medications, and write prescription for _____________ and contact lenses.
3. The Optician
   A. _________ and _________ prescription lenses and contacts.
   B. Completes a ______ to ______-year apprenticeship.
4. The Ophthalmoscope
   A. Used to view the __________ parts of the ________.
   B. The physician positions the ophthalmoscope so that ________ penetrates the ________ of the patient's eye and screens for ________ damage and ________ problems.
5. Evaluating the Status of the Patient's Pupils
   A. PERRLA is an acronym that stands for __________ __________, __________, __________ to __________, and _______________ and focus on objects at different ______________.
   B. Injuries to the brain may result in the patient having pupils of _________ size.

6. Visual Acuity

   A. Normal visual acuity, or clearness of vision, is referred to as ______ vision.
   B. Causes of errors in refraction
      i. The eyeball is too _________.
      ii. The eyeball is too _________.
      iii. The lens has _________ its ___________.
      iv. The _____ or ______ has an irregular ____________.

7. Myopia

   A. Myopia is a condition in which the eye sees _____ objects well but ______ objects appear _______.
   B. Occurs either because the eyeball is too ______ or because the ________ is too ______, and the light ________ do not reach the ________.

8. Strabismus

   A. Children with strabismus appear ____________ and may need to wear a __________ over the ________ ________ to ________ the weaker eye.
   B. If the ________ and _____________ are ineffective, surgery on the eye __________ may be necessary.

9. The Snellen Chart

   A. A person with normal vision can read the top line at ______ feet.
   B. To the ________ of each line is a ________ indicating that a person with normal vision can read the lines at decreasing distances of _____, _____, _____, _____, _____, and _____ feet.
   C. For preschool children or patients who are __________ or have a __________ barrier, the *Snellen E,* the ________ __, or pictorial charts are used.

10. Eye Abbreviations

    A. The abbreviation for the right eye is ______.
    B. The abbreviation for the left eye is ______.
    C. The abbreviation for both eyes is ______.

11. Steps for Using the Snellen Chart

    A. Determine the patient's ability to recognize __________.
    B. Place the patient ________ feet from the chart, either seated or standing, as long as the Snellen chart is at ________ level.
    C. Following office policies (regarding which eye to test first), have the patient cover the other eye with an __________.
    D. Instruct the patient to keep both eyes _________ even though one eye is covered.
    E. Use a pointer and point to the letters or appropriate symbols in _________ order.
    F. Starting with the _________ line, ask the patient to identify the letters on each line, and then proceed down the chart to the last line that the patient can read without ______.
    G. Observe for signs of _____________ or ____________ the head, which indicate difficulty identifying letters.
    H. Record the ______ numbers adjacent to the line that the patient can read without ________.
    I. Following testing of both eyes, clean the _________ with _________ and _________.

12. Steps for Testing for Near-Vision Acuity Using the Jaeger Card

    A. The patient reads the card held at a normal reading distance (________ to ________ inches).
    B. The card has a series of paragraphs in decreasing _________ of _________ with a _________ above each.
    C. Number one (_____) is next to the paragraph with the ____________ __________, and as the text becomes larger, the number ____________.
    D. Paragraph ______ represents 20/20 vision.

13. Color Vision Impairment
   A. Defects in color vision are __________, __________, or acquired through disease or injury.
   B. Changes in color vision may indicate diseases of the _______, _______ _______, or _______.
14. The Ishihara Test
   A. Screens for color vision _______.
   B. The patient is shown ________ color plates or pages and must correctly identify _______ to be considered to have color vision within a normal range.
15. Contrast Sensitivity
   A. Used to measure the patient's ability to distinguish faint __________ in shades of _______.
   B. Several new testing procedures have been used to test for contrast sensitivity, including the _______ _______ _______ and the _______ _______ _______.
16. Procedures and Diagnostic Tests Related to the Eye
   A. ______________________________
   B. ______________________________
   C. ______________________________
   D. ______________________________
   E. ______________________________
   F. ______________________________
   G. ______________________________
   H. ______________________________
   I. ______________________________
   J. ______________________________
   K. ______________________________
   L. ______________________________
   M. ______________________________
   N. ______________________________
17. Fluorescein Angiography
   A. This is the process of injecting ________, followed by a series of __________ of the _______ through dilated pupils.
   B. Provides diagnostic information about the blood flow in the ______.
   C. Detects _________ changes in diabetics and _________ _________.
   D. Identifies _________ in the macular area of the _________, determining whether there is _________ of the __________.
18. Radial Keratotomy
   A. Radial keratotomy is a surgical procedure that may be performed to correct ____________________.
   B. Incisions are made in the ________ to flatten it, thereby shortening the ________ so that ________ reaches the ________.
   C. Complications of surgery can lead to __________.
19. Steps for Irrigating the Eye
   A. The label of the irrigating solution must be checked _______ times to ensure that it is the correct _______ and _______ as ordered by the physician.
   B. The solution is brought to room temperature by _______ the bottle in a _______ _______ _______ or by standing the bottle in a ________ water _______.
   C. If both eyes are to be irrigated, then __________ separate sets of equipment must be used to prevent __________.
   D. Hold the syringe ___________ inch from the eye.
   E. Gently irrigate from the inner to the outer ________, or ________ of the eye, aiming at the ________ ________.

20. The Instillation of Eye Medication
    A. Only ________ or ________ medications can be used in the eye and they must be ________.
    B. Encourage patients to discard eye medications when the prescribed treatment time has been ____________.

21. Steps for the Instillation of Eye Medication
    A. Check the ________ of the medication, the ________ date, and the ________ three times.
    B. Ask the patient if he or she has any known ____________ to the medication.
    C. Position the patient with his or her headed tilted ________, with eyes looking ________.
    D. Pull down the ____________ ____________, exposing the ____________.
    E. Place the dropper about __________ inch above the __________ with your dominant hand.
    F. Insert the proper number of drops into the ________ of the conjunctiva. If ointment is used, apply as a thin strip from ________ to ________ canthus.
    G. Ask the patient to gently ________ the eye and ________ the eyeball.
    H. Dry the excess medication from the __________ canthus to the __________ canthus using __________ gauze.
    I. Explain to the patient that his or her vision may be __________.

II. The Study of the Ear

1. Steps for Irrigating the Ear
    A. Check the name, __________, and ________ date of the irrigating solution ________ times.
    B. Have the patient sit with the affected ear tilted slightly ____________.
    C. Place a towel over the patient's ____________ and ask the patient to hold the ____________ basin.
    D. Clean the __________ ear with a __________ cotton ball.
    E. Pour the warmed solution into a __________ basin and fill the syringe with ________ cc of solution.
    F. Aim the stream of flow toward the __________ of the ____________.

2. Steps for Instilling Ear Medication
    i. ____________________
    ii. ____________________
    iii. ____________________
    iv. ____________________
    v. ____________________
    vi. ____________________
    vii. ____________________
    viii. ____________________
    ix. ____________________
    x. ____________________
    xi. ____________________
    xii. ____________________

3. Steps for Performing Audiometric Testing
    i. ____________________
    ii. ____________________
    iii. ____________________
    iv. ____________________
    v. ____________________
    vi. ____________________
    vii. ____________________
    viii. ____________________
    ix. ____________________
    x. ____________________

xi. ____
xii. ____
xiii. ____
xiv. ____

4. Tests and Procedures for the Ear (Briefly explain each of the following.)
   A. Audiometric test: ______________________________
   B. Electrochochleography: __________________________
   C. Falling test: __________________________________
   D. Mastoid antrotomy: _____________________________
   E. Myringoplasty: ________________________________
   F. Otoplasty: ____________________________________
   G. Stapedectomy: ________________________________
   H. Tympanoplasty: _______________________________
   I. Rinne test: ___________________________________
   J. Weber test: ___________________________________

5. Examination of the Nose and Throat
   A. The physician uses a nasal ____________ to inspect the ____________ lining of the nose for signs of ______________ and ____________.
   B. Includes the use of a tongue ____________ to examine the ___________ for signs of ____________, enlarged ___________, and abnormalities of the tongue or ___________ ____________.

6. Signs and Symptoms of Nasal Problems
   i. ____
   ii. ____
   iii. ____
   iv. ____

7. Steps for Instilling Nasal Medication
   i. ____
   ii. ____
   iii. ____
   iv. ____
   v. ____
   vi. ____
   vii. ____
   viii. ____
   ix. ____
   x. ____
   xi. ____
   xii. ____
   xiii. ____
   xiv. ____
   xv. ____
   xvi. ____
   xvii. ____
   xviii. ____
   xix. ____
   xx. ____

KEY TERMINOLOGY REVIEW

Match the vocabulary term to the correct definition below.

a. acuity
b. astigmatism
c. audiogram
d. cerumen
e. cornea
f. decibel
g. frequencies
h. hyperopia
i. myopia
j. myringa
k. organ of Corti
l. otorhinolaryngologists
m. presbycusis
n. speculum
o. strabismus

1. ________ Impacted earwax or foreign matter in the ear.
2. ________ The medical term for the eardrum.
3. ________ Used by the physician to evaluate the patient's hearing.
4. ________ Any instrument that holds open an opening in the body to permit inspection.
5. ________ Visual and auditory sharpness.
6. ________ Also known as farsightedness.
7. ________ The clear, transparent covering of the eye.
8. ________ An eye disorder caused by weakness in the external eye muscles, resulting in the eyes looking in different directions.
9. ________ A refractive disorder in which irregularities in the curvature of the cornea cause light not to focus on the retina but instead to spread out over an area, causing overall blurring of vision.
10. ________ Also known as nearsightedness.
11. ________ Individual who specializes in treating conditions related to the ear, nose, and throat.
12. ________ The auditory nerve.
13. ________ The intensity of the sound.
14. ________ A decline in hearing acuity, a normal part of aging.
15. ________ Number of fluctuations per second of energy in the form of sound waves.

APPLIED PRACTICE

Follow the directions as instructed with each question below.

Activity 1: Read the following scenario and then answer the questions.

Shawn Collins, RMA, is working as a medical assistant at a local family practice. Rajan Avuri, a 17-year-old patient, is being seen for a driver's license eye examination. As part of the exam, Shawn tests Rajan's vision with a Snellen eye chart similar to the Snellen eye chart below. Shawn asks Rajan to cover his right eye and read line 8. Rajan reads the following letters from left to right: "D, E, F, P, O, T, E, C." Shawn asks Rajan to continue on and read line 9. Rajan reads the following letters from left to right: "L, E, P, O, D, R, O, T."

Shawn then asks Rajan to uncover his right eye and cover his left eye for assessment. Beginning with line 8, Rajan reads the following letters from left to right: "D, E, F, R, O, T, E, C." Rajan is not able to distinguish any letters on the lines below line 8.

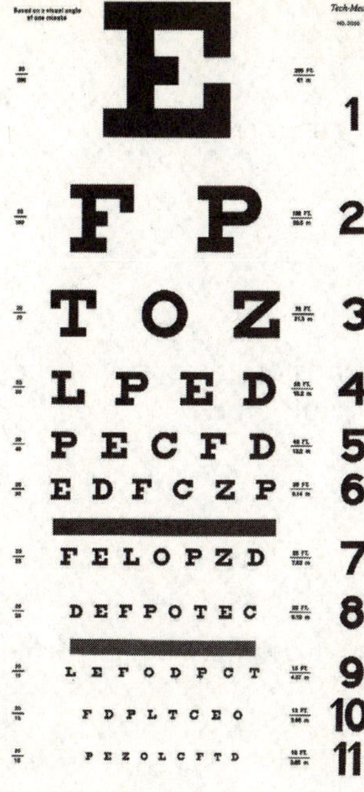

1. How should Shawn record Rajan's vision in his left eye? Explain your answer.

2. How should Shawn record Rajan's vision in his right eye? Explain your answer.

Activity 2

1. A 2-year-old child must have a myringotomy performed because the child has had reoccurring ear infections. Explain to the parents what this procedure entails.

LEARNING ACTIVITY: MULTIPLE CHOICE

Circle the correct answer to each of the questions below.

1. Which of the following specialists is not a medical doctor?
   A. Ophthalmologist
   B. Otorhinolaryngologist

C. Optometrist
D. None of the above

2. Which instrument measures intraocular pressure?

A. Ophthalmoscope
B. Tonometer
C. Slit lamp
D. Otoscope

3. The ability to distinguish colors depends on the cones of the _________, which react to light and permit us to see shades of red, green, and blue.

A. choroid
B. cornea
C. retina
D. iris

4. Which of the following surgical procedures may be performed to correct myopia?

A. Keratoplasty
B. Radial keratotomy
C. Phacoemulsification
D. None of the above

5. To be declared legally blind, a person must only be able to see at _______ feet what a normal person would see at 200 feet.

A. 20
B. 40
C. 50
D. 100

6. The most common type of color vision defect, which is inherited, is the inability to distinguish _________________________.

A. blue and yellow
B. blue and black
C. red and green
D. All of the above

7. The abbreviation AD (aurus dextra) is for _________________________.

A. both ears
B. the left ear
C. the right ear
D. None of the above

8. Which of the following instrument(s) is used in the office for ear examinations?

A. Otoscope
B. Tuning fork
C. Audiometer
D. All of the above

9. Sensorineural hearing loss is due to _________________________.

A. nerve damage
B. obstruction of sound waves
C. old age
D. None of the above

10. When instilling ear medication into a child's ear, the ear should be pulled _______________________.

   A. up and back
   B. down and back
   C. up
   D. Any of the above

CRITICAL THINKING

Answer the following questions to the best of your ability. Utilize the textbook as a reference.

1. You need to perform a Snellen visual acuity test and an Ishihara color vision test per the physician's orders. You do not have an occluder or the Ishihara plates. Which of the tests, if any, could you still perform using a different item and what replacement item(s) can you use?

____

____

____

____

____

2. As a medical assistant, how can you help patients with diminished visual or hearing capacities?

____

____

RESEARCH ACTIVITY

Utilize Internet search engines to research the following topics and write a brief description of what you find. It is important to utilize reputable websites.

1. Visit different websites that deal with vision and hearing loss. What information did you find that could be used to help families dealing with vision and hearing deficiencies? What websites did you find to be most useful? Could these websites be beneficial for staff members of an EENT practice. If so, why?

____

____

____

____

____

____

____

____

____

____

____

____

CHAPTER 40
Assisting with Life Span Specialties: Pediatrics

CHAPTER OUTLINE

General review of the chapter:

Assisting in Pediatrics
The Pediatric Office
The Pediatric Patient
Pediatric Office Visits and Procedures
Pediatric Diseases and Disorders
Child Safety Recommendations
Adolescence and Puberty
Eating Disorders

STUDENT STUDY GUIDE

Fill in the study guide below using both your textbook and notes from your instructor's lecture.

I. Assisting in Pediatrics

1. Specialists Who Treat Children
   A. Most pediatricians recommend that, at age _____, patients find a primary care physician.
   B. Primary care physicians and __________ also care for pediatric patients.
2. The Pediatric Office Reception Room
   A. Needs to be bright, _________, and interesting.
   B. Easy-to-clean __________ toys without tiny pieces are most practical.
   C. During office hours, toys should be _______________, as necessary, and put away to prevent falls.
   D. __________ toys should be done on a regular basis.
   E. Sick children should be brought __________ into an examination room.
3. Patient Safety in the Pediatric Office
   A. No child should be ___________ ___________ on an examination table.
   B. Three positions are used for carrying an infant
      i. ______________________________
      ii. ______________________________
      iii. ______________________________
4. Steps for Wrapping a Child for Restraint
   A. Speak to the child in __________, __________ tones.
   B. Place a____________ blanket or small sheet on the table and fold _________ the top corner.
   C. Place the child _______________ on the blanket, keeping one hand on the __________ to ensure safety.
   D. Wrap the ________ corner across the _________, covering the _________ arm, and tuck snugly under the ______ arm.

E. Wrap the _______ corner across the torso, covering the _______ arm, and tuck snugly under the _______.
F. To restrain the head, place yourself at the end of the table where the infant's head is located and place one hand on _______ side of the head.
G. Avoid sealing the _______ or touching the _______.

5. Developmental Checklist for 1 to 2 Month Olds
A. Able to _______ head when lying on the stomach.
B. Moves _______ and _______ in an energetic manner.
C. Likes to be held and _______.

6. Developmental Checklist for 2 to 3 Month Olds
A. Rolls _______ to the side when lying on the back.
B. Startled by _______ sounds.

7. Developmental Checklist for 3 to 4 Month Olds
A. Eyes follow _______ objects.
B. Able to hold head _______.
C. _______ objects in hands.
D. _______ out loud.
E. Rolls from _______ to _______.

8. Developmental Checklist for 4 to 5 Month Olds
A. Reaches for and _______ objects.
B. Stands _______ when held.
C. Turns toward the _______ of a voice.

9. Developmental Checklist for 5 to 6 Month Olds
A. Turns over from _______ to _______.
B. Sits with a _______ support.
C. Listens to _______ voice.

10. Developmental Checklist for 6 to 7 Month Olds
A. Can _______ an object from one hand to the other.
B. Can sit for a _______ minutes alone.
C. Is _______ at first with strangers.

11. Developmental Checklist for 7 to 8 Month Olds
A. Can sit steadily for _______ minutes.
B. Crawls on _______ and _______.
C. Grasps things with the _______ and the first _______ fingers.
D. Likes to be near the _______.

12. Developmental Checklist for 8 to 9 Month Olds
A. Responds to _______ _______.
B. Can stand for a _______ time holding onto support.
C. _______ with fingers.
D. Responds to _______.

13. Developmental Checklist for 10 to 12 Month Olds
A. Able to pull self up at side of crib or _______.
B. Can drink from a _______ when it is held.
C. Walks around holding onto _______.
D. Repeats a few _______.

14. Developmental Checklist for 12 to 15 Month Olds
A. Pulls _______ while walking.

B. Shows what he or she wants by ___________ and ___________.
C. Cooperates with ______________.

15. Developmental Checklist for 15 to 18 Month Olds

A. Can build a tower with ___________.
B. Can say ___________ words.
C. Drinks from a cup held in ___________ hands.

16. Developmental Checklist for 18 Months to 2-Year-Olds

A. Walks up and down ___________, alternating feet.
B. Says at least ___________ to ___________ words.
C. Sometimes uses ___________-word sentences.

17. Developmental Checklist for 2- to 3-Year-Olds

A. Can repeat ___________ numbers in a row.
B. Dresses self except for ___________.
C. Can build tower of ___________ blocks.

18. Developmental Checklist for 4- to 5-Year-Olds

A. Can repeat a simple ___________-word sentence.
B. Can wash hands and face ___________ help.
C. Can follow ___________ commands.

19. Growth from Infancy to Adulthood

A. The average infant weights about ___________ lbs. at birth.
B. By 6 months, that weight has ___________, and at a year, the child's length has ___________ and the weight has ___________.
C. From ages 5 to 10, the child grows _____ to _____ inches and gains _____ to _____ pounds yearly.
D. Adult proportions will not be reached until about age _____.

20. Failure to Thrive (FTT)

A. Children have __________ growth patterns.
B. A baby whose weight is under the ___________ percentile on the growth chart is in the failure-to-thrive syndrome category.
C. The most frequent cause of FTT is ___________ nutrition.

21. Obtaining a Blood Pressure Reading on a Child

A. Most pediatricians do not require a blood pressure measurement unless there are ___________ or ___________ disorders.
B. Some physicians require blood pressure readings on every patient regardless of age and others monitor blood pressure once a year after age _____.
C. A blood pressure cuff measuring no wider than __________-__________ of the child's upper arm must be used.

22. Steps for Measuring an Infant's Blood Pressure

i. ____
ii. ____
iii. ____
iv. ____
v. ____
vi. ____

23. Steps for Obtaining a Temperature with a Tympanic Thermometer

i. ____
ii. ____
iii. ____

iv. ______________________________
v. ______________________________
vi. ______________________________
vii. ______________________________

24. Steps for Obtaining a Temperature Reading Using the Axillary Method
    i. ______________________________
    ii. ______________________________
    iii. ______________________________
    iv. ______________________________
    v. ______________________________

25. Steps for Obtaining a Temperature Rectally by Using a Digital Thermometer
    i. ______________________________
    ii. ______________________________
    iii. ______________________________
    iv. ______________________________
    v. ______________________________
    vi. ______________________________
    vii. ______________________________
    viii. ______________________________
    ix. ______________________________

26. Steps for Measuring Heart Rate/Pulse by Apical Measurement
    i. ______________________________
    ii. ______________________________
    iii. ______________________________
    iv. ______________________________
    v. ______________________________
    vi. ______________________________

27. Normal Body Temperature
    A. Oral: ______°F (______°C)
    B. Aural: ______°F (______°C)
    C. Axillary: ______°F (______°C)
    D. Rectal: ______°F (______°C)

28. Normal Values for Respiration
    A. Infants: ____________
    B. Toddlers: ____________
    C. Preschool age: ____________
    D. School age: ____________
    E. Adolescents: ____________

29. Normal Values for Pulse
    A. Infants: ____________
    B. Toddlers: ____________
    C. Preschool age: ____________
    D. School age: ____________
    E. Adolescents: ____________

30. Normal Systolic and Diastolic Valves
    A. Infants: ____________ systolic, ____________ diastolic
    B. Toddlers: ____________ systolic, ____________ diastolic
    C. Preschool age: ____________ systolic, ____________ diastolic
    D. School age: ____________ systolic, ____________ diastolic

31. Height, Weight, and Head and Chest Circumference
   A. Infants should be weighted without a __________ to ensure that the most accurate weight is obtained.
   B. Height and weight are measured without __________.
   C. The measurement of the circumference of the __________ is part of each well-baby office visit until age __________.
   D. Rapid growth of the head may indicate __________.
   E. Head growth that falls below the normal percentile may indicate ____________.
   F. Normal head circumference at birth should be between _____ and _____ inches (_____ to _____ cm).
   G. Generally, the head and chest circumferences are equal at about _____ to _____ years of age.

32. Growth Charts
   A. Every patient should have a copy of the ________________________ growth chart as part of his or her permanent medical record.
   B. Individual growth graphs are available for boys and girls from birth to _____ months and _____ to _____ years.
   C. Once the measurements are obtained, the values are plotted according to the child's age and __________ and the __________ is obtained.

33. Evaluating a Child's Hearing and Vision
   A. Hearing tests are done in many hospitals at _________ as part of special federal and state programs to detect hearing difficulties at an early age.
   B. Early detection is important because _________ development depends on a child's ability to mimic sounds, word selection, and use of words.
   C. If the child tests below normal during the first test, it is repeated at about __________ weeks.
   D. At the yearly examination, visual acuity is measured for children ________ years and older using the ________ ________ chart.

34. Steps for Performing a Snellen Test on a Child
   i. ____
   ii. ____
   iii. ____
   iv. ____
   v. ____
   vi. ____
   vii. ____
   viii. ____
   ix. ____

35. Steps for Applying a Urine Collection Device on a Child
   i. ____
   ii. ____
   iii. ____
   iv. ____
   v. ____
   vi. ____
   vii. ____
   viii. ____
   ix. ____
   x. ____
   xi. ____

II. Pediatric Conditions and Disorders

1. The Common Cold
   A. Caused by more than __________ varieties of rhinovirus.
   B. In infants and children, there may be a _________ fever, nasal congestion, and __________.
   C. Children from age ________ to _________ may have _________ to _________ colds a year.
   D. Treatment usually includes use of ______________ medications to reduce fever.
   E. Due to recent studies, the use of _____________ and cough _____________ is not recommended by many physicians.

2. Strep Throat
   A. Strep throat is caused by group ____________ beta hemolytic _____________ *pyogenes*.
   B. The physician may order a throat ___________ to confirm that strep is the causative agent.
   C. Many pediatrician's offices perform these tests onsite with the use of a _______ _______ test.
   D. A child who has recurring strep throat infections may be a candidate for a ______________.
   E. Strep throat is treated with ___________.
   F. _____________ is the best defense for warding off upper respiratory infections.

3. Otitis Media
   A. Otitis media is an infection of the ____________ ear.
   B. It is due to colds, ___________, or other respiratory infections.
   C. Fluid builds up and applies pressure to the __________.
   D. Treatment includes _____________, ___________, and sometimes ___________.
   E. Children with chronic ear infections may require a ________________.

4. Croup
   A. Leads to a distinctive barking cough and _______________.
   B. There are two types of croup
      i. ______________________________
      ii. ______________________________

5. Bronchitis
   A. Bronchitis is an inflammation of the ____________.
   B. It is more common in children under ______ years old.
   C. Children with asthma and those exposed to ____________ smoke are at higher risk.
   D. Symptoms of bronchitis
      i. ______________________________
      ii. ______________________________
   E. Treatment for bronchitis
      i. ______________________________
      ii. ______________________________

6. The Respiratory Syncytial Virus (RSV)
   A. Can be spread by contact with upper respiratory ________________.
   B. Confirmation of RSV is the presence of __________ antibodies obtained from a _________ swab or __________ culture.

7. Asthma
   A. Asthma is the most common ___________ disease in children.
   B. Affects ______ out of ______ children, usually before age ______.
   C. Symptoms of asthma
      i. ______________________________
      ii. ______________________________
      iii. ______________________________
      iv. ______________________________
      v. ______________________________

8. Diarrhea
   A. Defined as ______ or more watery stools within ______ hours.
   B. May be caused by bacterial, ________, or parasitic infections; food ________; and medications.
   C. If it persists for more than ______ days, the child may need to be seen by the physician.
9. Colic
   A. Colic is severe ________________ pain in infants that occurs in both breast-fed and formula-fed babies.
   B. Cause is unknown, although some suspect ________________ of the digestive system.
   C. Symptoms of colic
      i. ________________
      ii. ________________
      iii. ________________
      iv. ________________
      v. ________________
   D. Treatment for colic
      i. ________________
      ii. ________________
10. Obesity
   A. Defined as being ______ over the patient's ideal weight with a body mass index greater than ________.
   B. Causes of obesity
      i. ________________
      ii. ________________
      iii. ________________
      iv. ________________
      v. ________________
11. Autism
   A. Autism is a __________ system disorder or group of disorders that begin in childhood.
   B. It is four times more frequent in __________.
   C. It is noticeable by age __________.
   D. Affects 1 in __________ children.
12. Possible Causes of Autism
   i. ________________
   ii. ________________
   iii. ________________
   iv. ________________
   v. ________________
   vi. ________________
13. Symptoms of Autism
   i. ________________
   ii. ________________
   iii. ________________
   iv. ________________
   v. ________________
   vi. ________________
14. Sudden Infant Death Syndrome (SIDS)
   A. Usually occurs during _________.
   B. It is the leading cause of death in children during the ______ year of life.
   C. The highest number of deaths occur between ______ and ______ months.
   D. More prevalent in ___________.

15. Probable Causes of Sudden Infant Death Syndrome
    i. ____________________
    ii. ____________________
    iii. ____________________
16. Risk Factors and Prevention Techniques for Sudden Infant Death Syndrome
    A. Risk factors
        i. ____________________
        ii. ____________________
        iii. ____________________
        iv. ____________________
        v. ____________________
        vi. ____________________
    B. Possible prevention techniques
        i. ____________________
        ii. ____________________
        iii. ____________________
17. Febrile Seizures
    A. Seizures can involve jerking arms and legs, loss of consciousness, and __________ of the child's body.
    B. After a seizure, the child may be ___________ and have a _____________.
    C. Not associated with __________.
18. Meningitis
    A. Meningitis is an inflammation of the _______________ surrounding the brain and the _______________.
    B. Usually results from an _____________ originating elsewhere in the body.
    C. Can be caused by viral or ____________ infection.
    D. _____________ meningitis is more common and is not life threatening.
19. Recommendations for the Meningitis Vaccination
    A. The _______________________________________ (ACIP) has made a recommendation regarding meningitis vaccinations.
    B. ACIP recommends that children ______ to _____ years of age, teens entering high school, and college freshmen receive the newly licensed ______________ vaccine.
20. Fifth Disease
    A. Fifth disease is also called _______________ _______________.
    B. It is a mildly contagious viral disease that occurs during springtime in children older than _____ years.
    C. Caused by ____________ B19.
    D. Symptoms of fifth disease (which last about a week)
        i. ____________________
        ii. ____________________
        iii. ____________________
21. Roseola
    A. Roseola is a common early childhood ________ infection characterized by the following
        i. ____________________
        ii. ____________________
    B. Treatment for roseola
        i. ____________________
        ii. ____________________
22. Hand, Foot, and Mouth Disease (HFM)
    A. HFM is a mild _________ infection.

B. Affects young children in daycare or nursery schools up to _____ years of age.
C. Usually caused by the ____________ virus.
D. Spread by the __________ route, saliva, or direct contact with __________.

23. Symptoms of and Treatment for Hand, Foot, and Mouth Disease
    A. Symptoms of HFM
        i. ______________________________
        ii. ______________________________
        iii. ______________________________
    B. Treatment for HFM
        i. ______________________________
        ii. ______________________________
        iii. ______________________________

24. Recommendations for General Child Safety
    A. Place smoke and ____________ detectors on every floor of the house.
    B. Use ___________ covers over electrical outlets.
    C. Keep _____ rails up on cribs.
    D. Place chemicals, cleaning products, and medications in a __________ cabinet.
    E. Teach all children how to dial _____.

25. Early Adolescence
    A. Early adolescence is considered ages _____ to _____.
    B. The leading cause of death is ___________________________.

26. Middle Adolescence
    A. Middle adolescence is considered ages _____ to _____.
    B. Conflicts with parents may ___________.

27. Eating Disorders
    A. Females suffer from eating disorders ______ frequently than males.
    B. ______ eating affects males and females equally.
    C. Some medical and _____________ treatments, including family counseling, are effective for some eating disorders.

28. Anorexia Nervosa
    A. Some anorexic patients lose weight by __________ dieting, _____________, taking _____________ or diuretics, or administering enemas.
    B. Patients with this condition are _____ times more likely to die than those without the illness.

29. Signs of Anorexia Nervosa
    i. ______________________________
    ii. ______________________________
    iii. ______________________________
    iv. ______________________________
    v. ______________________________
    vi. ______________________________
    vii. ______________________________

30. Treatment for Anorexia Nervosa
    i. ______________________________
    ii. ______________________________
    iii. ______________________________

31. Bulimia Nervosa
    A. Bulimic patients are ________ about their condition and deny that they have any problem with food.

B. Binging and ___________ may occur _______ times a week.
C. Patients have coexisting conditions, such as __________, ___________, and substance abuse problems.

32. Symptoms of Bulimia Nervosa
   i. ________________________________
   ii. ________________________________
   iii. ________________________________
   iv. ________________________________
   v. ________________________________
   vi. ________________________________

33. Eating Disorders Not Otherwise Specified (EDNOS)
   A. An EDNOS is an eating disorder that does not fit into the category of ________ or ________.
   B. Characterized by _______ eating episodes, which are reoccurring, leading to _________.
   C. This disorder is often associated with feelings of _______, guilt, depression, and other coexisting psychological disorders.
   D. Treatment is much the same as for bulimia, including the possible use of ____________ suppressants.

KEY TERMINOLOGY REVIEW

Match the selected key terms to their definitions below.

a. adolescence
b. amenorrhea
c. anorexia nervosa
d. BRAT diet
e. bronchiolitis
f. bulimia nervosa
g. croup
h. excoriation
i. failure to thrive (FTT)
j. febrile seizures
k. genitalia
l. hydrocephalous
m. meatus
n. microencephaly
o. myringotomy
p. pediatrician
q. purging
r. respiratory syncytial virus (RSV)
s. rhinovirus
t. sleep apnea
u. stridor
v. sudden infant death syndrome (SIDS)
w. tonsillectomy

1. ___________ The death with no known cause of an apparently healthy infant, usually before age 1.
2. ___________ A condition wherein patients binge eat and then either use self-induced vomiting, laxatives, diuretics, or all three to rid themselves of the large amounts of calories consumed.
3. ___________ A medical doctor who specializes in the treatment of newborns, infants, children, and adolescents.
4. ___________ Absence of menses.
5. ___________ A highly contagious virus that is the most common cause of bronchiolitis.
6. ___________ Excessive fluid around the brain.
7. ___________ The transition period between puberty and adulthood.
8. ___________ A method of losing weight by vomiting, taking laxatives or diuretics, or administering enemas.

9. ___________ "Noisy breathing," which is a possible symptom of viral croup.
10. ___________ Painful chafing or rawness of the skin.
11. ___________ The urinary tract opening.
12. ___________ Surgical removal of the tonsils.
13. ___________ The reproductive organs.
14. ___________ A syndrome identified when an infant gains insufficient weight according to the standardized baby growth charts.
15. ___________ A condition associated with a distorted sense of body image and the persistent quest for thinness.
16. ___________ An inflammation of the larynx and trachea.
17. ___________ Periods of absence of breathing during sleep.
18. ___________ A highly contagious condition with more than 200 varieties.
19. ___________ Often recommended by pediatricians for infants with diarrhea.
20. ___________ Present in some children with high fevers following a rapid spike in body temperature.
21. ___________ A procedure in which an incision is made into the eardrum and a tube is inserted through the eardrum to permit the drainage of fluid.
22. ___________ Symptoms include cold-like symptoms such as nasal and chest congestion and low-grade fever.
23. ___________ Head growth that falls below the normal percentile.

APPLIED PRACTICE

Read the scenario below and answer the questions that follow.

Scenario

Sandra Norwood has brought her daughter, Maya, into the office for her 6 month well-baby visit. Austin Shwartz is the medical assistant working with Ms. Norwood and Maya. From reading Maya's chart, Austin knows that Maya has had two doses of the following vaccines: HepB, Rota, DTaP, Hib, and PCV. *(Maya's chart entry for today's visit appears below.)*
Norwood, Maya
04-23-20XX

10/30/20XX, 9:30 A.M.
weight: 21 lbs., length: 27¼"
Head Circumference: 17½", Chest Circumference: 18"

CC: Mother states, "Maya is here for her 6 month checkup and immunizations."

A. Shwartz, RMA

Activity 1

1. Using the growth chart found in the textbook and the information noted above in the chart, determine the percentile for Maya's length-for-age and weight-for-age:
   a. Length-for-age percentile: ___________________
   b. Weight-for-age percentile: ___________________

Activity 2

> Kayla Jefferson, age 18 months, is being seen by Dr. Penningworth for a well-child check. The pediatrician is concerned about Kayla's size and developmental delays. He diagnoses her with failure to thrive.

1. Describe three possible signs and/or symptoms that might indicate developmental delays in the 18 months-old Kayla.

____

____

____

____

2. If the physician suspects and/or sees signs which might indicate that neglect or abuse caused the FTT, what steps might he or she take?

____

____

____

____

3. What federal law requires the physician to report abuse? Is a medical assistant responsible for reporting abuse? If so, how and to whom?

____

____

____

____

LEARNING ACTIVITY: TRUE/FALSE

Indicate whether the following statements are true or false by placing a T or an F on the line that precedes each statement.

______ 1. Injuries are the number-one cause of death in children.

______ 2. In California, carrying and undressing a pediatric patient is the responsibility of the parent.

______ 3. In some states, triaging can only be done by nurses and is considered to be beyond the scope of the medical assisting practice.

______ 4. Children mature at consistent rates; however, the stages that they pass through are variable, as are the age ranges.

______ 5. By 5 years old, the child reaches half his or her adult height.

______ 6. Abused children are at increased risk of suffering from low self-esteem and depression, and, as adults, they often are substance abusers and have eating disorders.

______ 7. Exposing the child to warm, moist night air is also frequently effective to combat the effects of croup.

______ 8. Most upper respiratory infections are spread easily by droplets from the nose or throat, or contaminated items handled by the infected person.

______ 9. A CDC survey found that 28% of high school students had suicidal thoughts and 8.3% had attempted suicide.

______ 10. EDNOS is characterized by binge eating episodes that are recurring and lead to obesity.

CRITICAL THINKING

Answer the following questions to the best of your ability. Utilize the textbook as a reference.

1. You have an order to obtain blood from a patient for a test. The patient is a 4½-year-old girl who is at the office with her father. She starts to get tears in her eyes when you approach, and the father tells her to quit that crying or he will tell the medical assistant to stick her a second time. What would you do?

2. You have a parent of a 3-month-old baby who calls in two to three times per day, extremely anxious and worried over every little thing and leaving messages with questions for the doctor. When you get the advice from the physician and return her calls, she keeps talking in detail for long periods of time. This is her first child, and she has no family in town to help her through this time of learning how to care for an infant. Everyone in the office is aware of her neediness, and many feel some annoyance at the amount of time and attention that this one patient requires. How would you handle the continuing phone calls? What would you do and/or say?

RESEARCH ACTIVITY

Utilize Internet search engines to research the following topics and write a brief description of what you find. It is important to utilize reputable websites.

1. To learn more about eating disorders and how they are treated, go online or use resources from your school or local library. Conduct research and then write a one-page essay on your findings and what you learned. Be sure to cite your resources.

CHAPTER 41
Assisting with Life Span Specialties: Geriatrics

CHAPTER OUTLINE

General review of the chapter:

The Aging Population
The Aging Process
Legal and Medical Decisions
Elder Abuse
Safety Guidelines for the Elderly Population

STUDENT STUDY GUIDE

Use the following guide to assist in your learning of the concepts from the chapter.

I. The Aging Process

1. A History of Gerontology
   A. The word "geriatric" is derived from the Greek word "__________," meaning "old age," and from "__________." meaning "physician."
   B. __________ illness is a major problem for the elderly.
2. Legislation to Benefit the Elderly
   A. 1935: __________________________________ was created under the Social Security Act.
   B. 1965: The Administration on Aging, the __________ __________ Act, Medicaid, and Medicare were created.
3. Groups of Elderly (Indicate the age range of the individuals in each of these categories.)
   i. Young-old: __________
   ii. Old: __________
   iii. Old-old: __________
   iv. Elite old: __________
4. Baby Boomers
   A. Baby boomers are persons born between ______ and ______.
   B. The oldest members of this group reach senior citizen status in ______.
   C. As of 2007, ______ of the U.S. population is between 44 and 62 years old.
5. Characteristics of Baby Boomers That Affect Health Care
   A. Have fewer ___________________ or have waited later than previous generations to start a _____________.
   B. Economic hardship, combined with advancing age and the deterioration of health, means that there will be an increased strain on __________ __________ for health care and prescription drug assistance.

6. Physical Changes That Accompany Aging: The Integumentary System
   A. Hair loses its color and becomes __________.
   B. Skin dries, becomes less __________, and __________ develop.
   C. Skin tears and bruises easily (called __________ __________).
   D. Fingernails and toenails __________.
   E. Reduced amount of __________.
   F. Increased sensitivity to __________.
   G. Age __________ become more common.
7. Physical Changes That Accompany Aging: The Nervous System
   A. Problems with __________
   B. Temperature __________ is off.
   C. Sensation of pain __________
   D. __________ sleep is shortened; there is more awakening during the night.
   E. Brain cells are lost, but intelligence is intact unless a __________ condition is present.
   F. Decreased sensitivity of __________ __________ for heat, cold, pain, and pressure
8. Physical Changes That Accompany Aging: The Sensory System
   A. It is more difficult to see __________ objects.
   B. Night vision may __________.
   C. __________ (clouding of the lens) are more common.
   D. Peripheral vision and depth perception __________.
   E. Smell and taste receptors are less __________.
9. Physical Changes That Accompany Aging: The Musculoskeletal System
   A. There is less muscle __________ and __________.
   B. Arthritis and __________ are more common.
   C. The body is more __________.
10. Physical Changes That Accompany Aging: The Urinary System
    A. The kidneys __________ in size.
    B. Urine production is less __________.
    C. __________ incontinence may develop.
11. Physical Changes That Accompany Aging: The Digestive System
    A. The primary __________ sensations of salty, sweet, and sour decrease.
    B. __________ increases; flatulence increases.
    C. Movement of food through the digestive tract __________ __________.
12. Physical Changes That Accompany Aging: The Cardiovascular System
    A. Blood vessels are less __________ and more __________.
    B. The heart may not pump as __________.
    C. Decreased __________ output and circulation.
13. Physical Changes That Accompany Aging: The Endocrine System
    A. Decrease in __________ and progesterone.
    B. Hot __________, __________feelings
    C. Higher levels of __________ and thyroid-stimulating hormone
    D. __________ gain
    E. __________ production is less efficient.
    F. Diabetes __________ is more likely.
14. Physical Changes That Accompany Aging: The Reproductive System
    A. Females: Ovulation and menstruation cease; the vaginal walls are __________ and __________.
    B. Males: The scrotum is less __________; the prostate gland may __________.

15. Diseases and Condition That Affect the Elderly (Briefly explain each disease and condition.)
   A. Alzheimer's disease and other dementias: ______________________
   B. Aortic aneurysm: ______________________
   C. Atrophic urethritis and vaginitis: ______________________
   D. Decubitus ulcers (bedsores): ______________________
   E. Benign prostatic hyperplasia: ______________________
   F. Cataracts: ______________________
   G. Chronic lymphocytic leukemia: ______________________
   H. Diabetes mellitus type 2: ______________________
   I. Glaucoma: ______________________
   J. Hypothyroidism: ______________________
   K. Osteoarthritis: ______________________
   L. Osteoporosis: ______________________
   M. Parkinson's disease: ______________________
   N. Prostate cancer: ______________________
   O. Shingles (herpes zoster): ______________________
   P. Stroke: ______________________
   Q. Urinary incontinence: ______________________
16. Considerations When Treating Elderly Patients
   A. Allow extra time for older patients to __________ __________ and __________ to questions.
   B. Do not __________ sentences for older patients or __________ a patient while talking about the patient to his or her family members or caregivers.
   C. Offer your __________ to patients when walking, and __________ them on and off the examination table as needed.
   D. Make sure that the __________ __________ is secure as patients get on and off the examination table.
   E. If you use a __________ scale in your office, assist patients onto and off of the platform and provide wall-mounted __________ for additional support.
17. Sensory Changes in the Elderly (Provide the word for the given definition.)
   A. __________ is an impairment of hearing that is associated with aging.
   B. __________ is the inability to focus on objects at close range, which reduces the ability of the elderly to interact with the environment around them.
18. Inquiring About Sensory Abilities
   i. ______________________
   ii. ______________________
   iii. ______________________
   iv. ______________________
19. Addressing Issues Associated with Aging
   A. Provide information on exercises that the elderly can perform at home while seated to increase __________ strength.
   B. Encourage eating proper amounts of __________ products to supply needed __________.
   C. Discuss __________ issues at home that can put the elderly patient at risk.
20. Mental Changes Observed in the Elderly
   i. ______________________
   ii. ______________________
   iii. ______________________
21. Mental Deterioration
   A. Mental deterioration is not a __________ part of aging.
   B. As people age, the risk of mental __________ increases.

C. Mental health is the capacity to cope __________ with life changes, manage life's __________, and achieve a state of __________ balance.
D. Brain __________ slows with aging.
E. For optimal mental health, the elderly should have a sense of __________ and feel that they are of __________ to society.

22. Cognitive Ability

A. Cognitive ability is the ability to think __________.
B. The __________ status of the mind is altered by health status, genetics, social factors, educational accomplishments, and physical activity.
C. Normally, an individual's personality does not change with age unless there is a __________ problem.

23. Three Types of Memory (Briefly describe each type of memory.)

A. Short-term memory: ______________________________
B. Long-term memory: ______________________________
C. Sensory memory: ______________________________

24. Memory

A. Aging does not necessarily mean a loss of __________ or __________ ability in the elderly.
B. With age, the ability to retrieve information from __________-__________ memory may be slower.
C. Physical exercise increases __________ flow and helps maintain blood supply to the brain, improving memory __________.

25. Learning

A. The ability to learn is not __________ by aging.
B. __________ memory (the ability to retain information while using other information) slows with age.
C. Keeping the brain active with games, puzzles, and other types of stimulation helps maintain __________ __________.

26. Sleep

A. Studies have shown that memories and information are __________ during sleep.
B. __________ physical rest delays the brain's response time.

27. The Four Areas of Memory Loss

i. ______________________________
ii. ______________________________
iii. ______________________________
iv. ______________________________

28. Suggestions for Dealing with Memory Loss

A. Encourage recalling distant memories.
   i. Caregivers can review with patients __________, __________, and __________.
B. Retaining new information
   i. Keep new information __________ and __________ it frequently.
   ii. If the information has more than __________ steps, break these steps down into smaller __________ so that they can be learned individually.
C. Remembering names
   i. Consistently __________-__________ yourself and what your intentions are.
D. Separating fact from fiction
   i. It is important to correct the patient in a __________ manner.

29. Addressing the Effects of Medications on Mental Abilities

A. Provide the patient or caregiver with a __________ organizer and a printed list of the __________ that he or she is taking and why he or she is taking them.
B. Warn the patient about possible food or drug __________ with written and __________ information.
C. When taking a patient history, specifically ask about __________-__________-__________ preparations, vitamins, and __________ supplements because the patient may not view these products as "medications."

30. Confusion in the Elderly

A. "Confusion" is the term used by physicians and health care providers to indicate that the person cannot:
   i. ______________________________
   ii. ______________________________
   iii. ______________________________
   iv. ______________________________
B. Acute confusion is characterized by symptoms that last for less than _____ months.
C. Chronic confusion is characterized by symptoms that persist for longer than _____ months.

31. The Three Categories of Confusion (Briefly explain each category.)

A. Systemic confusion: ______________________________
B. Mechanical confusion: ______________________________
C. Psychosocial/environmental confusion: ______________________________

32. Common Causes of Confusion

A. The most common cause of acute confusion is a __________ __________ __________ (UTI).
B. The confusion will be resolved with no __________ damage as soon as the infection has cleared.

33. Sundowners Syndrome

A. This is a type of confusion that occurs after sundown or at night in patients with __________________ or other forms of __________.
B. Tends to be more common in persons with __________ impairments.
C. Factors that may increase the incidence of Sundowners syndrome
   i. ______________________________
   ii. ______________________________
   iii. ______________________________
   iv. ______________________________
   v. ______________________________

34. Characteristics of Depression

   i. ______________________________
   ii. ______________________________
   iii. ______________________________
   iv. ______________________________

35. Facts About Depression

A. Depression in the elderly may be caused by ____________ ____________ that seem overwhelming.
B. Depression can be worsened by some ____________ interactions.

36. Dementia

A. Dementia is marked by a __________ loss of memory and other __________ functions.
B. Can occur at any __________, but is more frequently found in the elderly.

C. Currently, there are more than ______ different types of dementia.
D. Affects about __________ of people who are over age 65.
E. Onset is usually __________.
F. It is not a normal __________of aging.
G. It is irreversible unless caused by a treatable condition such as an __________ __________ or a thyroid dysfunction.
H. Half of all persons over ______ years of age have no signs of dementia.
I. Approximately half of all dementia patients suffer from __________ __________.

37. Causes of Dementia

i. ______________________________
ii. ______________________________
iii. ______________________________
iv. ______________________________

38. Symptoms of Dementia

A. Dementia gradually worsens at different rates over ______ to ______ years.
B. The first sign is usually __________.
C. The person has difficulty learning new __________.
D. The person may forget what he or she is __________.
E. He or she may forget the correct __________for __________ objects, have difficulty with time __________, and misplace items or put them in an inappropriate place.
F. The person may show a lack of __________, have mood swings, and demonstrate lack of initiative or disinterest in something that he or she previously __________ to do.

39. Alzheimer's Disease

A. Alzheimer's disease is a progressive disorder of the __________ __________ system that eventually destroys mental capacities.
B. Occurs more frequently in the __________.
C. Scientists have pinpointed several __________ abnormalities that are linked to the type of Alzheimer's disease that tends to run in families.
D. While there is a normal loss of some memory as people age, the memory loss associated with Alzheimer's disease is __________.

40. Diagnosing Alzheimer's Disease

A. Diagnoses of dementia and Alzheimer's disease are obtained by __________ other possibilities.
B. After ruling out possible causes, the patient should be given the __________ __________ __________ __________ to evaluate recall, writing, and math skills.
C. A significant portion of the Alzheimer's disease/dementia diagnosis depends on __________ revealed by the patient and family members or caregivers.

41. Symptoms of Alzheimer's Disease

i. ______________________________
ii. ______________________________
iii. ______________________________
iv. ______________________________
v. ______________________________
vi. ______________________________

42. Treatment of Alzheimer's Disease

A. During the early stages, medications, such as ____________, are purported to slow the progression of the disease.
B. Patients should not drink ____________, which can worsen the symptoms of Alzheimer's Disease.
C. Some depressed Alzheimer's patients may benefit from taking ____________ in the early stages.

D. Creating a soothing home environment, avoiding __________, and avoiding constantly correcting __________ all help to reduce the stress on Alzheimer's patients.

43. Caring for the Dementia Patient in the Medical Office

A. Always tell the patient what you are going to __________ and what to __________ next.
B. Speak to the patient __________ and in __________ terms, and be ready to repeat instructions.
C. Make __________ __________ with the patient and use appropriate body language.
D. Provide a warm smile and a __________ __________ on the arm to be encouraging.
E. Use the tactics of __________ and __________ when necessary.
F. Allow the patient to "__________ __________" and maintain his or her __________.
G. Take a __________ stand with the patient when necessary.

44. Steps for Communicating Effectively with the Elderly

A. Welcome the patient warmly and with a __________.
B. Face the patient, and speak __________ and __________ to him or her.
C. Treat the patient with __________.
D. If it appears that the patient does not comprehend, __________ using other words and simple gestures.
E. Allow sufficient time for the patient to __________ the information.
F. __________ the patient to the examination room and provide __________ if needed.

45. Obtaining Informed Consent

A. You may provide the family with information about how to proceed with obtaining it and identify a __________ __________ that is able to assist them.
B. __________ invalidates a power of attorney because a power of attorney implies the competency of the patient.

46. Advanced Medical Directives

A. Provide __________ or __________ formulated by the patient that express his or her desires with regard to terminal care.
B. May state whether or not __________ is desired.
C. Other directives should spell out the wishes of the patient if he or she degrades into a persistent __________ state.
D. These directives may indicate whether he or she wants medicine to be __________, except for pain relief, and whether he or she wants nutrition and __________ withheld.
E. In most states, unless the physician writes a specific order restating what the patient has expressed, a directive is not __________ on the staff and facility.

47. Forms of Elder Abuse

i. ______________________________
ii. ______________________________
iii. ______________________________
iv. ______________________________
v. ______________________________
vi. ______________________________

KEY TERMINOLOGY REVIEW

Match the vocabulary term to the correct definition below.

a. Ageism
b. Assisted-living facilities
c. Cognitive ability
d. Extended-care facilities
e. Geriatrician
f. Geriatrics

g. Gerontology

h. Medicare

i. Medigap insurance

j. Respite care

1. __________ A physician who diagnoses and treats diseases and conditions that mainly affect older patients.
2. __________ Offered by the American Association of Retired Persons (AARP) as a supplement to Medicare.
3. __________ Prejudice against and incorrect assumptions about an individual or individuals because of their age.
4. __________ The ability to think clearly, reason, and perceive is affected by many factors.
5. __________ The study of the process of aging and the effects of aging on people.
6. __________ Short-term care for the chronically ill.
7. __________ Facilities designed for residents who cannot live independently but do not require 24-hour care.
8. __________ The field of medicine that specializes in treating elderly patients.
9. __________ U.S. government insurance program for persons aged 65 and older and others with special conditions.
10. __________ Facilities that provide specialized care for the elderly.

APPLIED PRACTICE

Follow the directions as instructed with each question below.

1. Read the following scenario and answer the questions that follow.

> **Scenario**
>
> Fredrick Alamar, age 73, presents to your office today for a physical and a flu vaccination. Upon obtaining his weight, it is apparent that Mr. Alamar has lost 18 pounds since his last visit 2 months ago, which was shortly after his wife died. You make a note of this in his chart. Prior visits to the office have shown Mr. Alamar to be in fairly good health for his age. He only takes metoprolol succinate for hypertension. As you obtain his blood pressure, Mr. Alamar removes his sweater. You notice scratches and bruising on his lower back. He states "I fell after stepping out of the bathtub. I have been falling down a lot more lately and I don't seem to have any strength." After noting this in his chart, you excuse yourself from the examination room and inform the doctor of Mr. Alamar's changes since his last visit.

a. What are the likely causes of Mr. Alamar's significant weight loss?

____

____

b. What could be the cause of his recent lack of strength?

____

____

c. What things could be done to help Mr. Alamar at home?

____

____

d. The doctor may recommend a form of permanent care for Mr. Alamar. What options may be available for Mr. Alamar?

____

____

LEARNING ACTIVITY: MULTIPLE CHOICE

Circle the correct answers to each of the questions below.

1. Which of the following characteristics do baby boomers have that will affect health care and your role as a provider of health care?
   a. They are considered to be the best-educated generational group.
   b. They will be receiving less family assistance as they age because of fewer children.
   c. They may be caring for an ailing parent and a young child at the same time.
   d. All of the above

2. Which of the following is not an assistive device to aid older individuals?
   a. Handrails and grab bars
   b. Throw rugs
   c. Cane
   d. Bedside commode

3. Life expectancy is increasing due to _______________.
   a. better living conditions
   b. new medications
   c. better nutrition
   d. All of the above

4. Factors that affect how we age include _______________.
   a. genetics
   b. sports cars
   c. occupational hazards
   d. All of the above

5. Musculoskeletal system aging is characterized by _______________.
   a. decrease in muscle strength
   b. inability to see far distances
   c. increased risk of falling
   d. All of the above

6. Which of the following are true statements?
   a. Changes in sensorimotor abilities improve how the elderly interact with their environment.
   b. The loss of hearing, taste, smell, and mobility can lead to depression.
   c. The nervous system begins to speed up.
   d. All of the above

7. Urinary system changes that can occur with aging include _______________.
   a. thyroid hypofunction
   b. reduced ability to concentrate urine

c. faster waste removal by the kidneys
d. orthostatic hypotension

8. According to your textbook, which of the following does not accelerate the aging process?
   a. Disease
   b. Stress
   c. Depression
   d. Lack of social interaction

9. What factors are related to the mental health of aging populations?
   a. Capacity to cope effectively with life changes
   b. Sleep 8–10 hours per night
   c. Achieve a state of emotional balance
   d. All of the above

10. What might you do to find out if an elderly patient is receiving proper nutrition?
   a. Engage elderly patients in a discussion of favorite foods.
   b. Ask which restaurant is their favorite.
   c. Observe their teeth and oral hygiene.
   d. Ask when their last meal was.

CRITICAL THINKING

Answer the following questions to the best of your ability. Utilize the textbook as a reference.

1. Your patient is an 82-year-old woman who is in fairly good health, but she is worried about money. She states that Medicare doesn't pay for enough things, and she wonders if you know of any other resources for her. What can you suggest to this patient regarding medical costs?

____

____

____

____

2. Because your patient, Mr. Bjorklund, has diminished short-term memory, what can you do to ensure that any patient education you deliver will not be ignored because the patient forgot?

____

____

____

____

3. A 68-year-old patient named Mrs. Royer has come in today because she is depressed. She says she used to have lots of friends and family but now she is alone. Make a list of possible reasons that this patient feels so isolated.

____

____

____

____

RESEARCH ACTIVITY

Utilize Internet search engines to research the following topics and write a brief description of what you find. It is important to utilize reputable websites.

1. In addition to what is mentioned in your textbook, research additional "assistive aids" that can help elderly patients with their daily activities. What aids do you think might be the most helpful? Which would you be most likely to recommend to future patients? Why?

CHAPTER 42
Assisting with Minor Surgery

CHAPTER OUTLINE

General review of the chapter:

Ambulatory Surgery
Principles of Surgical Asepsis
Surgical Instruments
Surgical Assisting
Preparing the Patient for Minor Surgery
Postoperative Patient Care
Surgical Procedures Performed in the Medical Office

STUDENT STUDY GUIDE

Use the following guide to assist in your learning of the concepts from the chapter.

I. Surgical Asepsis

1. Ambulatory Surgery
   A. The patient is able to ________ into and out of the surgical facility on the same ________.
   B. Includes outpatient surgery, ___________ surgery, and office surgery.
   C. Hospitalization is not required unless __________ are expected.
2. Categories of Surgery (List and briefly explain each type.)
   i. ______________________________
   ii. ______________________________
   iii. ______________________________
   iv. ______________________________
   v. ______________________________
3. Medical Versus Surgical Asepsis
   A. Medical asepsis is the elimination of ______________ that have left the body.
   B. Surgical asepsis is the practice of creating and _________________ a sterile environment.
4. Principles of Surgical Asepsis
   A. Surgical asepsis is necessary for any ___________ procedure.
   B. Items required for surgical asepsis include sterile scrubs and sterile __________, as well as sterile technique when handling materials.
5. Guidelines for Surgical Asepsis
   i. ______________________________
   ii. ______________________________
   iii. ______________________________
   iv. ______________________________
   v. ______________________________

vi. ____
vii. ____

6. Steps for Surgical Hand Hygiene/Sterile Scrub
   A. Remove ____________ and dirt from behind the nails.
   B. Stand at the sink without allowing your body to ____________ it.
   C. Regulate running water to ____________, not ____________.
   D. Place hands under running water with hands pointed ____________.
   E. Vigorously scrub hands and wrists with a scrub brush for about ____________ minutes per hand.
   F. If performing a second lather, use ____________ minutes per hand.

7. Steps for Surgical Gloving
   i. ____
   ii. ____
   iii. ____
   iv. ____
   v. ____
   vi. ____
   vii. ____
   viii. ____
   ix. ____

8. Steps for Removing Gloves
   i. ____
   ii. ____
   iii. ____
   iv. ____

9. Sterile Packaging
   A. Packs are set up on a ____________ stand.
   B. The inside of the packet's wrapper is the ____________ field.

10. Steps for Opening a Sterile Pack
   i. ____
   ii. ____
   iii. ____
   iv. ____
   v. ____
   vi. ____
   vii. ____
   viii. ____
   ix. ____
   x. ____
   xi. ____
   xii. ____

11. Steps for Dropping a Sterile Packet onto a Sterile Field
   A. Assemble the equipment; check the ____________ date and the condition of the sealed packet.
   B. Locate the edge on the prepackaged item, and pull it apart by using the ____________ and ____________ of each hand.
   C. Do not let your fingers touch the ____________ of the packet.
   D. Pull the packet apart by securely placing the remaining ____________ fingers of each hand against the outside of the packet, one on each side.
   E. Holding the item securely about ______ to ______ inches away from the sterile field, gently drop the packet contents inside the sterile field.

12. Sterile Transfer
    A. Used to move items around the _______ field or to place instruments onto a ______ field.
    B. Must put on _______ gloves or use _______ forceps.

II. Sterile Instruments

1. Instruments Used in Minor Surgery
    i. ______________________________
    ii. ______________________________
    iii. ______________________________
    iv. ______________________________
    v. ______________________________

2. Cutting Instruments
    A. _________ or _________ are the terms used to name the instrument used to make an incision.
    B. The scalpel _________ must be inserted into the scalpel handle.
    C. Blades come in various sizes; the choice of blade depends on the type of __________ and _________.

3. Scissors
    A. The two primary uses of scissors are for ___________ and to cut _________.
    B. The ______ of the scissors vary; the choice of scissors depends on how they are to be used.

4. Types of Scissors (List each type of scissors and their use.)
    i. ______________________________
    ii. ______________________________
    iii. ______________________________
    iv. ______________________________

5. Forceps
    A. Forceps are used to grasp ________ or objects.
    B. Two-pronged forceps are used to clamp together tightly to prevent ___________.
    C. A ratchet clasp allows the forceps to close with different degrees of _________.

6. Types of Forceps (List the different types of forceps and briefly describe their use.)
    i. ______________________________
    ii. ______________________________
    iii. ______________________________
    iv. ______________________________
    v. ______________________________
    vi. ______________________________
    vii. ______________________________

7. The Speculum, Scope, Probe, Trocar, and Punch
    A. A speculum is an unlighted instrument inserted into a body ____________.
    B. An __________ is placed inside the scope to ____________ it into a canal, and then it is removed during visualization of the ____________ site.
    C. The probe is used to explore ________ and cavities; it usually has a curved, _______ point to facilitate insertion.
    D. A trocar is used to ________ fluids from cavities.
    E. The two parts of a trocar are a _________ and a ________.
    F. A punch is used to ____________ tissue for __________ or microscopic examination of the tissue in order to detect cancerous cells.

8. Disciplines That Use Specialized Instruments
   i. ______________________________
   ii. ______________________________
   iii. ______________________________
9. Absorbable Sutures
   A. Absorbable sutures are digested by tissue __________ and are absorbed by the body.
   B. Absorption usually occurs ______ to ______ days after insertion.
10. Types of Absorbable Sutures (List and briefly explain each type.)
   i. ______________________________
   ii. ______________________________
   iii. ______________________________
11. Nonabsorbable Sutures (List and briefly describe the characteristics of each type.)
   i. ______________________________
   ii. ______________________________
   iii. ______________________________
   iv. ______________________________
   v. ______________________________
   vi. ______________________________
12. The Size of Suture Material
   A. Measured by the __________ or __________.
   B. Stated in terms of __________.
   C. __________ in size with the number of zeros.
13. Suture Needles
   A. Available in various shapes, depending on where they are ______.
   B. Have either a __________ cutting point used for tissues that provide some resistance or a __________ noncutting point used for more __________ tissue.
14. The Straight Needle
   A. Used when the needle is pushed and pulled through the tissue without the use of a needle __________.
   B. Has an ______ that is threaded with the suture material.
15. The Curved Needle
   A. Allows the surgeon to go in and out of __________ where there is not enough room to maneuver a __________ needle.
   B. Requires a needle __________.
16. The Swaged Needle
   A. A swaged needle and suture materials are combined in ______ length.
   B. Because the suture material is attached to the needle, the material will not __________ off.
17. Steri-Strips™
   A. Steri-Strips are non__________ and are available in a variety of widths.
   B. Used instead of __________ when not much __________ is to be applied to a wound, such as on a small facial cut.
18. Staples
   A. Made of __________.
   B. Applied with a surgical __________.

19. Skin Adhesives
    A. Composed of ____________ adhesives that react with ____________ to create an instant, strong, flexible bond.
    B. Used to close ____________ or small surgical incisions.
20. Guidelines for Handling Instruments (List specific guidelines for instrument care.)
    i. ____________
    ii. ____________
    iii. ____________
    iv. ____________
    v. ____________
    vi. ____________

III. Preparing the Patient for Surgery

1. The Role of the Nonsterile Assistant
    A. ____________ the patient.
    B. Holds the vial of local __________ while the surgeon draws up the correct dosage into a syringe; __________ dressings.
2. Factors the That Make a Medical Assistant Valuable
    i. ____________
    ii. ____________
    iii. ____________
    iv. ____________
3. The Responsibilities of the Scrub Assistant
    A. Arranges the surgical __________ to meet the operating physician's preferences.
    B. __________ bodily fluids away from the operative site.
    C. __________ the incision area.
    D. __________ suture materials.
4. Guidelines for Sterile Techniques
    A. Immediately ________ if sterility is broken.
    B. __________ all instruments before passing them.
    C. Protect the surgeon from injury by __________ needles away from the surgeon.
    D. __________ the surgeon's needs by __________ the types of instruments used in a procedure.
    E. Place the __________ of the instrument into the surgeon's hand with a firm __________.
    F. When required to cut a suture, cut both ends at the same time, ______ to ______ inches above the knot.
5. Steps for Transferring Sterile Fluid into a Sterile Basin
    A. Check the ____________ on the solution and the sterile basin pack.
    B. Set up the sterile basin on the Mayo tray using the inside of the wrapper to create a ________.
    C. Remove the cap of the solution and place it on a clean surface with the outer edge ________ (inside facing up).
    D. Check the ________ on the solution bottle before pouring the solution.
    E. Pour a small amount of the liquid into a __________ ____________ for discarding.
    F. Pour from the bottle with the label held against the ______________ to protect the label from ____________.
    G. Hold the bottle about ____________ inches above the basin and pour slowly.
6. Steps for Assisting with Minor Surgery
    A. Open a set of ____________ gloves for the physician.
    B. Cleanse the vial of anesthetic with a ___________ alcohol swab and hold it ____________ in the palm of your hand with the label facing toward the ____________.

C. Collect and place all soiled instruments in a __________ out of the patient's view.
D. Place all soiled gauze sponges and dressings in a ________________.
E. Do not allow _________ items to remain on a sterile field.
F. Immediately _________ all specimens as they are obtained.
G. Periodically, check the patient's ____________ during the procedure.
H. Provide clear _________ and _________ postoperative instructions for the patient.
I. Send the ____________ to the laboratory with a _________________.

7. Steps for Disposing of Soiled Dressings

i. ____
ii. ____
iii. ____
iv. ____
v. ____
vi. ____

8. The Role of the Floating Assistant

i. ____
ii. ____
iii. ____
iv. ____
v. ____
vi. ____
vii. ____
viii. ____
ix. ____
x. ____
xi. ____
xii. ____

9. Proper Floating Technique During Surgery

A. Immediately report any _________ observations about the patient to the operating __________.
B. Use care not to touch the __________ while assisting.
C. Provide additional medications, such as local ________, that are needed during the procedure.

10. Guidelines for Providing Medication During a Procedure

A. Follow the correct procedure for ______________ the medication.
B. Clean the top of the vial/bottle with ___________.
C. Hold the vial/bottle upside down so that the physician can insert a sterile needle into the vial without touching the contaminated ___________ surface.
D. Do not hold the vial in front of your ___________.

11. Surgical Setup for a Typical Minor Surgical Procedure

i. ____
ii. ____
iii. ____
iv. ____
v. ____
vi. ____
vii. ____
viii. ____
ix. ____
x. ____
xi. ____

xii. ____________________
xiii. ____________________
xiv. ____________________

12. Methods for Preoperative and Postoperative Instructions
    i. ____________________
    ii. ____________________
    iii. ____________________
    iv. ____________________
    v. ____________________

13. Informed Consent
    A. Any invasive procedure with a scalpel, scissors, or other device requires __________ permission.
    B. Every attempt must be made to determine whether the patient actually __________ the explanation given.
    C. A medical assistant __________ witness the patient's signing of the consent form.

14. Anesthesia
    A. Anesthesia is the medication that causes the __________ or __________ loss of sensation.
    B. Used to block the __________ of surgery.
    C. Can relax __________, produce __________, calm __________, and cause sleep.

15. General Anesthesia
    A. Depresses the ____________________ to cause unconsciousness.
    B. Usually administered by __________ or ____________________.
    C. Sedatives and narcotics are usually administered ______________ before surgery.

16. Local Anesthesia
    A. Provides a loss of __________ in a particular area of the body without an overall loss of __________.
    B. Also referred to as a __________ anesthetic.
    C. Takes about ________ to ________ minutes to become effective and lasts from _____ to _____ hours.

17. Local Infiltration Anesthetic
    A. Injected directly into the ______ that will be operated on.
    B. Used for such procedures as removal of skin _________, skin suturing, and dental _________.

18. Epinephrine
    A. Epinephrine is a vasoconstrictor that causes the __________ blood vessels to _________.
    B. Often added to the local anesthetic when the physician is operating on the ______ and ______.

19. Nerve Blocks
    A. Administered by __________ into a nerve adjacent to the operative site.
    B. Used for surgery on __________, __________, and toes.

20. Topical Anesthetics
    A. Local pain control medications that are applied to the ______________ to produce a ______________ effect.
    B. Can be applied by drop, ____________, or swab.
    C. Commonly used in ____________ procedures.

21. Instructions for a Dry Shave
    A. To remove hair, __________ shavers are preferred to razor blades because they lessen the likelihood of accidental nicks in the skin.

B. Hair should be manually clipped as short as possible with _________.
C. The medical assistant should apply firm __________ to the skin with his or her ____________ hand.
D. Hair should be removed in the __________ of hair growth.

22. Instructions for a Wet Shave (List the steps for performing a wet shave.)
    i. ____
    ii. ____
    iii. ____
    iv. ____
    v. ____
    vi. ____
    vii. ____
    viii. ____

KEY TERMINOLOGY REVIEW

Match the vocabulary term to the correct definition below.

a. Ambulatory surgery
b. anesthesia
c. Biopsy
d. Cryosurgery
e. Debridement
f. Dehiscence
g. Eschar
h. Evisceration
i. Hyfrecator
j. Incisions
k. Invasive procedure
l. Mayo stand
m. Outpatient surgery
n. Scrub assistant
o. Sterile field
p. Surgical scrub

1. ______________ A scab.
2. ______________ Removal of dead tissue around wound edges using sterile technique.
3. ______________ Hand instruments to the surgeon.
4. ______________ Microscopic examination of tissue to detect cancerous cells.
5. ______________ A procedure in which the body is entered.
6. ______________ Separation of wound edges and protrusion of abdominal organs.
7. ______________ The process of removing microorganisms.
8. ______________ Surgery performed on a person who is admitted and discharged from a surgical facility on the same day.
9. ______________ A small portable table with enough room to hold an instrument tray.
10. ______________ The use of subfreezing temperatures to destroy tissue.
11. ______________ A specific area free of all microorganisms that will be the work area for a surgical procedure.
12. ______________ A miniature electrocautery unit.
13. ______________ Generally limited to procedures requiring less than 60 minutes to perform.
14. ______________ Medication that causes the partial or complete loss of sensation.
15. ______________ Separation of wound edges.

APPLIED PRACTICE

1. Identify each of the gynecological instruments as seen in the picture below.

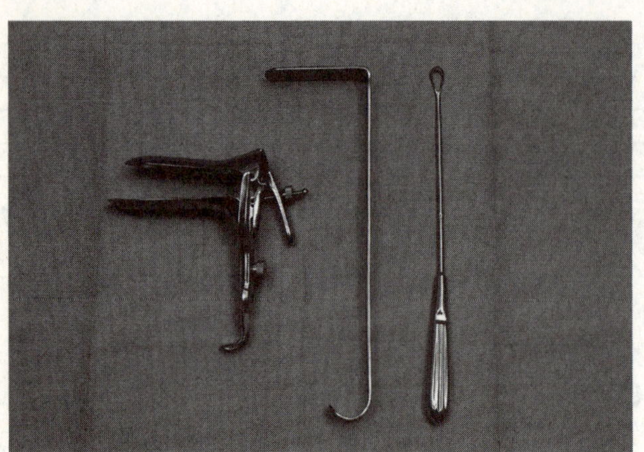

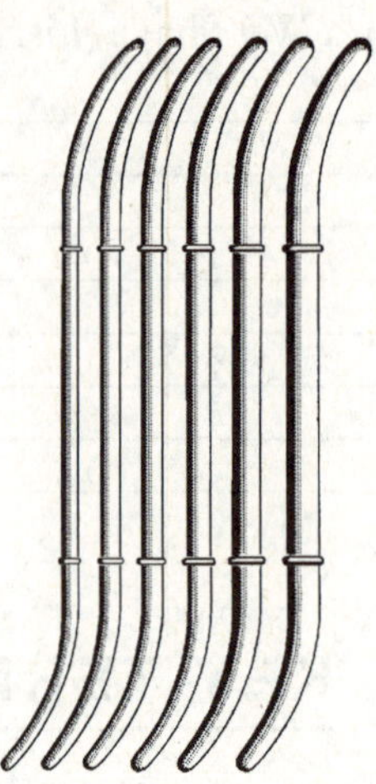

______ ______ ______ ______ ______

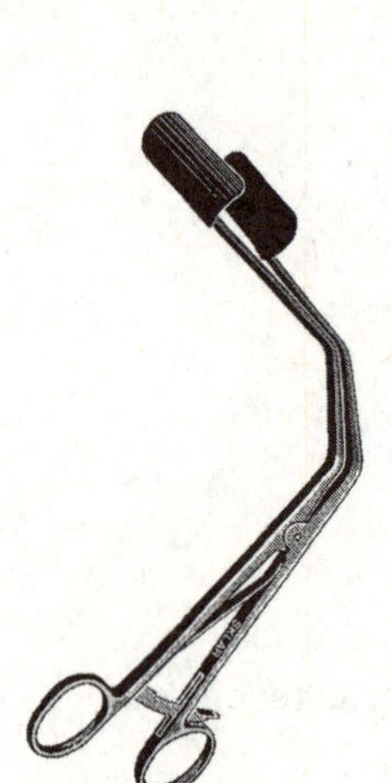

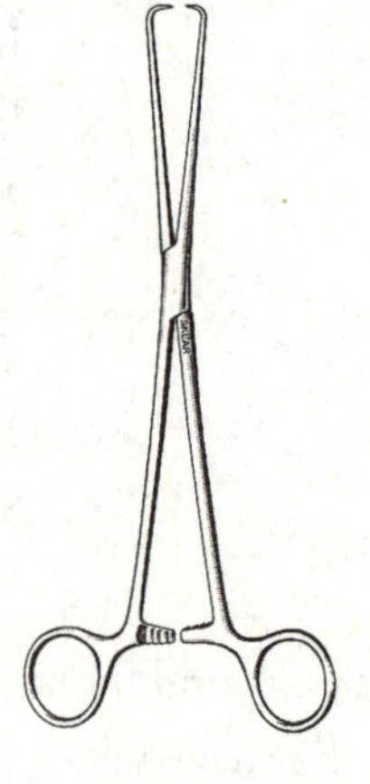

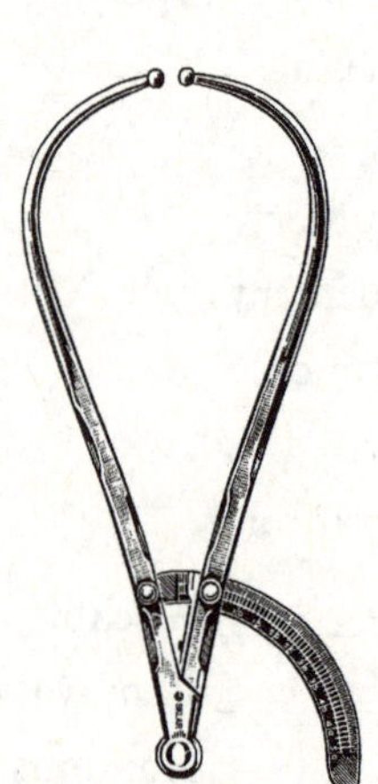

______ ______ ______

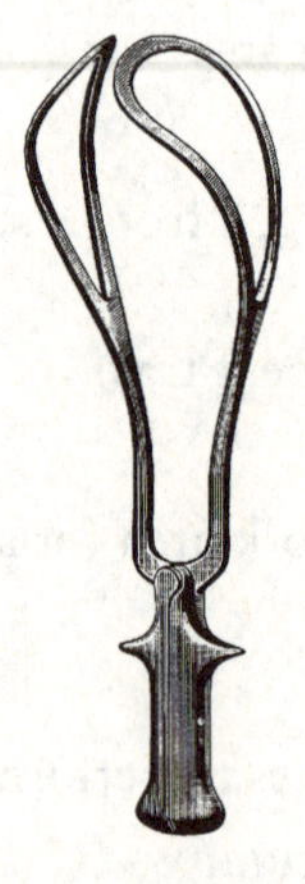

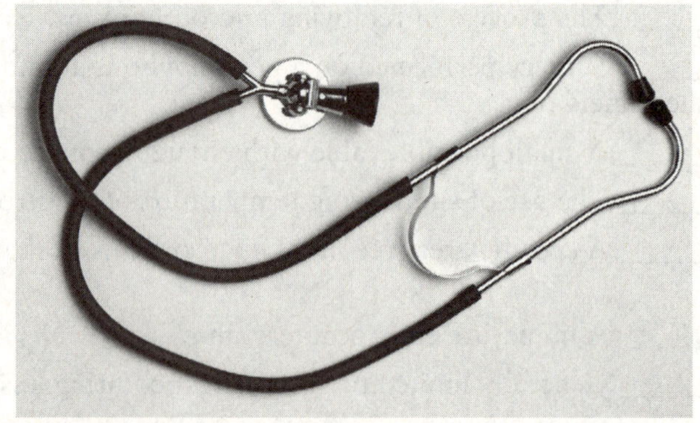

______ ______

2. Using the information from the following patient chart, correctly identify the instruments that you would prepare for an I&D (incision and drainage).

> Horsley, Will
> 10-26-1963
>
> 04/02/20XX_, 12:45 P.M.
> Wt: 175 lbs., T: 98.6°F, P: 104, BP: 118/78
> cc: Pt presents to office complaining of a cut that appears to be inflamed. Upon examination, the area sounding the cut is red and painful. The physician has requested that the patient be prepped for an I&D. I&D is successfully performed and the patient is discharged on antibiotics.
>
> Adam Bello, RMA

LEARNING ACTIVITY: MULTIPLE CHOICE

1. Which of the following types of drainage exhibit clear, watery drainage, such as the fluid in a blister?
   a. Serous drainage
   b. Sanguineous drainage
   c. Serosanguineous drainage
   d. Purulent drainage

2. Which of the following is an absorbable type of suture?
   a. Plain catgut
   b. Surgical catgut
   c. Chromic catgut
   d. All of the above

3. A wound that has torn edges in an irregular shape would be called a ____________________.
   a. puncture
   b. laceration
   c. abrasion
   d. incision

4. Which of the following forceps are used to grasp foreign bodies?
   a. Tissue
   b. Thumb
   c. Splinter
   d. Needle

5. The general classification of instruments is based on which of the following?
   a. Cutting
   b. Dissecting
   c. Grasping
   d. All the above

6. The three basic steps of skin preparation include all of the following except ________________.
   a. apply antiseptic solution to the surgical area
   b. scrub with an antiseptic soap and rinse
   c. air dry the skin prior to cleansing
   d. shave as necessary

7. Which of the following is not a sign of inflammation?
   a. Swelling
   b. Warmth
   c. Decreased drainage
   d. Pain

8. Sutures on the face are usually removed in ________________.
   a. 24–48 hours
   b. 3–5 days
   c. 5–7 days
   d. 7–10 days

9. Which of the following electrosurgery destroys tissue by creating a spark gap when the probe is inserted into unwanted tissue.
   a. Electrocoagulation
   b. Electrodessication
   c. Electrofulguration
   d. All of the above

10. Colposcopy is performed in which of the following cases?
    a. When an abnormal tissue development is observed by the physician during a routine pelvic examination
    b. When a Papanicolaou (Pap) smear result is in the abnormal range
    c. For magnified visualization
    d. All of the above

CRITICAL THINKING

Answer the following questions to the best of your ability. Utilize the textbook as a reference.

1. Patient instructions should be given both orally and in writing. Many errors can be made by the patient if instructions are not clear. Come up with a scenario of something harmful that could happen if a patient did not have any written instructions and did not remember the oral instructions provided by the physician or medical assistant.

   ____

   ____

   ____

   ____

2. During a sterile cyst removal procedure, the physician reaches up to scratch her head briefly. She is wearing a surgical cap and no visible bodily fluids are on her gloves. Take some time and think through this scenario. Has the sterile procedure been compromised? If so, indicate your thoughts in a paragraph.

   ____

   ____

   ____

   ____

RESEARCH ACTIVITY

Utilizing your textbook and Internet search engines research the following topics and write a brief description of what you find. It is important to utilize reputable websites.

1. Research one surgical procedure discussed in your textbook. Why is the procedure preformed? How is the procedure preformed? What instruments would be required to perform this procedure?

CHAPTER 43
Assisting with Medical Emergencies and Emergency Preparedness

CHAPTER OUTLINE

General review of the chapter:

Emergency Resources
Guidelines for Providing Emergency Care
Office Emergency Crash Kit
Medical Emergencies
Emergency Preparedness

STUDENT STUDY GUIDE

Use the following guide to assist in your learning of the concepts from the chapter.

I. Responding to a Medical Office Emergency

1. The Emergency Medical Services (EMS) System
   A. Established to provide ____________ care.
   B. Provides safe and prompt ____________ to an emergency facility.
2. Good Samaritan Laws
   A. These state laws protect a health care professional from ____________ while giving emergency care to an accident victim.
   B. The laws are in place to encourage ____________ to offer aid in emergency situations without fear of being prosecuted for ____________ injury or death.
3. The Chain of Survival
   i. ____
   ii. ____
   iii. ____
   iv. ____
4. The Medical Assistant's Emergency Response Primary Assessment
   A. Determine the patient's name, __________ __________, and gender.
   B. Determine whether the patient is ill or __________.
   C. Determine the patient's need for ____________________.
   D. Obtain a history of the __________.
   E. Gather the patient's __________ information.
   F. Determine the patient's __________.
   G. Do a __________ examination.
   H. Take the patient's __________ __________.

5. Items in an Emergency Crash Kit
   i. ______________________________
   ii. ______________________________
   iii. ______________________________
   iv. ______________________________
   v. ______________________________
   vi. ______________________________
   vii. ______________________________
   viii. ______________________________
   ix. ______________________________
6. The Medical Assistant and the Crash Kit
   A. The MA should do ________ checks of emergency supplies in the crash kit.
   B. Tasks involved in checking the crash kit include the following
      i. ______________________________
      ii. ______________________________
      iii. ______________________________
      iv. ______________________________

II. Medical Emergencies

1. General Guidelines for Emergency Care
   A. Access for the adult patient is initiated by calling 911 as soon as it has been determined that the patient is __________ and __________.
   B. In general, __________ __________ for an unresponsive adult.
   C. With children and infants, EMS access is made after __________ minutes of CPR.
2. The Heimlich Maneuver
   A. Stand __________ the patient with your feet slightly apart, placing __________ __________between the patient's feet and __________ to the outside.
   B. Place the ________ finger of one hand at the person's __________or belt buckle.
   C. Make a __________ with your other hand and place it, __________ side to the patient, above your other hand.
   D. Place your marking hand over your __________ fist and begin to give quick ______ and ________ thrusts.
   E. Continue to give thrusts until the object has been expelled or the patient becomes __________.
   F. Before administering the __________ breaths, open the airway with the __________-__________ chin lift and look for a foreign body in the patient's mouth and remove it if one is visible.
   G. __________ finger sweeps are no longer recommended and should not be performed.
   H. Continue with cycles of __________ compressions and __________ breaths until the foreign body is expelled or advanced medical personal arrive to relieve you.
3. Steps for Adult Rescue Breathing and One-Rescuer CPR
   A. __________ the patient and determine whether help is needed.
   B. Shout, "__________ __________ __________?" while gently shaking the patient's shoulders.
   C. If the adult patient is determined to be __________, activate EMS immediately by calling 911 and get an __________ if one is available.
4. Assessing the ABCs
   A. Airway: Perform a head-__________ chin __________, or, if a neck injury is suspected, a jaw __________.
   B. Look and feel for __________and __________movements.

C. If you are alone, begin the rescue sequence for ___ ________ and then attempt to call 911 yourself.
D. If you have a __________ mask, place it on the patient.

5. Performing Breaths
A. If breathing is absent, put on a __________ __________ and administer ______ ________ breaths.
B. If your breaths do not cause the chest to __________, look in the patient's mouth and remove the object if one is seen.
C. If no object is seen, make a second attempt to administer a _________ breath.
D. If the breaths cause the chest to __________, assess the patient's __________ by feeling for a pulse at the __________ __________.

6. Feeling a Pulse
A. If you feel a pulse, begin ______ _______.
B. Administer one breath every _____ seconds, or __________ every minute.
C. After _____ minute, reassess the patient for __________ and __________.

7. Performing Chest Compressions
A. If you do not feel a pulse, begin __________ __________.
B. Kneel at the patient's side and place your hand in the center of the __________ between the __________.
C. Place your other hand on __________ of the first hand, making sure to lift your __________ off the chest, using only the heels of your hands to administer compressions.
D. Keep your shoulders directly over your __________.
E. Compress the chest _____ to _____ inches; then allow the sternum to relax.
F. Do not lift your hands off the __________.
G. Continue to compress the chest a total of _______ times; then administer ______ breaths.
H. Repeat this sequence for __________ total cycles. Reassess the patient and continue CPR if necessary.

8. Steps for Infant or Young Child Rescue Breathing and One-Rescuer CPR
A. If the infant is determined to be __________, perform CPR for _____ minutes prior to activating _______ by calling 911; get an ________ if one is available.
B. Gently, with _____ fingers, tilt the patient's __________ and open the __________.
C. If breathing is absent, secure a __________ __________ over the patient's mouth and nose.

9. Administering Chest Compressions on a Child
A. Place __________ __________ in the center of the chest just below the nipple line.
B. Compressions should be made _______ to ______ the depth of the chest. Perform 30 quick compressions.
C. Give two more rescue breaths followed by ________ more compressions. Continue the __________ compressions and breaths.
D. After 2 minutes, leave the __________ and call 911 if you are still alone.
E. Continue compressions and breaths until the infant __________ or __________ arrives.

10. Automated External Defibrillation (AED)
A. Highly effective when used immediately after or within minutes of an adult __________ __________.
B. AED is not used on __________.

11. Symptoms of Respiratory Distress
i. ____
ii. ____
iii. ____
iv. ____

v. ____
vi. ____
vii. ____
viii. ____

12. Steps for Administering Oxygen
    A. Check the __________ __________ on the oxygen tank to make sure that it has enough oxygen in it.
    B. Start the flow of oxygen by opening the __________.
    C. Attach the __________ tubing to the flow meter.
    D. Adjust the oxygen __________ according to the physician's order.
    E. Hold the cannula tips over the _________ of your __________, without touching the skin, to determine whether oxygen is flowing.
    F. Place the tips of the __________ __________ into the patient's nostrils.
    G. Wrap the tubing behind the patient's __________.
    H. Instruct the patient to breathe normally through the __________and __________.
    I. Check the patient's oxygen level with an __________.
    J. Place the probe over the __________ finger and record the reading.
    K. If necessary, have the patient take a short __________ to verify that the oxygen flow rate is sufficient for activity.

13. Symptoms of Hyperventilation
    i. ____
    ii. ____
    iii. ____
    iv. ____
    v. ____
    vi. ____

14. Treatment for Hyperventilation
    A. Inform the physician and encourage the patient to __________ __________.
    B. Have the patient breathe into an __________ __________ (not connected to any oxygen), block one nostril, or breathe into a __________ __________.

15. Chest Pain
    A. The primary complaint will be pain in the ____________ or ______________ side of the chest, described as ______________, ______________, ______________, ____________, or aching.
    B. The pain may radiate to the __________ arm, to the __________, or up the neck.
    C. Sometimes the pain is brought on by ____________.

16. Care of Chest Pain
    A. Have the individual stop what he or she is doing and __________, feet __________ if possible.
    B. Ask a coworker to stay with the patient while you inform the __________ of the situation.
    C. Sometimes the pain is brought on by ____________.
    D. If oxygen is available, administer it according to office protocol by __________ cannula at _______ to ______ liters per minute until the physician or emergency personnel arrive.
    E. If the patient has previously been diagnosed with angia and has nitroglycerin tablets, insert __________ tablet under the ____________.
    F. Tablets may be administered every ______ minutes up to ________ doses.
    G. If the __________ is not relieved, inform the ___________ or EMS on the scene.

17. Shock
    A. Shock is the collapse of the __________ system caused by insufficient cardiac output.
    B. __________, shock can progress very rapidly to death.

18. Causes of Shock
   i. ___
   ii. ___
   iii. ___
   iv. ___
   v. ___
   vi. ___
   vii. ___
   viii. ___

19. General Signs of Shock
   i. ___
   ii. ___
   iii. ___
   iv. ___
   v. ___
   vi. ___
   vii. ___
   viii. ___
   ix. ___
   x. ___
   xi. ___
   xii. ___
   xiii. ___
   xiv. ___

20. Anaphylactic Shock
   A. Anaphylactic shock is a severe ___ ___ to a foreign substance, such as medications, bug bites, and latex gloves.
   B. Inform the physician immediately and call ___.
   C. The physician may order ___ and/or an ___.
   D. ___ is the most important factor in anaphylactic shock.

21. Signs of Insulin Shock or Diabetic Coma
   i. ___
   ii. ___
   iii. ___
   iv. ___
   v. ___
   vi. ___
   vii. ___
   viii. ___

22. Arterial Bleeding
   A. Arterial bleeding is usually copious, rapid, and ___ ___.
   B. Blood often spurts, echoing the ___
   C. Must be brought ___ ___ as soon as possible.
   D. Pressure applied directly over the ___ ___ may halt the flow of blood.
   E. If not successful, ___ ___ on the pressure points may be necessary.
   F. Elevating the injured part higher than the ___ may also slow the blood flow.

23. Bleeding from Veins and Capillaries
   A. Venous blood can usually be controlled with ___.
   B. Blood from the capillaries ___ rather than flows and can be halted with direct pressure.

24. Pressure Points

   A. Use pressure points if external bleeding cannot be stopped by __________ __________.
   B. Most often you will use the __________ and __________ pressure points.

25. Abrasions

   A. Occurs when the __________ __________ of skin is scraped away, leaving the underlying tissue exposed.
   B. Common terms for abrasions
      i. ____________________
      ii. ____________________
      iii. ____________________
      iv. ____________________

26. Avulsions

   A. An avulsion is a __________ __________ of skin or tissue.
   B. Usually occurs on __________ and __________.
   C. Cleanse minor avulsion wounds with __________ and __________ and return any skin flap to its normal position.
   D. Apply direct pressure, and then apply a dressing after __________ is controlled.

27. Amputation

   A. If body part has been __________, cleanse the __________ __________ with sterile saline.
   B. Wrap it with moist, sterile gauze. Seal it in a __________ __________; place the __________ __________ in a container on ice.
   C. Prompt medical attention and preservation of the __________ __________ enhance the chances for successful reattachment.

28. Lacerations

   A. A laceration is an __________ __________ in which the skin and underlying tissue are torn.
   B. Usually has __________ edges that may interfere with the healing process.
   C. If bleeding is __________, a physician should direct the cleansing process.
   D. Lacerations over a joint may require joint __________ for a few days while healing progresses.

29. Incisions

   A. An incision is a cut with smooth edges that is made with a knife or other __________ object.
   B. It is treated in the same manner as any __________.
   C. If there is damage to underlying __________, such as a tendon or ligament, surgical intervention is required.

30. Puncture Wounds

   A. A puncture wound is the result of a pointed __________ __________ penetrating the skin and tissue.
   B. Often the wound edges close, trapping __________ and __________ in the tissue.
   C. Depending on the nature of the pointed object, cleansing may consist of simply soaking the area, or may require invasive __________.
   D. After cleansing, a __________ is applied.

31. Impaled Objects

   A. The general rule is to leave the __________ in place until it can be safely removed by trained personnel.
   B. Control __________ and __________ the impaled object with a bulky dressing held in place with tape or bandages.
   C. __________ the area to prevent movement.

32. Soft Tissue Injuries

   A. Involves both the skin and __________ tissue.
   B. Avulsions, amputations, and __________ insults are considered soft-tissue injuries because tissue, as well as skin, is involved.
   C. Damage to the underlying tissue may involve __________ __________, __________, muscles, and __________ tissue.

33. Crush Injuries

   A. Result when force is applied to the __________.
   B. Depending on the area involved, the crush may be similar to the __________ of tissue or it may be so severe as to involve __________ and __________.
   C. Elevating the body part above the __________ and applying __________ are often the only intervention needed.
   D. With a more severe injury, the body part should be __________.
   E. Monitoring vital signs and observing __________ __________, __________, and __________ are essential to deciding whether more extensive intervention is needed.

34. Open Wounds (Define each type.)

   A. Superficial: ____
   B. Deep: ____

35. Open Wound Care

   A. Apply __________ __________ to the wound.
   B. If necessary, use a __________ dressing.
   C. Cleanse the wound from the __________ __________, beginning with vigorous irrigation using a disinfecting solution prescribed by the physician.
   D. Wipe the edges of the wound with sterile gauze in all directions, __________ from the wound.
   E. Cover with a __________ dressing and fasten the dressing in place.
   F. Make sure that you do not apply the bandage __________ __________, because it can restrict the blood flow out of the extremity, which may increase the bleeding instead of stopping it.

36. Applying a Triangular Bandage

   A. Keep the injured arm as __________ as possible.
   B. Carefully slide the triangular bandage under the __________ to be held.
   C. The two shorter sides should be pointing toward the __________, and the remaining longer edge should be parallel to the __________ __________ __________.
   D. Bring the __________ side up and over the arm.
   E. Tie the ends of the bandage behind and slightly to the __________ of the neck.
   F. Tuck the peak of the bandage in toward the __________ __________ of the bandage.

37. Applying a Figure 8 Bandage

   A. Place the __________ of one hand on one end of the bandage
   B. Anchor the bandage with your __________ __________, then complete one __________ around the extremity or body part.
   C. Continue to alternate wrapping above and below the __________ __________ or dressing, circling behind the __________ or dressing area until the injured area is covered adequately.
   D. If applying a bandage to a __________, ensure that the __________ are exposed to evaluate circulation.

38. Applying a Tubular Bandage (List the steps for applying this type of bandage.)

   i. ____
   ii. ____
   iii. ____

iv. ____________________
v. ____________________
vi. ____________________
vii. ____________________
viii. ____________________
ix. ____________________
x. ____________________

39. Epistaxis (Nosebleeds)
    A. Epistaxis is usually __________-__________ threatening.
    B. Tends to occur more commonly in __________ weather or under dusty conditions.

40. Caring for a Patient with a Nosebleed
    A. The physician will twist a __________ __________ and pack the patient's nose.
    B. A __________ __________ pack should be held against the bridge of the patient's nose.
    C. A patient may need an __________ procedure if the bleeding does not stop.

41. When to Worry About Persistent Nosebleeds
    i. ____________________
    ii. ____________________
    iii. ____________________
    iv. ____________________

42. Classification of Burns (Briefly explain each type.)
    A. First degree burns: ____________________
    B. Second degree burns: ____________________
    C. Third degree burns: ____________________

43. Caring for a Patient with First Degree Burns
    A. __________ water.
    B. Use __________ and __________, if ordered by the physician.

44. Caring for a Patient with Second Degree Burns
    A. Cool the burn with water as long as there are no __________ __________.
    B. __________ __________ use analgesic creams and ointments.
    C. Cover with a __________ __________ __________.
    D. Treat for __________, if necessary.

45. Caring for a Patient with Third Degree Burns
    A. Transport the patient to a __________ __________.
    B. Cover burns with __________, __________ __________.
    C. __________ the dead skin or damaged tissue (should be done only by a physician).
    D. Manage the pain with __________ as ordered by a physician.
    E. Separate the __________ or __________ with dry, sterile gauze on hand or foot burns.
    F. Do not remove __________ from the burned area.

46. Caring for a Patient with Upper Airway Burns
    A. Prompt __________ by the physician or EMS.
    B. Transport to a __________ center.
    C. Listen for __________ (noisy breathing).
    D. Administer __________ as ordered by the physician.

47. Caring for a Patient with Large Surface Area Burns
    i. ____________________
    ii. ____________________
    iii. ____________________

48. Hyperthermia: Heat Exhaustion

A. Extreme ______________ due to heat.
B. Occurs as the result of __________ and __________ depletion from the body.
C. Strenuous ____________ often preceded heat exhaustion.

49. Hyperthermia: Heat Stroke

A. Advanced heat exhaustion; body temperature __________
B. Many patients will not __________.
C. No __________ takes place, so the body stores heat in increasing amounts.
D. Eventually, the __________ cells begin to die and permanent damage or death may result.

50. Signs and Symptoms of Heat Exhaustion

i. ______________________________
ii. ______________________________
iii. ______________________________
iv. ______________________________
v. ______________________________
vi. ______________________________
vii. ______________________________
viii. ______________________________

51. Treating Heat Exhaustion

A. Move to a __________ environment.
B. Encourage patient to ____________.
C. Apply __________, ____________ compresses and give sips of water.

52. Signs and Symptoms of Heat Stroke

i. ______________________________
ii. ______________________________
iii. ______________________________
iv. ______________________________
v. ______________________________
vi. ______________________________
vii. ______________________________
viii. ______________________________
ix. ______________________________
x. ______________________________
xi. ______________________________
xii. ______________________________
xiii. ______________________________

53. Treating Heat Stroke

A. Remove the patient from __________ of heat.
B. __________ the victim's clothing.
C. __________ the body as quickly as possible by pouring ___________ water over the patient.
D. Contact __________ if physician is not available.

54. Hypothermia

A. Hypothermia is an __________ drop in body temperature.
B. Results from prolonged exposure to ___________ or ____________ water.

55. Signs and Symptoms of Hypothermia

i. ______________________________
ii. ______________________________
iii. ______________________________

iv. ______________________________
v. ______________________________

56. Treating Hypothermia
  A. Remove __________ and __________ clothes.
  B. Wrap the patient in __________ blankets.
  C. __________ packs may be used, but not directly on the __________.
  D. Sips of __________ liquid.
  E. __________ to treatment facility for assessment by a physician.

57. Convulsions (Seizures)
  A. Produced by __________ __________ activity in the brain.
  B. Characterized by __________ __________ __________ that alternate between the contraction and relaxation of muscles.

58. Caring for a Patient with Convulsions (Seizures)
  A. __________ spasms of the full body can restrict breathing.
  B. Patient may bite his or her __________, causing bleeding and swelling, which may obstruct the airway.
  C. Prevent __________.
  D. Pay close attention to what the patient is __________ so that you can __________ it later.

59. Fainting (Syncope)
  A. Fainting is a __________ loss of consciousness.
  B. Patient usually __________ and becomes __________, but should awaken and return to normal functioning within a minute.
  C. Patients seldom become __________ or have __________ as a result of simple fainting, but may be injured in the course of a fall.

60. Caring for a Patient Who Has Fainted
  A. If the patient fainted and there is no response, provide __________ if the physician orders this.
  B. Check the __________ and call for help.
  C. If the patient is breathing well but will not wake up, place him or her on the __________ side and notify the physician.
  D. If the physician is unavailable, contact __________.
  E. Obtain a full set of __________ and obtain a __________ reading if possible.

61. Fractures (Briefly explain both types.)
  A. Closed (simple): ______________________________
  B. Open (compound): ______________________________

62. Splinting Injuries
  A. Fractures of long bones require __________ by splinting to prevent joint movement __________ and __________ the fracture.
  B. __________ the fracture.
  C. Never try to __________ or __________ a bone in a compound fracture.

63. Sprains
  A. Occurs when __________, __________, or ligaments are torn.
  B. May be the result of trauma or cumulative __________ of the joint.

64. Strains
  A. A strain is often called a __________ __________.
  B. Occurs when a muscle or tendon is overextended by __________.
  C. The patient may be unable to use the __________.
  D. In the lower extremities, __________ __________ is painful and sometimes impossible.

65. Dislocation
    A. The bone is actually pulled away from the __________, stretching or tearing the __________ and tendons.
    B. A __________ is generally noted.
    C. Must be reduced and the bone __________ into the joint.
    D. Injured body parts should be __________ to prevent additional damage and to reduce pain.
    E. The application of __________ also helps with the pain and slows edema.

III. Emergency Preparedness

1. The Role of the Medical Assistant During an Emergency
    A. Be knowledgeable in the area of emergency __________.
    B. Know how to respond in the event of a __________ disaster, such as a terrorist event, and to a __________ disaster, such as a hurricane.
    C. Remaining __________ in the event of an emergency is paramount to the success of handling the emergency.

2. Preparing for an Earthquake
    A. Check for __________ around the facility.
    B. Identify safe places both __________ and __________.
    C. Educate yourself and your ______________.
    D. Have __________ supplies on hand.
    E. Develop an emergency __________ plan.

3. Checking for Facility Hazards
    A. Make sure that __________ are fastened securely to walls.
    B. Do not place large or heavy objects on the __________ __________.
    C. Store any breakable items in low, closed __________ equipped with locks.
    D. Avoid hanging __________ __________ on walls above where patients will sit or lie.
    E. Secure overhead __________ __________.
    F. Repair any defective __________ __________ or leaky gas connections.
    G. _______ water heaters to wall studs bolted to the floor.
    H. Repair __________ __________ in the ceilings or foundations.
    I. All __________ products should be stored in closed cabinets with locks, on the bottom shelf.

4. Safe Places to Go During an Earthquake
    A. Under sturdy __________
    B. Against an __________ wall
    C. Away from __________ that could shatter
    D. Away from __________ or furniture that could fall over
    E. If outside, stay away from __________, trees, telephone or __________ lines, overpasses, or elevated expressways.

5. Disaster Supplies
    i. ______________________________
    ii. ______________________________
    iii. ______________________________
    iv. ______________________________
    v. ______________________________

6. Warning Signs of a Tornado
    i. ______________________________
    ii. ______________________________
    iii. ______________________________

7. Safety During a Tornado
   A. Move to the basement of a building or the __________ __________ of a structure.
   B. If a basement is not available, it is advisable to seek shelter in a __________ or __________ hallway.
   C. Above all else, stay away from __________, __________, and outside walls.
   D. Avoid __________ and use the stairs to reach the lowest level of the facility.
8. Fire Preparedness
   A. Equip the office with properly working __________ __________ placed on every level of the building on the ceiling or high on the walls.
   B. Equip every room with a __________ detector and test and clean once per month.
   C. Know the __________ routes to use in the event of a fire.
   D. Ensure that __________ __________ are available if the office is located above the first level.
   E. Store __________ items in well-ventilated areas.
   F. Repair any __________ wiring to avoid a fire hazard.
   G. Locate __________ __________ throughout the office and train staff on their use.
9. Escaping a Fire
   A. If a person's clothes are on fire, that person should __________, __________, and __________ until the fire is extinguished.
   B. Check closed doors for __________ before opening.
   C. If the door is hot, it should not be __________, and another route of escape should be sought. If the door is cool, it should be __________ __________.
   D. When escaping a fire, __________ __________ under any smoke on the way to the exit and close doors as they are passed through to delay the spread of fire.
   E. Once out of the building, do not attempt to __________ until or unless the fire department declares that it is safe to do so.
10. In the Event of a Flood
    A. Listen to the radio for __________.
    B. Move to __________ ground.
    C. If there is time before evacuating, disconnect any __________ __________ and shut off utilities at their main valves.
    D. When evacuating, be careful not to walk through __________ water.
11. Preparing for a Hurricane
    A. Secure the windows using __________.
    B. Trees and shrubs around the office should be well __________.
    C. If the medical office is to be evacuated before a hurricane, listen to the radio or television for information provided by local __________ __________ __________.
    D. During the hurricane, listen to the __________ or __________ for information and prepare for high winds and possible flooding.
12. Types of Terrorist Attacks
    i. ______________________________
    ii. ______________________________
    iii. ______________________________
13. Questions to Ask If a Bomb Threat Is Made
    i. ______________________________
    ii. ______________________________
    iii. ______________________________
    iv. ______________________________
    v. ______________________________

14. Biological Threats (List and briefly explain each type.)

i. ______________________________

ii. ______________________________

iii. ______________________________

iv. ______________________________

15. In the Event of a Biological Attack

A. Be prepared to evacuate the area __________.
B. Wash with __________ and __________.
C. Contact the __________.
D. Listen to the radio for __________.
E. Remove and bag clothing if __________.

16. In the Event of a Nuclear Blast

A. Take cover as quickly as possible, __________ __________ if the building has a basement.
B. Remain in a safe location, listening to the radio for __________.
C. Do not look at the __________ or __________.
D. Lie flat on the ground with your head __________.
E. Seek __________ as quickly as possible.

17. The Role of the Medical Assistant in a Mock Environmental Exposure Event

A. Aid in __________ planning.
B. __________ patients to determine which patients require immediate attention.
C. Assist in __________-__________ response for wounded individuals.
D. Administer __________ and other vaccines under the direction of a physician.
E. Facilitate order and organization in the midst of __________.
F. Implement and follow through on an __________ safety plan.

KEY TERMINOLOGY REVIEW

Match words to their definitions.

a. Anaphylactic shock
b. Bandage
c. Crash cart
d. First responders
e. Heat exhaustion
f. Hyperglycemia
g. Hyperthermia
h. Hypoglycemia
i. Hypothermia
j. Intubate
k. Patent
l. Primary assessment
m. Rule of nines
n. Stat
o. Triage

1. __________ A prolonged exposure to extremely hot temperatures that results in an elevated body temperature.
2. __________ EMS providers trained to recognize medical conditions, initiate basic life support, and access other parts of the system.
3. __________ Inserting a tube into the trachea as an emergency airway.
4. __________ High blood sugar level.
5. __________ A severe allergic reaction that causes respiratory distress because of swelling of the upper airways.
6. __________ An unobstructed airway.

7. ____________ A useful tool for estimating body surface area.
8. ____________ A core temperature of below 95°F.
9. ____________ Resembles a large roll-around toolbox with drawers that can be used to store emergency equipment and medications. Sometimes called an emergency kit.
10. ____________ Assessing the emergency care needed by patients.
11. ____________ Immediate.
12. ____________ Extreme fatigue caused by heat, which occurs as the result of sodium and water depletion from the body.
13. ____________ Initial patient contact by a medical professional beginning with a few simple questions and a basic patient examination.
14. ____________ Low blood sugar level.
15. ____________ A strip of binding material used to hold a dressing in place.

APPLIED PRACTICE

Follow the directions as instructed with each question below.

Scenario A

Tasha Lopez, RMA, has recently been hired as a clinical medical assistant for a brand new family practice. She has been asked to stock the emergency medical box with drugs and make sure that it is ready in case of an emergency.

This is what she found:

- Atropine
- Diphenhydramine
- Furosemide
- Instant glucose
- Lidocaine
- Local anesthetics
- Normal saline
- Phenobarbital and diazepam
- Solu-Cortef
- Syrup of ipecac
- Verapamil

1. Based on the inventory list, what are some items that Tasha should add?

____

____

____

____

Scenario B

Sasha Daniels, CMA (AAMA), is employed at Community Urgent Care. A 47-year-old male patient has been brought to your facility. His right index finger was partially torn from his hand while he was working on a piece of farming machinery. His coworker has driven him to the medical facility.

1. What type of injury has this man sustained?

____

2. How should he be treated?

____

____

____

____

____

Scenario C

Later in the day at Community Urgent Care, Sasha encounters a 36-year-old female patient who is presenting with a liquid chemical burn covering the entire front and back of her right arm. Residue from the liquid chemical still remains on the patient's arm.

1. What will the first step likely be for treating this patient? Explain your answer.

____

____

____

____

2. Because the patient's skin was extremely sensitive to the chemical agent, the physician has diagnosed a second degree burn on the front and back of the patient's arm. According to the rule of nines, what percentage of her body has been affected?

____

LEARNING ACTIVITY: TRUE/FALSE

Indicate whether the following statements are true or false by placing a T or an F on the line that precedes each statement.

______ 1. An AED can be used on children ages 1 to 8 years old.

______ 2. Lock jaw is also known as an avulsion.

______ 3. A nosebleed that occurs after a head injury and does not stop should be considered a serious emergency until proven otherwise.

______ 4. In general, perform "CPR first" for unresponsive children and infants.

______ 5. Shock, the collapse of the cardiovascular system, is caused by insufficient cardiac output.

______ 6. Arterial bleeding is usually slow and pale red.

______ 7. Simple direct pressure with a dressing will usually stop bleeding from a soft tissue injury.

______ 8. Nosebleeds may be messy and embarrassing and are usually life threatening occurrences.

______ 9. The severity of a burn depends on the amount and depth of tissue injury.

______ 10. Once a seizure stops, especially a full-body seizure, it is normal for a patient to remain unconscious for as long as 2 hours.

FILL IN THE BLANK

Using words from the list below, fill in the blanks to complete the following statements.

105°F	EMS	Poisoning
Chemical	Immobilized	Prehospital
Contamination	Intact skin	Tendons
Darker in color	Irrigated	Tissue damage
Dislocations	Life threatening	Venous
Distal	Occluded airway	Water
Dressing	Perspire	

1. __________________ blood flows more slowly, is __________________, and can usually be controlled by direct pressure.
2. An individual experiencing heat stroke usually fails to __________________ and has a body temperature of __________________ or higher.
3. Internal bleeding occurs with __________________ and __________________.
4. Open wounds are seldom __________________, unless they penetrate the head, chest, throat, or abdomen.
5. A __________________ is a sterile covering placed directly over a wound to absorb blood and other body fluids, prevent __________________, and protect the wound from further trauma.
6. The __________________ was established to provide __________________ care and safe and prompt transportation from any location, including the medical office, to an emergency facility.
7. Musculoskeletal injuries involve bones, muscles, __________________ and ligaments and include fractures, __________________, sprains, and strains.
8. Respiratory and cardiac arrest may be caused by an __________________, electrocution, shock, drowning, heart attack, trauma, anaphylaxis, drugs, __________________, or traumatic head or chest injury.
9. Bone breaks can be complete, twisted, or splintered. The affected part is __________________ and examined for impaired circulation to the __________________ aspect.
10. Patients with __________________ burns should have the area __________________ immediately with large amounts of __________________.

CRITICAL THINKING

Answer the following questions to the best of your ability. Utilize the textbook as a reference.

1. A patient has presented to the front desk without an appointment and is obviously SOB, her lips and fingertips appear a bit cyanotic. How would you assess her treatment?

____

____

____

____

2. Your first job out of school is in an emergency care facility that has had an unfortunate number of lawsuits brought against it and its staff. What are your legal responsibilities as a medical assistant?

____

____

3. An 85-year-old man is choking on a hot dog. How will his advanced age affect your treatment of him?

RESEARCH ACTIVITY

Utilize Internet search engines to research the following topics and write a brief description of what you find. It is important to utilize reputable websites.

1. There is much to learn about how to face various types of emergencies. Select some emergencies that you know you may face on the job as a medical assistant. Then conduct research on these emergencies, utilizing the Internet or your school or local library. Write an essay on what you learned through your research. Be sure to cite your resources.

CHAPTER 44

The Clinical Laboratory

CHAPTER OUTLINE

General review of the chapter:

The Role of the Clinical Laboratory in Patient Care
Types of Clinical Laboratories
Clinical Laboratory Departments
Clinical Laboratory Personnel
Laboratory Safety Regulations
Laboratory Hazards
Quality Assurance
Laboratory Equipment
Laboratory Measurements and Equipment
The Clinical Laboratory and Patient Communication

STUDENT STUDY GUIDE

Use the following guide to assist in your learning of the concepts from the chapter.

I. The Clinical Laboratory

1. The Role of the Clinical Laboratory in Patient Care
   - i. ______________________
   - ii. ______________________
   - iii. ______________________
   - iv. ______________________
   - v. ______________________

2. The Outside Laboratory
   - A. Handles specimens collected from many types of __________.
   - B. Performs tests ranging from the __________ to the very __________.

3. The Reference Laboratory
   - A. Handles more __________ tests than an outside laboratory and those tests that are __________ requested.
   - B. Tests performed on a regular basis at a reference laboratory may provide more __________ results than tests performed a few times a year in an __________ laboratory.

4. The Physician's Office Laboratory
   - A. In the office laboratory, the doctor has the advantage of receiving the results more __________ than if the tests were done outside of the office.
   - B. Disadvantages
     - i. ______________________
     - ii. ______________________

5. Departments Within a Clinical Laboratory

   i. ______________________________
   ii. ______________________________
   iii. ______________________________
   iv. ______________________________
   v. ______________________________
   vi. ______________________________
   vii. ______________________________
   viii. ______________________________
   ix. ______________________________
   x. ______________________________
   xi. ______________________________
   xii. ______________________________

6. Personnel Within a Clinical Laboratory (Briefly describe the required training for each of the following persons.)

   A. Director of a Clinical Laboratory: ______________________________
   B. Clinical Laboratory Scientist (CLS) or Medical Technologist (MT): ______________________________
   C. Medical Laboratory Technician (MLT): ______________________________
   D. Medical Laboratory Assistant (MLA), Clinical Laboratory Assistant (CLA), Certified Medical Assistant (CMA), and Registered Medical Assistant (RMA): ______________________________
   E. Medical Assistant: ______________________________

7. Laboratory Safety Regulations

   A. Patients are entitled to __________ medical care and health care personnel deserve to work in a __________ environment.
   B. The accuracy and __________ of the test results are crucial to the health of the patient.

8. The Agencies and Committees That Set and Review Laboratory Safety Guidelines

   i. ______________________________
   ii. ______________________________
   iii. ______________________________
   iv. ______________________________
   v. ______________________________

9. The Occupational Safety and Health Administration (OSHA)

   A. Creates safeguards covering nearly every __________ in the United States.
   B. If no specific guidelines exist, then the "__________ __________ __________" must be followed.

10. Standard Precautions

   A. Developed by the ______________________________.
   B. Combine the major features of __________ precautions and __________ __________ isolation precautions into one set of recommendations.
   C. The CDC's precautions are enforced by __________.

11. The Clinical Laboratory Improvement Amendments (CLIA)

   A. Enacted by Congress in __________.
   B. States may have their own __________ __________ __________, but they must be at least as stringent as the federal government's regulations.
   C. Information regarding state __________ may be obtained from state health departments.

12. The Clinical Laboratory Improvement Amendments' Classification of Tests

   i. ____________________
   ii. ____________________
   iii. ____________________

13. Requirements for a Physician's Office Laboratory to Perform Waiver Tests

   A. Must __________ to perform these tests.
   B. Restricted to performing __________ of the more complex tests from Level I or Level II.
   C. Exempt from complying with CLIA __________ standards.
   D. May be subject to __________ __________ and investigations if test results are questioned or there are complaints against the laboratory.

14. Level I Tests

   A. Level I tests are moderately __________ and include __________ of specimens.
   B. Any laboratory that wishes to perform Level I tests must be headed by a __________/_____ or __________.
   C. All personnel must have training past __________ __________.
   D. The laboratory must perform ____________ testing and is subject to unannounced inspections.

15. Types of Level I Tests

   i. ____________________
   ii. ____________________
   iii. ____________________
   iv. ____________________
   v. ____________________
   vi. ____________________
   vii. ____________________

16. Level II Tests

   A. Level II tests include those which are highly __________.
   B. Laboratories that perform tests in this category are subject to unannounced __________, perform ____________ testing, and are headed by an _________ or _________ scientist.
   C. Tests may only be performed by ______________ personnel as specified in the CLIA 1988 standards.

17. Laboratory Safety Regulations

   i. ____________________
   ii. ____________________
   iii. ____________________
   iv. ____________________

18. Contents of the Material Safety Data Sheet (MSDS)

   i. ____________________
   ii. ____________________
   iii. ____________________
   iv. ____________________
   v. ____________________

19. Biohazards

   A. Biohazards have the potential to __________ others.
   B. Since 1992, all laboratories must have OSHA's __________ __________ __________ __________ __________ __________ in place.
   C. The CDC's ____________ ____________ must be employed when dealing with any infectious materials.

20. The Bloodborne Standards Requirements for Health Care Employers
    A. Review all new safety devices that lessen the risk of __________ to employees.
    B. Ask for safety input from employees on an __________ basis.
    C. Keep a detailed report of all __________ __________ incidents.
21. Addressing Fire and Safety Hazards in the Medical Office
    A. Have an awareness of the __________ plan and __________.
    B. Know the location of safety devices such as __________ __________, __________, and safety blankets.
    C. Remove __________ __________ properly.
22. Goals of a Quality Assurance Program
    A. Provide mechanisms for evaluating __________ __________ and policies.
    B. Identify and __________ problems.
    C. Ensure __________ and prompt reporting of results.
    D. Ensure that testing is performed by __________ persons.
23. CLIA Requirements for the Laboratory
    A. Evaluate the __________ of laboratory policies and procedures.
    B. Identify and __________ problems.
    C. Ensure reliable and __________ test results.
    D. Ensure the competence and __________ of staff.
    E. Take __________ __________ if errors are found.
    F. Integrate __________ __________ into future policies and procedures.
    G. Document employee __________ and assess __________ yearly after the first year.
    H. Maintain the ____________ and ____________ of patient samples during the entire testing process.
    I. Be subject to inspection every _____ years if performing moderate- or high-complexity tests.
24. Quality Control (QC) Programs in Clinical Laboratories
    A. Monitor the testing of patient __________ to ensure reliable and consistent results.
    B. Requirements (List the requirements of a QC program.)
        i. ____
        ii. ____
        iii. ____
25. Proficiency Testing
    A. May be performed on __________ __________, __________, __________, or urine.
    B. The samples will have a __________ of results similar to any group of patients.
26. Equipment Generally Found in a Physician's Office Laboratory
    A. An __________ is used to sterilize equipment or instruments that are used on patients or in certain test procedures.
    B. A ____________ is used to separate urine so that sediment can be examined under the microscope.
    C. A ________________ is used to separate whole blood samples into layers to measure a patient's hematocrit.
    D. A ____________ is a type of handheld photometer that is used to test glucose levels in patients.
27. Microscope
    A. Frequently used in the medical office to examine __________ __________ and various types of smears.
    B. It is an optical instrument that magnifies structures which are unseen by the ___________ eye for the purpose of counting, naming, or ________________.
    C. Better microscopes have better ___________.

28. The Process of Using and Cleaning a Microscope

A. Always carry the microscope with one hand on the ___________ and one hand under the ___________.
B. Make sure that the stage is in the __________ position before starting.
C. Clean objectives with __________ __________ starting with 10X and ending with oil immersion.
D. Turn on the light and rotate the nosepiece until the ________ _________ is directly over the slide.
E. Place the prepared slide on the __________.
F. Use the __________ __________ knob to raise the stage until the objective is close to the slide on the stage.
G. Look through the __________ and adjust the __________ __________ knob until the microscope field is seen (it is a round circle of bright light).
H. Use the __________ __________ knob to obtain a clearer image.
I. Open the __________ and adjust the __________ to focus if necessary.
J. Raise or lower the __________ to alter light refraction.
K. Change the objective to __________ and readjust as needed.
L. Move the objective and place a __________ of __________ on the slide before completing the turn to the oil immersion lens.
M. When focusing and examination is complete, lower the ___________ before removing the slide.
N. Turn off the __________.
O. Clean the __________ and objectives with __________ paper.
P. Clean the oil immersion lens with __________ cleaner.
Q. Unplug the __________ __________ and wrap it around the base.
R. Cover the microscope with a __________ __________.
S. Clean the __________ and store it.
T. Document __________ and __________ in the logbook.

29. Thermometers in the Medical Laboratory

A. Used to measure the temperature of various pieces of equipment, such as __________, __________, incubators, and __________ __________.
B. Must be maintained within __________ ranges.

30. Temperatures Routinely Associated with the Laboratory Environment (List both the Fahrenheit and Celsius temperature for each piece of equipment.)

A. Freezer: ______________________________
B. Autoclave: ____________________________
C. Refrigerator: __________________________
D. Incubator: ____________________________
E. Room: ________________________________

31. The Timing of Laboratory Tests

A. Tests must be timed __________ in order to provide accurate, meaningful test results.
B. Laboratory time is based on the ______-______ clock, or military time, to avoid the confusion that may result from using the A.M. and P.M. designations of ______ Mean Time.
C. The 24-hour clock uses __________ __________, with noon expressed as 1200 (twelve hundred hours) and midnight as 2400 (twenty-four hundred hours).
D. __________ __________ for 4:15 P.M. would be 1615 (sixteen-fifteen hundred hours), which is calculated by adding 4 hours and 15 minutes to 1200.

32. Laboratory Units of Measurement

A. A laboratory result must never be reported without a unit of ____________ after it
B. __________ __________ units are used most frequently in the laboratory.
C. The metric system is based on a decimal system combined with various designations.

i. ______________________________
ii. ______________________________
iii. ______________________________

33. Units Used to Express Laboratory Results

i. ______________________________
ii. ______________________________
iii. ______________________________

34. Abbreviations Commonly Used to Report Patients' Test Results

A. Gram: __________
B. Milligram: __________
C. Liter: __________
D. Milliliter: __________
E. Microliter: __________
F. Microgram: __________
G. Millimoles per liter: __________
H. Cubic centimeter: __________
I. Milligrams per deciliter: __________
J. Pint: __________
K. Quart: __________
L. Ounce: __________
M. Quantity not sufficient: __________

35. Measuring and Mixing Devices Used in the Laboratory

A. Beakers and flasks can be used to mix liquids but are not __________ measuring devices.
B. The __________ cylinder and the __________ flask are accurate measuring devices.

36. Pipettes

A. A __________ pipette is used for measuring and is marked with __________, which means "to deliver"; it will deliver that specific amount.
B. If a graduated pipette is marked with __________, "to contain", it must be emptied __________ to deliver the exact amount.
C. A __________ pipette is used for transferring liquid from one vessel to another.
D. A __________ pipette has graduations down to the tip and is used to make __________ __________ in the laboratory.
E. __________ are used to deliver very small amounts (microliters) of liquid; the __________ directions must be carefully followed.

37. The Phases of the Laboratory Testing Cycle (Briefly describe each phase.)

A. Preanalytical phase: ______________________________
B. Analytical phase: ______________________________

38. Tests Requiring Special Instructions

A. For most fasting tests, the fasting period is at least ______ hours.
B. Two-hour Postprandial (PP) or post cibum (pc) glucose means that the patient eats a __________ __________ of food for a meal and a blood glucose level is drawn exactly ______ hours after the completion of the meal.

39. Information Required on a Specimen Label

i. ______________________________
ii. ______________________________
iii. ______________________________

40. Steps for Correctly Completing a Laboratory Requisition

A. Check the patient's record for __________ or specific laboratory tests.
B. Verify which laboratory will be doing the testing and locate its __________ __________ form.

C. Complete the patient __________ section.
D. Complete the section that requires the physician's __________, __________, telephone number, and __________ number.
E. Complete the patient's __________ and __________ information.
F. Mark the appropriate boxes to indicate each __________ that is being ordered by the physician.
G. If a test is ordered that is not __________ on the requisition, write in the name of the test on the lines provided.
H. Indicate what __________ and __________ of specimen is to be tested.
I. Enter the patient's __________ on the requisition as needed.
J. If no diagnosis has been made, then __________ the patient's symptoms.
K. Complete the patient authorization to __________ and assign the benefits portion as needed.

41. Steps for Preparing a Specimen for Transport

A. Assemble the equipment and supplies needed to obtain the __________.
B. Perform __________ __________ and don gloves.
C. Obtain the required specimen after explaining the __________ to the patient.
D. Label the specimen with the patient's __________, the __________, the physician's __________, the __________ of collection, and other information required by the facility.
E. __________ the laboratory requisition, and complete the date and time that the specimen was obtained.
F. Process the specimens and, if they are not to be sent out until later in the day, store them according to laboratory __________ __________ requirements.
G. Attach the laboratory __________ securely to the specimen before sending.
H. Remove gloves and dispose of them in the __________ __________ container.
I. Record the specimen in the laboratory __________, indicating the date, the time of collection, the type and source of the specimen, the __________ ordered, where the __________ were sent, and the date that they were sent.

42. Steps for Monitoring and Following Up on Laboratory Test Results

A. Review incoming laboratory __________, and compare them with the __________ values provided by the analyzing laboratory.
B. Many laboratories highlight or indicate __________ results on the laboratory results sheet with an H or an L, for high and low, respectively.
C. Highlight any __________ results per facility policy.
D. Obtain the patient's __________ __________ and attach the new laboratory results and submit it to the __________ for review.

KEY TERMINOLOGY REVIEW

Match the vocabulary term to the correct definition below.

a. Aliquot
b. Analyte
c. Calibrate
d. Centrifuge
e. Certificate of Waiver Tests (WTs)
f. Clinical Laboratory Improvement Amendments (CLIA)
g. Compound microscope
h. Control samples
i. Diluent
j. Fasting
k. Hemolyzed
l. Icteric
m. Incubator
n. Outside laboratory

o. Photometer
p. Physician's office laboratory
q. Pipettes
r. Post cibum (pc)
s. Postprandial (PP)
t. Proficiency testing
u. Qualitative testing
v. Quantitative testing
w. Reagents
x. Reference library
y. Resolution
z. Turnaround time

1. __________ Instrument used to separate specimens into component layers.
2. __________ A microscope with two sets of lenses, oculars, and objectives.
3. __________ The patient must not consume any food for a prescribed number of hours prior to the collection of a specimen.
4. __________ After a meal.
5. __________ Analyzes for the presence or absence of a substance.
6. __________ Refers to the microscope's ability to distinguish clearly between two adjacent, but distinct, objects.
7. __________ The least complex and present the least risk if performed incorrectly.
8. __________ Bilious yellow-green color.
9. __________ Substances required for a chemical reaction or used to detect the presence of another substance.
10. __________ A laboratory in which some of the tests that the physician orders are performed right in the office.
11. __________ When red cells burst, causing serum to be a cherry-red color.
12. __________ Mandates that all laboratories that test human specimens must be regulated to ensure accurate patient test results.
13. __________ Some laboratory tests require the medical assistant do this to the machine or instrument prior to testing a specimen.
14. __________ Samples similar to the required testing specimen that have been previously tested and have a known value.
15. __________ It is either hospital-based or independent and handles specimens collected from many types of facilities.
16. __________ After a meal.
17. __________ An agent that dilutes a substance or solution to which it is added.
18. __________ Analyzes a specimen for the presence of a substance and the amount of the substance present.
19. __________ One of the various measuring and mixing devices that are employed in the laboratory.
20. __________ How long it takes for the test to be performed and the results generated, sent back to the physician for review, and added to the patient's chart.
21. __________ External quality control program that monitors the accuracy of test systems by comparing your results to results provided by a survey program of the College of American Pathologists or the American Association of Bioanalysts.
22. __________ The presence or absence of a substance.
23. __________ May be associated with a specific teaching hospital or medical school, or be independently owned.

24. __________ An instrument that measures light intensity.
25. __________ Used to maintain a specific temperature to achieve a specific result.
26. __________ A small portion of the whole.

APPLIED PRACTICE

Follow the directions as instructed with each question below.

1. Label the parts of the binocular microscope.

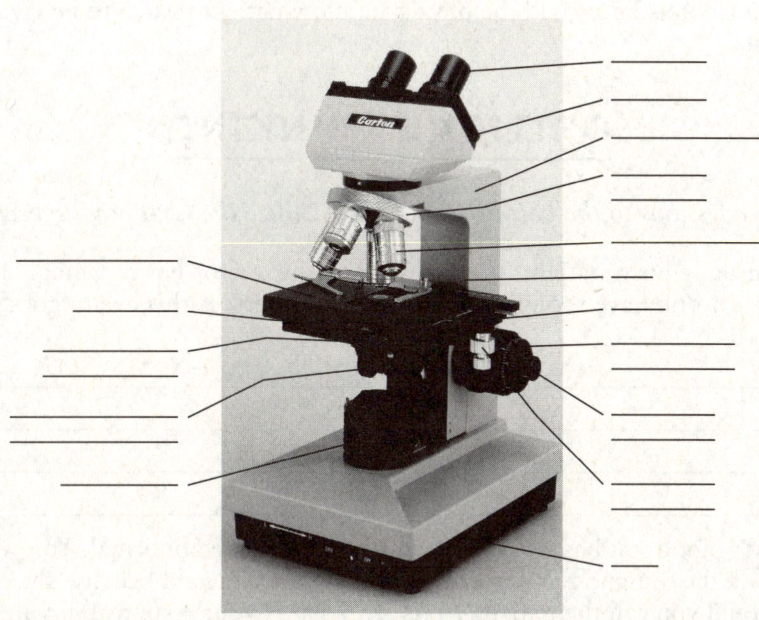

2. **Scenario**

   On your first day of work at a clinical laboratory, you are ordered to clean up any hazardous waste after each procedure and at the end of each day. How does your training prepare you for this task? What is the definition of hazardous waste? Briefly explain what you would do.

   ____
   ____
   ____
   ____
   ____
   ____

LEARNING ACTIVITY: TRUE/FALSE

Indicate whether the following statements are true or false by placing a T or an F on the line that precedes each statement.

_______ 1. A binocular microscope has one ocular lens.

_______ 2. The condenser is located on the substage of a microscope.

______ 3. Oil immersion is used with the 10X lens to increase the power to 100X.

______ 4. The United States uses the English system of measurement in everyday life.

______ 5. Measuring devices may be made of glass or plastic and be reusable or disposable.

______ 6. The laboratory testing cycle is divided into two phases: preanalytical and postanalytical.

______ 7. There are two focus knobs—one for low power and the other for high power.

______ 8. In tests such as the glucose tolerance test (GTT), specimen collection must be timed precisely in order to provide accurate, meaningful test results.

______ 9. When you are finished working with a microscope, you must clean the lenses with any soft cloth or paper.

______ 10. Under no circumstances will the physician allow patient results to be given to the patient by telephone.

CRITICAL THINKING

Answer the following questions to the best of your ability. Utilize the textbook as a reference.

1. The office is unusually busy, patients are crabby, and the doctor has repeatedly berated you for working too slowly. You have thought about cutting corners. Is this ever a good idea? Why or why not?

____

____

____

____

2. Michelle Oswald's blood test has returned and it is found to be abnormal. You were the medical assistant who took the test and felt especially close to Mrs. Oswald because she reminded you of your mother. Should you call the patient yourself? What is your responsibility in this case?

____

____

____

____

RESEARCH ACTIVITY

Utilize Internet search engines to research the following topics and write a brief description of what you find. It is important to utilize reputable websites.

1. To learn more about the agencies and committees that set and review safety guidelines affecting clinical laboratories, go online or utilize your school or local library to conduct further research. Write an essay on your findings and what more you learned beyond what is presented in the textbook about these agencies and committees and the guidelines established for laboratories. Be sure to cite your resources.

____

____

____

____

Chapter 45
Microbiology

CHAPTER OUTLINE

General review of the chapter:

Role of the Medical Assistant in Microbiology
Classifications of Microorganisms
Types of Microorganisms
Specimen Collection and Transportation
Diagnosing Infection
Microbiology Equipment and Procedures
Types of Specimens
Serology Testing

STUDENT STUDY GUIDE

Use the following guide to assist in your learning of the concepts from the chapter.

I. Introduction to Microbiology

1. Microorganisms: A Definition
   A. Microorganisms are also called __________.
   B. They are living organisms that can be seen only with a ____________.
   C. Harmless microorganisms can be found on your __________, in your digestive tract, and in your __________ tract.
   D. Microorganisms include ___________, viruses, __________, and bacteria.
2. Pathogens
   A. Pathogens are __________ microorganisms.
   B. Basic types of pathogens
      i. ______________________________
      ii. ______________________________
      iii. ______________________________
      iv. ______________________________
      v. ______________________________
      vi. ______________________________
3. What Microorganisms Need in Order to Grow
   i. ______________________________
   ii. ______________________________
   iii. ______________________________
   iv. ______________________________
4. Microbiology and Microorganisms
   A. Microbiology is the study of __________ __________ that cannot be seen with the naked eye.
   B. Microorganisms are the __________ __________ that microbiology studies.

5. The Role of the Medical Assistant in Microbiology
    i. ______________________________
    ii. ______________________________
    iii. ______________________________
    iv. ______________________________
    v. ______________________________
    vi. ______________________________
6. Classifications of Microorganisms (List the two classifications.)
    i. ______________________________
    ii. ______________________________
7. Retention of Dyes
    A. Bacteria are __________ by how they react to stain or dye.
    B. __________ stain is used for most gram-positive and gram-negative bacteria.
    C. Others use __________-__________ stain.
8. Hemolytic Properties
    A. One way in which to classify bacteria is by the bacteria's ability to __________ red blood cells in blood __________.
    B. A microbiologist observes the characteristics of a __________ of cells.
    C. The organism that causes __________ __________ is beta hemolytic.
9. Diseases Caused by Pathogenic Microorganisms
    i. ______________________________
    ii. ______________________________
    iii. ______________________________
    iv. ______________________________
    v. ______________________________
    vi. ______________________________
    vii. ______________________________
    viii. ______________________________
    ix. ______________________________
    x. ______________________________
    xi. ______________________________
    xii. ______________________________
    xiii. ______________________________
    xiv. ______________________________
    xv. ______________________________
    xvi. ______________________________
    xvii. ______________________________
    xviii. ______________________________
    xix. ______________________________
    xx. ______________________________
    xxi. ______________________________
    xxii. ______________________________
    xxiii. ______________________________
    xxiv. ______________________________
    xxv. ______________________________
    xxvi. ______________________________
10. Bacterium/Bacteria
    A. Bacteria are small, __________ microorganisms that are capable of rapid __________.
    B. Their reproductive ability explains how some infections become __________ in a short time and can be dangerous.

C. Bacteria may be named for their __________ (shape). (List the shapes.)

i. ______________________________
ii. ______________________________
iii. ______________________________

11. Cocci

A. Cocci are __________ bacteria that are arranged in various configurations.
B. Staphylococci are __________-__________, grape-like clusters of __________, some of which are pathogenic.
C. Nonpathogenic staphylococci are found on our __________ and in many of our body __________, or openings.

12. *Staphylococcus aureus* (*S. aureus*), or Staph

A. *S. aureus* is the major pathogen of this genus and may be found as __________ __________ in the nose and on the skin.
B. Causes __________, especially when __________ is lowered by a break in the skin or in the mucous membranes.
C. It is a common cause of ____________ infections and may also cause ____________, meningitis, and ____________ in persons who have reduced resistance.

13. Methicillin-Resistant *Staphylococcus aureus* (MRSA)

A. MRSA is a form of __________.
B. Tests are available to indicate the __________ or __________ of this enzyme and to help determine the most favorable treatment.

14. Streptococci

A. Streptococci are round, __________-__________ bacteria that are arranged in chains.
B. Some are ______________ and others are dangerous to humans.
C. They are part of the normal flora of the __________ __________ tract and skin.

15. Group A Beta-hemolytic Streptococcus Pyogenes

A. Cause a variety of diseases, varying from __________ to __________ __________.
B. Diseases caused by group A beta-hemolytic streptococcus pyogenes

i. ______________________________
ii. ______________________________
iii. ______________________________
iv. ______________________________
v. ______________________________
vi. ______________________________
vii. ______________________________
viii. ______________________________

16. Diplococci

A. Diplococci occur in __________.
B. Some diplococci are gram __________ and others are gram __________.
C. Diseases caused by diplococci

i. ______________________________
ii. ______________________________
iii. ______________________________
iv. ______________________________

17. Bacillus/Bacilli

A. __________-__________ bacilli may be pathogenic or nonpathogenic.
B. Some bacilli are gram __________ and others are gram __________.

C. Bacilli are responsible for a wide variety of illnesses. (List some of these illnesses.)
   i. ______________________________
   ii. ______________________________
   iii. ______________________________
   iv. ______________________________
   v. ______________________________
   vi. ______________________________

18. Gram-Negative Bacilli
   A. ______________ are a large family of gram-negative bacilli that are found mainly in the intestinal tract.
   B. Many of them will cause infections in other __________ in the body.
   C. One type, __________ __________, is most frequently associated with urinary tract infections.
   D. The group of __________ organisms is a major cause of foodborne illnesses worldwide.

19. *Helicobacter pylori* (*H. pylori*)
   A. *H. pylori* is a __________-__________ bacillus.
   B. It was discovered in the early __________.
   C. The organism is found in about __________ of the population and causes __________ symptoms in most individuals.
   D. It was discovered that *H. pylori* is the causative agent of __________ ulcers and a risk factor in __________ malignancy in some infected persons.
   E. The organism is responsive to a number of antibiotics, including ____________.
   F. The discovery of *H. pylori* led to major breakthroughs in treatment for __________.

20. Gram-Positive Bacilli
   A. May be found in __________ or singly and are __________ forming or __________ forming.
   B. Notable gram-positive bacilli
      i. ______________________________, which causes botulism
      ii. ______________________________, which causes tetanus

21. Vibrios
   A. Vibrios are __________-__________ bacilli.
   B. The main pathogen is *Vibrio cholerae*, whose __________ causes cholera.
   C. Cholera
      i. Characterized by profuse __________ stools, vomiting, leg cramps, ____________, and shock.
      ii. Caused by ingesting drinking water or eating __________ from water contaminated with infected urine, feces, or __________.

22. Spirilla and Spirochetes
   A. Spirilla and spirochetes are __________-shaped or __________-shaped organisms.
   B. They are __________ that are twisted in various shapes.
   C. They are classified as a separate category of __________.
   D. Some are nonpathogenic and are found in certain areas of the body and others, such as __________ __________, cause the sexually transmitted infection syphilis.
   E. *Borrelia burgdorferi*, a spirillum, was discovered in the mid-1970s to be the causative agent of __________ __________.

23. Mycobacteria
   A. Mycobacteria have a different type of material in the __________ __________ and can be stained only with an __________-__________stain.
   B. __________ __________ is the causative agent of tuberculosis, and *Mycobacterium leprae* is the cause of __________.

C. These organisms do not stain well with a __________ stain.
D. In a positive slide for __________-__________ __________ (AFB), the slender bacilli will appear pink when exposed to an acid-fast stain.

24. Rickettsia and Chlamydia
   A. Rickettsia is a bacterial parasite that lives in __________ and __________, which transmit the disease when they bite.
   B. Chlamydia
      i. Chlamydia is an __________ parasite, but it does not live in arthropod hosts.
      ii. It must invade __________ cells to reproduce.

25. Viruses
   A. Viruses are the smallest known __________ organisms.
   B. They depend on the __________ __________ of other organisms for growth.

26. Diseases Caused by Viruses
   i. ______________________________
   ii. ______________________________
   iii. ______________________________
   iv. ______________________________
   v. ______________________________
   vi. ______________________________
   vii. ______________________________
   viii. ______________________________
   ix. ______________________________

27. Types of Microorganisms: Protozoa
   A. Protozoa are __________-__________ organisms.
   B. Some are __________ and others are nonparasitic.
   C. They move with __________, or __________ feet.
   D. Diseases caused by protozoa
      i. ______________________________
      ii. ______________________________

28. Types of Microorganisms: Fungus/Fungi
   A. Fungi include parasitic and nonparasitic __________ and __________.
   B. They depend on other __________ __________ for nutrition.
   C. Reproduction occurs through __________.
   D. They feed on __________.

II. Specimen Collection and Testing Procedures
   1. Steps for Specimen Collection and Transportation
      A. __________ the patient properly.
      B. Follow the __________ carefully.
      C. Complete the label and __________ carefully.
      D. Maintain the appropriate environment and __________ to preserve the specimen.
   2. Information Required on a Specimen Label
      i. ______________________________
      ii. ______________________________
      iii. ______________________________
      iv. ______________________________
      v. ______________________________

3. Information for the Laboratory Requisition
   i. ______
   ii. ______
   iii. ______
   iv. ______
   v. ______
   vi. ______
   vii. ______
   viii. ______
   ix. ______
   x. ______
   xi. ______
4. Collection Devices
   A. The culturette system (List the items included.)
      i. ______
      ii. ______
5. Microbiology Equipment and Procedures
   A. Inoculating Equipment
      i. ______
      ii. ______
      iii. ______
   B. Culture Media
      i. ______
      ii. ______
      iii. ______
6. Common Culture Media
   i. ______
   ii. ______
   iii. ______
   iv. ______
   v. ______
   vi. ______
7. Microbiology Equipment and Procedures: Inoculating Media
   A. An inoculating ______ is used to create a ______ culture.
   B. After inoculation, a ______ dish is placed in an ______ to allow the organism to grow.
8. Microbiology Equipment and Procedures: Sensitivity Testing
   A. Determines which ______ will kill the ______.
   B. Tools include a ______ dish and ______ agar.
9. Steps for Performing a Direct Smear
   A. Perform hand ______ and don gloves.
   B. ______ the equipment.
   C. ______ a clean slide.
   D. ______ the slide.
   E. Allow the slide to air dry for ______ to ______ minutes.
   F. Hold the slide with ______ forceps and pass over the ______ flame.
   G. Slide is ready to be ______.

10. Steps for Preparing a Wet Mount Slide
    A. Perform __________ __________ and don gloves.
    B. __________ a dry slide.
    C. __________ the dry slide.
    D. Place a drop of __________ solution on top of the specimen.
    E. Place a __________ onto the smeared slide.
11. Gram Stain
    A. Used to differentiate, or separate, bacteria into two groups: gram __________ and gram __________.
    B. Different bacteria stain differently, depending on the __________ in their walls.
    C. Gram-positive bacteria retain the crystal __________-__________ color and gram-negative bacteria retain only the __________ __________ color.
    D. Gram stains must always be accompanied by a culture for __________ identification.
12. Throat Specimens
    A. One of the most __________ requested specimens in an office laboratory.
    B. Based on the __________ and __________ with which the patient presents, the physician will order a test to identify the pathogen involved and will begin treatment.
    C. Confirmation of __________ __________ is important because of its virulence and possible complications.
    D. When performing a throat culture, it is important not to touch the __________ of the mouth or the tongue with the __________ to avoid contaminating it.
13. The Sputum Sample
    A. Sputum is the __________ __________ that is expelled by coughing or clearing the bronchi.
    B. To obtain a sample, the patient must be carefully instructed to __________ __________, spitting the coughed up material into a sterile container.
    C. Explain to the patient that this should not be __________ from the mouth.
    D. The purpose of obtaining a sputum specimen is to isolate and diagnose diseases such as __________ __________, influenza, and __________.
14. The Urine Specimen
    A. For a culture it must be either a __________ specimen or a __________-__________ midstream sample (CCMS).
    B. Both methods provide __________ samples.
    C. Any other type of urine specimen would be contaminated by organisms in the container or on the __________ or __________ of the patient.
    D. In doctor's offices and smaller facilities, __________-__________ culture units are used.
    E. Often, urine cultures require a means to provide a __________ result of the number of microorganisms in the sample.
15. The Stool Specimen
    A. May be tested for __________, __________, or __________ infections; for the presence of occult blood; and for excessive amounts of fat __________.
    B. The method of collection varies with the __________ of __________ ordered.
    C. Fecal specimens must be free of __________ or __________ from the toilet and toilet tissue.
16. Occult Blood
    A. Patients are instructed to write their __________, __________, and __________ __________ on the label of the unit.
    B. Patients should close the unit and take it or __________ it to the doctor's office or the laboratory as requested.
    C. It is important to check the __________ __________ of any test kit before giving it to the patient.

17. The Stool Specimen for Ova and Parasites
    A. The presence of __________ organisms, such as ova and parasites, may be determined by testing feces or stool.
    B. The presence of ova, or __________, or other forms of a parasite indicates parasitic __________.
    C. Identification of the parasite aids in the selection of the __________ treatment.
    D. Commercial kits are available that provide containers for fresh stool specimen and two additional vials for preserved specimens, one containing __________ and the other containing __________ alcohol.
18. Wound Specimens
    A. Sterile swabs are used to obtain a specimen from a wound, __________, or __________ to test for pathogenic microorganisms.
    B. The procedure is similar to obtaining a __________ culture.
    C. Several specimens may be necessary from different __________.
    D. Be sure to __________ each specimen appropriately as to the source.
19. The Collection of Cerebrospinal Fluid (CSF)
    A. CSF is always treated as a __________ procedure.
    B. The procedure is __________ for the patient, and the specimen must be handled with care.
    C. Usually __________ tubes are collected under sterile conditions and are sent for testing.
    D. The __________ and __________ test should be performed before chemical and other tests using the second of the three tubes.
    E. Tubes one and three are more likely to be __________ because of the entry and removal processes of collection.
20. The Group A Strep Screen
    A. The group A strep screen is performed frequently in __________ __________.
    B. It is especially efficient in the __________ office because it is __________-__________ and can be done while the patient waits.
    C. The screen is an __________ __________ test for group A beta-hemolytic streptococci.
    D. There are many __________-__________ __________ ___ __________ __________ available that test for the extracted group A beta-hemolytic streptococcus antigen.

KEY TERMINOLOGY REVIEW

Without using any material from your textbook, write a sentence using the selected key terms in the correct context as related to the topics presented in Chapter 45.

1. *acid-fast stain*

   ____

   ____

2. *candidiasis*

   ____

   ____

3. *culturette*

   ____

   ____

4. *enteritis*

5. *exudates*

6. *facultative anaerobes*

7. *fixed*

8. *inoculated*

9. *microbiology*

10. *moniliasi*

11. *morphology*

12. *necrotizing fasciitis*

13. *normal flora*

14. *sequela*

15. *serology*

16. *spore*

17. *sputum*

18. *steatorrhea*

19. *subcellular*

20. *swabs*

APPLIED PRACTICE

Follow the directions as instructed with each question below.

1. Obtaining a stool specimen for ova and parasites versus for pinworms
   a. List the equipment and supplies needed for obtaining a stool specimen for ova and parasites.

   b. List the equipment and supplies needed for obtaining a stool specimen for examination for pinworms.

   c. Discuss the differences and similarities between the two procedures.

2. List the diseases that can occur from the following pathogens.

Body Location	Pathogen	Disease
Respiratory system	*Streptococcus pyogenes* *Corynebacterium diphtheriae* *Mycobacterium tuberculosis* *Haemophilus influenzae type B* *Streptococcus pneumoniae*	
Central nervous system	*Neisseria meningitidis* Polioviruses Rabies virus	
Genitourinary system	Herpes simplex viruses 1 and 2 *Candida albicans* (fungus) *Chlamydia trachomatis* *Escherichia coli*	
Integumentary system	*Staphylococcus aureus* *Varicella zoster* virus	
Gastrointestinal system	Hepatitis A, B, and C viruses *Salmonella enteritidis* *Escherichia coli*	
Circulatory system and blood, immune system	*Streptococcus pyogenes* *Staphylococcus aureus* *Plasmodium falciparum, P. vivax, P. malariae, P. ovale* Human immunodeficiency virus Epstein-Barr virus *Borrelia burgdorferi*	
Tissue	*Streptococcus pyogenes*	

LEARNING ACTIVITY: FILL IN THE BLANK

Using words from the list below, fill in the blanks to complete the following statements.

Note: Some terms are used in more than one statement.

agar
agglutination
cephalosporins
colony
culture medium
eukaryotic
feces
laboratory
lawn technique
methicillin-resistant
microorganisms
motility
organelles
ova
prokaryotic
seaweed
smear
Streptococci
viable
wet mount

1. The Group A Strep Screen is an antigen detection test for group A beta-hemolytic ______________ and follows the general procedure for antigen–antibody ________________ tests, which produce a clumping of cells.
2. Differences such as cell structure and the presence or absence of _________________ are used to classify organisms.
3. The "super bug" ____________-____________ *Staphylococcus aureus* (MRSA) produces an enzyme that makes the organism resistant to penicillin and _________________, which are normally used for treatment, and renders these antibiotics ineffective.
4. A _________________ is a thin layer of _________________ spread on a glass slide for identification purposes.
5. _________________ is a gelatinous substance made from seaweed that is added to a _________________ to provide nutrition and a semisolid surface on which microbes can grow.
6. _________________ cells have a nucleus and _________________ in the cytoplasm, while _________________ cells are simpler in structure, without a nucleus or organelles, such as bacteria.
7. A _________________ is a preparation in a liquid that will preserve the _________________ of the microbe.
8. The Mueller–Hinton agar is inoculated with the pure culture specimen in overlapping strokes in a technique called the _________________ or _________________ count.
9. Microorganisms must remain _________________ (capable of living) when they reach the _________________.
10. The stool or _________________ of the patient can be inspected for the presence of _________________ and mature forms of the worm.

CRITICAL THINKING

Answer the following questions to the best of your ability. Utilize the textbook as a reference.

1. A patient has been instructed to collect stool specimens to be tested for occult blood. You ask him to refrain from eating red meat or taking vitamin C for 3 days prior to testing for occult blood. Why? What other instructions does this patient need to follow in order to obtain an accurate test result?

____

____

____

____

2. Mrs. Chen is a 70-year-old woman from mainland China who has come to the clinic because of recent, sudden constipation. Mrs. Chen is shy and very hesitant to speak with a male medical assistant about her condition. How can the clinic help Mrs. Chen?

____

____

____

____

3. You are preparing a specimen smear for a microbiological examination by the doctor. You heat-fix the slide, but you realize that you have heated it too much because it has become hard to hold. What does this do to the specimen and what would you do?

____

____

RESEARCH ACTIVITY

Utilize Internet search engines to research the following topics and write a brief description of what you find. It is important to utilize reputable websites.

1. Methicillin-resistant *Staphylococcus aureus* (MRSA) has become a very real threat, not only to health care workers, but also to the general population. Visit www.cdc.gov and research the following topics:
   a. Provide a brief description of MRSA.
   b. What are some other multidrug-resistant organisms (MDROs)?
   c. In your opinion, what can be done to prevent the transmission of these organisms?

Chapter 46
Urinalysis

CHAPTER OUTLINE

General review of the chapter:

Asepsis
Collecting the Specimen
Routine Urinalysis
Urine Pregnancy Testing
Quality Control

STUDENT STUDY GUIDE

Use the following guide to assist in your learning of the concepts from the chapter.

I. Urinalysis

1. An Overview of Urinalysis
   - A. The purpose of performing a urinalysis
     - i. Checks for the presence of ____________ or ____________.
     - ii. Provides information about bodily ___________.
   - B. Properties of urine that are examined
     - i. ____
     - ii. ____
     - iii. ____
2. Types of Urinalyses: Routine Sample
   - A. Collected in a ____________ container.
   - B. Collected in the office or brought from ____________.
   - C. Used only for ___________ screenings.
3. Types of Urinalyses: Morning Sample
   - A. A morning sample is the most ________________ urine.
   - B. Collected ________________ upon on arising in the morning.
   - C. Used for __________ testing, urine ____________, and __________ examination.
   - D. The specimen should be brought in within _____ minutes to an hour after collection.
   - E. Refrigerate the sample if an examination cannot be done within _____ hours, or add a preservative.
4. Types of Urinalyses: Timed Specimen
   - A. Necessary for ____________ analysis of substances
   - B. Used to analyze _____________, ______________, and _____________.
5. Types of Urinalyses: Twenty-Four Hour Specimen
   - A. Collection begins after the patient __________ for the first time in the morning.
   - B. Every drop of urine is collected in a container for _____ hours.

C. Used to determine ________________________ rate, check specific __________ levels, and check for ______________ abnormalities.

6. Types of Urinalyses: Two-Hour Postprandial

 A. Collected _____ hours after a meal has been eaten.
 B. Used to screen for __________ that may be spilled into the urine once the blood levels exceed the __________ threshold.

7. Types of Urinalyses: Catheterized Specimen

 A. Used to collect a ___________ urine specimen.
 B. Collecting urine with the use of a catheter ensures that the specimen is free of ______________.
 C. The __________ and its surrounding tissues are cleaned to create a __________ field.
 D. A small, __________ tube is inserted through the __________ to the ___________.

8. Types of Urinalyses: Suprapubic Specimen

 A. A suprapubic puncture is performed using a __________ needle and syringe.
 B. Used for ___________ examinations.

9. A Review of Urine Chemistry

 A. Testing for chemical characteristics (List the substances for which urine is tested.)
 i. ____________________
 ii. ____________________
 iii. ____________________
 iv. ____________________
 v. ____________________
 vi. ____________________
 vii. ____________________
 viii. ____________________
 ix. ____________________

10. Reagent Strips

 B. The strip is dipped into the ___________ sample.
 C. Color changes indicate the presence and ____________ of substances in the urine.

11. Clinitests®

 A. Clinitests® are chemically treated tablets that are added to urine to determine the amount of _____________ in the urine.
 B. The tablets change color according to the ___________ in the urine.
 C. Checks for ________________, ___________________, ________________, and _____________.

12. Steps for Preparing a Urine Sample for Microscopic Analysis

 A. Perform the required ____________ and chemical tests.
 B. Place the urine in a ____________ tube and the tube into a ______________.
 C. Pour off the ____________________.
 D. Microscopically analyze the _____________ material.

13. Microscopic Analysis (List the formed elements in urine that are evaluated.)

 i. ____________________
 ii. ____________________
 iii. ____________________
 iv. ____________________
 v. ____________________

vi. ____________________

vii. ____________________

viii. ____________________

14. Calculating Formed Elements
    A. Examine under the ____________ power field.
    B. Locate ____________.
    C. Scan ____________ to ____________ fields.
    D. Note the number of cells, or ____________, in each field.
    E. Report the ____________ range of the observations.

KEY TERMINOLOGY REVIEW

Match the vocabulary term to the correct definition below.

a. Amorphous
b. Anuria
c. Bacturia
d. Crystals
e. Glomerulonephritis
f. Glycosuria
g. Hematuria
h. Ketones
i. Micturate
j. Occult
k. Oliguria
l. Parasites
m. Polyuria
n. Proteinuria
o. Renal threshold
p. Sediment
q. Specific gravity
r. Spermatozoa
s. Turbid
t. Urinalysis

1. __________ To urinate.
2. __________ The absence of urine.
3. __________ Excessive amounts of urine production.
4. __________ Blood in the urine.
5. __________ The male reproductive cell.
6. __________ Bacteria in the urine.
7. __________ It means that the urine is opaque and does not allow light to pass through.
8. __________ The term for the presence of abnormal sugar in the urine.
9. __________ The solid material that settles at the bottom of a test tube after centrifugation.
10. __________ Provides valuable information about many functions in the body, including kidney function.
11. __________ Formed by the precipitation of urinary salts when the pH, temperature, or concentration changes.
12. __________ The concentration at which a substance excreted by the kidneys, such as glucose, begins to appear in urine.
13. __________ The byproducts of fat metabolism.
14. __________ The weight of a substance in relation to the weight of the same amount of distilled water.
15. __________ Chemical material without shape.

16. __________ The presence of hidden blood in the urine.
17. __________ Organisms that live within other organisms.
18. __________ The presence of protein.
19. __________ Decreased amounts of urine production.
20. __________ A kidney disease that involves inflammation and lesions in the glomeruli.

APPLIED PRACTICE

Follow the directions as instructed with each question below.

1. Label the parts of the refractometer.

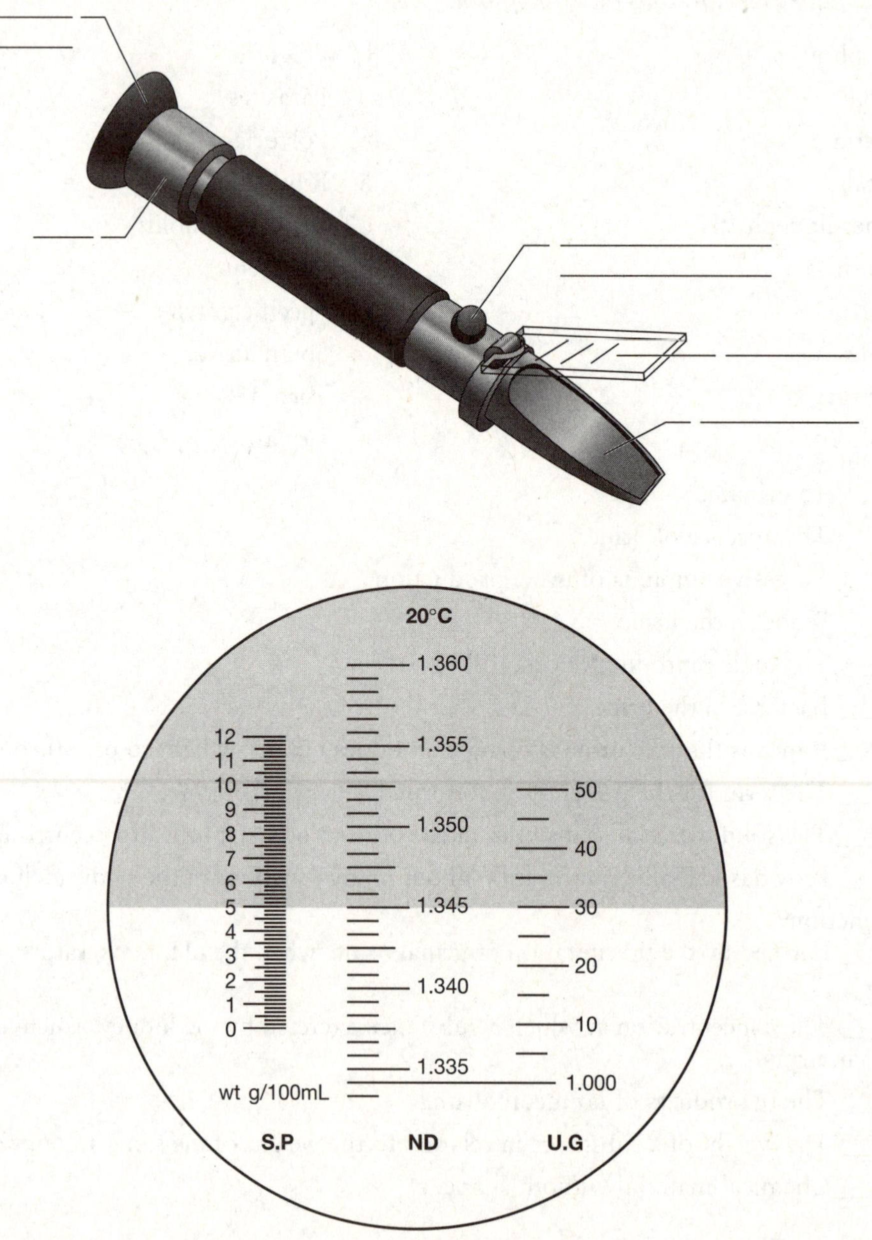

2. By each of the following microscopic images, note what is being seen in each urine sample.

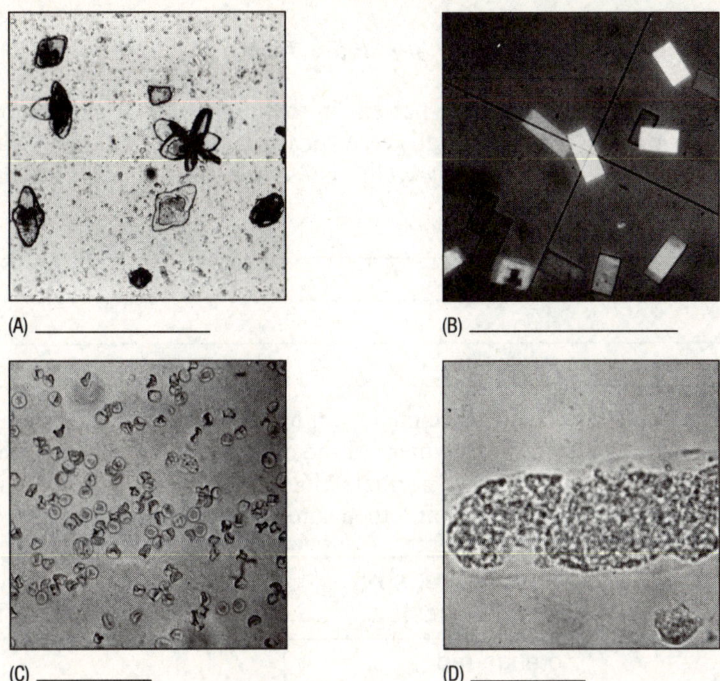

LEARNING ACTIVITY: FILL IN THE BLANK

Using words from the list below, fill in the blanks to complete the following statements.

acidity	organisms
alkalinity	overall
bile duct	physical
foreskin	positive
fruity	random
labia	slows

1. Urine samples provide valuable indicators of the __________ health of the patient.
2. A ___________ sample of urine is the most commonly collected type of urine specimen.
3. When collecting clean-catch specimens, be sure that the female patient understands how to clean the ___________ and the male knows how to clean the ____________.
4. Refrigeration of a specimen _________ the growth of bacteria and specimen deterioration, but does not stop it.
5. The ___________ characteristics of urine may be important diagnostic tools for the physician.
6. Individuals testing positive for ketones may have a ___________ odor to their urine.
7. The pH of a solution indicates __________ and __________.
8. If urobilinogen is not present, a _____ _________ obstruction may be present.
9. If a leukocyte test is positive, then a protein test should be ___________.
10. Microscopic examination identifies the type and approximate number of __________ present in a urine specimen.

CRITICAL THINKING

Answer the following questions to the best of your ability. Utilize the textbook as a reference.

1. You are to instruct a 68-year-old female patient in the collection of a 24-hour urine specimen. Explain this, in your own words, as if you were speaking to the patient. Avoid medical terms that the patient may not understand very well; also avoid treating the patient as if she were a child.

____

____

____

____

2. You have collected a clean-catch urine specimen from Mrs. Gonzalez, a long-time patient, and you have already performed the physical assessment of the color, odor, and clarity. The following are the results of your chemical testing. Fill in the normal value for each, circle those which are abnormal as if you were flagging them for the physician, and then state the possible reasons for the abnormal results.

Tests	Your Results on Mrs. Gonzalez	Normal Value	Possible Causes
Color	orange-red		
Clarity	cloudy		
pH	7.8		
Specific gravity	1.026		
Protein	++ or positive		
Glucose	0		
Ketones	0		
Bilirubin	0		
Urobilinogen	4		
Blood	+		
Leukocytes	++++		
Nitrite	0		

RESEARCH ACTIVITY

Utilize Internet search engines to research the following topics and write a brief description of what you find. It is important to utilize reputable websites.

1. To learn more about the Clinical Laboratory Improvement Amendments (CLIA) waived test, consult the Internet and/or use school or local library resources. Write an essay on what you learned from your research regarding CLIA and waived tests.

____

____

____

CHAPTER 47
Hematology

CHAPTER OUTLINE

General review of the chapter:

The Medical Assistant's Role
Blood Formation and Components
The Function of Blood
Blood Specimen Collection
Routine Blood Tests
Erythrocyte Sedimentation Rate
Phenylketonuria
Mono Testing
Blood Chemistry Panels

STUDENT STUDY GUIDE

Use the following guide to assist in your learning of the concepts from the chapter.

I. The Formation and Components of Blood

1. Blood Formation and Blood Components
   A. Blood cells originate from the ___________ ___________ cell.
   B. Blood cells mature into one of ___________ individual types of cells.
2. Red Blood Cells (RBCs)
   A. RBCs are formed in ____________ ____________.
   B. Contain _____________.
   C. Formation is controlled somewhat by ________________.
   D. They last for about _____ months and are continuously being reproduced in the body.
   E. The normal RBC range for a male adult is _____ to _____ million/mm^3.
   F. The normal RBC range for a female is _____ to _____ million/mm^3.
3. The Function of Hemoglobin
   A. Carries oxygen from the lungs to the ____________ of the body.
   B. Carries __________ __________ from the body back to the lungs, where it can be expelled with exhalation.
4. White Blood Cells (WBCs)
   A. WBCs are also known as ___________.
   B. Produced in the bone marrow from ____________ ____________.
   C. They are larger than ____________ blood cells.
   D. Their principal function is to ____________ against infection.
   E. The range of WBCs in an adult is _______ to _______ thousand/mm^3.

5. Leukocyte Classification
   A. Granulocytes (Briefly explain each.)
      i. Basophils: ____________________
      ii. Eosinophils: ____________________
      iii. Neutrophils: ____________________
   B. Agranulocytes
      i. Monocytes: ____________________
      ii. Lymphocytes: ____________________
6. Basophils
   A. Thought to be produced by the __________ __________.
   B. Produce __________.
   C. Patients who have had excessive exposure to radiation may have __________ basophils.
   D. Appear in tissues where an __________ __________ is occurring.
7. Eosinophils
   A. Assumed to be produced by the __________ __________.
   B. Detection of a large number of eosinophils can indicate a __________ condition or the presence of certain __________ conditions.
   C. Have granules that produce a __________ color on the laboratory-stained slide.
8. Neutrophils
   A. Divided into two categories: __________ neutrophils and __________ neurophils.
   B. The body reproduces neutrophils on an ongoing basis, and they only survive for __________ days.
   C. Reproduction is increased when __________ __________ is occurring.
   D. Neutrophils combat infection by __________.
   E. Phagocytosis is the process in which the __________ surrounds, swallows, and digests the __________.
9. Monocytes
   A. Formed in the __________ __________ from stem cells.
   B. Assist in __________.
   C. Ingest foreign particles or __________ that the neutrophils are unable to digest.
   D. Assist in cleaning up __________ debris that may have been left from the infection.
   E. An increase in monocytes is seen in patients who have certain diseases such as tuberculosis, typhoid, and __________ __________ __________ fever.
10. Lymphocytes
   A. Produced in the __________ __________ and in __________ __________ such as the spleen and lymph nodes.
   B. Produce __________ against foreign substances such as bacteria, viruses, and pollens.
   C. Are small and large and can proliferate into __________ and __________ cells.
   D. Lymphocytes do not have __________ and are nonsegmented.
11. Platelets (Thrombocytes)
   A. Formed in the __________ __________.
   B. Main function is to assist in the __________ of blood.
   C. Leads to formation of thrombin, which converts __________ to __________.
   D. Typically between __________ and __________ platelets/mm^3.
12. Solutes in the Plasma
      i. ____________________
      ii. ____________________
      iii. ____________________
      iv. ____________________

v. ______________________________
vi. ______________________________
vii. ______________________________
viii. ______________________________
ix. ______________________________
x. ______________________________

13. The Function of Blood

i. ______________________________
ii. ______________________________
iii. ______________________________
iv. ______________________________
v. ______________________________

II. Blood Specimen Collection

1. Steps for Quality Control When Collecting a Blood Specimen

A. __________ the request and __________ the test ordered.
B. Prepare the necessary __________ and work area.
C. Perform __________ __________ and don gloves.
D. Confirm that the patient has followed any __________ __________ requirements.
E. __________ the specimen properly, using the appropriate equipment and technique.
F. Use the appropriate __________ container and the correct preservatives.
G. Immediately label the specimen with the patient's __________, the date and __________ of collection, the test's name, and the __________ of the __________ who collected the specimen.
H. Follow the correct procedures for disposing of __________ __________ __________ and decontaminating the work area and equipment according to OSHA guidelines.
I. If the specimen is to be transported to an __________ __________, prepare it for transport in the proper container, with all of the appropriate information according to __________ guidelines.
J. The type and amount of the __________ required are determined by the __________ that will be performed.

2. Venipuncture

A. Used to collect __________ volumes of blood.
B. Three methods are used
   i. A vacuum tube is used for a __________ __________.
   ii. A syringe and needle are used if there is no __________ __________.
   iii. A butterfly is used for a __________ __________.

3. Vacuum Blood Tube Order for Filling

i. ______________________________
ii. ______________________________
iii. ______________________________
iv. ______________________________
v. ______________________________
vi. ______________________________
vii. ______________________________

4. Vacutainer® Color, Additive, and Function (Briefly explain each additive and function.)

A. Yellow
   i. The additive is ______________________________.
   ii. Prevents ______________________________.
   iii. Used for ______________________________.

B. Light blue
   i. The additive is ______.
   ii. Removes ______.
   iii. Used for ______.
C. Red
   i. Contains ______.
   ii. Used for ______.
D. Red marbled
   i. The additive is ______.
   ii. Enhances ______.
   iii. Used for ______.
E. Green
   i. The additive is ______.
   ii. Prevents ______.
   iii. Used for ______.
F. Light green
   i. The additive is ______.
   ii. Aids in ______.
   iii. Used for ______.
G. Lavender
   i. The additive is ______.
   ii. Removes ______.
   iii. Used for ______.
H. Pink, white, or royal blue
   i. The additive is ______.
   ii. Prevents ______.
   iii. Used for ______.
I. Gray
   i. The additive is ______.
   ii. Removes ______.
   iii. Used for ______.
J. Dark blue
   i. The additive is ______.
   ii. Detects ______.

5. Sites for Venipuncture
   i. ______
   ii. ______
   iii. ______

6. Patient Preparation
   A. Educate the patient properly ______ and ______ the procedure.
   B. Assemble the equipment ahead of time to show ______.
   C. Deal with ______ events professionally.
   D. Wear ______ for safety.

7. Steps for Obtaining Venous Blood with a Sterile Syringe and Needle
   A. Apply a tourniquet ______ to ______ inches above the antecubital space.
   B. ______ the vein, clean the venipuncture site with an ______ sponge, and then dry with clean gauze.
   C. Have the patient make a ______ and hold it shut until he or she is told to release it.
   D. Make sure that there is no ______ in the syringe and that the ______ moves freely.
   E. Remove the ______ ______ and insert the needle into the vein.
   F. Slowly pull back the syringe ______ until the proper amount of blood has been obtained.
   G. Instruct the patient to ______ his or her fist.

H. Release the __________ and withdraw the needle quickly.
I. Place a piece of cotton or gauze on the puncture site, and instruct the patient to maintain __________ on the site and to bend his or her arm.
J. Fill the appropriate __________ tubes to the proper level.

8. The Butterfly Method of Venipuncture
   A. Uses a needle that is attached to ______- to ______-inch tubing.
   B. The end of the tubing can be attached to the __________ or the __________ __________ tube holder.
   C. The butterfly method is used for __________ veins that are difficult to draw from with the standard vacuum container method or syringe and needle method.
   D. It is called the butterfly method because the needle on the end has a __________ portion that keeps the needle from turning and __________ the needle into the small vein.
   E. The needle used for the butterfly method is a small ______-, ______-, or ______-gauge needle.
   F. The drawback to performing the butterfly method is the __________.

9. Capillary Puncture
   A. Capillaries are the blood vessels between the __________ and the __________.
   B. __________ __________ and oxygen are exchanged at this level.
   C. Use this method to collect __________ amounts of blood.

10. Equipment and Supplies for Capillary Puncture
    i. ______________________________
    ii. ______________________________
    iii. ______________________________
    iv. ______________________________
    v. ______________________________
    vi. ______________________________
    vii. ______________________________
    viii. ______________________________
    ix. ______________________________
    x. ______________________________

11. Steps for Performing a Capillary Puncture
    A. Select the __________ or __________ finger on the nondominant hand; wipe with alcohol.
    B. Remove the plastic protective tip of the __________.
    C. Grasp the patient's hand and squeeze the finger gently 1 inch __________ the puncture site.
    D. Puncture with a quick, jabbing motion across the __________ to get a full blood drop.
    E. Wipe away the __________ __________ with gauze.
    F. Obtain the sample using a ________________ capillary tube.
    G. Apply clean gauze over the site and ask the patient to apply __________.

12. Routine Blood Tests
    i. ______________________________
    ii. ______________________________
    iii. ______________________________
    iv. ______________________________
    v. ______________________________
    vi. ______________________________
    vii. ______________________________
    viii. ______________________________

13. Recording Laboratory Test Results
    A. Methods by which results are received
       i. ______________________________
       ii. ______________________________

B. Contents of most lab reports include:
    i. ______
    ii. ______
    iii. ______

14. Equipment Used for Determining Blood Glucose
    i. ______
    ii. ______
    iii. ______
    iv. ______
    v. ______
    vi. ______
    vii. ______
    viii. ______
    ix. ______
    x. ______

15. Steps for Screening for Blood Glucose Level
    A. Identify the patient and make sure that the patient has ______, if required.
    B. Make sure that the ______ has been turned on for the required amount of time and has been ______ for accuracy according to the manufacturer's instructions.
    C. Perform a ______ blood puncture with a sterile lancet.
    D. Remove a plastic ______ ______ from the bottle without touching the chemically treated portion.
    E. After wiping away the first drop of blood with a ______ ______, gently touch the test strip to the second drop of blood that has formed on the patient's finger.
    F. Immediately ______ ______ for the duration specified by the manufacturer.
    G. Provide the patient with a ______ ______ ______ to hold over the puncture site after wiping the site with an alcohol sponge.
    H. Record in the patient's chart the number of ______ of glucose per ______ as displayed on the glucometer screen.

16. Normal Values for Common Laboratory Tests
    A. Total cholesterol: ______
    B. Glucose: ______
    C. Triglycerides: ______
    D. Creatinine: ______
    E. Uric acid: ______
    F. BUN: ______
    G. Sodium: ______
    H. Potassium: ______
    I. Chloride: ______
    J. CO_2: ______
    K. White blood cells: ______
    L. Red blood cells: ______
    M. Hemoglobin: ______
    N. Hematocrit: ______
    O. Sedimentation rate: ______
    P. Platelets: ______

17. Microhematocrit
    A. Provides the physician with information about the patient's ______ ______ cell volume.
    B. A ______ hematocrit indicates anemia or hemorrhaging.
    C. An ______ hematocrit indicates dehydration or polycythemia.
    D. A ______ hematocrit is 40–50% in males and 35–45% in females.

18. Performing a Microhematocrit
    A. Fill__________ capillary tubes three-quarters full.
    B. Seal one end with the __________ __________.
    C. Place the capillary tubes in the __________ with the sealed ends against the __________ __________.
    D. If more than one patient's blood is being tested, write down the __________ of the __________ that the patient's tube is in.
    E. Spin for 3 to 5 minutes at __________ rpms.
    F. After centrifuging, the sample will be separated into three layers.
        i. The top layer is __________.
        ii. The middle layer, or the buffy coat, is made up of __________ and __________.
        iii. The bottom layer is __________ __________.
    G. Remove the tubes immediately after the centrifuge __________. If the tubes are not removed immediately, the blood may begin to __________ __________.
    H. Use the __________ __________ by placing the sealing clay just below the zero line on both tubes. Then, on both tubes, match the __________ of the __________ with the 100 line.
    I. Read the results on both tubes directly below the __________ __________. Then add those results together and divide by ______.
    J. Discard the tubes into the __________ container.
    K. Record the value as a __________ on the patient's medical record.

19. Hemoglobin
    A. Low hemoglobin may indicate __________-__________ __________.
    B. Elevated readings are present in patients with __________ and in extreme situations, such as burns.
    C. Normal values for adult females are _____ to _____ g/dL, and for males, _____ to _____ g/dL.
    D. Can either be measured by an automated blood analyzer or manually by using a ________________.
    E. Typically, the __________ __________ is less accurate and not as reliable as the automated blood analyzer.

20. Equipment Used to Measure Hemoglobin
    i. ______________________________
    ii. ______________________________

21. Methods for Determining Hemoglobin Values
    i. ______________________________
    ii. ______________________________

22. White Blood Cells (WBCs)
    A. There are __________ types of WBCs, each with distinct characteristics.
    B. Count __________ WBCs, then express each cell type as a __________.
    C. Values may differ between __________ and __________ analyses.

23. Normal White Blood Cell Values for Adults
    A. Neutrophils: ________________
    B. Eosinophils: ________________
    C. Basophils: ________________
    D. Lymphocytes: ________________
    E. Monocytes: ________________

24. Red Blood Cells (RBCs)
    A. RBCs are ________ colored.
    B. They appear ________ with slightly ________ centers.
    C. They have no ________ or ________.

D. RBCs with nuclei are called __________.
E. Normal-looking RBCs are recorded as ______________________.

25. Performing a Manual Red Blood Cell Count
   A. Requires a small specimen sample to be __________ in a special solution.
   B. Place the sample in a _______________.
   C. Place the _______________ on a ____________ used to count RBCs and WBCs.
   D. The automated test for __________ is more common than __________ testing.

26. Differential White Blood Cell Count
   A. Determines the __________ of each type of WBC, RBC morphology, and platelet estimation.
   B. Performing this test __________ is a skill that requires practice to achieve proficiency.
   C. Testing is done using a microscope with a bright light and __________ magnification with an __________ __________ slide.
   D. Focus near the edge of the stained slide where the cells are __________ and where the cells are __________ layer thick.
   E. The test can also be performed by the __________ analyzer.

27. Preparing Slides for a Differential White Blood Cell Count
   A. Obtain a whole-blood sample using __________ as the anticoagulant of choice. Blood must be __________ thoroughly before testing.
   B. Using a dropper, place one drop of __________ __________ blood on the end of a clean, glass slide.
   C. Using the short side of another __________, __________ slide, back the slide to the drop of blood.
   D. Allow the blood to spread across the __________ side of the slide.
   E. Holding the spreader slide at a ____-__________ angle, spread the blood across the length of the slide.
   F. Use gentle, continuous pressure and a smooth gliding motion to create a __________.
   G. Notice that the smear has a __________ side that gradually changes to a __________ side.
   H. The thin side has a __________ edge, and the blood covers __________-__________ to __________-__________ the length of the slide.
   I. Allow the slide to air dry on a __________.
   J. Label the __________ edge of the slide with the patient's name and the date.
   K. Stain the slide using __________ staining method.
   L. Flood the slide with stain for exactly _____ seconds or the amount of time indicated by the manufacturer.
   M. Rinse with __________ water until the water runs clear.
   N. Allow the slide to __________ __________ before examining it under the microscope.
   O. __________ findings may need to be referred to a laboratory technician for analysis.

28. Platelets
   A. Platelets are about __________ the size of RBCs.
   B. They stain __________ and tend to appear in a clump.
   C. They appear to have a __________ __________ edge and contain small granules.
   D. There are typically between _____ and _____ platelets in one field of view.

29. The Erythrocyte Sedimentation Rate (ESR)
   A. The ESR is also called the __________ rate.
   B. Drawing a patient's ESR can be done using either the __________ or __________ method.
   C. When performing the _____________ method, the _____________ tube is calibrated in millimeters per hour.
   D. Depending on the type of method used, the __________ values may vary.
   E. The Wintrobe method indicates that the normal ESR in an adult female is _____ to _____ mm/hr; in an adult male, it is 0 to 9 mm/hr.

F. Increased values may indicate an ____________.
G. A person's ESR may also be elevated because of a variety of reasons, including __________, __________, and malignant tumors.
H. The sed rate is related to the condition of the red blood cells and the amount of __________ in the plasma.
I. When a sed rate test is conducted on a patient, the rate at which the RBCs __________ indicates the existence of possible conditions.

30. Phenylketonuria (PKU)
A. PKU is a __________ disease.
B. The unmetabolized portion of the __________ __________ phenylalanine accumulates in the bloodstream.
C. If undetected, it results in __________ __________.
D. The PKU test is always performed on __________ to determine the presence of the __________ protein phenylalanine.

31. Equipment for Performing a Phenylketonuria Test
i. ______________________________
ii. ______________________________
iii. ______________________________
iv. ______________________________
v. ______________________________

32. Testing for Mononucleosis (Mono)
A. The test is called the mononucleosis __________ test.
B. Used to help determine whether a patient has __________ __________.
C. Ordered with a ____________________ and a strep test.
D. Common in __________ patients who show symptoms of fever, headache, swollen glands, and fatigue.
E. If a patient has a positive mono test, an increased number of white blood cells, __________ __________, and symptoms, then the patient is diagnosed with infectious mononucleosis.
F. If the mono test is __________, but other symptoms exist, it may be too early to detect mono.

33. Equipment for Performing a Mononucleosis Spot Test
i. ______________________________
ii. ______________________________
iii. ______________________________
iv. ______________________________
v. ______________________________
vi. ______________________________
vii. ______________________________
viii. ______________________________
ix. ______________________________

34. Performing a Mononucleosis Spot Test
A. Perform a __________ stick on the patient.
B. Fill a __________ tube end to end, dispensing all of the blood into the test tube.
C. Slowly add _____ drop of __________ to the bottom of the test tube and mix.
D. Remove the __________ stick(s) from the container and recap the container immediately.
E. Place the __________ end of the test stick into the treated sample. Leave the test stick in the test tube.
F. Read the results at _____ minutes.
G. Positive results may be read as soon as the __________ __________ __________ appears.
H. Document the findings in the patient's record.
  i. Positive: A blue __________ line and a red __________ line is a positive result.
  ii. Negative: A red __________ line but no blue __________ line is a negative result.

KEY TERMINOLOGY REVIEW

Match the vocabulary term to the correct definition below.

a. Anemia
b. Antecubital space
c. Basophils
d. Capillaries
e. Carboxyhemoglobin
f. Electrolytes
g. Erythrocyte sedimentation rate (ESR)
h. Erythropoietin
i. Hematology
j. Hematopoiesis
k. Hemoglobin
l. Heparin
m. Lymphocytes
n. Microhematocrit
o. Monocytes
p. Mononucleosis
q. Oxyhemoglobin
r. Phenylketonuria
s. Platelets
t. Serum

1. __________ Blood carrying carbon dioxide.
2. __________ The formation of blood cells.
3. __________ The rate at which RBCs settle at the bottom of a tube.
4. __________ Deficiency of hemoglobin caused by a lack of RBCs.
5. __________ A crit performed on an extremely small quantity of blood.
6. __________ Plasma without the fibrinogen.
7. __________ The study of blood and the tissues that produce it.
8. __________ A contagious viral infection that frequently is spread through oral contact.
9. __________ Ionic solutions containing free ions.
10. __________ A depression in the front of the elbow, it is the most commonly used site for venipuncture.
11. __________ The WBCs produced in the lymphoid tissue, such as the spleen and the lymph nodes.
12. __________ The smallest of the body's blood vessels.
13. __________ The largest of WBCs, they have a nucleus that is shaped like a kidney bean.
14. __________ A congenital disease caused by a defect in the metabolism of the amino acid phenylalanine.
15. __________ A metalloprotein that aids in oxygen transportation in the RBCs.
16. __________ Hemoglobin-carrying oxygen.
17. __________ Like other white cells, these are thought to be produced by the bone marrow; they produce heparin.
18. __________ A substance that prevents clotting.
19. __________ A glycoprotein hormone that controls RBC production.
20. __________ The smallest cells found in the blood, they are formed in the bone marrow.

APPLIED PRACTICE

Follow the directions as instructed with each question below.

1. **Scenario**

Julie Turner is working as a clinical medical assistant. A patient, Hector Olanski, comes in for a blood draw. The physician's order reads as follows:

> **COOK FAMILY MEDICINE**
> (188) 555-1111
>
> Patient: Hector Olanski — DOB: 7-3-1938
> Date: 3-22-20XX
>
> Rx PTT and CBC
>
> Dx: (1) Heparin monitoring (E934.2)
> (2) Phlebitis of lower extremities (451.2)
>
> **Dr. Liam Cook**

While gathering supplies, Julie grabs a lavender-topped tube, a red-topped tube, and a light-blue-topped tube.

a. Did Julie collect the correct tubes for Mr. Olanski's blood draw? Why or why not? Explain your answer based on each of the tubes of blood that Julie collected.

____

____

____

____

b. What would be the correct order of draw?

____

____

____

c. Are there any additives in the tubes that Julie is using for the blood draw? If so, explain which additives are used (based on the color) and the action of the additive.

____

____

____

____

2. Fill in the label below according to how Julie should label each of Mr. Olanski's tubes of blood.

LEARNING ACTIVITY: TRUE/FALSE

Indicate whether the statement is true (T) or false (F).

_______ 1. Partially filled tubes, especially the light-blue-topped tube, can cause erroneous test results, resulting in the patient's blood needing to be redrawn.

_______ 2. Occasionally, uncontrollable bleeding can occur when the needle is withdrawn.

_______ 3. Capillary puncture is also called a fingerstick.

_______ 4. Blood analysis is not considered to be a routine tool of medicine.

_______ 5. Wait until all of the blood tubes have been collected before asking the patient to release his or her fist.

_______ 6. The National Committee for Clinical Laboratory Standards (NCCLS) has instituted a recommended order of draw to minimize the effects of additive carryover.

_______ 7. MCV, MVHV, and MCV are used to differentiate specific types of anemia.

_______ 8. When drawing blood, you should not promise the patient that the procedure will not hurt.

_______ 9. The functions of blood are transportation and hydration.

_______ 10. The liquid component of blood is called plasma.

CRITICAL THINKING

Answer the following questions to the best of your ability. Utilize the textbook as a reference.

1. A patient needs to have blood drawn for an ESR and a glucose level. The patient is extremely nervous and worried about the pain that she will experience with a blood draw and asks if you can "stick her finger" instead. Will that work in this scenario? Why or why not?

____

____

____

____

2. You have drawn three tubes of blood (gray-topped, lavender-topped, and green-topped). You filled the lavender-topped tube first, the gray-topped tube second, and the green-topped tube last. Is this the correct order of draw? If not, what could possibly happen because of this?

____

____

____

____

3. A patient has come in today for a blood draw to check her cholesterol level. She is 78 years old, has fragile skin, and her veins are impossible to see. Which method of phlebotomy would you use on this patient and why?

____

____

____

____

4. Your next patient for phlebotomy today is a 6-year-old child. What special considerations are appropriate for this patient?

RESEARCH ACTIVITY

Utilize Internet search engines to research the following topics and write a brief description of what you find. It is important to utilize reputable websites.

1. Visit the Clinical and Laboratory Standards Institute at www.clsi.org. Navigate through the website and identify reasons why the website would be beneficial for medical assistants working in a clinical or physician's office laboratory.

CHAPTER 48
Radiology

CHAPTER OUTLINE

General review of the chapter:

Radiology
Overview of Diagnostic Imaging
Preparing and Positioning the Patient
Diagnostic Imaging Procedures
Radiation Therapy
Nuclear Medicine
Safety Precautions
Radiographic Equipment
Processing X-ray Film
Storage and Records
Ownership of Film

STUDENT STUDY GUIDE

Use the following guide to assist in your learning of the concepts from the chapter.

I. Introduction to Radiology

1. Radiology
   A. Radiology is the branch of medicine that uses __________ substances, or matter that gives off __________.
   B. Uses various techniques for visualizing the __________ structures of the body for the diagnosis and treatment of disease.
   C. Divided into three specialties
      i. ______________________________
      ii. ______________________________
      iii. ______________________________
2. Radiology Personnel
   A. A __________ is a physician who specializes in radiology.
   B. A __________, or __________ technologist, makes diagnostic radiographs, or X-rays.
3. The Duties of a Radiological Technologist
   A. __________ patients for radiographic procedures.
   B. Determines the proper __________, __________, and __________ time for each X-ray.
   C. __________ radiographic equipment.
   D. Develops the __________.
   E. Assists the __________ with special procedures.

4. The Principles of X-rays

   A. Developed in 1895 by __________ __________ __________.
   B. X-rays are produced in a __________ __________ when electrons collide.
   C. This collision produces ______________ rays.
   D. X-rays coming from the tube form an X-ray __________.
   E. The radiation field is a cross section of the X-ray beam and the __________ of __________.
   F. The patient is placed between the tube that produces the X-ray __________ and the __________.

5. Characteristics of X-rays

   A. X-rays penetrate substances of different __________ to varying __________.
   B. Cause __________ of the substances through which they pass.
   C. Cause certain substances to __________.
   D. Travel in a __________ __________.
   E. Can __________ body cells.

6. Diagnostic Imaging

   A. Involves the use of the following
      i. ______________________________
      ii. ______________________________
      iii. ______________________________
      iv. ______________________________
      v. ______________________________

7. The Contrast Medium

   A. The contrast medium is a ____________ substance.
   B. Does not allow the __________ of X-rays.
   C. Include __________ (barium), __________, air, and gas.
   D. Administered orally, by __________ (parenterally), or by __________.
   E. Acts to convert an __________ or structure into an __________ area.

8. Contrast Medium Materials

   A. Barium sulfate
      i. Barium sulfate is a positive __________ ________.
      ii. Consists of a ______ compound mixed with water.
      iii. Used for ______________ examination.
   B. Iodine contrast compounds
      i. Used to form ___________ compounds.
      ii. Cannot be used on patients who are allergic to _________ **or** _________.
      iii. Interfere with _________ medicine.
   C. Negative contrast
      i. Appears ________ on X-rays.
      ii. Used to visualize the __________.

9. The Role of the Medical Assistant During Radiology Exams

   A. Schedules the __________.
   B. __________ the patient about the procedure.
   C. Explains to the patient any __________ required.
   D. Ensures that the patient is provided with an __________-__________ gown and drape.
   E. Requests that the patient remove all __________ materials.
   F. Assists the patient __________ and __________ the procedure.
   G. Provides __________-__________ instructions.
   H. Informs the patient about __________ to __________ the results.

10. X-ray Procedures That Require Special Preparation
    A. Angiogram: No __________ if the examination is in the morning or __________ if the examination is in the afternoon.
    B. Barium enema (Lower GI)
        i. Enemas are administered until the bowel return is __________ on the evening before the examination.
        ii. The doctor may order a rectal __________ in the morning or a __________ such as 2 oz. of castor oil or citrate of magnesia at 4:00 P.M. the day before the procedure.
        iii. The patient is to have clear liquids and __________ for dinner.
        iv. Nothing may be taken by mouth (NPO) after __________.
    C. Barium meal (Upper GI): NPO after __________.
    D. Cholecystogram (GB series)
        i. The patient may have a light supper of non-fatty food, such as __________ and __________ without __________ or oil, the evening before the procedure.
        ii. __________ tablets (prescribed by the physician) are taken with water after supper.
        iii. NPO except for water until after the __________ the following day.
    E. Computerized tomography (CT): NPO for _____ hours before the procedure if a __________ medium is used.
    F. Intravenous pyelogram (IVP)
        i. Three __________ tablets or 2 oz. of __________ __________at 4:00 P.M. the day before the procedure.
        ii. Eat a __________ supper.
        iii. __________ after midnight.
    G. Retrograde pyelogram
        i. Enemas are administered or ____________ are taken on the __________ before the procedure.
        ii. NPO for _____ hours before the procedure.
    H. Ultrasound: May require a full _________ or __________, depending on the type of ultrasound.

12. Steps for Assisting with a Radiological Procedure
    A. Check the X-ray examination __________.
    B. Check the necessary X-ray __________ as needed.
    C. Identify the patient and determine whether the patient has complied with the __________ __________.
    D. Explain the procedure to the patient, and then instruct the patient to remove __________ as necessary for the procedure.
    E. Ask the patient to remove all __________ and __________.

13. Anteroposterior (AP)
    A. The X-ray beam is directed from __________ to __________.
    B. The patient may be standing or __________.
    C. The patient's front will face the X-ray __________ and the patient's back will be near the __________ __________.

14. Posterioanterior (PA)
    A. The X-ray beam is directed from __________ to __________.
    B. The patient will be standing __________.
    C. The patient's __________ will face the X-ray equipment and his or her __________ will be near the film plate.

15. The Oblique Position
    A. The patient is turned at an angle to the film plate so that the X-ray beam can be directed at an area that would be hidden on an _____, _____, or __________ X-ray.

16. The Lateral Position
    A. The X-ray beam is directed toward __________ __________ of the body.
    B. In the right lateral (RL) position, the patient's right side is near the __________ __________ and the left side is near the __________ __________.
    C. In the left lateral (LL) position, the patient's __________ side is near the film plate.
17. The Axial Position
    A. The X-ray tube is angled to direct the X-ray beam along the __________ of the body or body part.
    B. With __________ angulation, the X-ray beam is directed at an angle from the feet toward the head.
    C. With __________ angulation, the X-ray beam is directed from the head toward the feet.
18. Information Required for Scheduling a Radiological Procedure
    i. ______________________________
    ii. ______________________________
    iii. ______________________________
    iv. ______________________________
    v. ______________________________
19. Beverages that May Be Restricted on an All-Liquid Diet
    i. ______________________________
    ii. ______________________________
    iii. ______________________________
    iv. ______________________________
    v. ______________________________
    vi. ______________________________
    vii. ______________________________
    viii. ______________________________
20. Guidelines for Sequencing Multiple Diagnostic Procedures
    A. Schedule all radiographic examinations and tests that do not require a __________ __________ and iodine intake first.
    B. Do CT scans of the __________ and __________ before performing procedures that require barium.
    C. CT procedures that require an IV contrast medium may be done __________ blood is drawn for the iodine uptake series.

II. Diagnostic Imaging Procedures
1. General Categories of Diagnostic Imaging
    i. ______________________________
    ii. ______________________________
    iii. ______________________________
    iv. ______________________________
2. Methods for Administering Contrast Media
    i. ______________________________
    ii. ______________________________
    iii. ______________________________
    iv. ______________________________
3. Radiological Imaging Procedures That Require Contrast Media
    i. ______________________________
    ii. ______________________________
    iii. ______________________________

4. Fluoroscopy Procedures
   A. Fluoroscopy is a __________ examination of a portion of the body or the functioning of an organ using a fluoroscope.
   B. Allows the radiologist to have __________ images.
   C. It is a __________ image that is seen on the fluoroscope and can be filmed using a radiograph (X-ray) to obtain a __________ record.
   D. __________ __________ are often used to better visualize organ functioning and abnormalities.
5. Gastrointestinal Series
   A. A gastrointestinal series is a __________ study of the __________ __________.
   B. Uses a __________ medium.
   C. Can involve an upper or lower __________ __________.
6. Patient Instructions for the Upper GI Series
   A. NPO after __________.
   B. No __________.
   C. Drink __________ __________ during the procedure.
   D. The procedure can last __________ hours.
   E. __________ eating can be resumed after the procedure.
   F. Drinking __________ after the procedure is important.
   G. Stool may be __________ for a few days.
7. Patient Instructions for the Lower GI Series
   A. __________-__________ diet a few days before the procedure
   B. _____-__________ diet the morning before the procedure.
   C. A __________ may be needed the day before the procedure.
   D. An __________ or barium sulfate is given, which the patient retains during the procedure.
   E. Prior to the end of the procedure, the enema is __________ and an X-ray of the __________ __________ is taken.
   F. A regular diet can be resumed, including a lot of __________.
   G. The patient may have __________ stools for 1 or 2 days following the procedure.
8. Intravenous Pyelogram (IVP)
   A. An IVP is an examination of the kidneys, __________, and bladder.
   B. The procedure takes about _____ to _____ hours.
   C. __________ is used.
   D. __________-__________ diet, including a lot of water the day before the procedure.
   E. _____ after midnight.
   F. A __________ with an enema the night before the procedure may be ordered.
9. Cholecystogram
   A. A cholecystogram is an examination of the __________.
   B. Requires a __________ medium.
   C. Utilized when __________ has not provided a definitive diagnosis.
   D. __________-__________ meal the night before the procedure with contrast medium pills.
   E. ________ after midnight.
   F. After the procedure, the patient is asked to eat a __________ meal. _____ hour later, another X-ray is taken.
   G. __________ may occur after the procedure.
10. Myelography
   A. Myelography is a fluoroscopic procedure used to visualize the __________ __________.
   B. Involves a __________ puncture.
   C. Used to detect __________ of the spinal cord or __________ disks.
   D. Typically done if a __________ or an __________ has not provided enough detail.

11. Pneumoencephalograph
    A. Performed by injecting __________ instead of a contrast medium after some cerebral spinal fluid has been removed.
    B. Allows visualization of the __________ of the brain.
12. Angiography
    A. Provides a visualization of the __________ __________ of blood vessels after a __________ material has been injected into the blood vessels.
    B. A contrast medium is injected into an __________ or __________ by way of a catheter, which is threaded through the vessel until it reaches the correct site.
    C. Because iodine is used as the contrast medium, the patient should be tested for an __________ to iodine before the procedure begins.
    D. The patient is monitored for a few hours after the procedure for any signs of __________ from the puncture site.
13. Cardiac Catheterization
    A. Cardiac catheterization is a form of ________________.
    B. Frequently performed to assess the status of the __________ __________.
    C. The catheter is inserted into the __________ artery and fed through the arteries until it reaches the heart.
    D. If obstructions are discovered, therapeutic interventions such as __________ __________ or stent insertion can take place to relieve a blockage of the coronary arteries.
14. Arthrography
    A. Used to produce an arthrogram, or image, of the inside of a __________.
    B. Helps diagnose abnormalities of the __________, tendons, __________, and cartilage of the knee, hip, or shoulder.
    C. The procedure involves injecting a local __________ followed by a contrast medium or __________, or both, into the joint.
    D. A ____________ is used to evaluate the functioning of the joint.
    E. The procedure usually takes about 1 hour, and the patient should be advised to expect some slight __________ and__________ for a day or two.
    F. The patient should be advised to __________ the joint during that time.
15. Procedures That Do Not Require Contrast Media
    Films of the following portions of the anatomy do not require contrast media
    i. ______________________________
    ii. ______________________________
    iii. ______________________________
    iv. ______________________________
    v. ______________________________
    vi. ______________________________
    vii. ______________________________
16. Mammography
    A. Mammography is a radiological examination of the __________ __________ of the breast.
    B. Identifies benign and malignant __________ (tumors).
17. Patient Instructions for Mammography
    A. Because of the effects that these products can have on the clarity of the test, prior to the procedure patients should be instructed not to use the following
       i. ______________________________
       ii. ______________________________
       iii. ______________________________
       iv. ______________________________

18. The Mammography Procedure

A. The patient stands in __________ of the X-ray equipment.
B. The technician positions the patient carefully in order to have all __________ __________ examined.
C. The patient should be instructed to follow the technician's directions regarding the placement of __________, __________, and __________ position.
D. Patients of __________ __________ are given a lead apron to wear during the procedure.
E. Each breast is __________ compressed by the equipment to spread the tissue for better viewing.
F. X-rays are directed at __________ into the breast tissue.
G. The procedure takes a __________ __________ for each view, with the entire procedure lasting about a half hour.
H. Patients may feel discomfort because of __________ during the breast compression.

19. Addressing Breast Lumps

A. If a __________ is detected, the patient should follow up immediately with further testing and not wait to see if the __________ disappears over time.
B. Many abnormalities detected on mammograms are __________ and present no danger to the patient.
C. Once a mammogram reveals __________ tissue, a breast biopsy should be done to confirm the type of mass detected.

20. Stereotactic Breast Biopsy

A. Less __________ and less __________ than previous types of biopsies.
B. The procedure is done with the patient lying __________ __________ with the breast compressed between two __________ with the suspicious mass centered in the window of a paddle.
C. A computer determines the precise positioning of the __________ __________.
D. A small sample of ______ is taken and sent for review by a pathologist.

21. Tomography

A. Allows for the penetration of __________ areas.
B. Tomography produces __________.
C. Computed tomography produces __________ scans.

22. Computed Tomography (CT)

A. Combines radiography with computer analysis of __________ __________.
B. An X-ray camera __________ completely around the patient, and the computer accumulates __________-__________ slices from each rotation of the camera.
C. The CT scanner consists of a __________ table with a remote control; the circular structure, or __________, that houses the X-ray equipment; and an __________ __________ with monitor and computer equipment.

23. The CT Procedure

A. The patient lies on a __________ table that slides into the scanner.
B. The procedure is painless, is __________, and requires no special preparation.
C. The computer calculates various factors to detect __________ __________, such as tumors; __________ displacement; and __________ accumulation.

24. Positron Emission Tomography (PET)

A. Examines the __________ __________ of the body.
B. The patient is injected with or inhales a __________ substance.
C. Used to assist in treating the following conditions
   i. ______________________________
   ii. ______________________________
   iii. ______________________________
   iv. ______________________________

25. Magnetic Resonance Imaging (MRI)

A. Provides a visual of internal __________, __________, and structures.
B. The image is __________-__________.
C. The hard portion of __________ __________ cannot be viewed.
D. Cannot be used on patients who have __________ or __________ clips on blood vessels.
E. No __________ radiation is used.
F. MRIs allow for the observation of organ __________.

26. Patient Instructions for Magnetic Resonance Imaging

A. Remove all __________, __________ __________, and metallic objects, such as watches, belts, hearing aids, and hairpins.
B. Identify which devices, if any, have been inserted into the patient's body, such as the following
   i. ____________________
   ii. ____________________
   iii. ____________________
   iv. ____________________
C. Leave __________ __________ or devices that contain metallic or __________ __________ strips outside the MRI chamber.
D. Use patient gown if patient's clothing has __________ or metal snaps.

27. Digital Radiology

A. Uses standard __________.
B. An image is projected onto a TV or __________ __________ screen.
C. Digital angiography is used for the cardiac and __________ arteries and head and neck angiograms.

28. Ultrasound/Sonography

A. Used __________-__________ __________ to view internal structures.
B. Provides __________ monitoring and the detection of abnormalities of the heart, liver, and kidneys.

29. Patient Preparation for the Ultrasound Examination

A. The patient should wear __________-fitting garments or clothing that is easy to remove because the procedure is performed over bare skin.
B. During a fetal ultrasound or pelvic ultrasound, the patient is instructed not to __________ right before the test because a full __________ displaces the intestines and allows for a better view of the uterus.
C. The patient may be asked to drink a __________ or more of water just prior to either of these examinations.
D. For an ultrasound of the __________ or __________, the patient may be asked not to eat for several hours before the procedure.

30. Radiation Therapy

A. Uses a specific dose of radiation to kill __________ cells.
B. Normal cells are altered, but will naturally __________.
C. Radiation therapy is also known by the following names:
   i. ____________________
   ii. ____________________
   iii. ____________________

31. Types of Rays Used in Radiation Therapy (Briefly explain each type.)

A. Alpha rays
   i. ____________________
   ii. ____________________

B. Beta rays
   i. ____________________
   ii. ____________________
C. Gamma rays
   i. ____________________
   ____
   ii. ____________________

32. Conditions That Are Treated with Radiation Therapy
   i. ____________________
   ii. ____________________
   iii. ____________________
   iv. ____________________
   v. ____________________
   vi. ____________________

33. Methods for Administering Radiation (Provide the name of each of the methods described.)
   A. __________ __________ __________ (ERT): Administering calculated doses of radiation to a specific site.
   B. __________ __________ __________ (IRT): Administering radiation through a sealed container that houses radioactive material; administering radiation through a liquid form via the patient's mouth or bloodstream; or administering radiation by instilling it into a body cavity.

34. Nuclear Medicine
   A. Nuclear medicine is also known as __________ imaging.
   B. Uses radioactive __________ to treat and diagnosis diseases.
   C. Involves the use of radioactive isotopes of __________, __________, and other elements.

35. Units of Radiation (Provide the name of each type of unit.)
   A. __________: Unit used to measure the amount of ionizing radiation absorbed.
   B. __________: Unit used to measure occupational exposure.
   C. Units used to measure the effects of radiation
      i. ____________________
      ii. ____________________
      iii. ____________________

36. The Effects of Overexposure to Radiation
   i. ____________________
   ii. ____________________
   iii. ____________________
   iv. ____________________
   v. ____________________
   vi. ____________________
   vii. ____________________

37. Primary Radiation
   A. Strikes the patient either for __________ reasons or for an X-ray examination.
   B. Once the primary __________ strikes the patient, it can then become __________ radiation as it bounces off the patient.

38. Guidelines for Maintaining the Personal Safety of the Medical Assistant and the Patient
   A. Wear a __________ __________ on outer clothing when exposed to any form of radiation.
   B. Ensure that the __________ is never covered.

C. Stay behind the __________ __________ in a __________-__________ room when X-ray equipment is being used.
D. Note the __________ or lighted display which indicates that X-ray equipment is in use.
E. Check the __________ on a routine basis.
F. Wear __________ devices if you are in the room when an X-ray is being taken.
G. Have periodic testing to ensure that there are no __________ __________ from radiation exposure.
H. Ask the __________ if he or she has had any recent exposure to X-rays.
I. Place a __________ __________ over the patient's abdominal and reproductive organs for patients who are of childbearing age or are pregnant.

39. The Darkroom
   A. Used for __________ film.
   B. Contain __________ or __________ safe lights.
   C. Should always be __________ when film is being processed.
   D. Film can be processed using either __________ or automated methods.
   E. Automated processing can take _____ seconds to _____ minutes, depending on the equipment being used.

40. Storage of X-ray Films
   A. Kept in containers that protect film from light, heat, __________ __________, and moisture.
   B. Stored in a dry, cool place in a __________ __________.
   C. Stored on end to prevent __________ __________ and where expiration dates can be viewed.
   D. Films should only be __________ with one hand.
   E. Processed films should be stored in __________ __________ and filed in film cabinets.

41. Ownership of the Film
   A. __________ reports can be sent to other physicians at the patient's request.
   B. Films can be loaned to __________ physicians if necessary.
   C. Films are a __________ __________ of the patient.

KEY TERMINOLOGY REVIEW

Match the vocabulary term to the correct definition below.

a. Angiography
b. Bucky
c. Claustrophobia
d. Collimator
e. Cumulative
f. Dosimeter
g. Fluoroscopy
h. Gantry
i. Grid
j. Nuclear medicine
k. Radioactive
l. Radiation
m. Radiographs
n. Radiologist
o. Radiology
p. Radiolucent
q. Radiopaque
r. Rem
s. Retrograde pyelography
t. Transducer
u. X-rays

1. __________ Procedure using a contrast medium whereby the actual function of a particular organ or structure can be visualized.
2. __________ A branch of medicine which uses radioactive substances or matter that gives off radiation (radiant energy) and various techniques to visualize the internal structures of the body for the diagnosis and treatment of disease.
3. __________ Device that both produces and senses ultrasonic waves.
4. __________ Fear of closed-in spaces.
5. __________ Used to protect patients from secondary or scatter radiation.
6. __________ Produced in a vacuum tube when electrons, traveling at the speed of light (186,000 miles per second), collide with a target made of specific materials such as tungsten.
7. __________ Inserting a catheter into the urinary tract through the bladder and into the ureters. The dye is then sent up the tube into the ureters and kidneys, and X-rays are taken to evaluate the function of the ureters, bladder, and urethra.
8. __________ Permitting greater penetration of X-rays.
9. __________ Radiant energy.
10. __________ A radiological procedure that involves the use of a contrast medium.
11. __________ A circular structure that houses the X-ray equipment.
12. __________ Allows fewer X-rays to pass through.
13. __________ A device that controls the size and shape of the X-ray field coming from the tube.
14. __________ The ability to give off radiation as the result of the disintegration of the nucleus in an atom.
15. __________ A type of grid composed of alternating strips of lead and radiolucent material.
16. __________ X-ray images.
17. __________ A film badge worn on the outer clothing of all personnel who work with or near radiological equipment.
18. __________ The roentgen equivalent in humans.
19. __________ A physician who specializes in radiology.
20. __________ A branch of medicine that uses radioactive isotopes in the diagnosis and treatment of disease.
21. __________ Exposure to radiation is added to the effects of all previous exposures.

APPLIED PRACTICE

Follow the directions as instructed with each question below.

1. Use information from the patient's chart listed below to answer the following questions.

> Epley, Marguerite V.
> 11-24-1941
>
> 3/18/20XX, 2:15 P.M.
>
> Ht: 5'5"   Wt: 115 lbs.   T: 98.6°F   P: 90 bpm   BP: 136/88
>
> cc: Pt. presents to office with rt. lower leg pain, after falling while getting out of her bathtub. Pt. rates the pain as a 6 on a scale of 1 to 10. Rt. lower leg appears to be swollen and without bruising at this time.
>
> Jerry Li, CMA (AAMA)

Scenario: Dr. Jefferson wants Jerry, the CMA (AAMA), to perform an X-ray of Ms. Epley's lower rt. leg. The order reads as follows:

> PT: Marguerite Epley DOB: 11/24/1941
>
> Rt. lower leg X-ray. AP and lateral views.
>
> Dx: R/O Fx *(Diagnosis: Rule out fracture)*

A. Dr. Jefferson ordered an AP view. What does this mean?

____

____

B. How do you think Jerry should position the patient for the lateral view?

____

____

C. List some of the protective barriers that Jerry would implement during the X-ray.

____

____

LEARNING ACTIVITY: FILL IN THE BLANK

Using words from the list below, fill in the blanks to complete the following statements.

allergic	front to back	safety precautions
carbon dioxide	high-frequency	sonography
childbearing age	iodine	stomach
contrast medium	liquid	ultrasound
dietary	negative	ultraviolet
education	pregnant	upper GI series

1. In preparation for an __________________, the patient should not eat or drink after midnight because the __________________ must be empty for this procedure.
2. The field of radiology uses X-rays, radioactive substances, and other forms of radiant energy such as __________________ rays.
3. A __________________ is a radiopaque substance that facilitates radiographic imaging of internal structures.
4. __________________ contrast media include air, __________________, and other gases.
5. In the anteroposterior view (AP), the central ray is directed from __________________.
6. Before an X-ray, any female of __________________ must be asked whether she could be __________________.
7. With regard to patient preparation and instructions for an IVP: This procedure should not be performed on a patient who is __________________ to __________________.
8. __________________, or __________________, is the use of __________________ sound waves to image internal structures.

9. Special ________________ restrictions in preparation for radiographic procedures often call for an all-________________ diet on the day before the procedure.
10. The medical assistant's role in medical imaging may involve patient preparation and ________________, scheduling, and following ________________.

CRITICAL THINKING

Answer the following questions to the best of your ability. Utilize the textbook as a reference.

1. You have placed a patient on the table for an X-ray and notice that the lead strip around the table has a few very small cracks in it. What should you do?

____

____

____

____

2. Mr. Abdul has come in for a cholecystogram. As you put the patient into the room, you ask him if he has followed the preparation instructions of taking iodine the day before and then NPO this morning. He looks surprised and then admits that he forgot to take the iodine. What would you do?

____

____

____

____

3. A patient comes to the front desk and does not have an appointment. She wants to get her original mammogram because she is moving to another state. What can you tell this patient?

____

____

____

____

RESEARCH ACTIVITY

Utilize Internet search engines to research the following topics and write a brief description of what you find. It is important to utilize reputable websites.

1. Research your state's laws regarding limited-scope radiography. Would you be allowed to practice limited-scope radiography as a medical assistant with proper training and supervision?

____

____

____

____

____

CHAPTER 49
Electrocardiography

CHAPTER OUTLINE

General review of the chapter:

Heart Structure and Function
The Electrocardiogram
Special Procedures

STUDENT STUDY GUIDE

Use the following guide to assist in your learning of the concepts from the chapter.

I. Heart Structure and Function

1. The Function of the Cardiovascular System

   A. Deoxygenated blood circulates through the body and discharges ______ ________, the waste product of cell metabolism, from the lungs.
   B. Blood circulates throughout the body and returns from the general circulation by way of the _________ and _________ vena cava, to the _______ atrium, moving in one direction from the heart.
   C. When the ________ atrium is full, the atrium ____________ and blood is pumped in the right ____________ through the _________ valve.
   D. Upon filling, the blood is pumped by the contraction of the right ______________ through the ____________ valves into the pulmonary artery going to the ________.
   E. Blood is then _____________ and returned to the left __________ through the four _________ veins.
   F. When that chamber is full, it contracts and blood is squeezed into the _______ ventricle through the _________ valve.
   G. In the ______ ventricle, blood enters the _______ semilunar valve and moves into all parts of the body except the _________.
   H. Blood travels to all parts of the body via the ________ and then goes into all other arteries.
   I. The heart muscle receives a supply of oxygen and nutrients through the _______ __________ system.

2. Heart Valves

   A. Act as gates to prevent the _____________ flow of blood.
   B. Open and shut in response to the changing __________ brought by cardiac contraction and _____________.

3. The Conduction System of the Heart

   A. The SA node normally serves as the ___________ of the heart.
   B. The normal rating of the SA node is ____________ beats per minute.
   C. The AV node will generate ________ beats per minute.

D. The bundle of His will generate less than ______ beats per minute.
E. The Purkinje system will generate rhythms in an ___________.

4. Heart Sounds Associated with Abnormal Conditions

A. Causes of heart murmurs
i. ______________________________
ii. ______________________________
iii. ______________________________

II. Performing an Electrocardiogram

1. The Electrocardiogram (EKG, also ECG)

A. The electrical charges created by the __________ system can be sensed throughout the body.
B. A normal cardiac cycle is one series of __________ waves.

2. Time and the Cardiac Cycle

A. The _______ wave represents the impulse that originated in the ______ node and spread through the _______.
B. The _______-_______ interval is the time from the beginning of _____ to the beginning of _____.
C. A _______-_______ interval that is too short means that the impulse has reached the ___________ through a shorter-than-normal pathway.
D. A _______-_______ interval that is too long means that possibly there is a ___________ delay in the _______ node.
E. The __________ complex represents the time necessary for the impulse to travel through the bundle of His, the bundle _________, and the __________ fibers to complete ____________ contraction.
F. The ST segment and the T wave represent ______________ of the ventricles.
G. The ST segment is normally _________ or only slightly ___________.
H. The T wave represents a part of the recovery of the ___________ after contraction.

3. The EKG Control Panel (Explain and/or provide important information about each part of the control panel.)

A. Main power switch: ______________________________
B. Record switch: ______________________________
C. Lead selector: ______________________________
D. Standard adjustment screw: ______________________________
E. Sensitivity control: ______________________________
F. Standard button: ______________________________
G. Stylus control: ______________________________
H. Stylus heart control: ______________________________
I. Marker: ______________________________

4. The EKG Paper

A. Paper is _______ sensitive and must be handled carefully.
B. If this paper is exposed to light for long periods, the _______ will fade with time.
C. Many newer models use an ____ ______to supply the stylus and provide a longer-lasting printout.
D. Paper records both _____ (horizontally) and ______ (vertically).

5. Time Markers on EKG Paper

A. Time markers are small ____________ with a light line and a larger ___________ with a _______ line.
B. The paper records both time and ___________.

6. Heart Rate: The 6-Second Method
   A. Begin at one ______-second marker and move to the right for two additional markers.
   B. Count the number of __________ complexes between the first and third markers.
   C. Add a ________.
7. Heart Rate: Count-off Method
   A. Locate a ________ complex close to a ______-mm line.
   B. Move to the next _____________ at the right or the left.
   C. Count how many ______-mm lines intersect the tracing before the next ______ complex.
   D. Count off at each ______-mm line.
   E. Stop counting when you reach the next ________ complex.
8. Heart Rate: Exact Calculations
   A. The paper moves at a standard speed of ______ mm/second = ______ mm/minute.
   B. Count the ____________ boxes between the two ______ complexes.
   C. Divide the number into ______.
9. Sensor Placement
   A. Sensors are placed in the following manner
      i. Over the ______ part of the inner aspect of ________ ________ ________
      ii. Over both upper ___________ or ___________, avoiding ___________
      iii. Chest electrodes are placed in ______ locations.
10. EKG Leads
    A. Each lead will record from a specific combination of _____________.
    B. By recording from different combinations of sensors, the ________ activity of the heart is seen from different ________.
11. Patient Preparation for an EKG
    A. Explain to the patient the _________ and _________ as well as what you will expect the patient to do.
    B. The surroundings should be ___________ and the table wide enough for adequate support.
    C. Patients will need to be bare to the _____________ so privacy should be provided for disrobing.
    D. Position patient in the ____________ or ____________ position.
    E. Jewelry, particularly _______ jewelry must be removed so that it does not interfere with the electrical current of the ECG.
    F. Prepare the skin where the _______ will be applied.
12. The EKG Recording
    A. Normally, the EKG recording is made in sensitivity 1 = 10 mm deflection per 1 mV of ____________.
    B. If the size is doubled, it is sensitivity _____________.
    C. If the size is cut in half, it is sensitivity _____________.
13. The Causes of Artifacts
    i. ____
    ii. ____
    iii. ____
    iv. ____
14. Mounting an EKG (List the steps.)
    i. ____
    ii. ____
    iii. ____
    iv. ____
    v. ____

15. Normal Sinus Rhythm (List the three distinct waves.)
    i. ____________________
    ii. ____________________
    iii. ____________________
16. Abnormalities Caused by Cardiac Pathology
    i. ____________________
    ii. ____________________
    iii. ____________________
    iv. ____________________
    v. ____________________
    vi. ____________________
    vii. ____________________
    viii. ____________________
    ix. ____________________
    x. ____________________
    xi. ____________________
    xii. ____________________

III. Electrocardiogram-related Diagnostic Procedures

1. Exercise Tolerance Testing
   A. Exercise tolerance testing is also called a ________ test or a ___________ test.
   B. Testing evaluates the heart's response during __________ exercise following a ______-lead EKG.
   C. May be used for the following reasons
      i. ____________________
      ii. ____________________
      iii. ____________________
      iv. ____________________
   D. Patient should be given instructions before test day to wear ______________ exercise or walking _________ and loose-fitting clothes.
   E. The physician evaluates the effect of exercise on the heart rate, ________ ________, and the EKG.
   F. The test may be stopped if the patient experiences _________ _____________ or complains of chest pain.
2. Placement of the Sensors for the Stress Test
   A. Sensors are all placed on the ____________.
   B. Arm and leg sensors are put at the ____________ line on the top of the _____ and on the ____________ line on the ____________.
3. Guidelines for the Stress Test
   A. The stress test is continued until _____% of the maximum target heart rate is achieved or the patient becomes ____________.
   B. The maximum target heart rate is calculated by using the following formula: ______________________________.
   C. For patients who have had a myocardial infarction, or a heart attack, the target heart rate is set lower at _____%.
4. The Use of Thallium
   A. Thallium is a ____________ used in nuclear medicine that emits _________ rays.
   B. Sometimes it is injected into the patient's ______________ during a stress test for a better understanding of perfusion, or blood flow, to the ____________.
   C. Normal perfusion of the ____________ is indicated by ___________ on the pictures.

5. Pharmacological Stress Testing
   A. In this test, no __________ is used. Instead, medication is given to the patient that causes the heart rate to climb to the ________ heart rate.
   B. The test is useful for patients with ____________ limitations or elderly persons who cannot perform enough exercise to elevate the heart rate.
6. Patient Safety During a Stress Test (List how patient safety may be maintained during the test.)
   i. ____________________
   ii. ____________________
   iii. ____________________
   iv. ____________________
7. The Holter Monitor
   A. The Holter monitor is used when the ______ is not conclusive or the ______ irregularity was not seen in the EKG.
   B. Patients should carry out all routine daily activities except for ________________ and ___________.
   C. Patients should avoid high-______________ areas.
8. Placement of the Holter Monitor (List the placement of each electrode.)
   i. ____________________
   ii. ____________________
   iii. ____________________
   iv. ____________________
   v. ____________________

KEY TERMINOLOGY REVIEW

Match the vocabulary term to the correct definition below.

a. Artifacts
b. Bradycardia
c. Coronary artery disease (CAD)
d. Einthoven's triangle
e. Electrocardiogram
f. Gallops
g. Heart rate
h. Holter monitor
i. Hyperventilating
j. Ischemic
k. Leads
l. Mediastinum
m. Murmurs
n. Multiple-gated acquisition (MUGA) scan
o. Pacemakers
p. Perfusion
q. Rhythm
r. Stress test
s. Tachycardia
t. Telemetry
u. Thallium
v. Wave

1. __________ The area where the heart is located in the thoracic cavity.
2. __________ A tracing, or recording, of electrical activity as it moves through the heart.
3. __________ The regularity of the occurrence of heartbeats.
4. __________ Movement away from the baseline.
5. __________ Any irregular or erratic markings on an EKG.
6. __________ A radioisotope that emits gamma rays and is used in nuclear medicine.

7. __________ Records cardiac activity while the patient is ambulatory for at least a 24-hour period.
8. __________ Blood flow to the myocardium.
9. __________ Blockage of the arteries that supply the heart muscle.
10. __________ Can be caused by damaged valves, regurgitation or backflow of blood through a valve, or high flow rates, all of which cause a kind of turbulence.
11. __________ When the heart is receiving less than the normal amount of blood flow.
12. __________ Involves an evaluation of the heart's response during moderate exercise while a 12-lead EKG is performed.
13. __________ A pictorial guide to placement of the EKG leads.
14. __________ A rapid heart rate.
15. __________ Heartbeats per minute.
16. __________ Electronic devices that help the heart maintain a normal rhythm.
17. __________ Performed to check blood flow in the myocardium.
18. __________ A slow heart rate.
19. __________ Involves using radio waves to transmit the heart's electrical activity to a central monitoring station.
20. __________ A variety of perspectives or angles.
21. __________ Excessively rapid breathing.
22. __________ An abnormal rhythm indicated by three distinct sounds in each heartbeat.

APPLIED PRACTICE

Follow the directions as instructed with each question below.

1. Identify the type of artifact shown in each of the following figures.

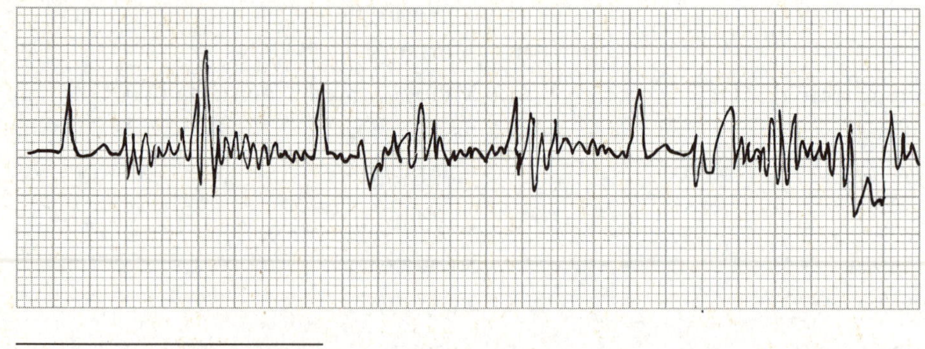

____

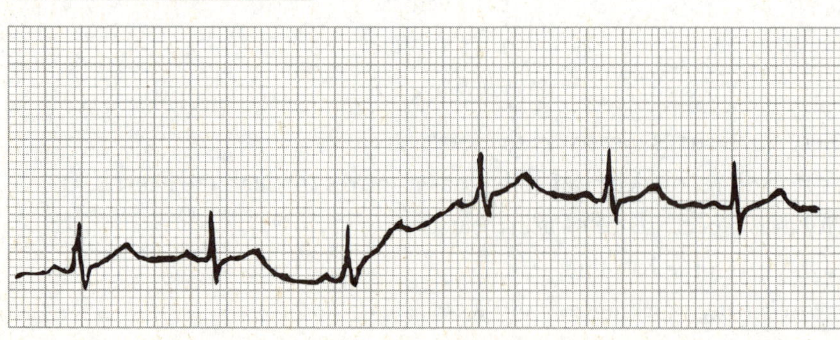

____

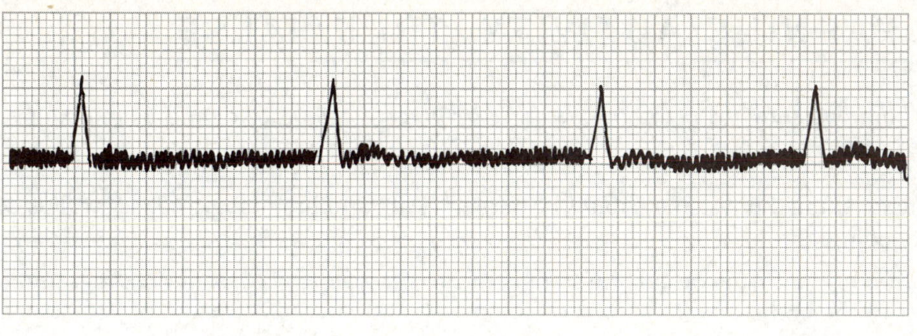

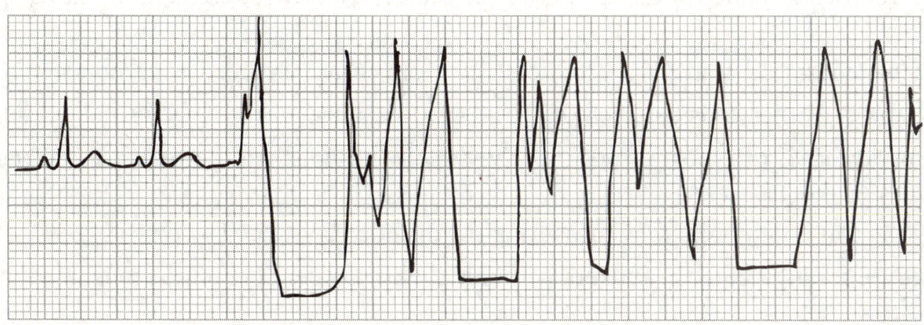

2. Using the figure provided, identify the placement of chest leads V1–V6.

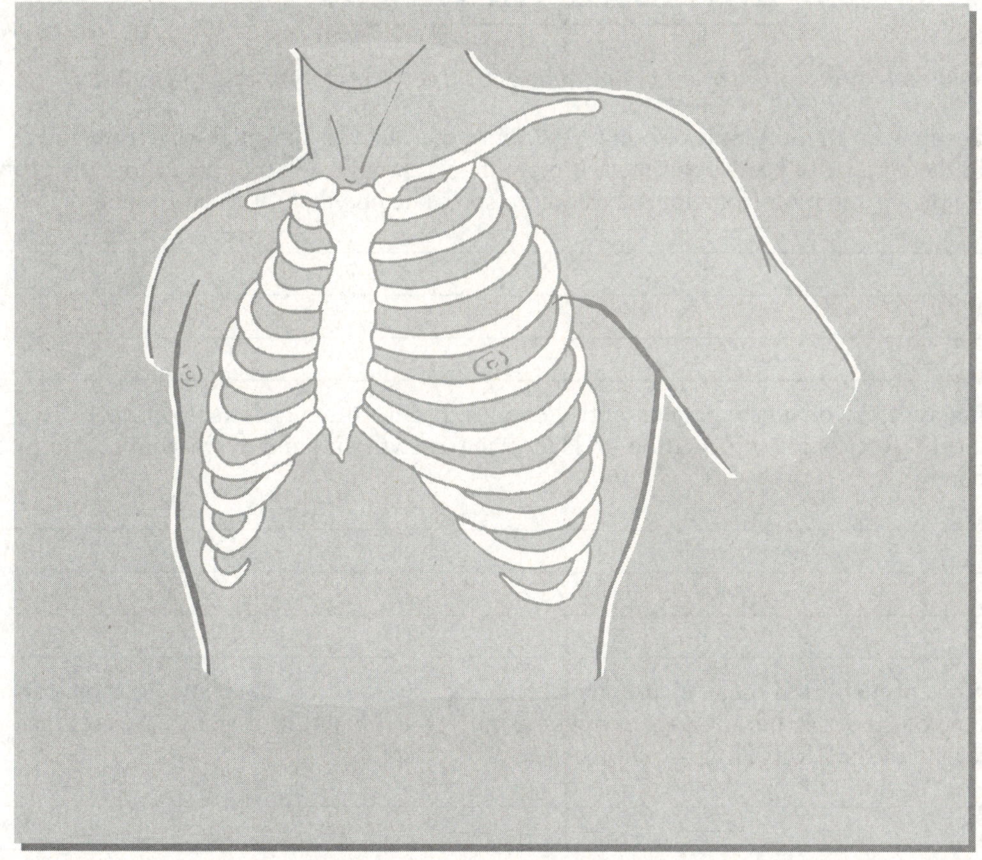

LEARNING ACTIVITY: TRUE/FALSE

Indicate whether the following statements are true or false by placing a T or an F on the line that precedes each statement.

_______ 1. All patients visiting a physician should have their heart and lungs assessed, regardless of their chief complaint.

_______ 2. The function of the cardiovascular system is to carry oxygen away from the lungs and to all the tissues of the body.

_______ 3. The blood that flows through the heart to the body is used for energy for the heart tissues.

_______ 4. Atrial and ventricular depolarization, plus atrial and ventricular repolarization, make up the cardiac cycle.

_______ 5. When completed, the 12-lead EKG produces a two-dimensional record of cardiac impulses.

_______ 6. Normally, the P–R interval is between 0.12 and 0.20 seconds.

_______ 7. A P–R interval that is too short means that the impulse has reached the ventricles through a longer-than-normal pathway.

_______ 8. The atrial rhythm is determined by measuring the distance between T waves.

_______ 9. The procedure for attaching the sensors will vary slightly, depending on the machine that you are using.

_______ 10. Pharmacological stress testing involves no exercise.

CRITICAL THINKING

Answer the following questions to the best of your ability. Utilize the textbook as a reference.

1. You are performing an EKG. As it is printing, you notice that there is a normal waveform and complex, but the number of beats per minute is more than 100 bpm. What do you think the problem could be? Use the information from your textbook to speculate on what the doctor might diagnose.

____

____

____

____

2. You are doing a history on a new patient, and she states that she often feels as if her heart has "skipped a beat." Review the information on identifying arrhythmias and dysrhythmias. Name and define this condition.

____

____

____

____

3. You need to perform an EKG on an elderly female patient, but she seems to be nervous or fearful. What are some of the signs that the patient might exhibit which might lead you to the conclusion that she is fearful of the EKG? How would that fear affect the EKG?

____

____

RESEARCH ACTIVITY

Utilize Internet search engines to research the following topics and write a brief description of what you find. It is important to utilize reputable websites.

1. Over the past 10 or more years, advancements have been made in addressing heart disease. Conduct research online to find out about some of the procedures and treatments that have been more recently discovered. Write an essay on your findings. Be sure to cite your resources.

Chapter 50
Pulmonary Function

CHAPTER OUTLINE

General review of the chapter:

- Pulmonary Function
- Pulmonary Disorders
- Pulmonary Function Tests
- Pulmonary Treatments

STUDENT STUDY GUIDE

Use the following guide to assist in your learning of the concepts from the chapter.

I. Pulmonary Functions

1. Pulmonary Functions
   - A. Pulmonology is the study and treatment of diseases of the ____________ system.
   - B. The primary function of the ____________ system is to transport ____________ to the lungs via the blood stream to all the cells in the body and carry ____________ products to the outside of the body for elimination.
2. The Purpose of Pulmonary Function Tests
   - A. __________ lung volume and capacity.
   - B. Assist in the __________ diagnosis of patients with suspected obstructive or restrictive pulmonary disease processes.
   - C. Assess the __________ of drug therapies.
3. Upper Respiratory Conditions
   - i. ____________________
   - ii. ____________________
   - iii. ____________________
   - iv. ____________________
   - v. ____________________
4. Lower Respiratory Conditions (Name the condition that is described.)
   - i. _____________ _____________: COPD, asthma, acute bronchitis, and emphysema
   - ii. _____________ _____________: Pneumonia, influenza, pleuritis, and Legionnaire's disease
   - iii. _____________ _____________: Cancer of the lungs, larynx, and other organs
   - iv. _____________ _____________: Pulmonary emboli, pneumothorax, and hemothorax
5. Signs and Symptoms of Respiratory Conditions
   - i. ____________________
   - ii. ____________________
   - iii. ____________________

iv. ____
v. ____
vi. ____
vii. ____

6. Examples of Pulmonary Disorders (Briefly explain each disorder.)
   A. Asthma: ____
   B. Chronic bronchitis: ____
   C. Cystic fibrosis: ____
   D. Emphysema: ____
7. Types of Pulmonary Function Tests
   i. ____
   ii. ____
   iii. ____
   iv. ____
   v. ____
8. Spirometry
   A. Spirometry is a noninvasive test that measures the ability of the lungs to __________.
   B. A diagnostic spirometer is used to evaluate the patient's ability to __________ during a maximum forced exhalation.
   C. The device measures and records the volume exhaled during a __________ length of time.
   D. Air movement is recorded on special paper with a __________ mark for each second and a __________ mark for each liter of oxygen.
   E. The patient must exhale as much air as possible and continue to exhale for ______ seconds for it to have been considered a satisfactory test.
   F. At least __________ efforts at exhalation must be demonstrated.
   G. In patients with healthy lungs, about _____% to _____% of air is exhaled in the first second.
   H. The values are often reported as a ratio: _____/_____.
   I. Patients with normal lungs may have a ratio of _____%.
9. Lung Volumes (briefly explain each type of measurement)
   A. Tidal Volume: ____
   B. Expiratory Reserve Volume: ____
   C. Inspiratory Reserve Volume: ____
   D. Residual Volume: ____
10. Lung Capacities (provide the name of each type of lung capacity explained)
   A. ________________________: Volume of the lungs at peak inspiration; equal to the sum of the four volumes.
   B. ________________________: Amount of air that can be exhaled following forced inspiration and including maximum expiration.
   C. ________________________: Maximum volume that can be inhaled after a normal expiration.
   D. ________________________: Volume of air left in the lungs after a normal expiration = ERV and RV
11. Volume Capacity Spirometry
   A. A diagnostic spirometer is used to evaluate the patient's ability to ventilate during a __________ __________ exhalation.
   B. This device measures and records the __________ __________ and the time required to complete the exhalation.
   C. Air movement is recorded on special paper with __________ __________ marks and __________ __________ marks.

12. Preparing a Patient for a Spirometry Test
    A. When the procedure is scheduled, a __________ explaining the test should be provided to the patient.
    B. Instruct the patient to refrain from smoking and eating a large meal for ______ to ______ hours and to not use __________ or __________ for 6 hours prior to the test.
    C. On arrival, again explain the test and the steps involved, and determine whether there are any reasons that the test should not be performed, such as __________, __________, or allergy.
    D. Weigh the patient and measure his or her __________ and __________ signs.
    E. __________ and __________ in simple terms what you would like the patient to do.
13. Patient Instructions
    A. If the patient has ill-fitting __________, ask that these be removed.
    B. Have the patient loosen any __________ clothing, ties, girdles, bras, or belts that could impede the test.
    C. The patient should be encouraged to sit because performing the test may cause __________-__________.
    D. The patient's feet should be __________ on the floor, legs __________, and head and chin slightly elevated for the entire procedure.
    E. If the patient prefers to __________ instead of sit, it is acceptable because it will not affect the results and the patient's comfort is important.
14. The Purpose of the Peak Flow Meter
    A. The peak flow meter is a portable, inexpensive handheld device used to measure how __________ __________ from the lungs in __________ __________ breath.
    B. It measures a patient's ability to move air __________ and __________ of the lungs over __________.
    C. It measures the __________ rate at which a patient exhales after taking a maximum breath.
    D. It helps the physician identify patterns of __________ __________ and determine the appropriate treatment.
15. Patient Use of the Peak Flow Meter
    i. ______________________________
    ii. ______________________________
    iii. ______________________________
16. The Role of the Medical Assistant
    A. Teaches the patient and family members the __________ for using the peak flow meter.
    B. Helps patients practice in the __________ until it is clear that they can perform the procedure correctly.
17. The Purpose of the Oximeter
    i. ______________________________
    ii. ______________________________
    iii. ______________________________
18. General Instructions for Using the Oximeter
    i. ______________________________
    ii. ______________________________
    iii. ______________________________
    iv. ______________________________
19. Arterial Blood Gases
    A. Arterial blood gases measure the amount of oxygen and carbon dioxide, and the _____ of the blood.
    B. They are helpful in evaluating breathing conditions such as __________ and __________.
    C. Provide information on the effectiveness of __________ treatment and the pH of the blood.

D. The pH of the blood must be stable, between __________ to __________, or the patient will be in a life-threatening situation.
E. The more carbon dioxide in the blood, the more __________ the blood pH becomes.
F. Usually drawn by respiratory specialists or _____ __________.
G. Arterial blood is drawn from the __________, __________, or arm after cleansing the site.
H. The specimen must be kept on __________ and tested immediately.
I. Direct pressure to the area is applied for _____ to _____ minutes to prevent bleeding.

20. Nebulizers

A. Deliver medication directly to __________ areas in the lungs.
B. The __________-__________ nebulizer is sometimes used to treat breathing difficulties.
C. If a handheld nebulizer is used, a small amount of __________ __________ medication is placed in the chamber.
   i. The patient is asked to put the nebulizer in his or her mouth and breathe deeply for _____ to _____ minutes.
   ii. A __________-__________ stream of air or oxygen passing through an opening creates the aerosol.
   iii. The aerosol is then delivered into the patient through either a ____________ or a ____________.

21. The Procedure for Using a Nebulizer

A. Note the patient's __________ data.
B. Assemble the handheld nebulizer and select a __________ or a __________ for delivery.
C. Using a mask can decrease the amount of the drug that reaches the lungs by about _____% to _____% because of __________ on the face.
D. The mask should be used only when the patient is __________ to take the treatment with a mouthpiece.
E. Measure the proper dosage of the drug and __________ into the nebulizer.
F. Set the gas flow to the nebulizer at _____ to _____ L/min.
G. Position the patient in a __________-__________ position.
H. Implement the therapy and encourage the patient to __________ __________ through the mouth.
I. Instruct the patient to deeply inspire periodically and to hold a breath for about _____ to _____ seconds.
J. When no aerosol is flowing, __________ treatment.
K. Monitor and evaluate the patient's __________ to the treatment.
L. Encourage the patient to __________ well, quantifying the amount and describing the type of sputum if the cough is productive.
M. Monitor the patient's pulse, breathing sounds, __________ __________ __________ rates, and blood oxygenation.

22. Inhalers

A. Used to deliver a measured amount of medication directly into the __________ __________ to dilate the airways.
B. One type of inhaler, a ________-________ __________ (MDI), holds about 200 doses of the prescribed medication in a pressurized container with an attached mouthpiece.
C. Patient __________ is very important because MDIs are frequently misused, resulting in inadequate treatment.
D. __________ __________ material is provided to the patient as well.

23. The Procedure for Using an Inhaler

A. The patient should put his or her the mouth over the mouthpiece of the inhaler and inhale when the medication container is __________ into the inhaler.
B. An extender is used to improve the __________ and to facilitate __________ of the medication.
C. A __________ of medication will be dispensed.

KEY TERMINOLOGY REVIEW

Match the vocabulary term to the correct definition below.

a. Chronic obstructive pulmonary disease (COPD)
b. Expiratory reserve volume (ERV)
c. Forced expiratory volume (FEV)
d. Forced vital capacity (FVC)
e. Functional residual capacity (FRC)
f. Inspiratory capacity (IC)
g. Inspiratory reserve volume (IRV)
h. Maximal midexpiratory flow (MMEF)
i. Oxygen saturation
j. Peak flow meters
k. Pulmonologist
l. Residual volume (RV)
m. Tidal volume (TV)
n. Total lung capacity (TLC)
o. Vital capacity (VC)

1. _________ The amount of air that can be forcibly inspired after a normal inhale.
2. _________ Measure the patient's ability to move air into and out of the lungs.
3. _________ The volume of air in liters that is forcefully exhaled in the first second of exhalation.
4. _________ The amount of air that can be inhaled after normal expiration.
5. _________ The oxygen content of the blood.
6. _________ The amount of air that can be exhaled following forced inspiration and including maximum expiration.
7. _________ The maximum volume of air expelled when the patient exhales as forcibly and quickly as possible following one inhalation.
8. _________ The average flow rate during the middle half of FVC.
9. _________ The volume of air left in the lungs at the end of an exhalation (around 1200 mL).
10. _________ The amount of air that can be forcibly exhaled after a normal exhalation.
11. _________ The amount of air inhaled or exhaled during normal breathing (about 500 mL).
12. _________ A specialist in lung diseases.
13. _________ The volume of the lungs at peak inspiration.
14. _________ A progressive, chronic, usually irreversible condition in which the lungs have diminished capacity for inhalation and exhalation.
15. _________ The amount of air remaining in the lungs after a normal expiration.

APPLIED PRACTICE

Follow the directions as instructed with each question below.

Scenario

It is a slow day at Fairview Family Practice where you are working as a clinical medical assistant. As you return files to the front office for filing, you see a woman rushing through the front door of the reception area. She states that her teenage son is in the car and suddenly began to have an asthma attack as they were driving. Two of your colleagues rush outside with the mother to assist in transporting the boy to an examination room. At the same time, you inform the physician of the situation. He asks that you gather the "necessary" supplies to assist him in assessing and treating the boy.

1. What signs and symptoms would the boy exhibit during a severe asthma attack?

____

____

____

2. What "necessary" supplies would you gather?

____

____

____

3. What steps might the physician take to assess and treat the boy?

____

____

____

LEARNING ACTIVITY: TRUE/FALSE

Indicate whether the following statements are true or false by placing a T or an F on the line that precedes each statement.

_______ 1. Pulse oximeters are not available in cordless models.

_______ 2. The respiratory system includes the trachea, bronchitis tubes, lungs, and alveoli.

_______ 3. Pharyngitis is a common upper respiratory condition.

_______ 4. The odor of cigarette smoke is possibly dangerous to patients, especially those with pulmonary problems.

_______ 5. Tuberculosis is considered to be an infectious disease of the blood.

_______ 6. Acute rhinitis is the most common URI.

_______ 7. The pulse oximeter uses an infrared light to measure oxygen in the tissues.

_______ 8. The acronym MMEF stands for minimum midexpiratory flow.

_______ 9. A peak flow meter can detect an asthma attack before symptoms occur.

_______ 10. Cyanosis and drumming of the fingertips are common symptoms of cystic fibrosis and are caused by low levels of oxygen in the blood.

CRITICAL THINKING

Answer the following questions to the best of your ability. Utilize the textbook as a reference.

1. A patient needs to start using an inhaler at home on a daily basis. The patient has rheumatoid arthritis and cannot hold the inhaler in the usual manner. What would you do or how would you teach this patient to use the inhaler?

____

____

____

____

2. You have a patient with obstructive lung disease who wants to know why he has a hard time breathing. This person has a form of COPD that doesn't allow him to exhale very much. Explain briefly here, as if explaining to the patient, why he feels so short of breath.

RESEARCH ACTIVITY

Utilize Internet search engines to research the following topics and write a brief description of what you find. It is important to utilize reputable websites.

1. Visit www.lungusa.org. What information do you think will be most useful with regard to patient education? What is "hidden" asthma and what age group does it commonly effect? How can this information be useful to patients?

CHAPTER 51
Physical Therapy and Rehabilitation

CHAPTER OUTLINE

General review of the chapter:

The Therapeutic Team
Rehabilitation
Patient Assessment
Conditions That Require Physical Therapy
Physical Therapy Methods
Adaptive Equipment and Devices
Diagnostic Testing

STUDENT STUDY GUIDE

Use the following guide to assist in your learning of the concepts from the chapter.

I. The Process of Rehabilitation

1. The Members of the Therapeutic Team
   i. ______________________
   ii. ______________________
   iii. ______________________
   iv. ______________________
   v. ______________________
   vi. ______________________
   vii. ______________________
   viii. ______________________
2. Places Where Members of the Therapeutic Team Work
   i. ______________________
   ii. ______________________
   iii. ______________________
   iv. ______________________
   v. ______________________
   vi. ______________________
   vii. ______________________
   viii. ______________________
3. Educational Requirements for Members of the Therapeutic Team

   A. Physiatrist (MD or DO)
      i. ____________ school graduate
      ii. ____-year residency in physical medicine
      iii. State ____________

B. Physical Therapist (PT):
   i. __________ degree
   ii. _____________ is required in all states.
C. Physical Therapy Assistant (PTA)
   i. ______-year accredited program or associate's degree plus ________.
   ii. ________ is required in all states.
D. Occupational Therapist (OT)
   i. _______ or ___________ degree and ________
   ii. Certification from the ____________________________
E. Occupational Therapy Assistant (OTA)
   i. ______- to ______-year certificate program or associate's degree and __________.
   ii. Licensure or ___________ is required by most states.
F. Massage Therapist
   i. _____-month to _____-year accredited message therapy program
   ii. Registration or __________ is required by most states.
G. Recreational Therapist (RT) or Certified Therapeutic Recreation Specialist (CTRS)
   i. Usually a ___________ degree plus an _________
   ii. Can be certified by the _________________________ or registration by the ________________.
H. Recreational Therapy Assistant (Activity Director)
   i. _____- to _____-year certificate program or ________ degree.
   ii. Can be certified by the ____.
I. Sports Medicine (Athletic Trainer, ATS)
   i. _______ or ______ degree
   ii. Can be certified by the ____.
J. Prosthetist/Orthotist
   i. ______ years of college
   ii. ______ years of supervised training

4. The Role of the Physical Therapist
   A. Receives special training in assisting patients through the use of __________ and __________ to regain body motion and strength.
   B. Skilled at using special equipment for __________ muscles and at measuring, fitting, and using __________ __________ such as crutches, walkers, and canes.

5. The Role of the Occupational Therapist
   A. Focuses on increasing the patient's ability to function within his or her own __________.
   B. Assists the patient by addressing areas that deal with __________ ____ __________ __________ (ADLs).

6. The Role of the Medical Assistant on the Therapeutic Team
   A. Carries out orders for treatments, such as the application of heat or cold __________ and exercise.
   B. Instructs the patient on how to appropriately apply heat or cold __________ at home.
   C. Demonstrates the use of assistive devices such as __________ and __________.

7. The Process of Rehabilitation
   A. Assists the patient in regaining a state of health and the __________ __________ of functioning possible.
   B. The __________ approach addresses every aspect of a patient's well-being, not just the present disease or injury.
   C. __________ are set for each patient by the professionals on the case and are suited to the individual patient's needs.
   D. The patient is assisted in resuming activities of __________ __________.

E. During rehabilitation, special attention should be paid to psychological problems, such as __________ and __________, that can occur from a feeling of loss of control over one's life.

8. Reasons for Receiving Rehabilitation

   i. ______________________________
   ii. ______________________________
   iii. ______________________________
   iv. ______________________________

9. The Physician's Assessment of a Patient for Rehabilitation

   A. __________ and __________ the patient's limbs and joints to evaluate muscle strength and flexibility.
   B. Evaluates the patient's __________ for clues to specific problems.
   C. Evaluates the patient's __________ to assess symmetry.

10. Conditions That May Require Physical Therapy (Provide the name of each condition described.)

   A. __________: The removal of an extremity because of injury or disease
   B. __________: The inflammation of a joint that usually causes pain and swelling
   C. __________: Damage to the skin from first, second, or third degree burns that result in strictures, decreased mobility, and stiffness
   D. _____ __________ _______: Damage to the superficial layer of skin or the outer layer of the epidermis with no scarring, but resulting in erythema
   E. _____ __________ _____: Damage that extends through the epidermis and into the dermis, causing vesicles and scarring
   F. _____ __________ _______: Damage to the full thickness (the epidermis and dermis) and into the underlying layers of the skin with scarring
   G. __________ __________: Diseases of the circulatory and cardiac systems
   H. __________ __________: A nonprogressive paralysis caused by defects in the brain or birth trauma
   I. __________ __________ (CVA): Hemorrhaging or clotting in the brain that can result in unconsciousness or paralysis (stroke)
   J. __________ __________: An inflammatory disease of the central nervous system, generally strikes adults between the ages of 20 and 40; causes progressive weakness and numbness
   K. __________ __________: A wasting disease of the muscles
   L. __________: A disease that results in a reduction of bone mass, which frequently occurs in postmenopausal women; can result in back pain and fractures
   M. __________: Paralysis of the lower portion of the body
   N. __________ __________: A chronic nerve disease with fine tremors, a slow gait, muscular weakness, and rigidity
   O. __________: An acute viral disease that causes an inflammation of the gray matter of the spinal cord, resulting in paralysis in some cases; it has been brought under partial control through vaccinations
   P. __________: Paralysis of all four extremities of the body
   Q. __________ __________: A form of arthritis with inflammation of the joints, swelling, stiffness, and pain

11. Physical Therapy Methods

   i. ______________________________
   ii. ______________________________
   iii. ______________________________
   iv. ______________________________
   v. ______________________________
   vi. ______________________________

vii. ___

viii. ___

12. Massage

    A. Involves using one's hands to ___ or apply ___ to parts of a patient's body.
    B. Performed to promote muscle relaxation, improve ___ ___, and reduce tension.
    C. Can help to restore ___ and decrease pain.
    D. Considered a form of ___ exercise.

13. Categories of Massage Practiced by Massage Therapists (Provide the name of the type of massage described.)

    A. ___ or ___ massage: Most commonly used in the United States, includes stimulating blood circulation through the soft tissues.
    B. ___ ___ massage: Used to release chronic patterns of tension or pain by applying massage and pressure at deeper levels.
    C. ___ ___ massage: Concentrates finger pressure directly to individual muscles to release "trigger points," or knots in the muscles.

14. Exercise Therapy

    A. Conducted to maintain or ___ fitness.
    B. Can help increase or establish lost ___ ___, improve circulation, relieve stress, correct posture issues, and increase ___.
    C. Twenty to thirty minutes, ___ times a week is recommended for healthy adults.

15. Types of Exercises (Provide the name of the type of exercise described.)

    A. ___: Strengthens the cardiopulmonary system.
    B. ___: Maintains uniform (unchanging) tension or tones the muscles upon stimulation.
    C. ___: Involves contractions with muscles fixed in place so that the tension occurs without noticeable movement.
    D. ___: Results in muscle elongation.

16. Range-of-Motion Exercises (Describe each of the following types of exercises.)

    A. Active range of motion (AROM): ___
    B. Passive range of motion (PROM): ___
    C. Active assist range of motion (AAROM): ___

17. Types of Body Movements Used in a Range-of-Motion Assessment

    i. ___
    ii. ___
    iii. ___
    iv. ___
    v. ___
    vi. ___
    vii. ___
    viii. ___
    ix. ___
    x. ___
    xi. ___
    xii. ___
    xiii. ___
    xiv. ___

18. Guidelines for Performing Range-of-Motion Exercises
    A. Perform each exercise __________ times unless otherwise ordered by the physician.
    B. The patient should attempt to do as much as he or she is able without __________.
    C. No body part should be forced beyond the __________ range.
    D. No exercise should bring on __________.
    E. If joints are __________ or swollen, the exercise should not be performed.
    F. Limbs should be supported at the __________ when exercising.
19. The Benefits of Applying Heat
    i. ______________________________
    ii. ______________________________
    iii. ______________________________
    iv. ______________________________
    v. ______________________________
20. Methods for Applying Moist Heat
    i. ______________________________
    ii. ______________________________
    iii. ______________________________
    iv. ______________________________
    v. ______________________________
    vi. ______________________________
    vii. ______________________________
21. Methods for Applying Dry Heat
    i. ______________________________
    ii. ______________________________
    iii. ______________________________
    iv. ______________________________
    v. ______________________________
22. Methods for Applying Cold
    i. ______________________________
    ii. ______________________________
    iii. ______________________________
    iv. ______________________________
23. Other Physical Therapy Methods (Explain how both types work.)
    A. Ultraviolet radiation: ______________________________
    B. Ultrasound: ______________________________

II. Adaptive Equipment and Devices
   1. An Overview of Adaptive Equipment and Devices
      A. Equipment is used to assist recovery from physical __________ or __________.
      B. Includes wheelchairs, walkers, canes, crutches, and special furniture, such as __________ chairs and __________ chairs.
      C. __________ aids or __________ assistive devices are designed to enable the patient to ambulate.
      D. Other devices, including braces, casts, traction, prostheses, splints, and slings, are used to manipulate the patient's damaged __________ and __________.
   2. Crutches
      A. Allow the patient to walk without placing weight on the __________ __________.
      B. __________ is transferred to the arms and hands.
      C. Made from __________ or __________ and should have a __________ tip at the end to prevent slipping on a smooth floor surface.

3. The Three Most Common Types of Crutch
   A. Axillary crutch
      i. A tall crutch with a __________ and ______ that reaches from the ground to under the __________.
      ii. Commonly used for patients who have sustained a ___________.
   B. Lofstrand (forearm crutch)
      i. A single aluminum tube with an ___________ that fits snugly around the patient's forearm and uses a handgrip for weight bearing.
      ii. Allows the patient to release the _________ to use the hand while still having the crutch held in place by the ___________ for support.
   C. Canadian or elbow crutch
      i. A variation of the _____________ that extends farther up the arm.
4. Axillary Crutch Measurement
   A. Measurement has to be determined carefully to prevent pressure damage to the ______.
   B. If crutches are too long, the patient may develop a condition known as ______ _______, resulting in muscle weakness in the arm, wrist, and hand.
   C. Back pain, nerve damage, and injury to the ______ and palms of the hands can occur if the crutches are improperly fitted.
5. Steps for Measuring Axillary Crutches
   A. Have the patient wear ___________ __________ and stand straight.
   B. Place the crutch tips _______ to _______ inches to the side and _______ to _______ inches in front of each foot.
   C. Adjust the crutch, using the bolts and nuts at the sides of the crutch, so that the axillary crutch bars are _________ _________ widths below the axillae.
   D. Next, adjust the handgrips so that the patient can flex his or her elbows at a ____-degree angle when the crutch is in place and the patient's hands are on the hand bars.
6. The Four-Point Gait
   A. The four-point gait is a __________ and __________ gait.
   B. Used when a patient can __________ __________ on both legs.
   C. Considered the safest of all gaits because the patient always has __________ points of support in contact with the ground at all times.
   D. Used for patients who may have muscular __________ and some lack of __________.
7. The Three-Point Gait
   A. Used when one leg is __________ than the other or when there is no weight bearing on one leg.
   B. Patient must have good __________ coordination and __________ strength.
   C. To use this gait, the patient must be able to support his or her __________ __________ on one leg.
   D. Have the patient move both crutches and the __________ leg forward and then move the __________ leg forward while his or her weight is balanced on both crutches.
8. The Two-Point Gait
   A. The two-point gait is __________ than the four-point gait.
   B. Used by the patient who can bear some weight on both __________ and has good __________.
   C. Occurs when a crutch and the opposite foot are moved __________ at the same time.
9. Swing Gaits
   A. Used by patients who have severe leg disabilities such as __________ or __________.
   B. They may use either of the two swing gaits (Name the two swing gaits described.)
      i. __________-_____ __________: The patient moves the crutches forward, lifts his or her body, and then swings the legs up to the same point.

ii. __________-__________ __________: The patient moves the crutches forward, as in the swing-to gait, and then swings the legs past the crutches.

10. Procedure for Sitting with Crutches
    A. The patient should face __________ and then __________ into a straight-back chair with arm rests until the back of his or her legs touch the chair seat.
    B. Crutches should be placed in the hand on the __________ side of the body, opposite the __________ leg.
    C. The patient should grasp the __________ __________ with the other hand and lower him- or herself gently into the chair.

11. Procedure for Standing with Crutches
    A. The patient should place the crutches in the hand on the ______ side of the body to use as support.
    B. The patient should move or __________ his or her body forward in the chair.
    C. The patient should grasp the chair arm with the free hand on the __________ side.
    D. The patient should push up to a __________ position.

12. Canes
    A. Used by patients who have muscle or bone weakness on __________ __________ or need assistance with balance.
    B. Two common types of canes are the __________ cane and the __________-__________ cane.
    C. All canes should have __________ tips to prevent slipping.

13. Walkers
    A. Walkers are assistive devices made of __________.
    B. Provide a base of support for patients who need help with __________ and __________.
    C. Should be adjusted to the patient's height and reach just below the patient's __________.
    D. A stationary walker must be picked up by the patient, moved forward, and then used as a base of support while the patient walks into it. This requires strong __________ __________ development.
    E. A walker with wheels can be used by patients who have good __________ and __________.

14. Wheelchairs
    A. Wheelchairs are hand manipulated or __________ __________.
    B. Many patients __________ their own wheelchairs.

15. Considerations When Transferring a Patient from a Wheelchair
    A. Always think of moving a patient as the process of ____________ him or her from one place to another.
    B. In many cases, the patient is __________ with the techniques necessary for the transfer and will be able to assist the medical assistant.
    C. A patient who is paralyzed on one side of the body (hemiplegia) or who has a general weakness can be moved from a wheelchair by __________ the patient so that he or she can use the __________ leg to assist you.
    D. Explain to the patient that this __________ technique is used to prevent __________ to the patient and to the individual assisting with the transfer.

16. Braces
    A. Braces are one type of __________ used to support weakened body parts, correct deformities, and prevent joint movement.
    B. May be made out of metal, plastic, or __________ and are customized to the patient's needs and anatomy.

C. To wear this type of assistive leg device, the brace is placed in the patient's __________, the patient's __________ is inserted, and a __________-and-__________ strap is used to hold the brace in place.
D. Any orthotic positioned over a __________ __________ must be padded to avoid skin breakdown.

17. Casts

A. Applied over a __________ to protect the skin.
B. Fiberglass and plastic casts dry quickly, while a __________ of __________ cast may take up to _____ hours to dry.
C. Made from a variety of __________ materials that the physician will mold to fit the body part.
D. A cast can be considered to be a form of __________ bandage.
E. Casts are generally applied using a wet __________-__________ material around a __________ liner and cotton padding over the limb. As the cast dries, it becomes hard.
F. Newer __________ fiberglass materials are being used to form casts that are lighter in weight than a plaster cast.

18. Assisting in Cast Placement

A. Use caution when handling fiberglass materials by wearing protective __________ or an __________ shield.
B. It may be necessary to hold the limb at the __________ areas as the cast is being applied.
C. Remember to handle a damaged limb __________.
D. After the cast has been applied, it must be left __________ during the drying process.
E. The limb may need to be supported on a __________ at this time.
F. The patient should be cautioned against __________ around until the cast is dry.
G. The cast may become __________ or even __________ during the drying process. This is normal.
H. The patient's limb should not become __________ or __________ once the cast has been applied.
I. Check the __________of the cast and report any changes to the physician.
J. The medical assistant should make frequent checks of the patient's __________.

19. Cast Issues That the Patient Should Report

i. ______________________________
ii. ______________________________
iii. ______________________________
iv. ______________________________
v. ______________________________
vi. ______________________________
vii. ______________________________
viii. ______________________________
ix. ______________________________

20. Traction

A. Traction is a method of ________ or ________ in ____ directions.
B. Used to __________ fractures and correct __________.
C. Reduces __________ of the __________ or other musculoskeletal conditions.

21. Two Types of Traction

A. Skeletal traction
   i. Performed on __________.
   ii. Applied by the physician to the patient's bone by inserting a __________ or __________ through the bone.
B. Skin traction
   i. Done by the physical therapist by attaching __________ and strips of __________ to the skin.

ii. __________ are then attached to the material and tension is applied to reduce painful muscle spasms.
iii. This type of traction can be set up in a patient's __________.

22. The Prosthesis

A. A prosthesis is an artificial replacement for a __________ body part.
B. A benefit of immediate fitting is that the patient is able to begin __________ the next day.
C. The decision to select a specific type of fitting rests with the physician and must include an assessment of the patient's overall __________, age, and __________ to learn to use the new limb.

23. The Elements of a Neuromuscular Evaluation

i. ____
ii. ____
iii. ____
iv. ____
v. ____

24. Electromyography (EMG)

A. Consists of using an electromyograph to test the __________ __________ in the muscles.
B. Most often performed when a patient complains of muscle __________ or __________.
C. Consists of electrodes, an __________ to visually produce the waves of muscle activity, an __________, a loudspeaker, an electrical stimulator, and a camera.
D. The patient may receive sedation before this test is conducted, because the stimulation from the __________ __________ can be painful.
E. Consists of inserting a __________-__________ needle electrode through the skin and into a muscle and then sending a small amount of electrical current into the muscle.
F. The procedure permits the physician to examine __________ parts of muscles.
G. Abnormal results are found in conditions such as __________ __________ __________ (ALS), muscular dystrophy, and peripheral nerve damage.
H. The electrical activity of the muscle that is recorded on graph paper or on film is known as an __________ (EMG).

25. Surface Electromyography (SEMG)

A. Involves less __________ for the patient.
B. The results are less __________.
C. In this test, electrodes are attached to the __________ of the body to detect electrical activity.
D. Electrical stimulation with __________-__________ current is helpful to stimulate the nerves that supply muscles.
E. An electrical current is applied using __________ __________ electrodes.
F. This is a passive means of stimulating muscles when a patient cannot _______ because of injury or disease.

26. Transcutaneous Electric Nerve Stimulation (TENS)

A. TENS is another way of using __________ __________ in physical medicine.
B. A TENS unit is attached to the patient at the __________ area, and a __________ dose of current is sent to the muscle to help control intractable pain when medication has not been effective.
C. TENS units may be used at __________.

27. Evoked Potential Studies

A. The study of the responses within the brain to __________ __________ such as light, sound, and touch is called an evoked potential study.
B. The tests are considered __________ because no equipment or needle is inserted into the body.

C. Two types of evoked potential studies (Name the type described.)

i. ________________ ____________ ____________ ____________ (BAER): Used to assess the auditory nerve pathways. Useful in diagnosing auditory tumors and lesions.

ii. ________________ ____________ ____________ (SEP): Used for diagnosing nerve function defects in peripheral nerves (e.g., in the legs).

KEY TERMINOLOGY REVIEW

Without using your textbook, write a sentence using the selected key terms in the correct context as discussed in material covered in Chapter 51.

1. *ambulation*

____

____

2. *atrophy*

____

____

3. *contracture*

____

____

4. *diathermy*

____

____

5. *effleurage*

____

____

6. *erythema*

____

____

7. *exudate*

____

____

8. *friction*

____

____

9. *goniometer*

____

____

10. *heat hydrotherapy*

____

____

11. *hemiplegia*

12. *holistic*

13. *massage*

14. *modalities*

15. *orthotist*

16. *petrissage*

17. *physiatrist*

18. *physiatry*

19. *prosthesis*

20. *prosthetist*

21. *range of motion (ROM)*

22. *rehabilitation*

23. *Reiki*

24. ***suppuration***

25. ***tapotement***

APPLIED PRACTICE

Follow the directions as instructed with each question below.

1. Read the following scenario and answer the corresponding questions.

Scenario

It is a busy Monday morning, and you are working as a clinical medical assistant at an orthopedic office. Rachel Dade, an administrative MA, has just informed you that an emergency appointment was just scheduled for Li Chen, a teenager who injured his lower leg while participating in a soccer game during gym class. While he is currently en route to the office, his parents have arrived and are insisting that he be treated using traditional Chinese medicine. Explain how you would address their wishes and traditions.

2. Create a diagram of the four-point gait as a tool for explaining the use of crutches to an 8-year-old child.

LEARNING ACTIVITY: TRUE/FALSE

Indicate whether the following statements are true or false by placing a T or an F on the line that precedes each statement.

_______ 1. Bones are classified according to structure, including flat, round, short, and long.

_______ 2. The three-point gait requires good coordination and muscle strength.

_______ 3. Bursitis is a form of arthritis.

_______ 4. Diathermy is useful in treating muscular disorders, tendonitis, arthritis, and bursitis.

_______ 5. In order to have access to a wheelchair, patients must be able to drive an automobile.

_______ 6. Cryotherapy is using cold for therapeutic purposes.

_______ 7. Prolonged use of a brace may weaken muscles.

_______ 8. Casts are made of plaster, plastic, fiberglass, and metal.

_______ 9. The immediate fitting of a prosthesis involves fitting the patient immediately after the limb is removed, sometimes before leaving the operating room.

_______ 10. There are four types of crutches: axillary, Lofstrand or forearm, Canadian or elbow, and bipedal crutches.

CRITICAL THINKING

Answer the following questions to the best of your ability. Utilize the textbook as a reference.

1. Review the case study at the beginning of this chapter in the textbook. Explain why it is important that Samra wheel Sylvia to the examination room rather than have Sylvia wheel herself.

____

____

____

____

2. Without looking back at the material, imagine that you are working in an orthopedic office and a 19-year-old college football player has been brought into the clinic by his coach. He has been seen by the doctor, and X-rays have been taken and looked at by the doctor. He was diagnosed with a strain and you are preparing him for application of a cast by the technician. The patient insists that he has a sprain, not a strain, and asks that you explain to him the difference between the two. From your memory of the material, write your answer. Then check the book and write a correct answer if yours differs.

____

____

____

____

3. A patient calls in and has questions after reading her cast care written instructions. She asks how she is supposed to bathe or take a shower. What patient education/instructions would you give her?

____

____

____

____

RESEARCH ACTIVITY

Utilize Internet search engines to research the following topics and write a brief description of what you find. It is important to utilize reputable websites.

1. Research new materials and advances being made in prosthetics. What information do you find most interesting and why?

Chapter 52
Math for Pharmacology

CHAPTER OUTLINE

General review of the chapter:

Mathematics Review
Weights and Measures
Drug Calculations
Rules for Conversion
Calculating Pediatric Dosages

STUDENT STUDY GUIDE

Use the following guide to assist in your learning of the concepts from the chapter.

I. Math for Pharmacology

1. Weights and Measures Used to Calculate Medication Doses
   A. Most physician and facilities have moved to the ________ system when calculating medication doses.
   B. The medical assistant must be familiar with both the apothecary and metric systems because occasionally, medications do appear in the ___________ system.
2. The Apothecary System
   A. The dry weight measurement is based on the __________.
   B. ____________ numerals are used when numbering in the apothecary system.
   C. It is important to note that the unit of measurement in the apothecary system is placed before the __________ number.
3. Rules for Writing an Apothecary Notation
   A. The unit or ________________ comes before the ___________.
   B. Use fractions to designate amounts less than _______.
4. The Metric System
   A. Metric system prefixes (Indicate the value of each.)
      i. Kilo = ____
      ii. Hecto = ____
      iii. Deka = ____
      iv. Deci = ____
      v. Centi = ____
      vi. Milli = ____
      vii. Micro = ____
5. Guidelines for Converting Within the Metric System
   A. No change is required to change milliliters into ______ ______________ because they are equal to each other.

B. To convert liters to milliliters, ______ the liters by ______ or move the decimal point ______ places to the ___________.

C. To convert milliliters to liters, ______ the milliliters by __________ or move the decimal point _______ places to the ______.

6. Metric System Dosages

A. In the metric system, the dosage is written as a __________ number first, followed by the unit of measurement.

B. Commonly used equivalents for the apothecary and metric systems include the following

i. Apothecary 1 gr = Metric ____

ii. Apothecary 5 gr = Metric ____

iii. Apothecary 10 gr = Metric ____

iv. Apothecary 15 or 16 gr = Metric ____________________________________

v. Apothecary 15 or 16 m = Metric ____________________________________

7. The Ratio Method of Calculating Dosages

A. A ratio establishes a relationship between two ______________.

B. The proportion resulting from the fraction ½—or the ratio—could be _________ = ½, or _________.

C. The symbol _____ is used for the unknown quantity.

8. Cross Multiplying

A. Multiply the _____ number on the _____ side of the equals (=) sign by the _____ number on the _____ side of the equals sign.

B. The ______ number on the _____ is multiplied by the _____ number on the ________.

C. Then divide both sides by the number with the _____.

9. The Formula Method

A. The calculation formula

i. Available _________ is the __________ of the drug in stock.

ii. Available ____________ is the ______________ of the drug in the container.

iii. Ordered _______ is the physician's order.

iv. The amount to be given is the ______________ quantity.

10. D/H × Q Formula

A. D = ____

B. H = ____

C. Q = ____

11. Guidelines for Conversion

A. To change grains to grams, divide by ________.

B. To change ounces to cubic centimeters or milliliters, multiply by ________.

C. To change grains to milligrams, multiply by ________.

D. To change kilograms to pounds, multiply by ________.

E. To change cubic centimeters or milliliters to ounces, divide by ________.

F. To change drams to milliliters, multiply by ________.

G. To change cubic centimeters or milliliters to minims, multiply by ________ or ________.

H. To change minims to cubic centimeters or milliliters, divide by ________ or ________.

I. To convert drams to grams, multiply by ________.

12. Clark's Rule for Calculating Pediatric Doses

A. Doses are based on the _______ of the child.

B. This rule is followed by dividing the child's ________ by ________ ________ and then multiplying that number by the adult dose.

13. Fried's Rule for Calculating Pediatric Doses
    A. Fried's assumption is that a ________-year-old child could take an adult dose.
    B. The formula uses ______ months in the denominator as the equivalent for ________ years.
14. Young's Rule for Calculating Pediatric Doses
    A. To use this formula, divide the child's age in years by the age plus ______.
    B. Multiply this number by the ______ dose to determine the correct pediatric dosage.
15. West's Nomogram Method of Drug Calculation
    A. This method can be used for both _________ and children.
    B. The chart is frequently found in _________ offices, medical textbooks, and dictionaries.
16. The Body Weight Method for Calculating Pediatric Doses
    A. Uses calculations based on the patient's weight in ______________.
    B. This is done by calculating the safe drug dosage in ____________ and then multiplying that amount by the child's weight in __________.

KEY TERMINOLOGY REVIEW

Use the key terms found at the beginning of the chapter to finish the sentences below.

1. The bottom number in a fraction is called the ________________.
2. _____________ is the study of medications and drugs, including their forms, intentions for use, and effects.
3. A __________ is a comparison between two numbers.
4. When writing a decimal number less than 1, you must apply the ________________.
5. ________________ is the preferred method for calculating pediatric dosages, particularly for oncology and critical care patients and underweight children.
6. The top number in a fraction is called the ______________.
7. The ________________ is based on a calculation of the child's height and weight, and is expressed in square meters (m^2).
8. The ______________________ states that it is never appropriate to include a zero after a whole number.
9. The _______________ is the most commonly used conversion system for dosage calculations.
10. _________________ is the method used to calculate dosages for children who are over 1 year of age.
11. The _______________ is considered to be the oldest system of measurement.
12. An _____________ occurs when not enough medication is given to achieve the desired effect.
13. The two numbers in a fraction are separated by a _________________.
14. Taking too much medication could result in an ___________.
15. _______________ is used to calculate medications for children under the age of 1.
16. When there are two ratios to compare, they may be set up as a ____________.
17. A _______________ is made up of both a whole number and a fraction.
18. _____________ is the most common law used in the calculation of drug dosages for children.

APPLIED PRACTICE

Complete the following exercises.

1. Basic Math Review: *Do not use a calculator.*
   a. Addition
      1. 18 + 49 = ________
      2. 142 + 730 = ________
      3. 1799 + 283 = ________
      4. 7839 + 943 + 41 = ________
      5. 28845 + 83 = ________
   b. Subtraction
      1. 75 − 52 = ________
      2. 429 − 81 = ________
      3. 1648 − 379 = ________
      4. 612 − 419 = ________
      5. 3527 − 274 = ________
   c. Multiplication
      1. 9 × 3 = ________
      2. 32 × 5 = ________
      3. 815 × 4 = ________
      4. 711 × 30 = ________
      5. 3780 × 210 = ________
   d. Division
      1. 150/15 = ________
      2. 1152/12 = ________
      3. 450/60 = ________
      4. 327/6 = ________
      5. 825/50 = ________
2. Dosage Calculations
   A. The physician orders digoxin 0.125 mg to be given to a patient. On hand is a vial of digoxin marked 250 mcg/mL. How much should the medical assistant administer?

   ____

   ____

   B. The physician orders 500 mg of metformin to be given to a patient. On hand is a bottle of metformin that reads 1000 mg/tablet. How much should the medical assistant administer?

   ____

   ____

   C. The physician orders 125 mg of a medication. On hand is a bottle of the same medication that reads 500 mg/5 mL. How much should the medical assistant administer?

   ____

   ____

   D. The medication that the physician ordered reads 20 mg/kg/day. Your patient weighs 220 lbs. The physician wants the patient to take the medication BID in equal doses. How much will the patient be given for each dose?

   ____

   ____

   E. The physician orders 40 mg of furosemide to be given to a patient. On hand is a bottle of furosemide that reads 20 mg/tablet. How much should the medical assistant administer?

   ____

   ____

LEARNING ACTIVITY: MULTIPLE CHOICE

Circle the correct answer to each of the questions below.

1. If the doctor orders 4 mg of a certain medication, and the vial states that there are 2 mg in 1 cc, how many cc's would you give to deliver 4 mg?
   a. 2 cc
   b. 4 cc
   c. 6 cc
   d. ½ cc

2. If the doctor orders 1 dram of medication to be given and the vial states that there is 1 mg in 1 cc, you must ____.
   a. give 1 cc
   b. ask the doctor how to determine the number of cc's
   c. ask the pharmacy
   d. convert from the apothecary system to the metric system and then calculate the dosage

3. When adding and subtracting fractions ____.
   a. you do not always need to have a common denominator
   b. to obtain the common denominator, you must multiply the entire fraction by the correct multiplier
   c. subtract the numerators; the denominator remains the same
   d. All of the above

4. When converting an improper fraction to a mixed number ______________________________.
   a. divide the numerator by the denominator
   b. the remainder, if any, is then placed over the denominator to form the fractional component of the mixed number
   c. reduce the fractional component to its simplest form
   d. All of the above

5. To accurately write an apothecary notation, the following rules should be applied:
   a. The unit or abbreviation comes after the amount.
   b. Use lowercase Roman numerals to express whole numbers 1 through 10, 15, 20, and 30.
   c. Use fractions to designate amounts greater than 1.
   d. The symbol *ss* is used to designate the fraction ¾.

6. Metric conversions are simply accomplished by multiplying or dividing by __________.
   a. 100
   b. 500
   c. 1000
   d. None of the above

7. The apothecary measurement of 5 gr is equivalent to __________________________using the metric system.
   a. 65 mg, or 0.065 g
   b. 325 mg, or 0.33 g
   c. 650 mg, or 0.67 g
   d. 4 mL

8. The apothecary measurement of 3.5 fl oz is equivalent to ______________________ using the metric system.
   a. 100 mL
   b. 200 mL
   c. 500 mL
   d. 15 mL

9. The measurement of 60 gtts (drops) is equivalent to the common household measurement of ____________________.
   a. 1 teaspoon (tsp)
   b. 1 tablespoon (T)
   c. 1 oz.
   d. 2 oz.

10. Which of the following factors should be considered when calculating the correct dose of a drug?
   a. Patient's age
   b. Patient's weight
   c. Patient's current health
   d. All of the above

CRITICAL THINKING

Answer the following questions to the best of your ability. Utilize the textbook as a reference.

1. You have received a physician's order to administer 1 mg of a medication to a patient. It is a medication that is injected into the muscle. As soon as you have given the medication, you realize you measured 1 mL instead of calculating 1 mg. What would you do?

____

____

____

____

2. An established patient has come in to ask for a new prescription for a medication that she has taken for many years because she is out of refills. The physician is not in the office today, but after checking the medical record and noting that it is the patient's usual medication, the medical assistant calls in a new prescription to the pharmacy and makes a note to have the doctor write the order in the chart when she returns. Is this an appropriate action for the MA, since she used critical thinking to check the chart and felt sure that the physician would approve it? Explain your answer.

____

____

____

____

RESEARCH ACTIVITY

Utilize Internet search engines to research the following topics and write a brief description of what is found. It is important to utilize reputable websites.

1. Visit www.rxlist.com. Navigate through the site and determine how the information on this site could be best used by patients. How could a patient benefit from this website?

CHAPTER 53
Pharmacology

CHAPTER OUTLINE

General review of the chapter:

Drug Names
Regulations and Standards
References
Legal Classifications of Drugs
Drug Abuse
General Classes of Drugs
Routes and Drug Administration
Frequently Administered Drugs
Side Effects of Medications
Drug Interactions
Drug Use During Pregnancy
Reading and Writing a Prescription
Abbreviations Used in Pharmacology

STUDENT STUDY GUIDE

Use the following guide to assist in your learning of the concepts from the chapter.

I. Pharmacology

1. The Generic Name
   A. The generic name is typically noted in ___________ letters.
   B. Considered to be the drug's ___________ name.
   C. A generic drug must meet the requirements of the corresponding ___________ name drug.
   D. Typically priced _________ than __________ name drugs.
2. The Brand Name
   A. The brand name is typically noted in ___________ letters.
   B. It is also called the ____________ name.
   C. It is often a drug's most _____________ name.
3. Drug Resources (List the available resources.)
   i. ______________________________
   ii. ______________________________
   iii. ______________________________
   iv. ______________________________
   v. ______________________________

4. Drug Classifications (List the three classifications.)
   i. ______________________________
   ii. ______________________________
   iii. ______________________________
5. Controlled Substances
   A. Must always be kept in a __________ cabinet.
   B. Must be labeled according to __________ specifications.
   C. All narcotics should be tracked on a ___________ log.
6. Commonly Stocked Injectables Drugs (List the injectable drugs that are typically stocked.)
   i. ______________________________
   ii. ______________________________
   iii. ______________________________
   iv. ______________________________
   v. ______________________________
   vi. ______________________________
   vii. ______________________________
   viii. ______________________________
   ix. ______________________________
   x. ______________________________
   xi. ______________________________
   xii. ______________________________
   xiii. ______________________________
   xiv. ______________________________
   xv. ______________________________
   xvi. ______________________________
   xvii. ______________________________
   xviii. ______________________________
7. The Medication Logbook
   A. Contains a complete list of all ______ medications, including sample products.
   B. Contains the name of each medication, the _______ on hand, and the ________ date.
   C. Contains a section for the patient's name, the ________, the date and time of ____________, and the medical assistant's initials.
8. Form DEA 224
   A. Used by physicians to register with the ______________________________.
   B. Allows physicians to _____________, ______________, or _____________ controlled substances.
   C. Renewal is required every ______ years.
9. Commonly Abused Drugs
   i. ______________________________
   ii. ______________________________
   iii. ______________________________
   iv. ______________________________
   v. ______________________________

10. Steps to Take When Drug Abuse Is Suspected
    i. ______
    ii. ______
    iii. ______

II. Routes and Drug Administration

1. Methods for Drug Administration: Parenteral
    i. ______
    ii. ______
    iii. ______
    iv. ______
    v. ______
    vi. ______

2. Methods for Drug Administration: Nonparenteral
    i. ______
    ii. ______
    iii. ______
    iv. ______
    v. ______
    vi. ______
    vii. ______
    viii. ______

3. Checklist for Administering Medication
    A. Be sure that you have the correct ______.
    B. Check and ______ that you have the correct ______ as ordered.
    C. Check that you are giving the correct ______.
    D. Make sure that you are using the correct ______.
    E. Make sure that you are giving it at the right ______.
    F. Be sure that the correct ______ is provided.

4. Examples of Side Effects of Medications: Anaphylactic Shock
    A. Anaphylactic shock is a Life-______ reaction to a drug, food, or insect bite.
    B. Symptoms of anaphylactic shock
        i. ______
        ii. ______
        iii. ______
        iv. ______
        v. ______

5. Drug Interactions
    A. Factors that contribute to a patient's reaction
        i. ______
        ii. ______
        iii. ______
        iv. ______
        v. ______
        vi. ______

6. Method of Administration
   A. The method of administration affects the rate at which the body _________ the medication.
   B. The method is chosen according to the ___________ ___________.
7. Intolerance to Medication
   A. Common symptoms
      i. ______________________________
      ii. ______________________________
      iii. ______________________________
8. Drug Use During Breast Feeding
   A. Contraindicated medications
      i. ______________________________
      ii. ______________________________
      iii. ______________________________
      iv. ______________________________
      v. ______________________________
      vi. ______________________________
9. Guidelines for the Administration of Medications
   A. Medications/drugs can only be administered to a patient under the supervision of a ____________ physician.
   B. The order must be written and ____________ on the patient's medical record by the ____________.
   C. Medications must be checked _______ times before administration.
   D. All narcotics must be ______________ in a record maintained for that purpose.
   E. Medication labels should be clean and ____________.

KEY TERMINOLOGY REVIEW

Match the correct medical term with the definition listed below.

a. Adverse effects
b. Bioequivalent
c. Brand name
d. Broad-spectrum
e. Contraindicated
f. Drug abuse
g. Drug dependency
h. Drug Enforcement Administration (DEA)
i. Drug tolerance
j. Generic name
k. Habituation
l. Idiosyncratic
m. Inscription
n. Lethal
o. Over-the-counter (OTC)
p. Pharmacists
q. Pharmacology
r. Prophylactically
s. Proprietary name
t. Side effects
u. Signa (sig.)
v. Subscription
w. Superscription
x. Synthetic
y. Toxic

1. __________ The use of a drug improperly or wrongly.
2. __________ Nonprescription drugs.
3. __________ Dependence on a drug.
4. __________ Equivalent to what is sometimes called the "official" or "nonproprietary" name of a drug.
5. __________ Adverse effects that may cause death.
6. __________ The Latin term for label.
7. __________ Having the same strength and action.
8. __________ This name is often the most familiar name for a specific drug.
9. __________ A decrease in the effectiveness of a drug as the body gets used to having the drug in the system.
10. __________ One who relies on the medication or uses the medication for psychological support has a __________________.
11. __________ Contains the patient's name, address, age, and date on the top line.
12. __________ Drugs used to prevent the onset of a condition.
13. __________ The name given to a drug by a specific manufacturer.
14. __________ Undesirable effects from a drug.
15. __________ Medications that are so dangerous for the infant that the mother must stop breastfeeding while she is taking them.
16. __________ Specially trained and licensed professionals who prepare and dispense drugs.
17. __________ The dose cannot always be increased because some drugs can become harmful or __________________ in excessive amounts.
18. __________ Require the patient to discontinue the medication because the negative effects outweigh the benefit of taking the medication.
19. __________ Side effects or adverse effects that are specific to the individual.
20. __________ Medications created in a laboratory by artificial means.
21. __________ The agency of the federal government responsible for enforcing drug control.
22. __________ Tells the pharmacist how to mix the drug and how much to provide to the patient.
23. __________ The study of medications and drugs, including their forms, intentions for use, and effects.
24. __________ Antibiotics are effective against a wide range of microorganisms.
25. __________ Gives the name of the medication, the actual ingredients, and the dosage.

APPLIED PRACTICE

Complete the following exercises.

1. It is important for patients to understand the instructions when taking medications. If a patient has a difficult time understanding the English language, it is important to overcome this communication barrier. List the various methods that you might use to overcome this barrier.

____

____

____

____

2. On the right-hand side of the table below, explain the use for each drug listed.

Name	Use
Adrenergic	
Adrenergic blocking agent	
Analgesic	
Anesthetic	
Antacid	
Antianxiety	
Antiarrhythmic	
Antibiotic	
Anticoagulant	
Anticonvulsant	
Antidepressant	
Antidiabetic	
Antidiarrheal	
Antidote	
Antiemetic	
Antifungal	
Antihelminthic	
Antihistamine	
Antihypertensive	
Anti-inflammatory	
Antineoplastic	
Antipruritic	
Antipyretic	

(continued)

(*Continued*)

Name	Use
Antiseptic	
Antitussive	
Astringent	
Bronchodilator	
Cardiogenic	
Cathartic	
Contraceptive	
Decongestant	
Diuretic	
Emetic	
Expectorant	
Hemostatic	
Hypnotic	
Hypoglycemic	
Immunosuppressant	
Laxative	
Miotic	
Muscle relaxant	
Mydriatic	
Narcotic	
Purgative	
Psychedelic	
Sedative	
Stimulant	
Tranquilizer	
Vaccine	
Vasodilator	
Vasopressor	
Vitamin	

LEARNING ACTIVITY: MULTIPLE CHOICE

Circle the correct answer to each of the questions below.

1. Which of the following is not included in Schedule II drugs?
   a. marijuana
   b. morphine
   c. cocaine
   d. Dilaudid

2. An injection into the fatty tissue under the skin is a(n) ________________ injection.
   a. intramuscular
   b. Z-track
   c. subcutaneous
   d. intradermal

3. The medication abbreviation for twice a day is ________________.
   a. b.i.d.
   b. t.i.d.
   c. prn
   d. q2h

4. The drug acetaminophen is also known as ________________.
   a. Tylenol
   b. Motrin
   c. iso-butyl-propanoic phenolic acid
   d. All of the above

5. The PDR is divided into six sections. The first white section ________________________.
   a. contains an alphabetical listing of the generic and brand names of each product
   b. contains an alphabetical listing by category or classification of generic and brand names
   c. contains current information regarding pharmaceutical manufacturers
   d. provides product identification and color photos of tablets and capsules listed alphabetically by the manufacturer

6. OTC medications are regulated by the ________________.
   a. AMA
   b. FDA
   c. CSA
   d. CMS

7. Schedule III drugs have ____________________________________.
   a. the highest potential for addiction and abuse
   b. moderate to low potential for addiction and abuse
   c. lower potential for addiction and abuse
   d. the lowest potential for addiction and abuse

8. Which of the following are common controlled substances?
   a. anabolic steroids
   b. butabarbital
   c. chloral hydrate
   d. All of the above

9. How often should the medical assistant review the inventory to ensure that a sufficient supply of all drugs is available and that no medication has expired?
   a. once a day
   b. once a week
   c. every other week
   d. once a month

10. Which of the following is the abbreviation meaning "before meals".
    a. Aa
    b. Ac
    c. ba
    d. ante

CRITICAL THINKING

Answer the following questions to the best of your ability. Utilize the textbook as a reference.

1. A patient has finished seeing the doctor, and on her way out she asks the medical assistant for a sample of Motrin, which is an OTC medication. The MA gives her two packages but does not document this and does not ask the doctor, because the MA felt that, since Motrin is an OTC medication, getting it without an order would be appropriate. Is this appropriate and if not, why?
   ____
   ____
   ____
   ____

2. When administering medications to children, what considerations should be given?
   ____
   ____
   ____
   ____

RESEARCH ACTIVITY

Utilize Internet search engines to research the following topics and write a brief description of what you find. It is important to utilize reputable websites.

1. Visit the FDA website at http://www.fda.gov/. Navigate through the site to learn more about this organization and the information provided on this site. Write an essay on what you learned by visiting the site.
   ____
   ____
   ____
   ____
   ____
   ____
   ____

CHAPTER 54

Administering Medications

CHAPTER OUTLINE

General review of the chapter:

Medication Administration
Equipment Used for Medication Administration
Administration Procedures: OSHA Standards
Charting Medication Administration
Sites for Intramuscular Injections
Subcutaneous Injections
Intradermal Injections
Intravenous Therapy
Immunizations
Reconstituting a Powdered Medication for Administration

STUDENT STUDY GUIDE

Use the following guide to assist in your learning of the concepts from the chapter.

I. The Administration of Medication

1. Nonparenteral Methods (Name and briefly explain each of the nonparenteral routes that can be used to provide medication to patients.)
   - i. ______________________: ____
   - ii. ______________________: ____
   - iii. ______________________: ____
   - iv. ______________________: ____
   - v. ______________________: ____
   - vi. ______________________: ____
   - vii. ______________________: ____
   - viii. ______________________: ____
2. The Tuberculin Syringe
   - A. ________- to _________-gauge needle.
   - B. Used to perform tuberculosis and __________ testing.
3. The Insulin Syringe
   - A. ________- to _________-gauge syringe
   - B. Injected into the __________, __________, or thigh.
4. Needles
   - A. The larger the needle, the ____________ is the gauge.
   - B. Needle length varies from _______ to _______ inches.
   - C. Larges needles are ________- to ________-gauge and are used in __________ care.
   - D. Needle length varies, depending on the _____ used and the area to be injected.

5. Considerations Regarding Syringes and Needles
   A. There is a puncture-proof ____________, or cover, on the needle.
   B. Never handle an un____________ needle.
   C. Any dirty or used needles should never be handled or ____________.
6. Single-dose or Multiple-dose Vials
   A. These are the most common forms for ____________ medications.
   B. They are glass vials with ____________ stoppers to protect the medication inside.
7. Withdrawing Medication from an Ampule
   A. Snap ____________ and ____________ finger gently against tip of ampule.
   B. ________________ neck of ampule.
   C. Use __________ between ampule and thumbs when breaking ampule.
   D. Insert the ________________________ and withdraw fluid.
8. Prefilled Cartridge Injection Systems
   A. Uses a prefilled, ___________-dose cartridge that fits in a special cartridge holder.
   B. The system is convenient because medications do not have to be ______ up prior to injection.
   C. The cartridge holders are __________ and long lasting.
9. OSHA
   A. Stands for ____.
   B. Provides guidelines for the ____________ of contaminated needles and syringes.
   C. Outlines follow-up procedures for health care workers who are stuck with ___________ needles.
10. The Biohazard Sharps Container
   A. All medical offices must have a ___________ proof, rigid, ___________ container labeled with an ___________ biohazard sticker for the disposal of sharps.
   B. These containers should be replaced and disposed of properly when ___________ full.
11. Charting Medications
   A. Parenteral medications and oral medications are charted using the same documentation (List the information that should be provided.)
      i. ____
      ii. ____
      iii. ____
      iv. ____
      v. ____
      vi. ____

II. Injection Methods

1. The Deltoid Muscle
   A. Works well for __________-volume injections only.
   B. The muscle is found by measuring _____ finger widths _________ the _________ process of the shoulder.
   C. Do not give shots in the __________ of the arm.
   D. Use a _________-gauge needle.
   E. For smaller arms, use a _________-gauge, ______-inch needle.
2. The Vastus Lateralis Muscle
   A. In infants, the vastus lateralis muscle lies _______ the greater ___________ of the _________.
   B. In adults, the vastus lateralis muscle extends from the ________ of the anterior _______ to the middle of the lateral __________ one handbreadth above the _________.
3. The Dorosgluteal Muscle
   A. Patient should lie _________ and point toes __________.
   B. Draw an imaginary line from the greater trochanter of the ___________ to the posterior superior ___________ spine.

4. The Ventrogluteal Muscle
   A. Place the palm of the ________ hand on the greater trochanter and the ________ finger on the superior __________ crest.
   B. Inject in the space between the ________ and ________ fingers.
   C. Give the injection at a ______-degree angle.
5. Subcutaneous Injections
   A. Used for ____________ doses of ______________ medications.
   B. Used in the __________, the upper back, the ____________, and the thighs.
   C. Given at a ______-degree angle.
6. Intradermal Injections
   A. Common sites for giving an intradermal injection include the ________ chest and ________ back, as well as the __________ forearm.
   B. Because just the top level of skin is entered, a small ___________, or bubble, that contains the injection fluid appears on the skin.
   C. Do not ____________ the area after giving the injection.
7. The Tuberculin Skin Test
   A. Administered __________________.
   B. Performed to determine whether a patient has developed an immune response to the bacterium that causes ______________.
   C. The test cannot tell if the infection is __________ or __________.
8. Tuberculin Skin Test Results
   A. Redness alone at the skin test site is a __________ reaction.
   B. A firm __________ is a __________ reaction to the skin test.
9. Intravenous (IV) Therapy
   A. This process involves administering fluids and solutions directly into a patient's __________.
   B. Medical assistants must consult their state ________ act before attempting any IV procedure.
10. How to Prepare an IV Tray (list the steps)
    i. ____
    ii. ____
    iii. ____
    iv. ____
    v. ____
    vi. ____
    vii. ____
    viii. ____
    ix. ____
    x. ____

III. Immunization

1. Antibodies and Immunity
   A. Antibodies are __________ substances that are produced by __________ in the spleen, lymph nodes, and tissues.
   B. Can react in response to __________ or foreign substances.
   C. Produced __________ by the human body when one becomes ill.
2. Childhood and Adolescent Immunizations
   A. Every year, a new recommended childhood and adolescent immunization schedule is produced by the ______________________________, the CDC's ________________ ________________, and the American Academy of Family Physicians.
   B. Indicates the recommended ______________ for immunizations.

3. The Hepatitis B Vaccine
   A. Hepatitis B is spread by the ____________ virus.
   B. Transmitted by contaminated ____________ in blood.
   C. A child will receive a total of ____________ doses before he or she is 24 weeks old.
4. The Diphtheria Vaccine
   A. Given to children in __________ doses.
   B. The __________ dose is given between ______ and _____ years of age.
   C. Diphtheria is diagnosed through a ______ culture.
   D. The symptoms are _________, _________, and _________ __________.
5. The Pertussis Vaccine
   A. Pertussis is caused by ___________, directly and indirectly transmitted.
   B. Only _____________ vaccination is needed before the child is immune to the disease.
6. The *Haemophilus influenzae* Type B Conjugate Vaccine
   A. _____ out of _________ children in the United States under 5 years of age gets Hib disease.
   B. Caused by a _____________ that is spread through the ___________.
7. The Hepatitis A Vaccine
   A. Hepatitis A affects the ___________.
   B. Spreads through personal contact or by eating _____________ food or drinking water.
   C. The vaccine is given to children over ___ years old.
8. The Poliovirus Vaccine
   A. Has been available since ___________.
   B. Polio is caused by a ___________.
   C. Spreads through contact with ___________.
9. Reconstituting a Powdered Medication for Administration
   A. Medications supplied in a powdered form generally have a __________ shelf life.
   B. In order to be injected, these powdered medications must be reconstituted with diluents, usually ________________.
10. Steps for Reconstituting a Powdered Medication for Administration (List the steps.)
    i. ____
    ii. ____
    ____
    iii. ____
    ____
    iv. ____
    v. ____
    vi. ____
    vii. ____
    viii. ____
    ____

KEY TERMINOLOGY REVIEW

Complete the following sentences using the key terms found at the beginning of the chapter.

1. The _______________ site is most commonly used for large volume, deep intramuscular injections or irritating, viscous (thick) medications.
2. _________________ are used for dispensing oral medication into the respiratory tract.
3. Meningitis is a result of _________________.

4. ____________________ administration means administering a medication through an injection.
5. An alcohol pad or cotton pad must be used to hold the vial to prevent glass cuts when opening ____________________.
6. The ______________ vaccine, until very recently, was not licensed for children under the age of 2 years.
7. There are two types of polio vaccines: _______________ and _________________.
8. The _____________ injection is commonly used for allergy skin tests in which a minute amount of material is injected within the top layer of skin to determine a patient's sensitivity.
9. _____________ is a disease of the nervous system and is caused by a bacterium that enters the body through a break in the skin.
10. Hepatitis ______ is the most common type of hepatitis in the United States.
11. ____________, also known as whooping cough, is a respiratory disease that is most common in children under age 4.
12. ________________ are given to humans to decrease the susceptibility to disease.
13. ________________, or chickenpox, is one of the most common childhood diseases.
14. The ____________ site is considered safer than the dorsogluteal site because there are no major nerves or blood vessels in this muscle.
15. A _______________ injection is given just under the skin in the fat (adipose) tissue.
16. The ____________, or thickness, of the medication being given also determines the gauge of the needle.

APPLIED PRACTICE

Complete the following exercises.

1. On the figure below, label each part of the syringe.

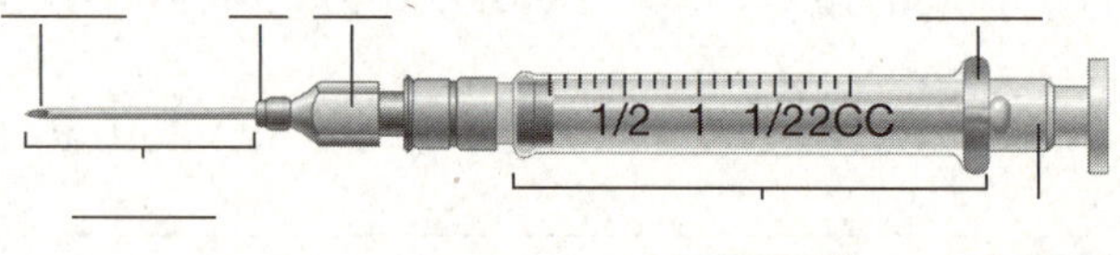

2. To demonstrate your knowledge regarding the angle of insertion for intramuscular, subcutaneous, and interdermal injections, indicate on the figure provided which angles represent each type of injection. In addition, provide the names of each of the layers of the skin.

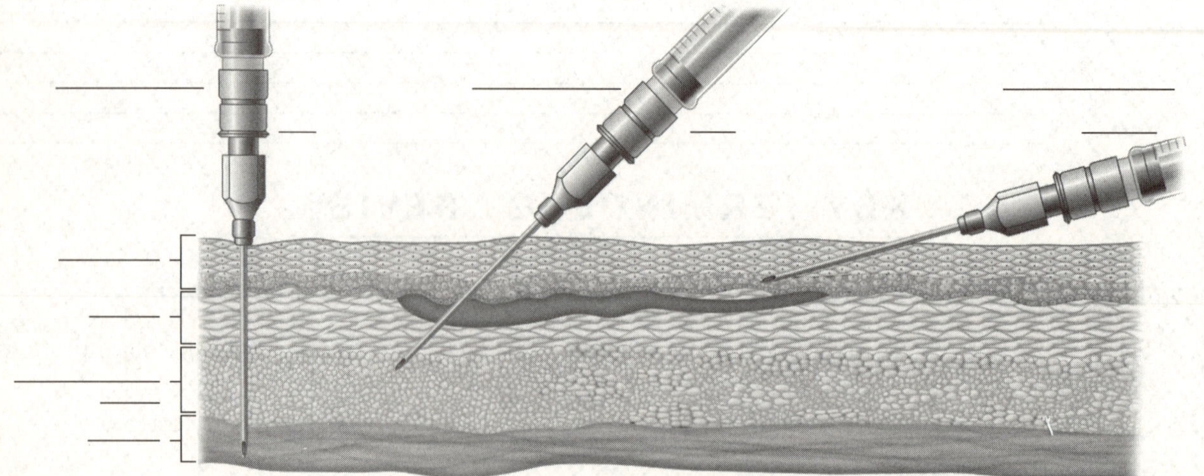

LEARNING ACTIVITY: TRUE/FALSE

Indicate whether the following statements are true or false by placing a T or an F on the line that precedes each statement.

_______ 1. Artificially acquired active immunity develops in response to receiving vaccinations with active organisms.

_______ 2. The deltoid muscle is located on the lower outer surface of the upper arm.

_______ 3. Transmission of diphtheria is by direct and indirect contact.

_______ 4. Hepatitis B, a form of viral hepatitis, is highly contagious and can be fatal.

_______ 5. Immunity can be either genetic or acquired.

_______ 6. Intramuscular injections are usually given with 25- or 26-gauge needles.

_______ 7. Many liquid medications are prescribed for the pediatric patient because of the ease of administration.

_______ 8. The MMR is given in three doses.

_______ 9. Oral medication is swallowed; it enters the body through the tissues of the gastrointestinal system and is then slowly absorbed into the body.

_______ 10. The vastus lateralis muscle is on the outer portion of the upper thigh and is part of the quadriceps.

_______ 11. When giving a medication using the Z-track method, you need to pull the skin upwards prior to inserting the needle.

CRITICAL THINKING

Answer the following questions to the best of your ability. Utilize the textbook as a reference.

1. Explain why IV infusion of medication is the most dangerous method to administer medication and MUST be the right medication, strength, and amount. Errors with this route can cause serious problems. All routes of medication administration MUST be done accurately, but there are specific reasons why this route is riskier than the others.

____

____

____

____

2. Although a very small of amount of bubbles or air injected into the muscle or the subcutaneous tissue would not be harmful, *the medical assistant must never let this happen*. Explain why it is not acceptable to have even tiny bubbles within the medication inside the syringe.

____

____

____

____

RESEARCH ACTIVITY

Utilize Internet search engines to research the following topic. It is important to utilize reputable websites.

1. Some parents believe that it is not necessary to immunize their children. To learn more about this issue, conduct research online and then write an essay on your findings. Conclude with a synopsis of what you believe about the necessity of immunizations for children. Be sure to cite your sources.

Chapter 55
Patient Education

CHAPTER OUTLINE

General review of the chapter:

Patient Education
How Adults Learn
Teaching Methods and Strategies
Developing a Teaching Plan
Learning Environment
Teaching Resources
Patient Issues
Health and Wellness
Mind–Body Connection
Teaching the Patient

STUDENT STUDY GUIDE

Use the following guide to assist in your learning of the concepts from the chapter.

I. Teaching Methods and Strategies

1. The Responsibilities of the Medical Assistant When Teaching the Patient
   A. Be prepared to educate the patient on behaviors that might _________ the health of the patient.
   B. Prepare the patient for a _________.
   C. Improve _________ with therapy or medication.
   D. Educate the patient about his or her own _________ behaviors.
2. Activities and Techniques for Teaching
   i. ______________________________
   ii. ______________________________
   iii. ______________________________
   iv. ______________________________
   v. ______________________________
3. Guidelines for Creating a Community Resource Brochure
   A. Identify __________ __________ that are available to help patients with disease prevention or health promotion, such as smoking cessation or weight loss.
   B. Research information found in a __________ __________, newspaper, or website.
   C. Create an attractive ____________ for distribution to patients that includes the name, location, telephone number, and services offered by the resources.
   D. After the brochure has been polished, obtain approval from the __________ __________ or physician before distributing the brochure to patients.

4. Information to be Included in a Public Relations Brochure
   i. ______________________________
   ii. ______________________________
   iii. ______________________________
   iv. ______________________________
   v. ______________________________
   vi. ______________________________
   vii. ______________________________
   viii. ______________________________
5. Motivational Incentives for Adult Patients
   i. ______________________________
   ii. ______________________________
   iii. ______________________________
   iv. ______________________________
   v. ______________________________
6. Roadblocks to Effective Patient Learning
   i. ______________________________
   ii. ______________________________
   iii. ______________________________
7. Communications and Language Roadblocks
   i. ______________________________
   ii. ______________________________
   iii. ______________________________
   iv. ______________________________
   v. ______________________________
   vi. ______________________________
   vii. ______________________________
   viii. ______________________________
   ix. ______________________________
   x. ______________________________
   xi. ______________________________
8. The Effects of Cultural Influences
   i. ______________________________
   ii. ______________________________
   iii. ______________________________
   iv. ______________________________
   v. ______________________________
   vi. ______________________________
9. The Effects of the Patient's Stage of Development
   A. Attitudes and ____________ have a powerful impact on learning readiness.
   B. Some patients may ____________ education because of previous negative experiences.
   C. In addition, illness affects people in different ways; ____________ and ____________ can be obstacles to learning.
10. Ways to Overcome Roadblocks
   A. Create a learning ____________ that encourages patient readiness.
   B. Consider ____________ the session if the patient is not feeling well at the time.
11. Lecture
   A. The advantages of lecturing include efficiency and the absence of limits on the ____________ of patients.

B. The disadvantage of lecturing is that there is no _________ in which to handle an individual patient's confusion.

12. Role-Playing

   A. Definition: The patient participates in a _________ _________ in which he or she acts out a story.
   B. Advantages
      i. ____________________
      ii. ____________________
   C. Disadvantages
      i. ____________________
      ii. ____________________

13. Case Problems

   A. Definition: Apply _________ to real situations.
   B. Advantages: They are believable and concrete instead of _________.
   C. Disadvantages: Significant _______ may be missing, and effectiveness depends on the _______.

14. Demonstration/Return Demonstration

   A. Definition: _________ patients how to do something, and then _________ has them do the same procedure.
   B. Advantages
      i. ____________________
      ii. ____________________
   C. Disadvantages
      i. ____________________
      ii. ____________________
   D. Usefulness
      i. ____________________
      ii. ____________________

15. Contracting

   A. Definition: Sets up goals with clear ___________ and ___________ for the patient.
   B. Advantages
      i. ____________________
      ii. ____________________
      iii. ____________________
   C. Disadvantages
      i. ____________________
      ii. ____________________
      iii. ____________________
   D. Usefulness
      i. ____________________
      ii. ____________________

16. The Use of a Significant Other

   A. Definition: Teaches a close _________/_________ the same information that the patient is being taught.
   B. Advantages
      i. ____________________
      ii. ____________________
   C. Disadvantages
      i. ____________________
      ii. ____________________
      iii. ____________________

D. Usefulness
   i. ______________________________
   ii. ______________________________
   iii. ______________________________

17. Past Experiences
   A. Definition: Build on what has been __________ in the past instead of creating a new set of knowledge.
   B. Advantages
      i. ______________________________
      ii. ______________________________
   C. Disadvantages
      i. ______________________________
      ii. ______________________________
   D. Usefulness
      i. ______________________________
      ii. ______________________________

18. Group Teaching
   A. Definition: Brings together patients who have common __________ needs.
   B. Advantages
      i. ______________________________
      ii. ______________________________
      iii. ______________________________
   C. Disadvantages
      i. ______________________________
      ii. ______________________________
      iii. ______________________________
      iv. ______________________________
   D. Usefulness
      i. ______________________________

19. Programmed Instruction
   A. Definition: ______________________________
   B. Advantages
      i. ______________________________
      ii. ______________________________
      iii. ______________________________
      iv. ______________________________
   C. Disadvantages
      i. ______________________________
      ii. ______________________________
      iii. ______________________________
      iv. ______________________________
   D. Usefulness
      i. ______________________________
      ii. ______________________________

20. Simulations (Games)
   A. Definition: Create a __________ __________ for learning purposes.
   B. Advantages
      i. ______________________________
      ii. ______________________________
      iii. ______________________________

C. Disadvantages
   i. ______________________________
   ii. ______________________________
   iii. ______________________________

21. Tests of Knowledge
   A. Definition: The patient is given __________ __________ that are related to his or her knowledge of the subject.
   B. Advantages
      i. ______________________________
      ii. ______________________________
      iii. ______________________________
   C. Disadvantages
      i. ______________________________
      ii. ______________________________
      iii. ______________________________

22. Printed Handouts
   A. Definition: Brochures or instruction sheets are printed for the purpose of __________ knowledge to the patient.
   B. Advantages
      i. ______________________________
      ii. ______________________________
   C. Disadvantages
      i. ______________________________
      ii. ______________________________

23. Diagrams
   A. Definition: Diagrams are __________ of concepts in __________ form.
   B. Advantages
      i. ______________________________
      ii. ______________________________
      iii. ______________________________
   C. Disadvantages
      i. ______________________________
      ii. ______________________________

24. Models
   A. Definition: Models are __________ __________ of an object that is produced in a substance such as clay or plaster.
   B. Advantages
      i. ______________________________
      ii. ______________________________
   C. Disadvantage: ______________________________

25. Film
   A. Definition: In this context, a film is considered to be a video, __________ __________, or moving picture.
   B. Advantages
      i. ______________________________
      ii. ______________________________
   C. Disadvantages
      i. ______________________________
      ii. ______________________________
      iii. ______________________________

26. Helpful Materials to Use When Teaching Children
    A. Children may need to see a treatment or procedure performed on a ___________ before tolerating it well.
    B. Many children like to ___________ equipment that will be used on them, such as a ___________ or a blood pressure cuff.
    C. Older children may wish to see videos about their upcoming __________ or other treatments.
27. Considerations for Teaching the Visually Impaired
    A. Visually impaired patients may not be able to read written instructions unless the type is __________ __________, and some may not be able to read it at all.
    B. The medical assistant may need to make __________-__________ instructions of information that is usually written.
    C. Be sure to clear ___________ from the office that might impede the patient, and make sure to hold the patient's hand to lead him or her to examinations and procedures.
28. Considerations for Teaching Non–English-Speaking Patients
    A. When the appointment is made, ask the patient if he or she would like to have an ______________ present.
    B. The patient may prefer to bring a relative who ___________ ___________.
    C. Be sure to get the patient's permission to discuss ___________ ___________ with relatives.
    D. Send __________ __________ home with the patient.
    E. If a large percentage of patients in the office speaks a particular language other than English, it may be helpful to create brochures in __________ __________.
    F. Consider __________ and __________, as well as the patient's likes and dislikes, to promote compliance.
29. Changes That Affect the Elderly Learner
    i. ____
    ii. ____
    iii. ____
    iv. ____
30. Methods to Be Considered When Teaching the Elderly
    A. Use handouts with ___________ ___________, and use video and audiovisual displays.
    B. __________-__________ slides are preferable to a fast video or movie because the slide can be stopped to reinforce learning.
    C. __________-__________ can be useful as long as the patient's energy level can be maintained.
    D. __________ __________ should be included in the teaching process whenever possible.
    E. The elderly person is accustomed to being in ____________ and may not wish to learn anything new if he or she does not see the ___________ of doing so.
31. Considerations for Creating a Teaching Plan
    A. Patients may not be honest and open in a busy place where they lack ___________.
    B. It is ideal if patient education can take place in a __________-__________ room with privacy.
    C. Sometimes placing patient education materials in racks in examining rooms allows patients to take brochures ___________.
    D. If a medical assistant is teaching a patient how to use equipment, then that equipment should be ___________ for the patient.
    E. If the patient asks a question that the medical assistant cannot answer, the MA should admit that he or she does not know the answer and __________ __________ to the patient with the answer to the question.
    F. Teaching resources are available for ___________, or the MA can develop ___________ for the office.
    G. Patients have different ___________ styles, and the teaching should match the patient's preferred style.

32. Ways to Help Patients Be More Compliant

   A. Ensure a __________ relationship is formed between the patient and the health care provider, physician and other staff such as the medical assistant.
   B. Convey to the patient the knowledge that he or she needs to make __________ decisions about health care.
   C. Reinforce learning and reduce __________ by working out a __________-__________ plan with regular evaluation of progress.
   D. This plan should include an __________ stating what the patient should be able to do, as well as a __________ indicating when the objective should be accomplished.

II. Patient Education

1. The Mind–Body Connection

   A. __________are released when patients are happy.
   B. Characteristics of these proteins
      i. They have __________ properties.
      ii. The benefit __________ functioning.
      iii. They boost __________ to disease.
   C. Negative feelings such as fear, anger, and grief can cause certain symptoms (List these symptoms.)
      i. Increase in __________
      ii. Tightening of the __________
      iii. __________ response

2. The Reality of Pain

   A. Pain is an unpleasant __________ and __________ experience.
   B. Patients respond differently to pain, depending on their tolerance and __________ __________.
   C. It is important for the medical assistant not to put a __________ value on the patient's pain.
   D. Pain can be __________ and __________.
   E. Sometimes pain is __________, meaning that it is felt in an area other than where it actually occurred.
   F. It is important for the medical assistant to assure the patient that pain __________ is possible.

3. Considerations for the Various Aspects of Pain

   A. Pain is a __________ experience for the patient.
   B. Pain is what the patient __________ it as.

4. The Long-Term Effects of Chronic Pain

   i. __________
   ii. __________
   iii. __________
   iv. __________
   v. __________
   vi. __________
   vii. __________
   viii. __________
   ix. __________
   x. __________
   xi. __________
   xii. __________

5. Teaching about Nutrition (list the elements contained in MyPyramid, developed by the United States Department of Agriculture)

   i. __________
   ii. __________

iii. ______________________________
iv. ______________________________
v. ______________________________

6. Teaching about Exercise
   A. Before starting any exercise program, a patient should consult the _________ to confirm that it is safe for the patient to exercise.
   B. Some patients with heart or respiratory problems may need to have a _________ exercise plan.
   C. Patients need to be taught to _________ and _________ _________ properly, and how to exercise without becoming injured.
7. Ways to Reduce Stress
   i. ______________________________
   ii. ______________________________
   iii. ______________________________
   iv. ______________________________
   v. ______________________________
   vi. ______________________________
8. Methods for Stopping Smoking
   A. Use nicotine or _________ therapy.
   B. Utilize various _________ substitutes.
   C. Choose the right _________ to quit smoking.
   D. Seek _________ support to help stop smoking.
   E. _________ in support groups.
   F. Receive information about _________ rates.
9. Preparing a Patient for a Cast Application
   A. Explain that casts are applied for the purpose of _________ a broken bone or muscle strain and sprain.
   B. A cast may be applied after a _________ _________ on a limb to immobilize the area until healing takes place.
10. Supplies Used for Cast Application
    i. ______________________________
    ii. ______________________________
    iii. ______________________________
    iv. ______________________________
    v. ______________________________
    vi. ______________________________
    vii. ______________________________
11. Assisting the Physician with Cast Application
    A. It may be necessary to hold the limb at the _________ _________ as the cast is being applied.
    B. Remember to handle a _________ _________ gently
    C. After the cast has been applied, it must be left _________ during the drying process.
    D. The limb may need to be supported on a _________ at this time.
    E. The patient should be cautioned against moving around until the cast is _________.
    F. The cast may feel _________ or even _________ during the drying process.
12. Observations That Patients Should Report
    A. _________ that is restricted by the cast.
    B. Pain as a result of the cast _________ the skin.

C. Excessive __________ under the cast
D. __________ or __________ in the fingers or toes.
E. Discolored __________ or __________
F. __________ of the limb around the edge of the cast
G. __________ soaking through the cast
H. A __________ __________ coming from the cast

13. Types of Casts (Describe each type.)
    A. Short arm cast (SAC): ____________________
    B. Long arm cast (LAC): ____________________
    C. Long and short leg casts: ____________________

14. Patient Cast Care
    A. Clean the cast with a __________ __________.
    B. Do not __________ or __________ the cast. If the edge seems sharp, apply __________ __________ to the sharp edge or use a nail file to trim it down.
    C. Elevate the extremity with the cast on it to reduce __________ and __________.
    D. Observe the fingers and toes for __________ __________, temperature changes, pain, tingling, or decreased sensation.
    E. Allow the cast material to __________ by exposing it to the air and keeping it uncovered, even during the night. If you apply pressure to the cast before it is dry, you can damage the __________ underneath.
    F. Do not try to __________ under the cast by putting objects into the cast. This will result in broken skin that can lead to infection.
    G. When decorating a cast, use only __________-__________ paints or marking pens; otherwise, the cast will not be able to __________.
    H. Call the physician's office if you smell a __________ odor coming from the cast, lose __________ or blood flow beyond the cast, feel a burning sensation, or notice blood coming from the cast.
    I. After being sure that the patient understands the __________ of cast care, the medical assistant must document the teaching in the patient's chart.

15. Equipment Needed for Cast Removal
    i. ____________________
    ii. ____________________
    iii. ____________________
    iv. ____________________
    v. ____________________

16. Procedure for Cast Removal
    A. After performing hand hygiene and draping the patient, explain the process to the patient.
       i. The __________ vibrates and does not __________.
       ii. The patient may feel some __________ and __________.
       iii. The patient may be shocked to see that the skin under the cast has become __________ and the muscle tone has decreased, and may need some reassurance that physical therapy will improve the functioning and appearance of the limb.
    B. The medical assistant should stand near the __________ and hand him or her the necessary equipment as requested.
    C. After the cast is removed, the medical assistant should do the following
       i. ____________________
       ii. ____________________
       iii. ____________________
       iv. ____________________

KEY TERMINOLOGY REVIEW

Complete the sentence by selecting the correct key term, as found in Chapter 55 of your textbook. A few of the sentences will use one or more key terms.

1. The education process begins with ____________, or ____________ of the patient's needs.
2. _____________ pain is pain that continues over time; ____________ pain can occur after surgery.
3. Some patients with heart or respiratory problems may need to have a modified exercise __________.
4. _____________—not following a physician's orders—can seriously jeopardize a patient's health and recovery.
5. If a patient is unable to complete a teaching plan, be sure to ____________ this in the patient's chart.
6. _________________ the plan involves actually teaching the patient what to do.
7. Some procedures that require small-muscle ______________, such as flossing the teeth and opening medication bottles, are almost impossible for elderly persons with arthritis.
8. ________________ are the goals of patient education.

APPLIED PRACTICE

Explain how you would handle the following scenario.

Scenario

Ethan is an RMA working at a pain management clinic. He often conducts patient education seminars on proper medication administration and methods of pain management. Today, Ethan is working with Aidan Baker, a child who had a below-the-knee right leg amputation, and who is also deaf. Explain how you would approach a child with special needs.

____

____

____

____

LEARNING ACTIVITY: MULTIPLE CHOICE

Circle the correct answer to each of the questions below.

1. What is the main difference between adult and child learning?
   a. The child expects milk and cookies afterward.
   b. The adult needs self-directed learning.
   c. The adult is stubborn and will tend to refuse most new knowledge.
   d. The child is likely to cry throughout most of the teaching session.

2. Which of the following is essential to an exercise program?
   a. Attractive warm-up clothes
   b. Stretching

c. Health club membership
d. A running partner

3. Which of the following is not part of a prevention program?

   a. Meditating
   b. Routine immunizations
   c. Smoking cigars instead of cigarettes
   d. Jogging

4. Which of the following should be part of an effective teaching plan?

   a. Understanding desired outcomes.
   b. Behaving in a commanding, authoritative way.
   c. Using sarcasm and ironic comments when the patient is slow.
   d. Offering private lessons.

5. Which of the following should *not* be an aspect of teaching older adults?

   a. Understanding that older adults may take longer to process new information.
   b. Keeping instructions to the point and providing clear written materials.
   c. Not talking down to an adult.
   d. Keeping a bowl of favorite candies nearby for reinforcement.

6. Which of the following is conducive to a proper learning environment?

   a. The reception area
   b. A private examination room
   c. The hallway
   d. The front desk

7. Which of the following is *not* an appropriate teaching resource?

   a. Audiocassette
   b. Videos
   c. Pamphlets
   d. Personal websites

8. The long-term effects of chronic pain can include ______________________________.

   a. a feeling of helplessness
   b. decreased sleep
   c. lowered self-esteem
   d. All of the above

9. When educating patients with regard to dieting and weight loss, what information should *not* be included?

   a. Successful fad diets
   b. Information regarding how to read food labels
   c. Copies of MyPyramid
   d. All of the above should be given.

10. Which of the following is *not* a phase of patient education?

    a. Implementation
    b. Documentation
    c. Production
    d. Planning

CRITICAL THINKING

Answer the following questions to the best of your ability. Utilize the textbook as a reference.

1. **Scenario**

   a. Imagine that you are a family member of a patient with chronic pain and are going with him or her to an office visit. You know that the patient is truly in pain and is not a drug seeker. What do you think you would say or do if the medical assistant or any staff member gave the impression, through body language only, that he or she did not believe that the patient had as much pain as the patient indicated?

   ____

   ____

   ____

   ____

   ____

   b. What do you think you would say or do if the medical assistant did not make eye contact, was not warm and caring, and did not chat at all, except to ask the required questions, and then hurried out when the patient started to ask a question?

   ____

   ____

   ____

   ____

   ____

   c. What do you think you would say or do if the medical assistant would talk over the medication treatment, not with you, but only with the patient, stating that the patient alone needs to be able to handle his or her medications?

   ____

   ____

   ____

   ____

   ____

2. **Scenario**

   You are a new medical assistant, and the physician has asked you to go into the examination room and give patient teaching to Mrs. McCarty about her rheumatoid arthritis pain management plan. The physician has written in the chart what the plan is but you are not very familiar with rheumatoid arthritis. Would you (a) try to do the best you can, (b) ask another MA to tell you what to do or how to do it, or (c) ask the patient to wait while you research office policy manuals and the Internet to figure it out? Choose one of the options and then explain your reasoning.

   ____

   ____

   ____

   ____

   ____

3. **Scenario**

   You are a medical assistant at an OB/GYN office. The physician has recently put you in charge of creating a list of resources and materials to be used in a patient education library. What patient education topics would you include in an OB/GYN resource library? List at least three topics and explain why you chose them.

RESEARCH ACTIVITY

Utilize Internet search engines to research the following topics and write a brief description of what you find. It is important to utilize reputable websites.

1. Choose a topic for patient education and search the Internet for reputable information. List at least five reputable websites that could be used for patient education. Also, list at least five items of special interest that you learned.

CHAPTER 56
Nutrition

CHAPTER OUTLINE

General review of the chapter:

Nutrition
Dietary Guidelines

STUDENT STUDY GUIDE

Use the following guide to assist in your learning of the concepts from the chapter.

I. Nutrition

1. Diet and Nutrition (Provide the name of the professional who is described.)
   A. __________: A professional who provides information on foods and nutrition
   B. __________: A professional who promotes good health through proper diet and the use of diet in the treatment of disease
2. Digestion
   A. The actual process the body undergoes when it converts food into _________ __________ that can be absorbed into the blood and used by the body tissues and organs.
   B. The actual digestive process is accomplished by physically breaking down, diluting, dissolving, and chemically splitting into _________ __________, the food substance we consume.
3. Major Nutrient Classes
   i. ______________________________
   ii. ______________________________
   iii. ______________________________
   iv. ______________________________
   v. ______________________________
   vi. ______________________________
4. Carbohydrates
   A. Carbohydrates include the following
      i. ______________________________
      ii. ______________________________
      iii. ______________________________
   B. Carbohydrates are stored in the body as ______________.
5. Carbohydrates for Health
   A. __________ carbohydrates are ideal foods for a healthy diet.
   B. They are generally low in __________, high in __________, and a good source of vitamins and minerals.
   C. Excess carbohydrates are stored as __________ (after the small amount of glycogen stores fill up).

6. Carbohydrate Consumption Recommendations
   A. Only __________ of calories from refined sugar
   B. Approximately __________ to __________ of calories from carbohydrates
7. Sources of Carbohydrates
   i. ____________________
   ii. ____________________
8. Fats
   A. Fats are also called __________.
   B. They do not dissolve in __________.
   C. Some fat is needed in the diet for __________ __________.
   D. Fats are a major __________ source for the body.
   E. Found in animal and __________ food products.
   F. Provide taste, consistency, and __________ to foods.
9. Saturated Fats
   A. Produced by __________ sources.
   B. They have many __________ effects on the body.
   C. No more than ______ of the daily caloric intake should come from saturated fat.
   D. Reducing these fats can help __________ the risk of disease.
10. Unsaturated Fats
   A. Polyunsaturated fat is found in ______________ and fish oils.
   B. Monounsaturated fat can lower ________________ levels and ________________.
11. How Fats Benefit the Body
   A. Serve as a __________ energy source.
   B. Help __________ fat-soluble vitamins.
   C. Provide some __________ to foods.
   D. Satisfy the __________.
   E. __________ the skin and internal tissues.
   F. Are __________ for energy use after the meal.
12. Fat Consumption Recommendations
   A. Only __________ of calories should come from saturated fat.
   B. Less than ___________ of total calories should come from fat.
13. Sources of Fats (List the sources for each of the following fats.)
   A. Saturated Fats: ____________________
   B. Polyunsaturated Fats: ____________________
   C. Monounsaturated Fats: ____________________
14. Protein
   A. Forms the __________ of every cell.
   B. Formed from __________ of amino acids.
   C. Protein is needed by the body to accomplish the following
      i. ____________________
      ii. ____________________
      iii. ____________________
15. Reading Food Labels
   A. __________ products are the only foods that provide complete proteins (all nine essential amino acids).
   B. Combining certain __________ proteins can add up to a complete protein.

16. Water
    A. Water has no __________ value.
    B. The human body is __________ to __________ water.
    C. __________ holds more water.
    D. __________ holds less water.
    E. The water content is __________ in males than in females and __________ with age.

17. Sources of Water
    i. ______________________________
    ii. ______________________________
    iii. ______________________________

18. The Functions of Water
    A. Carries _________ and nutrients to cells.
    B. Regulates body _____________.
    C. Prevents ____________.
    D. Replaces water lost through perspiration, respiration, ___________, and ____________.
    E. Removes waste products from _________.
    F. Protects _________ and tissues.

19. The Amount of Water Needed Varies Because of the Following Factors
    i. ______________________________
    ii. ______________________________
    iii. ______________________________
    iv. ______________________________
    v. ______________________________
    vi. ______________________________
    vii. ______________________________

20. Vitamin Classifications
    A. Water-soluble vitamins (Provide examples of water-soluble vitamins.)
        i. ______________________________
        ii. ______________________________
        iii. ______________________________
        iv. ______________________________
        v. ______________________________
        vi. ______________________________
        vii. ______________________________
        viii. ______________________________
        ix. ______________________________
    B. Fat-soluble vitamins (Provide examples of fat-soluble vitamins.)
        i. ______________________________
        ii. ______________________________
        iii. ______________________________
        iv. ______________________________

21. Requirements for Vitamins
    A. Several conditions increase the requirement for vitamins beyond the usual recommended amounts.
        i. ______________________________
        ii. ______________________________
        iii. ______________________________
        iv. ______________________________

22. Sources of Vitamins: Vitamin B1 (thiamine)

i. ______________________
ii. ______________________
iii. ______________________
iv. ______________________
v. ______________________
vi. ______________________

23. Sources of Vitamins: Vitamin B2 (riboflavin)

i. ______________________
ii. ______________________
iii. ______________________
iv. ______________________
v. ______________________
vi. ______________________

24. Sources of Vitamins: Vitamin B6

i. ______________________
ii. ______________________
iii. ______________________
iv. ______________________
v. ______________________
vi. ______________________

25. Sources of Vitamins: Vitamin B12

i. ______________________
ii. ______________________
iii. ______________________
iv. ______________________
v. ______________________

26. Sources of Vitamins: Niacin

i. ______________________
ii. ______________________
iii. ______________________
iv. ______________________
v. ______________________

27. Sources of Vitamins: Biotin

i. ______________________
ii. ______________________
iii. ______________________

28. Sources of Vitamins: Folacin (folic acid)

i. ______________________
ii. ______________________

29. Sources of Vitamins: Pantothenic acid

i. ______________________
ii. ______________________

30. Sources of Vitamins: Vitamin C

i. ______________________
ii. ______________________
iii. ______________________

31. Sources of Vitamins: Vitamin A

i. ______________________
ii. ______________________
iii. ______________________
iv. ______________________

32. Sources of Vitamins: Vitamin D

i. ______________________
ii. ______________________
iii. ______________________
iv. ______________________
v. ______________________
vi. ______________________

33. Sources of Vitamins: Vitamin E

i. ______________________
ii. ______________________
iii. ______________________

34. Sources of Vitamins: Vitamin K

i. ______________________
ii. ______________________
iii. ______________________
iv. ______________________

35. Minerals

A. Minerals are __________ substances that are of neither plant nor animal origin.
B. They are found throughout the body, but mainly in __________ and __________.

36. Mineral Classifications

A. Macrominerals (List the minerals that are classified as macrominerals.)

i. ______________________
ii. ______________________
iii. ______________________
iv. ______________________
v. ______________________
vi. ______________________
vii. ______________________

B. Microminerals (List the minerals that are classified as microminerals.)

i. ______________________
ii. ______________________
iii. ______________________
iv. ______________________
v. ______________________
vi. ______________________
vii. ______________________
viii. ______________________
ix. ______________________
x. ______________________
xi. ______________________
xii. ______________________

37. Sources of Minerals: Calcium

i. ______________________
ii. ______________________
iii. ______________________

iv. ____________________
v. ____________________
vi. ____________________

38. Sources of Minerals: Copper
i. ____________________
ii. ____________________
iii. ____________________
iv. ____________________
v. ____________________

39. Sources of Minerals: Fluorine
i. ____________________
ii. ____________________
iii. ____________________

40. Sources of Minerals: Iodine
i. ____________________
ii. ____________________
iii. ____________________

41. Sources of Minerals: Iron
i. ____________________
ii. ____________________
iii. ____________________
iv. ____________________
v. ____________________
vi. ____________________

42. Sources of Minerals: Magnesium
i. ____________________
ii. ____________________
iii. ____________________
iv. ____________________
v. ____________________
vi. ____________________
vii. ____________________

43. Sources of Minerals: Phosphorus
i. ____________________
ii. ____________________
iii. ____________________
iv. ____________________
v. ____________________
vi. ____________________

44. Sources of Minerals: Potassium
i. ____________________
ii. ____________________
iii. ____________________
iv. ____________________
v. ____________________

45. Sources of Minerals: Sodium
i. ____________________
ii. ____________________
iii. ____________________

iv. ____
v. ____
vi. ____

46. Cholesterol
    A. Cholesterol is normally found in and is __________ by the body.
    B. It is __________ for the __________ of bodily systems, such as the nervous system, and for the formation of cell membranes and many hormones.
47. Sources of Cholesterol
    A. The _____________ body.
    B. Animal _____________.
    C. Your _____________ produces most of the cholesterol in your body (1000 mg/day).
48. Cholesterol in the Body
    A. Cholesterol moves into and out of the body cells within __________.
    B. ___________-____________ ____________ (HDLs) carry cholesterol away from the bloodstream.
    C. ___________-___________ ___________ (LDLs) carry most of the cholesterol into the bloodstream.
49. Cholesterol and Disease
    A. An increase in cholesterol is linked to an increase in the following diseases
        i. ____
        ii. ____
50. Dietary Guidelines for Americans
    i. ____
    ii. ____
    iii. ____
    iv. ____
    v. ____
51. Calories
    A. Food intake is measured in terms of the __________ that food produces.
    B. Calorie: A measurement of a unit of ______ that provides _______.
52. Caloric Requirements
    A. All food (except water) generates ________ in the body.
    B. The daily caloric requirement is based on the following
        i. ____
        ii. ____
        iii. ____
        iv. ____
    C. Men generally need more __________ than women.
    D. Women require more calories during __________ and __________.
53. Dietary Modification
    A. Common conditions that necessitate dietary modification
        i. ____
        ii. ____
        iii. ____
        iv. ____
        v. ____
    B. Common dietary modifications
        i. ____
        ii. ____

iii. ____________________
iv. ____________________
v. ____________________
vi. ____________________
vii. ____________________
viii. ____________________
ix. ____________________
x. ____________________
xi. ____________________
xii. ____________________

54. Patient Education
   A. Diet __________ should be carefully explained to the patient.
   B. Patients are often referred to a __________ __________ (RD) who will discuss the therapeutic diet with the patient.
   C. The medical assistant will often provide __________ education for patients in the medical office.
   D. __________ __________ are often associated with dietary modification and should be included in patient education.

55. The Clear Liquid Diet
   A. Contains no __________ __________ or milk products.
   B. Frequently required before certain __________ __________, examinations, or surgery.
   C. The patient must not remain on a clear liquid diet for __________ periods.
   D. Foods included in a clear liquid diet
      i. ____________________
      ii. ____________________
      iii. ____________________
      iv. ____________________
      v. ____________________

56. The Full Liquid Diet
   A. Prescribed for patients who are unable to chew and/or digest solid food because of the following conditions
      i. ____________________
      ii. ____________________
      iii. ____________________
   B. Often prescribed as the next step after a __________ __________ diet.
   C. Foods included in a full liquid diet
      i. ____________________
      ii. ____________________
      iii. ____________________
      iv. ____________________
      v. ____________________
      vi. ____________________

57. The Mechanical Soft Diet
   A. Recommended for patients who have __________ __________ or difficulty swallowing.
   B. Recommended for patients who are recovering from __________.
   C. Foods included in a mechanical soft diet
      i. ____________________
      ii. ____________________
      iii. ____________________
      iv. ____________________
      v. ____________________

vi. ______________________________
vii. ______________________________

58. The Bland Diet
   A. Contains no seasonings or __________ that are irritating.
   B. Prescribed for patients who have __________ problems or allergies.
   C. Eliminates foods that are __________ __________ (e.g., cabbage).
   D. Eliminates __________ and spices.
   E. Eliminates foods that are high in __________.
   F. Foods included in a bland diet
      i. ______________________________
      ii. ______________________________
      iii. ______________________________
      iv. ______________________________
      v. ______________________________

59. The BRAT Diet
   A. BRAT stands for __________, __________, __________, and __________.
   B. Prescribed for __________ __________ who are experiencing vomiting, nausea, and diarrhea.

60. The High-Protein Diet
   A. Recommended for patients who are recovering from __________ __________.
   B. Aids in __________.

61. The Diabetic Diet
   A. Considerations for placing a patient on a diabetic diet
      i. ______________________________
      ii. ______________________________
      iii. ______________________________
      iv. ______________________________
      v. ______________________________
   B. Often uses a __________ __________ system to allow patients to select preferred foods.
   C. Foods are grouped into the Food Pyramid categories (List the categories.)
      i. ______________________________
      ii. ______________________________
      iii. ______________________________
      iv. ______________________________
      v. ______________________________
      vi. ______________________________

62. The High-Residue/Fiber Diet
   A. Used to treat patients with __________ __________.
   B. Dietary fiber may provide protection against the following diseases or conditions
      i. ______________________________
      ii. ______________________________
      iii. ______________________________
      iv. ______________________________
      v. ______________________________
      vi. ______________________________
      vii. ______________________________
      viii. ______________________________
   C. May __________ cholesterol.
   D. The recommended daily intake of fiber is ______ to ______ grams per day.
   E. Fiber is not found in __________ products or __________ products.

63. The Low-Residue Diet

A. The low-residue diet is often called a __________-__________diet.

B. It is useful for patients with the following conditions

i. ____________________

ii. ____________________

iii. ____________________

iv. ____________________

C. Foods included in a low-residue diet

i. ____________________

ii. ____________________

iii. ____________________

iv. ____________________

v. ____________________

vi. ____________________

vii. ____________________

64. The Low-Fat/Cholesterol Diet

A. Aimed at keeping fat content between _____ and _____ grams of fat per day.

B. The average American diet contains between _____ and _____ grams of fat per day.

C. May reduce the risk of colon, breast, and __________ cancer; __________ __________; and __________.

D. Foods included in a low-fat/cholesterol diet

i. ____________________

ii. ____________________

iii. ____________________

iv. ____________________

v. ____________________

65. The Low-Sodium/Salt Diet

A. Used for patients with _____________ and heart or kidney disease.

B. Recommended for patients on _____________-_____________ diets in order to reduce water retention.

66. Guidelines for a Low-Sodium/Salt Diet

A. Mild Restriction: __________ to __________ mg of sodium per day

i. Allow __________ __________ of table salt per day.

ii. Limit foods that contain salt, including __________ foods.

B. Moderate Restriction: _______ to _______ mg of sodium per day

i. Allow __________ __________ of table salt per day.

ii. No processed and __________ foods with salt.

iii. No salt in food __________.

iv. This is the most __________ low-sodium/salt diet.

C. Severe Restriction: __________ mg of sodium per day

i. Limit ___________ ___________ ___________, including salt in cooking.

ii. Use only ___________-___________ products.

iii. Increase the intake of ___________ ___________ and ___________.

iv. Read ___________ carefully.

67. The Caloric Content Diet

A. Often prescribed as a ___________-___________ ___________ for persons affected by excess weight.

B. Helps to prevent and control the following diseases or conditions

i. ____________________

ii. ____________________

iii. ____________________

C. The ___________-___________ diet uses a balance of the five food groups and low-fat foods.
D. Guidelines for a low-calorie content diet
   i. ____
   ii. ____
   iii. ____
   iv. ____
   v. ____
   vi. ____
E. Caloric intake should total _______ calories.
F. Keep a ___________ ___________.

68. Healthy Food Choices: Eat Less Fat
   A. Eat ___________ and fish more often.
   B. Prepare all meats by roasting, broiling, or ___________.
   C. Trim off all ___________ fat.
   D. Remove the ___________ from all poultry.
   E. Avoid adding ___________ during cooking.
   F. Eat fewer ___________-___________ foods.
   G. Drink skim or ___________-___________ milk.

69. Healthy Food Choices: Eat More High-Fiber Foods
   A. Choose dried beans, ___________, and ___________ more often.
   B. Eat whole-___________ ___________, cereals, and crackers.
   C. Eat more ___________, both raw and cooked.
   D. Try ___________-___________ foods such as oat bran, barley, brown rice, bulgur, and wild rice.

70. Healthy Food Choices: Use Less Salt
   A. Reduce the amount of ___________ that you use in cooking.
   B. Try not to put ___________ on food at the table.
   C. Eat fewer ___________-___________ foods such as canned soups, ham, hot dogs, pickles, sauerkraut, and foods that taste salty.

71. Healthy Food Choices: Eat Less Sugar
   A. Avoid ___________ ___________, syrup, honey, jam, jelly, candy, sweet rolls, fruit canned in syrup, regular gelatin, desserts, pie, cake with icing, and other sweets.
   B. Avoid ___________ soft drinks.
   C. Choose fresh fruit or fruit canned in ___________ ___________ or water.
   D. If desired, use non-caloric ___________ instead of sugar.

72. Exercise
   A. Activity helps to ___________ the fat in the diet so that it is not stored in the body.
   B. Patients should be cleared by a ___________ before exercising.
   C. Keep exercise programs ___________.

KEY TERMINOLOGY REVIEW

Match the vocabulary term to the correct definition below.

a. Calorie
b. Cholesterol
c. Digestion
d. Hydrogenation
e. Lactating
f. Lactose
g. Lipids
h. Macrominerals
i. Metabolism
j. Minerals

k. Monosaccharides
l. Nutrients
m. Polysaccharides
n. Recommended Dietary Allowances (RDAs)
o. Refined sugars
p. Vitamins

1. __________ Process whereby unsaturated (liquid) fat can be converted into a solid fat.
2. __________ The sum of all physical and chemical changes that take place within the human body.
3. __________ Recommendations for the amount of protein, vitamins, and minerals that Americans should try to eat for good nutrition (developed by the Food and Nutrition Board of the National Academy of Sciences).
4. __________ Simple sugars.
5. __________ Producing milk.
6. __________ Fatlike material that is essential for the function of bodily systems.
7. __________ Trace minerals, including calcium, magnesium, phosphorus, sodium, potassium, chlorine, and sulfur.
8. __________ Starches that are reduced to glucose during the digestive process and transported into the blood.
9. __________ Processed sugars that have been extracted and concentrated from natural sources.
10. __________ The process the body undertakes when it converts food into chemical substances that can be absorbed into the blood and used by the body tissues and organs.
11. __________ Fatty acids that can be chemically classified as saturated or unsaturated.
12. __________ Organic substances that are essential for metabolism, growth, and development of the body.
13. __________ Organic and inorganic chemical substances found in foods that supply the body with the elements necessary for the process of metabolization.
14. __________ Inorganic elements that are of neither animal nor plant origin.
15. __________ A measurement of a unit of heat that provides energy.
16. __________ The combination of glucose and galactose that is found in animal milk.

APPLIED PRACTICE

Follow the directions as instructed with each question below.

Scenario

Emily is a medical assistant working for Dr. Wynn. Melody Hoffstettler is the first patient of the day. Melody has been unable to control her eating for most of her life and has come for help with this issue. Dr. Wynn suggests that Emily begin by explaining the revised Food Guide Pyramid as a way to begin the conversation.

1. Pretend that you are Emily and write as if you were talking to Melody.

____

____

____

____

____

____

2. Draw and explain MyPyramid in such a way that Emily will understand and feel encouraged and confident.

LEARNING ACTIVITY: TRUE/FALSE

Indicate whether the following statements are true or false by placing a T or an F on the line that precedes each statement.

_______ 1. Energy released from the metabolization of proteins, fats, and carbohydrates is measured in units of kilograms.

_______ 2. The key to a balanced diet is to eat a variety of foods in the correct amount.

_______ 3. Reducing the intake of fat can also reduce the risk of certain types of cancer.

_______ 4. A good postoperative diet is the full liquid diet.

_______ 5. Children are placed on the BRAT diet when they behave like one.

_______ 6. A person's religion can play a role in his or her nutrition.

_______ 7. In a heart-healthy diet, avoid tuna packed in oil.

_______ 8. Carbohydrates are the body's primary source of energy and are found primarily in breads, cereals, pasta products, rice, fruit, and potatoes.

_______ 9. Vitamins are not sources of energy, but they are required for good health.

_______ 10. Minerals constitute 11% percent of the body.

CRITICAL THINKING

Answer the following questions to the best of your ability. Utilize the textbook as a reference.

1. Mr. McNeill is experiencing constipation and has called for advice on how to deal with this. Recall what you have read in this chapter of your textbook and use your common sense to list a few things that might help. After you have done this, check the book and review any items that you may not have learned yet.

____

____

____

____

2. The patient, Millie Stewart, is chatting while you are getting her ready for an examination. She tells you that she has tried every kind of diet and many have worked well and rapidly, but the weight always comes back. Ms. Stewart explains that she has decided that she is just supposed to be 20 pounds overweight and she is not going to diet any more; she is going to enjoy her food and her life. How would you respond to her?

RESEARCH ACTIVITY

Utilize Internet search engines to research the following topics and write a brief description of what you find. It is important to utilize reputable websites.

1. Visit www.mypyramid.gov. Using the information that you find on the website, develop a diet plan for yourself or for one of your patients.

Chapter 57
Mental Health

CHAPTER OUTLINE

General review of the chapter:

Psychology
Psychological Disorders
Substance Abuse Disorders
Treatments
Developmental Stages of the Life Cycle
Mind–Body Connection
Maslow's Hierarchy of Needs
Heredity, Environmental, and Cultural Influences on Behavior
Emotions
Motivation
Stress
Assisting the Patient with a Terminal Illness

STUDENT STUDY GUIDE

Use the following guide to assist in your learning of the concepts from the chapter.

I. Psychological Disorders and Treatments

1. The Psychologist
   A. Usually has a ______________ in psychology.
   B. Usually administers psychological tests, performs ______________, or does research.
   C. Cannot ______________ medication

2. The Psychiatrist
   A. Can order and perform ________________ ________________ (ECT) and perform psychotherapy as well.
   B. Can ______________ medications.

3. Abnormal Psychology
   A. Abnormal psychology is the study of behavior that ______________ from the normal.
   B. Manifestations of abnormal psychology.
      i. ____
      ii. ____
      iii. ____
      iv. ____
      v. ____

4. Mental Disorders
   A. Caused by ______________ changes to the brain, such as those suffered in depression, but exclude substance abuse and other disorders that are primarily behavioral.
   B. Defined as any behavior or emotional state that causes the following
      i. ______________________________
      ii. ______________________________
      iii. ______________________________
5. Anxiety and Cognitive Disorders (Provide examples of each type of disorder.)
   A. Anxiety disorders
      i. ______________________________
      ii. ______________________________
      iii. ______________________________
   B. Cognitive disorders
      i. ______________________________
      ii. ______________________________
      iii. ______________________________
      iv. ______________________________
6. Disorders Diagnosed in Infancy and Childhood
   i. ______________________________
   ii. ______________________________
   iii. ______________________________
7. Dissociative Disorders
   A. Dissociative __________ is a condition in which important events cannot be remembered after a traumatic event.
   B. Dissociative __________ __________ (multiple personality disorder) is a condition in which two or more personalities or identities are present in one person.
8. Eating Disorder
   A. Abnormal eating ____________.
   B. Distorted body ____________.
   C. Fear, ____________, and ___________ characterize these disorders.
9. Factitious Disorders
   A. These are characterized by physical and/or psychological symptoms that are ____________ ____________ by the patient, which the patient knows are not real.
   B. Patients __________ to be sick (or sicken others) to get attention.
10. Impulse Control Disorder
    A. An impulse control disorder is an inability to __________ an impulse to perform some act that is __________ to the individual or others.
    B. These may include __________ gambling, stealing (kleptomania), __________ __________ (pyromania), or having violent rages.
11. Personality and Mood Disorders
    A. Personality disorders
       i. Personality disorders are inflexible __________ __________ that cause distress or the inability to function.
       ii. These include paranoid, __________, and __________ disorders.
    B. Mood disorders (Provide examples of this type of disorder.)
       i. ______________________________
       ii. ______________________________
       iii. ______________________________

12. Schizophrenia and Other Psychotic Disorders

    A. Characteristics of psychotic disorders
    B. i. ______________________________
       ii. ______________________________
       iii. ______________________________

13. Sexual and Gender Identity Disorders (List these types of disorders.)

    i. ______________________________
    ii. ______________________________
    iii. ______________________________

14. Anxiety Disorders

    A. Anxiety disorders are mild emotional disturbances that impair __________.
    B. Patients suffering from anxiety disorders are able to tell the difference between __________ and __________.
    C. Anxiety is a __________ feeling of apprehension, worry, uneasiness, or dread.
    D. A certain amount of anxiety is normal, but when it impairs __________, it is an anxiety disorder.
    E. Anxiety disorders are treated with __________, which decrease anxiety.

15. Phobias

    A. The fear of leaving the home and going out is called __________.
    B. __________ is the fear of spiders.
    C. __________ is the fear of enclosed spaces.

16. Cognitive Disorders

    A. Impair the ability of a patient to think __________.
    B. Delirium, particularly if related to __________ __________, can be transient and usually is treated by easing the person into __________ from substances, or treating the __________ cause.
    C. Dementia is a progressive disease that robs the patient of __________-__________ memory, while frequently leaving __________-__________ memory intact.
    D. New medications have been developed to treat dementia, but __________ must be early to be successful.

17. Developmental Disorders

    A. Sometimes disorders appear before age ______.
    B. Include __________ __________ (such as Down syndrome) and __________ disorders (such as antisocial behavior).
    C. Developmental delays are usually treated by __________ the potential of the patient with rehabilitation.
    D. Rehabilitation is usually successful at improving the quality of life for the patient with developmental delays, but will not usually increase the __________ quotient.
    E. Autism, also called __________ __________, has a range of symptoms.
    F. Some patients with __________ __________ (a milder form of autism) may be highly intelligent, but may not seek social contact.
    G. Other patients may be totally absorbed in their own world, hypersensitive to outside stimuli, and engage in __________-__________ behaviors such as rocking back and forth.

18. Dissociative Disorders

    A. Cause a person to withdraw from reality and dissociate, at least temporarily, from the life issues that cause him or her __________.
    B. If the person attempts to flee the life that he or she is living to assume another identity in another place, it is called __________ __________.
    C. __________, or forgetting events, is frequently present with dissociative disorders.

D. Dissociative identity disorder, formerly called ___________ ___________ ___________, is a severe dissociative disorder in which the patient assumes multiple personalities.
E. Contrary to frequent depictions of patients with this disorder in the media, these patients have usually been severely ___________ and assume multiple personalities as a defense mechanism to protect themselves.

19. Eating Disorders

A. __________ __________ is a psychiatric disorder in which the patient, starved for affection, starves literally as well, while believing that he or she is overweight.
B. __________ __________ is usually found in slightly overweight persons who seek to control their lives by overeating, then purging with laxatives or vomiting.
C. Medications to increase the appetite can be used, but __________ __________ therapy is usually indicated.

20. Hypochondriasis

A. Hypochondriasis is a disorder in which the patient is preoccupied with fears of having, or the idea that one has, a __________ __________, based on a misinterpretation of one of more bodily signs or symptoms.
B. With this disorder, it is important to rule out __________ __________.
C. Therapy would then be directed toward improving the patient's __________ and decreasing anxiety.

21. Impulse Control Disorders

A. Attention-deficit/hyperactivity disorder, an impulse-control disorder, is thought to be a problem with either the _______-____________ ____________ or dopamine processing.
B. Although controversial, it is currently treated with ______________ that help the patient to focus better.
C. Other impulse control disorders include ______________ ______________, stealing, and setting fires.

22. Mood Disorders

A. Mood disorders are _____________ _____________ or _____________, including a pervasively negative world view.
B. Depression
   i. Depression is a mood disorder that is characterized by a ___________ of ___________ in life's pleasures.
   ii. Can be life-threatening when accompanied by ______________ thoughts.
   iii. It is a serious mental illness that affects ________________ million people in the United States.
   iv. One out of _____________ women and one out of _____________ men will be diagnosed with depression in their lifetime.

23. Symptoms of Depression

i. ____
ii. ____
iii. ____
iv. ____
v. ____
vi. ____
vii. ____
viii. ____

24. Bipolar Disorder

A. Patients with __________ may not stop to eat, rest, relate to others, or sleep.
B. Bipolar disorder is characterized by periods of __________ __________ from excessive mania to profound depression.

C. Mania is characterized by __________ __________, flight of ideas, weight loss, and cognitive lack of focus.
D. Medication therapy is targeted usually at the __________ __________, but antidepressants can sometimes be helpful with the depression phase caused by __________ following the manic phase.

25. Personality Disorders

A. Usually treated with __________ __________ with a psychologist.
B. Unlike the other disorders, which may necessitate __________ therapy, talk therapy is the treatment of choice for entrenched personality disorders.

26. Psychotic Disorders

A. Psychotic disorders are severe mental disorders that interfere with a patient's __________ of __________ and his or her ability to cope with the demands of daily living.
B. Psychoses must be treated with __________ medications.

27. Somatoform Disorders

A. Occur when ______________ mental illness is displaced into bodily complaints.
B. ______________ can be used to decrease anxiety and improve the effectiveness of talk therapy.

28. Factitious Disorders

A. The patient creates ____________ to seek attention.
B. Sometimes a patient with a factitious disorder might ____________ another person, such as a spouse or child, in order to get attention.
C. If the person injures him- or herself, the disorder is ______________ syndrome.
D. If another person is injured by the patient in order to get attention, the condition is known as ____________ ____________ ____________ ____________.
E. __________ __________ therapy is preferred over medication for this group of disorders.

29. Dealing with Substance Abuse Patients

A. Carefully document visits to the physician's office so that ____________ ____________ can be traced.
B. Notify the physician if ____________ ____________ is suspected.
C. Never give a patient ______________ access to medications in the medical office.

30. Psychotherapy

A. Psychotherapy is a method for treating __________ __________ by cognitive rather than physical means.
B. Includes psychoanalysis, humanistic therapies, and __________ and __________ therapy.
C. __________ __________ therapy helps the patient to change the way that he or she both thinks and acts.
D. For some impulse behaviors, the therapist extracts a ____________ from the patient, using a contract in order to stop the behavior.
E. The goal of psychotherapy is to help the patient __________ with life.

31. Psychoanalysis

A. Psychoanalysis is a method for obtaining a __________ account of the past and present emotional and mental experiences from the patient in order to determine the source of the problem and to eliminate the effects.
B. It is a system developed by __________ __________ that encourages the patient to discuss repressed, painful, or hidden experiences with the hope of eliminating or minimizing the current problem.
C. Because psychotherapy can be lengthy, __________-__________ payers frequently limit the number of visits that a patient can have with a psychoanalyst.

32. Humanistic Therapies
   A. Humanistic therapies are also called __________-__________ or nondirective therapies.
   B. The therapist does not __________ into the patient's past when using these methods.
   C. The patient is helped to feel better by building __________-__________ and a feeling that he or she is respected.
   D. This therapy was pioneered by __________ __________.

33. Family and Group Therapy
   A. Family and group therapy is __________ focused.
   B. The therapist places __________ __________ on the patient's past history and places a strong emphasis on having the patient state his or her goals and then finding a way to achieve them.
   C. Usually led by a specialist in this kind of therapy, and frequently led by someone who has __________ substance abuse.

34. Electroconvulsive Therapy (ECT)
   A. ECT is a controversial treatment in which __________ are placed on one or both sides of the patient's head and a brief electrical current is administered, causing a seizure.
   B. A low level of __________ is used in modern ECT.
   C. The patient is given a __________ __________ and anesthesia prior to administration of the current. This helps prevent violent __________ __________.
   D. Advocates of this treatment say that it is a more effective way to treat __________ __________ than the use of drugs.

35. Antipsychotic Drugs (List the major antipsychotics that can be used.)
   i. ______________________________
   ii. ______________________________
   iii. ______________________________
   iv. ______________________________

36. Antidepressant Drugs
   A. __________ __________ inhibitors, such as Prozac, Effexor, Paxil, and Zoloft, are frequently prescribed because they have fewer side effects.
   B. __________ __________ inhibitors (MAO inhibitors) require a special diet and are thus infrequently prescribed.
   C. __________ antidepressants are nonaddictive, but they can produce unpleasant side effects such as dry mouth, weight gain, blurred vision, and nausea.

37. "Minor" Tranquilizers
   A. Minor tranquilizers include ______________ and ______________.
   B. They are classified as ______________ and are prescribed for anxiety.
   C. They are the ______________ effective methods for treating emotional disorders.
   D. Patients may develop a problem with ______________ after taking these drugs for an extended time. (They begin to need larger doses.)
   E. In general, antidepressants are preferred to tranquilizers for treating ______________ disorders.

38. Lithium
   A. Used successfully to calm patients who suffer from ______________ ______________ (depression alternating with manic excitement).
   B. Patients on lithium need to be carefully monitored because too much of this drug is ______________ and too little is ______________.
   C. ________________ levels should be regularly monitored to prevent overdosing or underdosing.

II. Understanding Patients and Their Needs

1. The Developmental Stages of the Life Cycle
    i. ____________________
    ii. ____________________
    iii. ____________________
    iv. ____________________
    v. ____________________

2. The Prenatal Period
    A. Throughout this period, the __________ of the body, as well as the organs, are formed.
    B. At this time, development is influenced by the __________ and __________.

3. The Infancy Period
    A. This period of vast changes occurs from childbirth until __________.
    B. During this time, an infant gains __________ ability, along with coordination.
    C. The infant will also develop __________ and sensory skills.
    D. During this period, the infant will express basic emotions and feelings, develop __________ or __________, and become attached to caregivers.

4. The Childhood Period
    A. Ages __________ to __________ are considered to be early childhood.
        i. During a child's preschool years, his or her __________, physical, and __________ capabilities will grow rapidly.
        ii. The concept of __________ begins to develop, as does socialization.
    B. Ages ________ to ________ are considered to be middle childhood.
        i. During middle childhood, a child starts to know his or her world, think __________, and make major advances in reading and writing.
        ii. Moral and __________ development progress rapidly.

5. The Adolescence Period
    A. Ages ________ to ________ are considered to be early adolescence.
        i. During this time, the beginning of __________ __________ thinking and sexual maturation take place.
        ii. The early adolescent wants more __________ from his or her parents and, as a result, starts to form companionships with friends.
    B. Late adolescence occurs from ages ________ to ________.
        i. The psychosocial task of __________ identity is achieved.

6. The Adulthood Period
    A. Early adulthood
        i. Occurs during a person's __________ and __________.
        ii. During this time, there are the challenges of making a __________ __________, achieving intimacy, and accomplishing vocational success.
    B. Middle adulthood
        i. Occurs during a person's __________ and __________.
        ii. Achieving vocational success, plus social and __________ responsibility, occurs during this period.
        iii. At some point during this period, a person's __________ changes, as does his or her emotional status.
    C. Late adulthood
        i. Occurs from age _________ until death.
        ii. During this period, many __________ are made.
        iii. A person's __________ capabilities change, as do his or her relationships with others.
        iv. Life __________ and __________ are reported by many during this life stage.

7. Maslow's Hierarchy of Needs
   A. Developed by __________ __________.
   B. Maslow believed that a person could not move to a __________ __________ until his or her basic, lower level needs were met.
8. Levels of Maslow's Hierarchy of Needs
   A. Level I: __________ needs such as food, water, and shelter
   B. Level II: __________ needs, which include physical safety, as well as security related to employment
   C. Level III: __________ needs, which include having a sense of belonging to a group and the need for social interaction
   D. Level IV: __________-__________, which includes having a sense of self-worth and pride
   E. Level V: __________-__________, which occurs when the individual achieves all that he or she is capable of achieving and experiences a sense of accomplishment
9. The Role of Heredity and Environmental and Cultural Influences on Behavior
   A. Some people believe that __________ influences behavior more than the environment.
   B. Others believe that the __________ influences behavior more than heredity.
   C. Each one of these factors has been determined to be essential for __________, because each factor can interact with the other.
   D. Before you can __________ effectively with a patient from another culture, you should understand the terms "bias," "prejudice," and "stereotyping."
10. How to Communicate When a Language Barrier Exists
   A. Avoid using __________ __________ if possible.
   B. Determine whether the patient __________ you.
   C. Never use __________.
   D. Be aware of your __________ communication, as well as that of the patient.
   E. Determine whether __________ __________ should be direct or indirect.
   F. __________ __________ can show a variety of emotions, such as sadness, anger, confusion, and happiness.
11. Predisposing Factors for Stress
   i. ______________________________
   ii. ______________________________
   iii. ______________________________
   iv. ______________________________
   v. ______________________________
12. Stress
   A. Can be emotional, ________________, or physical.
   B. It can also be ________________, economical, or social.
   C. Can be energizing, ________________, or exhausting.
   D. Medical research has shown that a certain amount of stress is not a ________________ ________________.
   E. The body's reaction to stress determines whether it is good stress or bad stress (______________________).
   F. Stress has also been implicated in various ________________.
13. Methods for Coping with Stress
   A. Develop a strong ____________ ____________, including family and friends.
   B. Find a balance between ____________ and the fear of failure.
   C. Eat ____________ meals.
   D. Avoid ____________ ____________ such as smoking and drinking.
   E. Engage in __________ exercise such as walking, jogging, dancing, biking, and swimming.

F. Look outward to develop a social interest by understanding other people's ______________ and needs.
G. Try to see the ______________ in situations.
H. Limit the number of activities to a ______________ few.

14. Encountering a Patient with Stress
    A. After allowing the patient to discuss the stress and stressors, assess the patient's __________ of the topic of stress.
    B. Next, determine the appropriate reading, language, and educational level of the patient so that you can select and prepare __________ for use in teaching the patient about stress.
    C. After you gather all of your __________ and __________, you will be ready to provide the patient with information about stress.
    D. When you have completed __________ the patient, you will need to document it in the patient's medical record.

15. Defense Mechanisms
    A. Operate at a ____________ ____________ to manage anxiety by denying, misinterpreting, or distorting reality.
    B. Often hinder ____________-____________ by preventing a person from being sensitive to anxiety.
    C. Can be helpful in dealing with ______________.
    D. The consistent use of certain defenses leads to the ______________ of either good or self-destructive behavior patterns.

16. Compensation and Denial
    A. Compensation
        i. Definition: ______________________________
        ii. Purpose: ______________________________
    B. Denial
        i. Definition: ______________________________
        ii. Purpose: ______________________________

17. Displacement and Identification
    A. Displacement
        i. Definition: ______________________________
        ii. Purpose: ______________________________
    B. Identification
        i. Definition: ______________________________
        ii. Purpose: ______________________________

18. Intellectualization
    A. Definition: ______________________________
    B. Purpose: ______________________________

19. Introjection
    A. Definition: ______________________________
    B. Purpose: ______________________________

20. Minimization and Projection
    A. Minimization
        i. Definition: ______________________________
        ii. Purpose: ______________________________
    B. Projection
        i. Definition: ______________________________
        ii. Purpose: ______________________________

21. Rationalization and Reaction Formation
    A. Rationalization
        i. Definition: ____
        ii. Purpose: ____
    B. Reaction formation
        i. Definition: ____
        ii. Purpose: ____

22. Repression
    A. Definition: Resorting to an earlier, more ______________ level of functioning that is characteristically less demanding and responsible.
    B. Purpose: Allows a person to return to a point in development when ______________ and dependency were needed and accepted with comfort. Protects a person from a __________ ______________ until he or she has the resources to cope with it.
    C. An unconscious mechanism by which ___________ ___________, feelings, and desires are kept from becoming conscious; the __________ material is denied entry into consciousness.

23. Sublimation and Substitution
    A. Sublimation
        i. Definition: ____
        ii. Purpose: ____
    B. Substitution
        i. Definition: ____
        ii. Purpose: ____

24. Undoing
    A. Definition: An action or words designed to cancel some ____________ ____________, impulses, or acts in which the person relieves guilt by making reparation.
    B. Purpose: Allows a person to appease ______________ ______________ and atone for ______________.

25. Dealing with Patients Who Have a Terminal Illness
    A. Listen to the patient express his or her fears and concerns rather than offer ____________ ______________ for recovery.
    B. Death is a ____________ process that everyone must face.
    C. People have various ways of coping with their own death based on a variety of influences, including culture, religion, __________ __________, and age.
    D. The terminally ill patient and his or her family may have already established a very personal approach or method for handling ____________ and ____________.
    E. If the patient wishes to discuss his or her approaching death, the medical assistant should be ready to ____________.

26. Stages of Grief
    A. Denial
        i. Denial is a __________ to believe that dying is taking place.
        ii. In this stage, the patient (or family member) may need time to __________ to the __________ of the approaching death.
        iii. This stage cannot be __________.
    B. Anger
        i. At this stage, the patient may be angry at everyone and may express this intense anger at God, his or her own family, and even __________ __________ __________.
        ii. The patient may take this anger out on the person __________ to him or her.
    C. Bargaining
        i. The third stage of grief involves attempting to __________ __________ by making promises in return.

ii. The patient may bargain with __________.

iii. The patient may also indicate a need to __________ at this stage.

D. Depression

i. This stage is marked by a ____________ ____________ over the loss of health, independence, and eventually life.

ii. There is the additional sadness of leaving loved ones __________.

iii. The grieving patient may become ___________.

E. Acceptance

i. In the acceptance stage, there is a sense of __________ and __________.

ii. The patient may make comments such as "_____________________________."

KEY TERMINOLOGY REVIEW

Match the vocabulary term to the correct definition below.

a. Adolescence
b. Adulthood
c. Bias
d. Childhood
e. Compulsions
f. Electroconvulsive therapy (ECT)
g. Hierarchy of needs
h. Infancy
i. Motivation
j. Obsessions
k. Personality disorders
l. Prejudice
m. Psychiatrist
n. Psychiatry
o. Psychologist
p. Psychology
q. Psychopathic disorders
r. Psychotherapy
s. Stress
t. Stressor
u. Terminal illness
v. Tolerance

1. _________ Procedure occasionally used in cases of prolonged major depression.
2. _________ Include narcissistic (self-centered), paranoid (abnormally concerned that people will hurt the patient), antisocial (not concerned with laws and other people), histrionic (dramatic), and borderline (impulsive) behaviors.
3. _________ A branch of medicine that deals with the diagnosis, treatment, and prevention of mental disorders.
4. _________ When a person favors a certain belief or attitude.
5. _________ The science of behavior and the human thought process.
6. _________ An illness expected to end in death.
7. _________ A theory that people have special needs and move through various levels in achieving satisfaction in life.
8. _________ Occurs between childhood and adulthood.
9. _________ A preformed and unfavorable belief or attitude toward a certain culture or group with little or no information about the culture or group.
10. _________ One who is trained in the methods of psychological analysis, therapy, and research.
11. _________ A stimulus that drives us to act.
12. _________ A method for treating mental disorders by cognitive rather than physical means.

13. __________ A medical doctor who has chosen to specialize in psychiatry.
14. __________ Divided into early, middle, and late.
15. __________ The body's reaction to the world around it.
16. __________ The second period of childhood development.
17. __________ Repetitive acts performed to relieve anxiety.
18. __________ A real or imaginary event that causes stress.
19. __________ Persistent thoughts.
20. __________ Disorders that affect about 1% of the population and that are characterized by a lack of empathy, narcissism, impulsivity, and antisocial reactions, such as breaking the law and manipulating others.
21. __________ The last period of childhood development.
22. __________ A condition that creates a need for larger and larger doses of medication.

APPLIED PRACTICE

Follow the directions as instructed with each question below.

Scenario

As a medical assistant working in a medical office, you will encounter patients who are frightened, depressed, and angry. On this particular day, Timothy Smither seems to be quite angry about the procedure that he is to undergo, especially because the doctor is late in keeping the appointment.

1. How should you act when you encounter a patient that is experiencing anger?

____

____

2. How can you help that patient?

____

____

LEARNING ACTIVITY: FILL IN THE BLANK

Using words from the list below, fill in the blanks to complete the following statements.

absence	delusions	reality
addiction	diagnose	schizophrenia
antidepressants	hallucinations	statistical
bipolar	neurotransmitters	stereotyping
capacity to cope	prenatal period	withdrawal symptoms
characteristics	psychopharmacology	
conception	psychotic	

1. A __________________ disorder has two poles: depression and mania.
2. ____________ is a physiological need for a substance, which in its absence causes ____________.

3. ___________________ is a psychotic disorder marked by a variety of symptoms, including _________________ (fixed false beliefs), __________________ (false sensory perceptions), disorganized and incoherent speech, severe emotional abnormalities, and withdrawal into an inner world.
4. ___________________ is the study of the effects of drugs on the mind and brain, particularly the use of drugs in treating mental disorders.
5. The Diagnostic and __________ Manual of ___________________ IV (DSM-IV) is the reference manual used by mental health providers to diagnose a wide range of mental disorders.
6. ___________________ is the formation of negative beliefs or attitudes concerning the specific ___________________ of a person or group and then their unfair application to an entire population.
7. The first period of childhood development is the ___________________, which covers the process from ___________________ until birth.
8. Mental wellness is not necessarily a(n) ___________________ of mental problems but instead a ___________________ in healthy ways with the pressures of daily living.
9. ___________________ alter the patient's mood by affecting the levels of ___________________ in the brain.
10. ___________________ disorders are severe mental disorders that interfere with a patient's perception of ___________________ and his or her ability to cope with the demands of daily living.

CRITICAL THINKING

Answer the following questions to the best of your ability. Utilize the textbook as a reference.

1. If a patient mentions to you that she has been thinking about suicide recently and asks you not to tell the doctor because she would "never really do it," what would you say or do? The answer is not in the book, but use knowledge from what you have learned in your program so far and your thoughts to formulate a few sentences for your answer.

____

____

____

____

2. You have a female patient who is 4 months old, and the mother has come in today for test results on the infant. The infant was diagnosed with mental retardation and the mother was told by the physician that there is no treatment that will help the child. The mother is upset and wants to know why there is no treatment available when modern medicine can transplant hearts and do brain surgery. What will you tell her?

____

____

____

____

RESEARCH ACTIVITY

Utilize Internet search engines to research the following topics and write a brief description of what you find. It is important to utilize reputable websites.

1. Visit the Mental Health America website at www.nmha.org.
   a. What information do you find to be most helpful on this website?
   b. How could patients with mental health issues benefit from this website?
   c. In what ways could you become involved with Mental Health America?

CHAPTER 58
Professionalism

CHAPTER OUTLINE

General review of the chapter:

Professional Skills in the Workplace
Workplace Communication
Critical Thinking
Teamwork
Managing Priorities
Persistence
Professional Image
Lifelong Learning

STUDENT STUDY GUIDE

Use the following guide to assist in your learning of the concepts from the chapter.

I. Professionalism

1. Office Systems
   A. A system is a ___________ interacting group of people who function with an organized set of doctrines and __________ typically recorded in a formal policy and procedures manual.
   B. Having a clear understanding of managers' expectations makes the system function __________.
   C. If a medical assistant does not know how to perform a procedure, an admission must be made to his or her __________ in order that the medical assistant can receive the needed training.
2. Communication
   A. Communication is perhaps the most important ____________ skill.
   B. Many problems can be solved by having effective communication ____________ among team members.
3. Active Listening
   A. While a patient is speaking, if the medical assistant is already beginning to formulate an answer instead of listening, some ____________ information may not be heard.
   B. If the physician is giving an order and the medical assistant is thinking of something else, the results can be ___________.
   C. Instead of making __________ about what is being said, a medical assistant with good professional skills will focus on the ___________ and will ask for clarification if needed.
4. The Key to Presenting Difficult Concepts
   A. Seek ____________ from the listener to make sure that he or she understands.
   B. When communicating with a patient, always take into account the ____________ and ____________ of the patient.
   C. Use a different _____________ depending on the age and mental capacity of the patient.

5. Critical Thinking
   A. For proper decision making, the medical assistant needs to retrieve ____________ facts and events, add ____________ to the thinking process, and act in the appropriate manner.
   B. Involves differentiating ____________ from ____________ or opinion.
6. Insurance Billing and Critical Thinking
   A. The medical assistant must advocate for the patient with the patient's ____________ company through a maze of complicated rules for ____________.
   B. Thinking critically can improve ____________ from the ____________ company to the medical practice and greatly relieve the burden on the patient.
7. Laboratory Results and Critical Thinking
   A. Although the medical assistant should never diagnose a patient, it is the medical assistant's responsibility to bring ____________ results to the physician's attention.
   B. A critically thinking medical assistant will take in all information before forming a ____________.
8. Value Judgments
   A. A medical assistant must make value judgments on a ____________ basis.
   B. Critical thinking should become so ____________ that the medical assistant is comfortable with value judgments.
9. Teamwork in the Medical Setting
   A. Teamwork is a critical workplace ____________.
   B. All medical assistants need to understand how the team functions and be prepared to share ____________.
   C. The medical assistant should practice only within his or her own ____________ of practice.
10. Diversity in the Medical Office
    A. It is in everyone's best interest that ____________, stereotypes, and prejudices be put aside.
    B. Holding grudges or ____________ beliefs can prevent the team from functioning smoothly.
11. Managing Priorities
    A. Patient priorities may be managed by a combination of an efficient ____________ and a ____________ system.
    B. Because the medical assistant is versatile, he or she may be asked to do ____________ tasks over a short length of time.
    C. If a medical assistant is distracted by family issues or other personal problems, it can be detrimental and have a ____________ impact on job performance.
12. Stress Management (Explain how each of the following techniques help with stress management.)
    A. Aromatherapy: ____________
    B. Biofeedback: ____________
    C. Deep breathing: ____________
    D. Distraction: ____________
    E. Exercise: ____________
    F. Guided imagery: ____________
    G. Hypnosis: ____________
    H. Humor: ____________
    I. Meditation and prayer: ____________
    J. Music: ____________
    K. Relaxation: ____________
    L. Slow breath counting: ____________
    M. Water therapy: ____________
    N. Heat: ____________

O. Cold: ______________________________

P. Pressure: ______________________________

13. Time Management

A. Requires the ability to ____________ what the important tasks are and to complete them on ____________.

B. One of the main responsibilities of the office manager or medical assistant is to manage all of the ____________ office functions.

C. Before establishing a time management system, it is important to define office ____________ with the physician.

14. Professional Dress (List what constitutes professional attire.)

i. ______________________________

ii. ______________________________

iii. ______________________________

iv. ______________________________

v. ______________________________

vi. ______________________________

vii. ______________________________

viii. ______________________________

KEY TERMINOLOGY REVIEW

Match the vocabulary term to the correct definition below.

a. Affective

b. Aromatherapy

c. Biofeedback

d. Cognitive

e. Diversity

f. Encounter note

g. Guided imagery

h. Lifelong learning

i. Persistence

j. Psychomotor

k. Soft skills

l. System

1. ____________ means "variety".
2. ____________ is a type of therapy that utilizes biological information in order to relieve stress.
3. ____________ involves taking a few minutes to imagine being in some relaxing place, which can cause your body to relax in response to that stimulus.
4. ____________, which utilizes pleasant smells such as lavender, has been shown to decrease stress.
5. Although ____________ knowledge is important, using facts learned is the goal of learning.
6. ____________ is the quality of being able to stay on task longer than the usual time when necessary, even after others might have given up.
7. ____________ skills are behaviors that come from feelings and emotions and are truly important in the medical office.
8. ____________ refers to coordination of mind and body.
9. An ____________ is documentation of the patient's visit to the physician's office.
10. A ____________ is a regularly interacting group of people who function with an organized set of doctrines and principles.
11. ____________ is the process of continuing to learn throughout one's life.
12. ____________ are those skills necessary for the smooth functioning of the workplace.

APPLIED PRACTICE

Scenario

John Summers is an office manager at Hillcrest Family Medicine. The physicians at the office have voiced concern to John regarding the lack of professionalism among the office staff. They have asked John to conduct a staff meeting to focus on the importance of professionalism. The physicians have asked that John highlight five qualities of a professional in a health care setting.

1. What five qualities do you think John should choose to discuss during the staff meeting? Explain why. The physicians have also asked John to decide upon appropriate consequences for unprofessional behavior.

____

____

____

____

____

____

____

____

____

____

____

____

____

____

____

2. How do you think John should handle this request by the physicians? What consequences do you think would be appropriate for unprofessional behavior?

____

____

____

____

____

____

____

____

LEARNING ACTIVITY: TRUE/FALSE

_______ 1. It is very important that the medical assistant always engage in passive listening.

_______ 2. When communicating in the health care environment, accuracy is more important than brevity.

_______ 3. Critical thinking involves differentiating fact from fiction or opinion.

_______ 4. The first step in resolving conflicts is to seek to understand the situation.

_______ 5. If two workers are in conflict, it may be wise to ask a peer to resolve the conflict.

_______ 6. The office manager generally has most of the control over the tasks presented in the office.

_______ 7. Urgent tasks are not necessarily important tasks.

_______ 8. Stress can be caused by pain.

_______ 9. In the busy medical office, many tasks may have to be deferred to a later time.

_______ 10. It is not the medical assistant's job to question laboratory results that do not seem to be consistent with the patient's presentation.

CRITICAL THINKING

Answer the following questions to the best of your ability. Utilize the textbook as a reference.

1. In preparation for his externship, Stefan Marquise has been assigned to write an essay on barriers to professionalism in the health care setting. What information should Stefan include in his essay?

____

____

____

____

____

2. A very angry patient asks to talk with the office manager. The patient explains to the office manager that she overheard two staff members discussing the test results of another patient, who happens to be her sister-in-law. How should the office manager handle this situation?

____

____

____

____

____

3. Karen, the office manager, has noticed that a medical assistant, Charles, has been answering his cell phone while at work; as well as checking his e-mail between patients. Today, Charles's wife came to the office to talk with Charles during the busy morning hours. How should Karen address Charles's unprofessional behavior?

____

____

____

____

____

RESEARCH ACTIVITY

Utilize Internet search engines to research the following topics and write a brief description of what you find. It is important to utilize reputable websites.

1. Type the word "professionalism" into an Internet search engine. What are some of the most interesting and helpful results that are returned with your search?

Chapter 59
Externship and Career Opportunities

CHAPTER OUTLINE

General review of the chapter:

What Is an Externship or Practicum?
Preparing for the Certification Examination
The Job Search
The Résumé
The Cover Letter
The Interview
Follow-up After the Interview
What Does the Employer Want?

STUDENT STUDY GUIDE

Use the following guide to assist in your learning of the concepts from the chapter.

I. Preparing for the Externship and Certification Examination

1. The Externship Experience

   A. Refers to a situation in which one leaves the classroom and works, without __________, in a health care setting under the supervision of someone at the site.
   B. Offers the student an opportunity to get __________-__________-__________experience.
   C. Can be as short as __________ weeks or as long as one semester of school.
   D. Schools that are accredited by the Council on Accreditation of Allied Health Education Programs (CAAHEP) in conjunction with the AAMA require an externship of a minimum of _________ hours.
   E. The American Medical Technologists require a similar experience, which is known as a __________.
   F. Both professional organizations expect the graduates to have had actual __________ experiences in a real-world medical office in order to be certified.
   G. The externship experience should provide the medical assistant with ample experience in both __________ and __________ skills.
   H. Ideally, the practicum or externship experience is carefully monitored by the clinical instructor or __________/__________ coordinator so that any problems that may arise can be addressed.

2. Employer Expectations of Externs

   i. ______________________________.
   ii. ______________________________.
   iii. ______________________________.
   iv. ______________________________.
   v. ______________________________.

3. The Benefits of Participating in an Externship
   A. Having the opportunity to see how a physician's office, ____________________________ ____________, or clinic operates on a day-to-day basis.
   B. Being exposed to a variety of different ____________ in a work setting.
   C. Gaining additional experience using skills (List the skills that you might use.)
      i. ____
      ii. ____
      iii. ____
   D. Learning how to budget your _____________ and ______________ your workday, school day, and home life.
4. Areas Evaluated in the Externship
   i. ____
   ii. ____
   iii. ____
   iv. ____
   v. ____
   vi. ____
   vii. ____
   viii. ____
5. Possible Requirements for the Externship
   A. _____________ insurance.
   B. A physical examination and immunizations, including immunizations for ____________ and _____________.
   C. A _____________ skin test.
   D. Consideration of ____________ and ____________ issues.
   E. Errors are to be reported _____________ to the supervisor without alarming the patient.
   F. ____________ must be maintained.
6. The Role of the Preceptor
   A. Provides additional ____________ and ____________ for the student by observing the performance of particular skills.
   B. Provides a ____________, ____________ ____________ for the student, usually at the midpoint and end point.
   C. Looks for continual ______________ in skills as the student gains confidence.
   D. The student should make every attempt to establish a ______________, or a comfortable working relationship, with the preceptor.
7. Areas Covered on a Typical Evaluation Form
   i. ____
   ii. ____
   iii. ____
   iv. ____
   v. ____
   vi. ____
   vii. ____
   viii. ____
   ix. ____
   x. ____
   xi. ____
   xii. ____
   xiii. ____
   xiv. ____
   xv. ____

8. Evaluating of the Externship Experience (What questions could you ask yourself in order to evaluate your externship experience?)

   i. ______________________________
   ii. ______________________________
   iii. ______________________________
   iv. ______________________________

9. The AAMA Certification Exam

   A. Given at numerous __________ __________ throughout the United States.
   B. Available only to medical assistants who have completed a __________-__________ program in medical assisting.
   C. The Certified Medical Assistant (CMA) examination is a comprehensive test that includes the following

      i. ______________________________
      ii. ______________________________
      iii. ______________________________

10. Major Areas Tested on the CMA (AAMA) Examination

   A. General

      i. ______________________________
      ii. ______________________________
      iii. ______________________________
      iv. ______________________________

   B. Administrative

      i. ______________________________
      ii. ______________________________
      iii. ______________________________
      iv. ______________________________
      v. ______________________________

   C. Clinical

      i. ______________________________
      ii. ______________________________
      iii. ______________________________
      iv. ______________________________
      v. ______________________________

11. The Registered Medical Assistant (RMA) (AMT) Certification Exam

   A. Given as a computer-based test or a __________-__________-__________ test at various times throughout the year.
   B. Eligibility to take this examination is based on having either __________ __________ of work experience or a combination of training and work experience.

II. Getting Hired

1. Preparing for Your Job Search

   i. ______________________________
   ii. ______________________________
   iii. ______________________________
   iv. ______________________________

2. The Six Most Common Job Search Mistakes

   i. ______________________________
   ii. ______________________________
   iii. ______________________________
   iv. ______________________________

v. ____
vi. ____

3. Where to Search for Jobs
   i. ____
   ii. ____
   iii. ____
   iv. ____
   v. ____
   vi. ____
   vii. ____
   viii. ____
   ix. ____
   x. ____
   xi. ____

4. Writing a Résumé
   A. Typed on 8½" × 11", good-quality __________ or off-__________ paper.
   B. Do not use __________ colored paper.
   C. Should be neatly typed and __________ free.
   D. Always use a __________ __________ to prepare your résumé so that you can easily update it.
   E. Always have a backup copy of your résumé stored on a disk, __________ __________, or other type of storage device.
   F. __________ your résumé to make sure that it is error free.

5. Standard Items on a Résumé
   i. ____
   ii. ____
   iii. ____
   iv. ____
   v. ____
   vi. ____
   vii. ____

6. The Heading
   A. Your name, address, and telephone number are prepared as a __________ __________ at the top of the page.
   B. If you have a cellular phone number and an __________ __________, this information can also be included.
   C. When this information is printed in slightly __________ type than the rest of the text, it stands out and provides an easy reference for the reader.

7. The Objective
   A. Listing an objective lets the reader know your ____________ goals.
   B. When you write your objective, it should be ____________ and to the point with regard to what you want in a career.
   C. Your objective may need to be ____________, depending on where you are sending your résumé.

8. Education
   A. If you are still a student or are a recent graduate with limited work experience, list your education first, in __________ __________ order, beginning with the most recent school/program.
   B. Add any educational experiences that you have had, such as ____________, ____________, and courses.

9. Employment
   A. List your work experience in the __________ chronological order.
   B. Include externship or practicum experience with a brief description of your __________.
10. Professional Organizations and Memberships
   A. Belonging to a professional organization can be a wonderful experience. It helps you to stay __________ on topics related to your career.
   B. Being a member and participating in an __________ shows your dedication, commitment, and loyalty to your chosen career field.
   C. Many schools have organized a __________ __________ __________.
   D. For a yearly fee, students or graduates can also obtain membership in the __________ or the __________ __________ __________.
11. Credentials
   A. Include information about your professional credentials, such as __________ (AAMA) certification or __________ (AMT) registration.
   B. If you do not have any credentials, __________ __________ include this section on your résumé.
12. References
   A. The references section should never include the name, address, and phone number of the __________ you will be using.
   B. You need to indicate only that references are __________ __________ __________.
13. Items NOT to Be Included on a Résumé
   i. ______________________________
   ii. ______________________________
   iii. ______________________________
   iv. ______________________________
   v. ______________________________
   vi. ______________________________
   vii. ______________________________
   viii. ______________________________
14. Considerations Regarding Your References
   A. State at the __________ of your résumé that references will be furnished upon request.
   B. Type on a separate piece of paper a list of at least __________ references with their addresses and phone numbers.
   C. Names of references are generally not included on the __________ __________.
   D. Obtain permission to use a __________ as a reference.
   E. It is wise to include the names of __________, as well as personal references.
15. Characteristics of the Cover Letter
   A. The cover letter should be __________.
   B. It is not a __________ of everything that is in your résumé.
   C. Explain what you can do for the employer and why your qualifications are a good __________ for their requirements.
   D. Be sure to include an address and __________ __________ where you can be reached.
   E. Do not add __________ comments or additional information to your cover letter.
   F. Always review the __________ of the employer's name and address carefully for accuracy.
   G. If you have word-processing capability, you may wish to __________ several __________ cover letters that you can then access from your computer and add the appropriate heading.

16. Common Mistakes to Avoid When Writing a Cover Letter
    A. Failing to ____________ the letter to a specific person in the organization.
    B. Failing to clearly state the ____________ for which you are applying.
    C. Sending a cover letter that is too long. ____________ ____________ works best.
    D. Sending a letter that is poorly ____________ or has spelling or typographical errors.
    E. Always send the ____________ cover letter, never a copy.
17. Reference Materials for Interviewing (List some reference materials that you can use to prepare for an interview.)
    i. ______________________________
    ii. ______________________________
    iii. ______________________________
    iv. ______________________________
18. Dressing for the Interview: What to Avoid
    i. ______________________________
    ii. ______________________________
    iii. ______________________________
    iv. ______________________________
    v. ______________________________
    vi. ______________________________
    vii. ______________________________
    viii. ______________________________
    ix. ______________________________
    x. ______________________________
    xi. ______________________________
19. Dressing for the Interview: What to Wear
    i. ______________________________
    ii. ______________________________
    iii. ______________________________
    iv. ______________________________
    v. ______________________________
    vi. ______________________________
    vii. ______________________________
    viii. ______________________________
20. Guidelines for the Interview
    A. Provide a copy of your résumé and references to the ____________.
    B. Never give dishonest or ____________ answers.
    C. Know what questions are ____________ from being asked in an interview.
    D. Do not make ____________ or ____________ the focus of the first interview.
    E. Be ____________ when the interview is over.
21. The Ten Most Common Errors Committed When Interviewing
    i. ______________________________
    ii. ______________________________
    iii. ______________________________
    iv. ______________________________
    v. ______________________________
    vi. ______________________________
    vii. ______________________________
    viii. ______________________________
    ix. ______________________________
    x. ______________________________

22. Documentation for Completing an Application

    i. ______________________________
    ii. ______________________________
    iii. ______________________________
    iv. ______________________________
    v. ______________________________

23. After the Interview

    A. Always send a letter thanking the interviewer for his or her ______________.
        i. It is a good opportunity to again express your ______________ in the position.
        ii. Be meticulous about proofreading your letter for mistakes. It may be your final ______________ ______________ with the interviewer before the decision to hire is made.
    B. You may wish to call the office a few days later to ask about the ______________ made on filling the position.
    C. If you are offered a position and decide not to accept it, you would use the same ______________ when turning down an offer as you would use when accepting one.

24. Six Basic Skills That Employers Want

    i. ______________________________
    ii. ______________________________
    iii. ______________________________
    iv. ______________________________
    v. ______________________________
    vi. ______________________________

25. Characteristics That Employers Want to See in a Medical Assistant

    i. ______________________________
    ii. ______________________________
    iii. ______________________________
    iv. ______________________________
    v. ______________________________

KEY TERMINOLOGY REVIEW

Match the vocabulary term to the correct definition below.

a. Application
b. Blind ad
c. Certification examination
d. Cover letter
e. Externship
f. Personal assessment
g. Practicum
h. Preceptor
i. Professional reference
j. Proofread
k. Résumé

1. ______________ A summary of your credentials, including your employment history, experience, training, and education.
2. ______________ An examination needed to become a Certified Medical Assistant and that is offered by the AAMA throughout the year.
3. ______________ Does not identify the institution or facility that placed the ad.

4. _______________ An opportunity that provides the medical assistant with ample experience in both administrative and clinical skills.
5. _______________ Refers to a situation in which one leaves the confines of the classroom and works, without payment, in a physician's office, hospital, or other health care setting.
6. _______________ Statement of someone who has either worked with you or has known you for a period of time.
7. _______________ Making sure that your résumé and cover letter are error free in content and typing.
8. _______________ Includes personal information and previous work experience.
9. _______________ Self-evaluation of strengths and weaknesses.
10. _______________ Provides additional instruction and guidance for a student by observing the performance of particular skills.
11. _______________ Intended to introduce you and your résumé to the recipient.

APPLIED PRACTICE

Assume that you are a recent medical assisting graduate preparing to enter the workforce.

1. You have recently received a phone call for an interview for Mountain View Health Care Center. How will you research the medical facility prior to your interview and why is this important?

____

____

____

____

2. Considering your current wardrobe, which outfit would you choose to wear to your interview and why?

____

____

____

____

3. Practice writing a cover letter to go along with your application. Submit your letter with your completed workbook materials.

LEARNING ACTIVITY: MULTIPLE CHOICE

Circle the correct answer to each of the questions below.

1. The _______________ is a fellow medical assistant who will serve as a resource for the student medical assistant during the externship.

   a. office manager
   b. mentor
   c. physician
   d. None of the above

2. Which of the following is a responsibility of the student medical assistant during the externship?
   a. Be on time
   b. Dress appropriately
   c. Act in a professional manner
   d. All of the above

3. Circle the answer that should not be part of an interview.
   a. Have a specific job in mind when you interview so that you project self-assurance.
   b. Prepare responses should the interviewer ask you difficult questions or ask you to describe yourself.
   c. Show off your legs.
   d. Carry extra copies of your résumé.

4. When a student medical assistant has a concern about something at the externship site, to whom should the student bring the problem?
   a. The medical assisting program director
   b. A coworker
   c. The student's spouse
   d. The dean of the college

5. Which of the following may be a reason that a medical assistant may not be called for an interview?
   a. The résumé contains typographical errors.
   b. The résumé contains grammatical errors.
   c. The résumé contains crossed-out words and handwritten corrections.
   d. All of the above.

6. A résumé should ideally be _________ pages in length.
   a. 2–3
   b. 1–2
   c. 3–4
   d. 4–5

7. A thank you note should be sent to the potential employer after an interview within _____________ days.
   a. 1–2
   b. 2–3
   c. 3–5
   d. 6–8

8. Which of the following are places that a medical assistant might look for employment?
   a. The newspaper
   b. The local medical assisting program
   c. An employment agency
   d. All of the above

9. Which of the following is an interview "don't"?
   a. Requesting parking validation.
   b. Arriving a bit early.

c. Taking notes.
d. All of the above.

10. Which of the following is an appropriate dress code for an applicant going to a job interview?
    a. Casual attire
    b. Business suit
    c. Scrubs
    d. Any of the above

CRITICAL THINKING

Answer the following questions to the best of your ability. Utilize the textbook as a reference.

1. Willie Harrison is finishing his medical assisting training and is preparing for his externship experience. Willie's wife asks him what he will be doing during his externship. How might Willie answer her question?

   ____

   ____

   ____

   ____

2. Joann Felmer is a student in an administrative medical assisting course. She has been given an assignment to describe the benefits of the externship experience for the student medical assistant. How might Joann answer this question?

   ____

   ____

   ____

   ____

3. Corey Rubatino, CMA (AAMA), has recently been hired to work for Dr. Joe Cresanti. On Corey's first day, he has been asked by Dr. Cresanti to describe what is meant by practicing within his scope of practice. How might Corey answer this question?

   ____

   ____

   ____

   ____

4. Maggie Levinski, RMA, is the program director in an accredited medical assisting program. She is attempting to add new externship sites to the program roster. When Maggie meets with someone from a potential site, she is asked to explain the benefits of the externship to the site. How might Maggie answer this question?

   ____

   ____

   ____

   ____

RESEARCH ACTIVITY

Utilize Internet search engines to research the following topics and write a brief description of what you find. It is important to utilize reputable websites.

1. Using the Internet and other sources, locate prospective job opportunities for medical assistants in your area. Which jobs interest you most? Explain why.

APPENDIX
Competency Check-Offs

Affective Behaviors

Affective behaviors are very important to the role of medical assisting. These behaviors display sensitivity to the patient, convey an understanding of laws and regulations, and also provide an overall professional component to the medical assisting profession.

The weighed competencies that are found in the student workbook vary slightly from the competencies found in the textbook. The competencies within the student workbook have placed an emphasis on these affective behaviors by showing them in a ***bold and italicized*** font. Not all procedures will have affective behaviors; affective behaviors will primarily be addressed during a procedure that involves direct patient contact.

Your instructors will be expecting to see these behaviors demonstrated during the performance of a procedure, as necessary. Failure to exhibit these affective behaviors will result in a loss of points associated with the point value of the given step. It is essential to review the weighted competencies found in the workbook prior to being tested and graded.

Name: ______________________________

Date: ______________________________

Procedure 5-1:

Effective Listening Skills

Objective: Use effective listening skills to obtain chief complaint from patient.

Supplies: Patient history form

Affective Behaviors: Affective behaviors provide a professional approach to a skill that enhances the patient encounter. These behaviors may also display sensitivity to a patient's rights and enhance communication. Pay close attention to these skills, which will be in ***bold, italicized*** font.

Notes to the Student

____

____

____

____

____

____

Skills Assessment Requirements

Read and familiarize yourself with the procedure; complete the minimum practice requirements. Document each MPR using proper charting technique. Complete each procedure within a reasonable amount of time, with a minimum of 85% accuracy.

Name: ____________________

Date: ____________________

POINT VALUE
✦ = 3–6 points
✶ = 7–9 points

		PRACTICE TRIAL	GRADED TRIAL # 1	GRADED TRIAL # 2	NOTES
1. ✦	Identify patient.				
2. ✶	***Smile and establish eye contact.*** *Explain why this is important.*				
3. ✦	Seat the patient in the appropriate area.				
4. ✶	***Focus full attention on patient.*** Ask patient the reason for current appointment.				
5. ✦	Ask open-ended questions.				
6. ✶	Do not interrupt the patient. ***Provide feedback by paraphrasing what the patient said.***				
7. ✦	***Observe the patient for signs of needing to give more information.***				
8. ✦	***Restate the chief complaint before leaving the patient. Conclude the patient interview in appropriate manner.***				
9. ✶	Document the chief complaint with 100% accuracy.				

Name: ______________________________

Date: ______________________________

Document: Enter the appropriate information in the chart below.

Grading

Points Earned	_______		
Points Possible	_______	66	66
Percent Grade (Points Earned/Points Possible)	_______		
PASS:	_______	❑ YES ❑ NO ❑ N/A	❑ YES ❑ NO ❑ N/A

Instructor Sign-Off

Instructor: ______________________________ **Date:** ______________

Name: ______________________________

Date: ______________________________

Procedure 5-2:

Assisting the Hearing-Impaired Patient

Objective: Use effective communication skills to assist a hearing-impaired patient prepare for a physical examination.

Supplies: None

Affective Behaviors: Affective behaviors provide a professional approach to a skill that enhances the patient encounter. These behaviors may also display sensitivity to a patient's rights and enhance communication. Pay close attention to these skills, which will be in ***bold, italicized*** font.

Notes to the Student

____

____

____

____

____

____

Skills Assessment Requirements

Read and familiarize yourself with the procedure; complete the minimum practice requirements. Document each MPR using proper charting technique. Complete each procedure within a reasonable amount of time, with a minimum of 85% accuracy.

Name: ______________________________

Date: ______________________________

POINT VALUE
✦ = 3–6 points
✶ = 7–9 points

		PRACTICE TRIAL	GRADED TRIAL # 1	GRADED TRIAL # 2	NOTES
1. ✦	Identify patient.				
2. ✦	Reduce external noise as much as possible.				
3. ✶	***Smile, establish eye contact, and face the patient.*** *Explain why this is important.*				
4. ✦	***Speak slowly and do not shout.***				
5. ✦	Provide careful explanation of the procedure.				
6. ✦	***Provide paper and pen for the patient to use if desired.***				
7. ✦	Use written information to reinforce message for the patient.				
8. ✦	Have patient repeat your response to ensure accuracy of message, if possible.				
9. ✦	***Give directions using actions as well as words.***				
10. ✦	***Be sensitive to patient's needs. Employ an empathetic, professional attitude.***				
11. ✦	Notify physician of patient's concerns.				

Name: ___________________________

Date: ___________________________

Document: Enter the appropriate information in the chart below.

Grading

Points Earned	______		
Points Possible	______	69	69
Percent Grade (Points Earned/Points Possible)	______		
PASS:	______	❑ YES ❑ NO ❑ N/A	❑ YES ❑ NO ❑ N/A

Instructor Sign-Off

Instructor: ___________________________ **Date:** ___________________

Name: ______________________________

Date: ______________________________

Procedure 6-1:

Handling a Fire in the Medical Office

Objective: Respond to a fire in the medical office.

Supplies: Policy and procedures manual; evacuation maps of the office

Affective Behaviors: Affective behaviors provide a professional approach to a skill that enhances the patient encounter. These behaviors may also display sensitivity to a patient's rights and enhance communication. Pay close attention to these skills, which will be in ***bold, italicized*** font.

Notes to the Student

____

____

____

____

____

____

Skills Assessment Requirements

Read and familiarize yourself with the procedure; complete the minimum practice requirements. Document each MPR using proper charting technique. Complete each procedure within a reasonable amount of time, with a minimum of 85% accuracy.

Name: ______________________________

Date: ______________________________

POINT VALUE
✦ = 3–6 points
✶ = 7–9 points

		PRACTICE TRIAL	GRADED TRIAL # 1	GRADED TRIAL # 2	NOTES
1. ✶	As soon as a fire is discovered, call 911 or the local fire department, following the same procedure as practiced during fire drills.				
2. ✦	Activate the established mechanism for signaling fire within the office. This may mean pulling the alarm, calling a code over the intercom, or taking other action.				
3. ✦	Calmly and quickly assist in getting all patients out of the office in an orderly manner, following the exit routes on the posted evacuation maps, and using the stairs, if applicable.				
4. ✦	If the fire is contained, attempt to extinguish it using the fire extinguisher. However, if the fire is not contained, valuable time should not be spent attempting to extinguish it.				
5. ✦	The individual charged with ensuring that all rooms are cleared should quickly go through the office to confirm that no one is left behind.				
6. ✦	After each room is evacuated, close the door.				
7. ✦	Staff and patients should gather away from the building at the predetermined area.				

Name: ______________________

Date: ______________________

Document: Enter the appropriate information in the chart below.

Grading

Points Earned	________		
Points Possible	________	45	45
Percent Grade (Points Earned/Points Possible)	________		
PASS:	________	❑ YES ❑ NO ❑ N/A	❑ YES ❑ NO ❑ N/A

Instructor Sign-Off

Instructor: ______________________ **Date:** ______________________

Name: ______________________________

Date: ______________________________

Procedure 6-2:

Housekeeping Using OSHA Guidelines

Objective: Safely clean and disinfect contaminated surfaces.

Supplies: Prepared spill kit; gloves; 1:10 bleach/water solution; dustpan; broom; sharps container; biohazard bag or container

Affective Behaviors: Affective behaviors provide a professional approach to a skill that enhances the patient encounter. These behaviors may also display sensitivity to a patient's rights and enhance communication. Pay close attention to these skills, which will be in ***bold, italicized*** font.

Notes to the Student

____

____

____

____

____

____

Skills Assessment Requirements

Read and familiarize yourself with the procedure; complete the minimum practice requirements. Document each MPR using proper charting technique. Complete each procedure within a reasonable amount of time, with a minimum of 85% accuracy.

Name: ______________________________

Date: ______________________________

POINT VALUE
✦ = 3–6 points
✶ = 7–9 points

		PRACTICE TRIAL	GRADED TRIAL # 1	GRADED TRIAL # 2	NOTES
1. ✶	Prior to performing any housekeeping procedures, ensure the appropriate PPE has been applied.				
2. ✦	For any wet spills, use the prepared spill kit according to package directions.				
3. ✶	Immediately after exposure to infectious materials, clean and disinfect contaminated surfaces with a 1:10 bleach/water solution. All surfaces must be decontaminated on a regular schedule. This schedule must be posted, signed by the person who performs the decontamination, and kept with OSHA records.				
4. ✦	Properly bag contaminated clothing and laundry in leak proof, labeled biohazard bags. Contaminated laundry should not be handled or washed at the medical office or with any uncontaminated clothing.				
5. ✦	Replace a damaged biohazard bag by placing a second bag around the first. Do not remove infectious material from the damaged bag.				
6. ✶	Biohazardous waste must be removed by a licensed waste disposal service and incinerated or autoclaved before it is placed in a designated landfill area.				
7. ✦	Use puncture-proof, sealable, biohazard sharps containers for all needles and sharps, such as razors and glass pipettes.				

Name: ______________________________

Date: ______________________________

POINT VALUE
✦ = 3–6 points
✶ = 7–9 points

		PRACTICE TRIAL	GRADED TRIAL # 1	GRADED TRIAL # 2	NOTES
8. ✦	Place each sharps container close to the work area, and ensure that each container remains upright.				
9. ✦	Replace a sharps container when it is two-thirds full.				
10. ✦	Seal and label each sharps container before placing it with the biohazardous waste for removal by the disposal service.				
11. ✦	In the event of broken glass, use a dustpan or other mechanical device, such as a hemostat or another type of forceps, to pick it up. Never pick up broken glass with hands.				
12. ✦	Properly dispose of any PPE used during housekeeping. Failure to do so may result in an OSHA citation.				
13. ✶	Perform hand hygiene both before and after using gloves.				

Name: ______________________________

Date: ______________________________

Document: Enter the appropriate information in the chart below.

Grading

Points Earned	______		
Points Possible	______	90	90
Percent Grade (Points Earned/Points Possible)	______		
PASS:	______	❑ YES ❑ NO ❑ N/A	❑ YES ❑ NO ❑ N/A

Instructor Sign-Off

Instructor: ______________________________ **Date:** ______________

Name: ____________________

Date: ____________________

Procedure 7-1:

Answering the Telephone and Placing Calls on Hold

Objective: Ensure that the telephone is answered in a professional manner and, if necessary, that patients are placed on hold appropriately.

Supplies: Message pad, pen, notepad

Affective Behaviors: Affective behaviors provide a professional approach to a skill that enhances the patient encounter. These behaviors may also display sensitivity to a patient's rights and enhance communication. Pay close attention to these skills, which will be in ***bold, italicized*** font.

Notes to the Student

____

____

____

____

____

____

Skills Assessment Requirements

Read and familiarize yourself with the procedure; complete the minimum practice requirements. Document each MPR using proper charting technique. Complete each procedure within a reasonable amount of time, with a minimum of 85% accuracy.

Name: ____________________

Date: ____________________

POINT VALUE
✦ = 3–6 points
✶ = 7–9 points

		PRACTICE TRIAL	GRADED TRIAL # 1	GRADED TRIAL # 2	NOTES
1. ✶	Answer the telephone by at least the third ring, with the mouthpiece 1 to 2 inches from your mouth.				
2. ✦	***Smile and speak clearly, using inflection, a pleasant tone, and a moderate rate of speech.***				
3. ✦	Answer using the greeting your office prefers (e.g., "Thank you for calling Dr. Smith's office. This is Carlos. How may I help you?").				
4. ✶	At this point, callers will typically identify themselves. If not, ask callers to identify themselves and then verify the information against the patient's medical record.				
5. ✶	Listen to the caller closely to identify the reason for the call. Act accordingly while providing excellent customer service.				
6. ✦	While speaking with one caller, another incoming line may ring. When this occurs, notify the current caller that another line is ringing and ask if he or she can hold. Wait for the caller's response, and then place the call on hold.				
7. ✦	Answer the second call following the procedures described, ask the second caller if he or she can hold, wait for a response, and then place the second call on hold. (If the second call is an emergency, do not ask the person to hold and assist the caller immediately.)				

Name: ______________________________

Date: ______________________________

POINT VALUE
✦ = 3–6 points
✶ = 7–9 points

		PRACTICE TRIAL	GRADED TRIAL # 1	GRADED TRIAL # 2	NOTES
8. ✦	Return to the first call, ***thank the caller for holding,*** and continue assisting the person.				
9. ✦	Once the first call is completed, return to the second call, ***thank the person for holding,*** and continue assisting that caller.				
10. ✦	If the caller asks to speak with another employee who is not readily available and it is necessary to place the call on hold, check back with the caller approximately every 30 seconds.				
11. ✦	Once the first call is completed, return to the second call, thank the person for holding, and continue assisting that caller.				
12. ✦	If the caller asks to speak with another employee who is not readily available and it is necessary to place the call on hold, be sure to check back with the caller approximately about every 30 seconds.				

Name: ______________________

Date: ______________________

Document: Enter the appropriate information in the chart below.

Grading

Points Earned	_______		
Points Possible	_______	81	81
Percent Grade (Points Earned/Points Possible)	_______		
PASS:	_______	❏ YES ❏ NO ❏ N/A	❏ YES ❏ NO ❏ N/A

Instructor Sign-Off

Instructor: ______________________ **Date:** ______________________

Name: ___________________________________

Date: ___________________________________

Procedure 7-2:

Taking a Telephone Message

Objective: Ensure that the correct and relevant information is retrieved when taking a telephone message.

Supplies: Message form or pad with carbon or carbonless for duplicates; pen

Affective Behaviors: Affective behaviors provide a professional approach to a skill that enhances the patient encounter. These behaviors may also display sensitivity to a patient's rights and enhance communication. Pay close attention to these skills, which will be in ***bold, italicized*** font.

Notes to the Student

____

____

____

____

____

____

Skills Assessment Requirements

Read and familiarize yourself with the procedure; complete the minimum practice requirements. Document each MPR using proper charting technique. Complete each procedure within a reasonable amount of time, with a minimum of 85% accuracy.

Name: ______________________________

Date: ______________________________

POINT VALUE
✦ = 3–6 points
✶ = 7–9 points

		PRACTICE TRIAL	GRADED TRIAL # 1	GRADED TRIAL # 2	NOTES
1. ✦	***Smile prior to answering the telephone and, in a warm voice, properly answer the telephone.***				
2. ✦	Use a message form or pad with a carbon copy to keep a record of the message.				
3. ✦	Record the date and time of the call.				
4. ✶	Record the caller's full name, date of birth, and telephone number. (Always ask the caller to spell his or her name.)				
5. ✦	Document for whom the message is intended.				
6. ✶	Document the complete message. Avoid using abbreviations, other than accepted medical abbreviations. Include symptoms, such as temperature, rash, emesis, as well as duration of symptoms.				
7. ✦	***Thank the patient for calling and, prior to hanging up the telephone, ask if he or she has any other questions.***				
8. ✦	Write your initials to indicate that you took the message.				

Name: ______________________________

Date: ______________________________

Document: Enter the appropriate information in the chart below.

Grading

Points Earned	_______		
Points Possible	_______	54	54
Percent Grade (Points Earned/Points Possible)	_______		
PASS:	_______	❑ YES ❑ NO ❑ N/A	❑ YES ❑ NO ❑ N/A

Instructor Sign-Off

Instructor: ______________________________ **Date:** ____________________

Name: ______________________________

Date: ______________________________

Procedure 7-3:

Taking a Prescription Refill Message

Objective: Ensure that correct information is acquired when refilling a patient's prescription.

Supplies: Message form, pad, or paper; pen

Affective Behaviors: Affective behaviors provide a professional approach to a skill that enhances the patient encounter. These behaviors may also display sensitivity to a patient's rights and enhance communication. Pay close attention to these skills, which will be in ***bold, italicized*** font.

Notes to the Student

____

____

____

____

____

____

Skills Assessment Requirements

Read and familiarize yourself with the procedure; complete the minimum practice requirements. Document each MPR using proper charting technique. Complete each procedure within a reasonable amount of time, with a minimum of 85% accuracy.

Name: ______________________

Date: ______________________

POINT VALUE
✦ = 3–6 points
✶ = 7–9 points

		PRACTICE TRIAL	GRADED TRIAL # 1	GRADED TRIAL # 2	NOTES
1. ✶	Document the patient's name.				
2. ✦	Document the patient's telephone number.				
3. ✶	Document the name and dosage of the medication. Ask the caller to spell the name of the medication if you are unclear about what the caller is saying.				
4. ✦	Document how long the patient has been on the medication.				
5. ✦	Document the patient's symptoms and why the prescription is still needed.				
6. ✶	Ask for the patient's date of birth and weight (if the patient is a child).				
7. ✦	Ask for the name and telephone number of the pharmacy and the prescription number.				
8. ✦	Let the caller know you will give the message to the physician and you will call back if the prescription cannot be refilled.				
9. ✦	Attach the telephone message to the patient's medical record and give both to the physician to review.				

Name: ______________________________

Date: ______________________________

Document: Enter the appropriate information in the chart below.

Grading

Points Earned	_______		
Points Possible	_______	63	63
Percent Grade (Points Earned/Points Possible)	_______		
PASS:	_______	❏ YES ❏ NO ❏ N/A	❏ YES ❏ NO ❏ N/A

Instructor Sign-Off

Instructor: ______________________________ **Date:** ____________________

Name: ______________________________

Date: ______________________________

Procedure 7-4:

Placing a Conference Call

Objective: Allow for a discussion over the telephone among three or more parties.

Supplies: Telephone numbers of participating parties

Affective Behaviors: Affective behaviors provide a professional approach to a skill that enhances the patient encounter. These behaviors may also display sensitivity to a patient's rights and enhance communication. Pay close attention to these skills, which will be in ***bold, italicized*** font.

Notes to the Student

____

____

____

____

____

____

Skills Assessment Requirements

Read and familiarize yourself with the procedure; complete the minimum practice requirements. Document each MPR using proper charting technique. Complete each procedure within a reasonable amount of time, with a minimum of 85% accuracy.

Name: ______________________________

Date: ______________________________

POINT VALUE
✦ = 3–6 points
✶ = 7–9 points

		PRACTICE TRIAL	GRADED TRIAL # 1	GRADED TRIAL # 2	NOTES
1. ✦	Gather the telephone numbers of all participants before beginning the call.				
2. ✶	Determine the time that everyone will be available for the conference call. You may have to call people in advance to determine a convenient time. Be aware of time zone differences when arranging conference calls.				
3. ✦	Dial "0" for operator and give the operator the name and telephone number (area code first) for each person to be called.				
4. ✦	When the operator has placed the call and all participants are on the line, tell the participants to begin.				
5. ✦	Hang up when you have ensured that the conference has started.				

Name: ______________________________

Date: ______________________________

Document: Enter the appropriate information in the chart below.

Grading

Points Earned	_______		
Points Possible	_______	33	33
Percent Grade (Points Earned/Points Possible)	_______		
PASS:	_______	❑ YES ❑ NO ❑ N/A	❑ YES ❑ NO ❑ N/A

Instructor Sign-Off

Instructor: ______________________________ **Date:** ____________________

Name: ______________________________

Date: ______________________________

Procedure 8-1:

Opening the Office

Objective: Prepare and set up the office to receive patients and operate efficiently.

Supplies: Checklist of opening office procedures; office keys for rooms and files; message form or pad; master list of scheduled patients

Affective Behaviors: Affective behaviors provide a professional approach to a skill that enhances the patient encounter. These behaviors may also display sensitivity to a patient's rights and enhance communication. Pay close attention to these skills, which will be in ***bold, italicized*** font.

Notes to the Student

____

____

____

____

____

____

Skills Assessment Requirements

Read and familiarize yourself with the procedure; complete the minimum practice requirements. Document each MPR using proper charting technique. Complete each procedure within a reasonable amount of time, with a minimum of 85% accuracy.

Name: ______________________________

Date: ______________________________

POINT VALUE ✦ = 3–6 points ✶ = 7–9 points		PRACTICE TRIAL	GRADED TRIAL # 1	GRADED TRIAL # 2	NOTES
1. ✦	Arrive at least 30 minutes prior to the first scheduled appointment.				
2. ✦	Turn on the lights in the patient reception area before the first patient arrives.				
3. ✦	Check that the heating or air conditioning and computers are working properly.				
4. ✶	Observe overall reception room for safety hazards such as frayed electrical cords, slippery floor, or torn carpeting. Place a warning sign near any safety hazard and report it immediately to the office manager.				
5. ✦	Check magazines and recycle or discard any that are torn, damaged, or outdated.				
6. ✦	Check for level of cleanliness of housekeeping services and report inadequate services.				
7. ✦	Unlock file rooms or cabinets where records are kept.				
8. ✶	Take calls from the answering machine or answering service. Handle any that need immediate attention.				
9. ✦	Unlock any money that may be used for the day. Count and balance the money to make sure that the amount is the same as it was the day before, when the office was being closed.				
10. ✦	Unlock the outer office door.				

Name: ______________________________

Date: ______________________________

POINT VALUE
✦ = 3–6 points
✶ = 7–9 points

		PRACTICE TRIAL	GRADED TRIAL # 1	GRADED TRIAL # 2	NOTES
11. ✶	Compare the master list of all patients who will be seen during the day against the patient records that were pulled during the previous office hours. Make phone calls to gather any laboratory test information that is missing from the record. Provide the physician(s) and nurse(s) with a copy of the list of any laboratory test information that you have called for but that has not yet been received.				
12. ✦	Type and place a list of all patients who will be seen that day on the physician's desk or other designated area.				

Name: ______________________

Date: ______________________

Document: Enter the appropriate information in the chart below.

Grading

Points Earned	_______		
Points Possible	_______	81	81
Percent Grade (Points Earned/Points Possible)	_______		
PASS:	_______	❑ YES ❑ NO ❑ N/A	❑ YES ❑ NO ❑ N/A

Instructor Sign-Off

Instructor: ______________________ **Date:** ______________

Name: ____________________

Date: ____________________

Procedure 8-2:

Collating Records

Objective: Prepare medical records of scheduled patients for review by the physician.

Supplies: Master lists of scheduled patients; charts and records of scheduled patients

Affective Behaviors: Affective behaviors provide a professional approach to a skill that enhances the patient encounter. These behaviors may also display sensitivity to a patient's rights and enhance communication. Pay close attention to these skills, which will be in ***bold, italicized*** font.

Notes to the Student

Skills Assessment Requirements

Read and familiarize yourself with the procedure; complete the minimum practice requirements. Document each MPR using proper charting technique. Complete each procedure within a reasonable amount of time, with a minimum of 85% accuracy.

Name: ______________________________

Date: ______________________________

POINT VALUE
✦ = 3–6 points
✶ = 7–9 points

		PRACTICE TRIAL	GRADED TRIAL # 1	GRADED TRIAL # 2	NOTES
1. ✦	Print or copy the day's appointment schedule.				
2. ✦	Pull all of the medical records of patients who are scheduled to be seen.				
3. ✦	In each record, review the patient's last appointment and make note of any results that should have been received, including laboratory tests, x-ray results, consultation notes, and other tests.				
4. ✶	If any of the results are not in the patient's chart, call the appropriate places to retrieve the results. You may take oral results, but request that the results be faxed to the office as soon as possible.				
5. ✦	Make a list of all results that have been received by phone and any that are outstanding. Let the physician know what remains outstanding.				
6. ✦	Add all received information to each chart for the physician to review and sign off on.				

Name: ____________________

Date: ____________________

Document: Enter the appropriate information in the chart below.

Grading

Points Earned	_______		
Points Possible	_______	39	39
Percent Grade (Points Earned/Points Possible)	_______		
PASS:	_______	❏ YES ❏ NO ❏ N/A	❏ YES ❏ NO ❏ N/A

Instructor Sign-Off

Instructor: ____________________ **Date:** ____________________

Name: ______________________________

Date: ______________________________

Procedure 8-3:

Registering a New Patient

Objective: Accurately complete a registration form for a new patient.

Supplies: For paper-based charts: registration form, pen, clipboard, private area; for electronic medical records: computer and possibly online access

Affective Behaviors: Affective behaviors provide a professional approach to a skill that enhances the patient encounter. These behaviors may also display sensitivity to a patient's rights and enhance communication. Pay close attention to these skills, which will be in ***bold, italicized*** font.

Notes to the Student

____

____

____

____

____

____

Skills Assessment Requirements

Read and familiarize yourself with the procedure; complete the minimum practice requirements. Document each MPR using proper charting technique. Complete each procedure within a reasonable amount of time, with a minimum of 85% accuracy.

Name: ______________________________

Date: ______________________________

POINT VALUE
✦ = 3–6 points
✶ = 7–9 points

		PRACTICE TRIAL	GRADED TRIAL # 1	GRADED TRIAL # 2	NOTES
1. ✦	Gather the supplies.				
2. ✦	Verify that the patient has not been seen in the office before.				
3. ✶	Obtain and record the following information from the patient: • Full name spelled correctly • Date of birth • Home address, including zip code • Telephone number, including area code • Cell phone number, including area code • Marital status • Employer • Employer address • Employer telephone number • Social Security number • Insurance information, including group number • Insurance subscriber's name • Insurance co-payment amount (photocopy both sides of the insurance card) • Name of the patient's guardian, if applicable • Name of the person responsible for payment • Address of the person responsible for payment • Telephone number of the person responsible for payment • Photocopy of the patient's photo ID, such as a driver's license or military ID				

Name: ______________________________

Date: ______________________________

POINT VALUE
✦ = 3–6 points
✶ = 7–9 points

		PRACTICE TRIAL	GRADED TRIAL # 1	GRADED TRIAL # 2	NOTES
4. ✦	Once the preceding information has been documented, ***review everything with the patient to ensure accuracy.***				
5. ✶	Ask the patient to read and sign the HIPAA privacy notification form. This form may vary from office to office, but the information it contains is the same.				
6. ✦	For patients who are unable to complete the form themselves, document within the record that the patient verbally provided the documented demographic information, verify everything for accuracy, and have the patient sign in the appropriate area. The receptionist completing the form should also sign and date it.				

Name: ______________________

Date: ______________________

Document: Enter the appropriate information in the chart below.

Grading

Points Earned	_______		
Points Possible	_______	42	42
Percent Grade (Points Earned/Points Possible)	_______		
PASS:	_______	❑ YES ❑ NO ❑ N/A	❑ YES ❑ NO ❑ N/A

Instructor Sign-Off

Instructor: ______________________ **Date:** ______________________

Name: ______________________________

Date: ______________________________

Procedure 8-4:

Closing the Office

Objective: Secure the office properly during nonoperating hours.

Supplies: Checklist of office closing procedures; blank deposit forms and envelope/ pouch; office keys for rooms and files

Affective Behaviors: Affective behaviors provide a professional approach to a skill that enhances the patient encounter. These behaviors may also display sensitivity to a patient's rights and enhance communication. Pay close attention to these skills, which will be in ***bold, italicized*** font.

Notes to the Student

____

____

____

____

____

____

Skills Assessment Requirements

Read and familiarize yourself with the procedure; complete the minimum practice requirements. Document each MPR using proper charting technique. Complete each procedure within a reasonable amount of time, with a minimum of 85% accuracy.

Name: ______________________________

Date: ______________________________

POINT VALUE
✦ = 3–6 points
✶ = 7–9 points

		PRACTICE TRIAL	GRADED TRIAL # 1	GRADED TRIAL # 2	NOTES
1. ✦	Leave at least 15–30 minutes at the end of the day to close the office.				
2. ✦	Check all records used during the day for any orders that may have been missed. In addition, make sure that every visit is posted and billed.				
3. ✶	Pull, review, and collate records for patients who will be seen during the next day. Place the collated records with the charge slips attached and the master list of the next day's scheduled patients together in the appropriate place. Also, make a copy of the master list of patients for each physician.				
4. ✦	Either deposit in a bank or lock in the office safe all money received from patient payments. It is wise to have the person designated to make the daily bank deposit vary the time of deposit. Many offices now use a courier for this task. For purposes of quality control, the person completing the bank deposit and the person making the deposit should not be the same. Both people should be bonded.				
5. ✦	Lock all files and file rooms, physician offices, and other individual offices within the medical practice.				

Name: ______________________________

Date: ______________________________

POINT VALUE
✦ = 3–6 points
✶ = 7–9 points

		PRACTICE TRIAL	GRADED TRIAL # 1	GRADED TRIAL # 2	NOTES
6. ✦	Turn off electrical equipment and appliances. *Note:* Some equipment such as an incubator, fax machine, and computer may require 24-hour operation.				
7. ✦	Check all examination rooms to make sure they are clean and supplied for the next day. *Note:* This step may be done by the medical assistant who was in charge of rooming patients that day.				
8. ✦	Straighten the reception room. Put away all magazines and pick up toys.				
9. ✦	Activate the answering service before leaving. Know the name of the physician who is accepting emergency calls, or is on call, until morning. Remind the physician who is on call.				
10. ✶	Activate the security system if there is one. Always double-check to make sure the door is locked.				

Name: ______________________________

Date: ______________________________

Document: Enter the appropriate information in the chart below.

Grading

Points Earned	______		
Points Possible	______	66	66
Percent Grade (Points Earned/Points Possible)	______		
PASS:	______	❏ YES ❏ NO ❏ N/A	❏ YES ❏ NO ❏ N/A

Instructor Sign-Off

Instructor: ______________________________ **Date:** ______________

Name: ______________________________

Date: ______________________________

Procedure 9-1:

Scheduling Established Patients

Objective: Use an appointment scheduling system to efficiently schedule patients.

Supplies: Pencil or pen (if preferred by office management); appointment schedule book or computerized scheduling system

Affective Behaviors: Affective behaviors provide a professional approach to a skill that enhances the patient encounter. These behaviors may also display sensitivity to a patient's rights and enhance communication. Pay close attention to these skills, which will be in ***bold, italicized*** font.

Notes to the Student

____

____

____

____

____

____

Skills Assessment Requirements

Read and familiarize yourself with the procedure; complete the minimum practice requirements. Document each MPR using proper charting technique. Complete each procedure within a reasonable amount of time, with a minimum of 85% accuracy.

Name: ______________________________

Date: ______________________________

POINT VALUE
✦ = 3–6 points
✶ = 7–9 points

		PRACTICE TRIAL	GRADED TRIAL # 1	GRADED TRIAL # 2	NOTES
1. ✦	Understand the scheduling system used in your office.				
2. ✦	When scheduling manually, use a pencil so that appointments can be erased to make changes as needed. *Note:* Some offices prefer the use of black or blue ink instead of pencil.				
3. ✦	If using computerized scheduling, be sure the scheduling system is open.				
4. ✶	Before scheduling patients, set up a matrix by blocking out all time periods when the physician is not available for appointments (due to hospital rounds, vacations, etc.). Ideally, matrix setup or appointment blocking on the computer is done three months ahead of time.				
5. ✦	Schedule appointments by beginning with the first empty appointment in the morning or early in the afternoon, and then fill in the day. Do not schedule appointments at the end of the day with large open gaps in between.				
6. ✦	When scheduling manually, print the patient's full first and last name next to the appropriate time on the schedule. Add Jr. for Junior and Sr. for Senior if two patients in a family have the same name.				

Name: ______________________

Date: ______________________

POINT VALUE
✦ = 3–6 points
✶ = 7–9 points

		PRACTICE TRIAL	GRADED TRIAL # 1	GRADED TRIAL # 2	NOTES
7. ✦	If using computerized scheduling, search for the correct patient. Some systems allow searching by the patient's Social Security number or medical record number. This decreases the chances of pulling up the wrong patient if you have more than one patient with the same name.				
8. ✦	When scheduling manually, ask the patient for a current work and home telephone number, including area code. Write these numbers next to the patient's name. If using computerized scheduling, verify that the telephone numbers in the system are correct. If they are incorrect, immediately take the time right to update them. Correct contact information is necessary if the office needs to contact the patient prior to the appointment.				
9. ✦	Record the reason for the visit on the schedule using accepted medical abbreviations only.				
10. ✶	Allow the correct amount of time for the appointment. If an appointment will take more than the minimum time allotted on the schedule, use an arrow to indicate that the patient will be using two or three blocks of time. In some offices a line is drawn across the time blocks.				

Name: ______________________

Date: ______________________

POINT VALUE ✦ = 3–6 points ✶ = 7–9 points		PRACTICE TRIAL	GRADED TRIAL # 1	GRADED TRIAL # 2	NOTES
11. ✦	***Once the appointment is recorded, repeat to the patient the date, time, and any special instructions.***				
12. ✦	If the patient is in the office while you are scheduling the appointment, ***record the appointment on a reminder card and hand the card to the patient***.				

Name: ______________________________

Date: ______________________________

Document: Enter the appropriate information in the chart below.

Grading

Points Earned	_______		
Points Possible	_______	78	78
Percent Grade (Points Earned/Points Possible)	_______		
PASS:	_______	❑ YES ❑ NO ❑ N/A	❑ YES ❑ NO ❑ N/A

Instructor Sign-Off

Instructor: ______________________________ **Date:** ____________________

Name: ______________________

Date: ______________________

Procedure 9-2:

Scheduling a New Patient Appointment

Objective: Schedule the first visit for a new patient.

Supplies: Pencil or pen (if preferred by office management); appointment schedule book or computerized scheduling system

Affective Behaviors: Affective behaviors provide a professional approach to a skill that enhances the patient encounter. These behaviors may also display sensitivity to a patient's rights and enhance communication. Pay close attention to these skills, which will be in ***bold, italicized*** font.

Notes to the Student

Skills Assessment Requirements

Read and familiarize yourself with the procedure; complete the minimum practice requirements. Document each MPR using proper charting technique. Complete each procedure within a reasonable amount of time, with a minimum of 85% accuracy.

Name: ______________________________

Date: ______________________________

POINT VALUE
✦ = 3–6 points
✶ = 7–9 points

		PRACTICE TRIAL	GRADED TRIAL # 1	GRADED TRIAL # 2	NOTES
1. ✦	Assemble necessary appointment scheduling equipment.				
2. ✶	Obtain the patient's full legal name and correct spelling, birth date, full address, telephone contacts (home, office, cell), and e-mail address.				
3. ✦	Record the patient's chief complaint and symptoms.				
4. ✶	Request the name of the patient's insurance carrier and insurance policy number.				
5. ✦	Ask how the patient was referred to the medical office (physician referral, friend, colleague, insurance company, etc.).				
6. ✦	Ask the patient if he or she has a preference for morning or afternoon appointments.				
7. ✦	Attempt to accommodate the new patient's request for a preferred appointment time.				
8. ✦	Confirm the day, date, and time of the appointment, and ***have the new patient repeat the information for verification and mutual understanding.***				
9. ✦	Inform patients that they need to arrive 15 to 30 minutes prior to their scheduled appointment time to allow them ample time to enter the data requested on the initial history form.				

Name: ______________________________

Date: ______________________________

POINT VALUE
✦ = 3–6 points
✶ = 7–9 points

		PRACTICE TRIAL	GRADED TRIAL # 1	GRADED TRIAL # 2	NOTES
10. ✦	Provide the new patient with directions to the office.				
11. ✶	Inform the new patient of all materials to bring for the first visit (i.e., insurance verification, photo identification, list of current medications, past medical records, current lab, x-rays, and other medical reports, as necessary).				
12. ✦	***Welcome and thank the new patient by name for selecting your medical office.***				
13. ✦	Forward all information as discussed with the new patient by mail if there will be enough time between the day the appointment was made and the actual appointment date.				
14. ✦	Document new patient information in a new medical record.				

Name: ______________________________

Date: ______________________________

Document: Enter the appropriate information in the chart below.

Grading

Points Earned	______		
Points Possible	______	93	93
Percent Grade (Points Earned/Points Possible)	______		
PASS:	______	❏ YES ❏ NO ❏ N/A	❏ YES ❏ NO ❏ N/A

Instructor Sign-Off

Instructor: ______________________________ **Date:** ______________

Name: ______________________________

Date: ______________________________

Procedure 9-3:

Arranging a Referral Appointment

Objective: Schedule a referral appointment for a patient.

Supplies: Patient chart; telephone; paper; pen; Rolodex or physician directory; physician request for referral information

Affective Behaviors: Affective behaviors provide a professional approach to a skill that enhances the patient encounter. These behaviors may also display sensitivity to a patient's rights and enhance communication. Pay close attention to these skills, which will be in ***bold, italicized*** font.

Notes to the Student

____

____

____

____

____

____

Skills Assessment Requirements

Read and familiarize yourself with the procedure; complete the minimum practice requirements. Document each MPR using proper charting technique. Complete each procedure within a reasonable amount of time, with a minimum of 85% accuracy.

Name: ____________________

Date: ____________________

POINT VALUE
✦ = 3–6 points
✶ = 7–9 points

		PRACTICE TRIAL	GRADED TRIAL # 1	GRADED TRIAL # 2	NOTES
1. ✦	Gather supplies.				
2. ✦	Open patient chart for insurance information and physician request for referral.				
3. ✦	Place call to physician's office to whom the patient is being referred.				
4. ✦	***Identify yourself and the physician on whose behalf you are calling***. Let the office know you are calling to schedule a referral appointment.				
5. ✦	Before providing the patient's name and so on, verify that the practice accepts the patient's medical insurance. If so, continue with the call. If the office does not accept the patient's insurance, ***thank the practice for its time*** and notify the physician. The physician will then recommend another physician for the patient referral.				
6. ✶	Once it has been determined that the office accepts the patient's insurance, provide the following information: patient's name, address, telephone number, and reason for referral.				

Name: ______________________

Date: ______________________

Document: Enter the appropriate information in the chart below.

Grading

Points Earned	______		
Points Possible	______	39	39
Percent Grade (Points Earned/Points Possible)	______		
PASS:	______	❏ YES ❏ NO ❏ N/A	❏ YES ❏ NO ❏ N/A

Instructor Sign-Off

Instructor: ______________________ **Date:** ______________

Name: ______________________________

Date: ______________________________

Procedure 9-4:

Scheduling Inpatient Surgical Procedures

Objective: Perform the proper procedure for scheduling inpatient surgical procedures.

Supplies: Patient's chart, patient's insurance card, notepad, pen, written instructions for patients (if required)

Affective Behaviors: Affective behaviors provide a professional approach to a skill that enhances the patient encounter. These behaviors may also display sensitivity to a patient's rights and enhance communication. Pay close attention to these skills, which will be in ***bold, italicized*** font.

Notes to the Student

____

____

____

____

____

____

Skills Assessment Requirements

Read and familiarize yourself with the procedure; complete the minimum practice requirements. Document each MPR using proper charting technique. Complete each procedure within a reasonable amount of time, with a minimum of 85% accuracy.

Name: ______________________

Date: ______________________

POINT VALUE
✦ = 3–6 points
✶ = 7–9 points

		PRACTICE TRIAL	GRADED TRIAL # 1	GRADED TRIAL # 2	NOTES
1. ✦	Review the patient's chart for the most current information.				
2. ✦	Verify with the physician the type of procedure that you are scheduling for the patient.				
3. ✦	Determine the category of the surgical procedure (routine, elective, or urgent).				
4. ✶	Find out the name of the surgeon who will perform the procedure. Obtain the surgeon's scheduling preference. Get the estimated length of the procedure.				
5. ✦	Gather the following information on the patient and/or chart: name, age, sex, and other pertinent information; current diagnosis; special preoperative orders and patient instruction; and insurance information.				
6. ✦	Obtain preauthorization from the patient's insurance company, if required.				
7. ✦	Contact the surgery scheduler.				
8. ✶	Record the surgery scheduling information in the patient's chart. Record the surgery information on the appropriate physician's schedule.				
9. ✦	Contact other members of the surgical team as the surgeon requests or per office procedure.				
10. ✶	***Give the patient instruction on special preparation, other instructions, and admission requirements. Provide written instructions, if available.***				

Name: ______________________________

Date: ______________________________

Document: Enter the appropriate information in the chart below.

Grading

Points Earned	______		
Points Possible	______	69	69
Percent Grade (Points Earned/Points Possible)	______		
PASS:	______	❏ YES ❏ NO ❏ N/A	❏ YES ❏ NO ❏ N/A

Instructor Sign-Off

Instructor: ______________________________ **Date:** ______________

Name: ______________________________

Date: ______________________________

Procedure 9-5:

Scheduling Outpatient Surgical Procedures

Objective: Schedule outpatient surgical procedures.

Supplies: Telephone, patient's insurance card, notepad, pen, written instructions for patient

Affective Behaviors: Affective behaviors provide a professional approach to a skill that enhances the patient encounter. These behaviors may also display sensitivity to a patient's rights and enhance communication. Pay close attention to these skills, which will be in ***bold, italicized*** font.

Notes to the Student

____

____

____

____

____

____

Skills Assessment Requirements

Read and familiarize yourself with the procedure; complete the minimum practice requirements. Document each MPR using proper charting technique. Complete each procedure within a reasonable amount of time, with a minimum of 85% accuracy.

Name: ______________________________

Date: ______________________________

POINT VALUE ✦ = 3–6 points ∗ = 7–9 points		PRACTICE TRIAL	GRADED TRIAL # 1	GRADED TRIAL # 2	NOTES
1. ✦	Review the patient's chart for the most current information. Make sure the chart contains the physician's notes and orders regarding the surgical procedure.				
2. ✦	Verify with the physician the type of procedure for which you are to schedule the patient and gather the following information from the physician: • Category under which the surgical procedure falls (i.e., routine, elective, urgent) • Name of the surgeon who will perform the procedure • The surgeon's scheduling preference for this type of procedure • Estimated length of time for the procedure				
3. ✦	Gather the following information from the patient and the patient's chart: • Patient's full name, age, sex, and any other pertinent identification or information • Physician's current diagnosis for the patient • Any existing allergies • Special preoperative orders and patient instructions • Patient's insurance information • Days/times patient is available for surgery				

Name: ____________________

Date: ____________________

POINT VALUE
✦ = 3–6 points
✶ = 7–9 points

		PRACTICE TRIAL	GRADED TRIAL # 1	GRADED TRIAL # 2	NOTES
4. ✶	Obtain preauthorization from the patient's insurance company, if required.				
5. ✦	According to the facility policy, contact the outpatient scheduler at the local hospital or clinic and identify yourself and your office.				
6. ✦	Instruct the facility about the type of procedure and the amount of time the physician expects to need the operating room.				
7. ✶	Notify the facility of the date and time chosen.				
8. ✶	Create a patient instruction sheet that includes the date and time of the procedure and any necessary preoperative instruction.				
9. ✦	Document the conversation in the patient chart.				
10. ✶	Document the scheduled surgery on appropriate physician's schedule.				

Name: ______________________________

Date: ______________________________

Document: Enter the appropriate information in the chart below.

Grading

Points Earned	_______		
Points Possible	_______	72	72
Percent Grade (Points Earned/Points Possible)	_______		
PASS:	_______	❑ YES ❑ NO ❑ N/A	❑ YES ❑ NO ❑ N/A

Instructor Sign-Off

Instructor: ______________________________ **Date:** ____________________

Name: ______________________________

Date: ______________________________

Procedure 11-1:

Composing a Business Letter

Objective: Compose a business letter using proper guidelines.

Supplies: Computer or typewriter; office stationery

Affective Behaviors: Affective behaviors provide a professional approach to a skill that enhances the patient encounter. These behaviors may also display sensitivity to a patient's rights and enhance communication. Pay close attention to these skills, which will be in ***bold, italicized*** font.

Notes to the Student

____

____

____

____

____

____

Skills Assessment Requirements

Read and familiarize yourself with the procedure; complete the minimum practice requirements. Document each MPR using proper charting technique. Complete each procedure within a reasonable amount of time, with a minimum of 85% accuracy.

Name: ______________________________

Date: ______________________________

POINT VALUE
✦ = 3–6 points
✶ = 7–9 points

		PRACTICE TRIAL	GRADED TRIAL # 1	GRADED TRIAL # 2	NOTES
1. ✦	Gather all necessary information and supplies.				
2. ✦	Determine the reason for the correspondence.				
3. ✦	Make a list of all points you need to cover in the letter.				
4. ✦	Arrange the items in a logical manner. Make sure that the letter has all parts—a beginning, a middle, and an end.				
5. ✦	Use a natural style of writing and a positive tone.				
6. ✦	Pay attention to spelling, punctuation, and grammar.				
7. ✦	Produce a rough draft; once the draft is satisfactory, compose the final letter.				
8. ✦	Proofread for mistakes.				
9. ✶	Obtain necessary signatures. Include any enclosures as indicated.				

Name: ______________________________

Date: ______________________________

Document: Enter the appropriate information in the chart below.

Grading

Points Earned	_______		
Points Possible	_______	57	57
Percent Grade (Points Earned/Points Possible)	_______		
PASS:	_______	❑ YES ❑ NO ❑ N/A	❑ YES ❑ NO ❑ N/A

Instructor Sign-Off

Instructor: ______________________________ **Date:** ____________________

Name: ______________________________

Date: ______________________________

Procedure 11-2:

Proofreading Written Documents

Objective: Proofread a written document correctly within the time limit set by the instructor.

Supplies: Ruler, pencil, piece of paper, computer

Affective Behaviors: Affective behaviors provide a professional approach to a skill that enhances the patient encounter. These behaviors may also display sensitivity to a patient's rights and enhance communication. Pay close attention to these skills, which will be in ***bold, italicized*** font.

Notes to the Student

____

____

____

____

____

____

Skills Assessment Requirements

Read and familiarize yourself with the procedure; complete the minimum practice requirements. Document each MPR using proper charting technique. Complete each procedure within a reasonable amount of time, with a minimum of 85% accuracy.

Name: ______________________________

Date: ______________________________

POINT VALUE
✦ = 3–6 points
✶ = 7–9 points

		PRACTICE TRIAL	GRADED TRIAL # 1	GRADED TRIAL # 2	NOTES
1. ✦	Draft bulleted list of points to be made within the document.				
2. ✦	Check the list to see if it flows in a logical order.				
3. ✦	Key the document using proper grammar and correct spelling.				
4. ✶	Review the document to ensure all points are covered.				
5. ✦	Run computer spelling and grammar checks and consider the suggestions made.				
6. ✦	Use a ruler, pencil, or edge of a piece of paper to follow each line as you proofread.				
7. ✦	Check for missing and repeated words.				
8. ✦	Verify the spelling of proper names and titles. Verify numbers in dates, figures, and time (hours of the day).				
9. ✦	Check where the word breaks occur.				
10. ✶	Proofread at least twice. If still unsure, ask a coworker to review the document.				
11. ✦	Check the general appearance of the letter for spacing and format.				
12. ✦	Print the document.				

Name: ______________________________

Date: ______________________________

Document: Enter the appropriate information in the chart below.

Grading

Points Earned	______		
Points Possible	______	78	78
Percent Grade (Points Earned/ Points Possible)	______		
PASS:	______	❑ YES ❑ NO ❑ N/A	❑ YES ❑ NO ❑ N/A

Instructor Sign-Off

Instructor: ______________________________ **Date:** ______________

Name: ______________________________

Date: ______________________________

Procedure 11-3:

Opening and Sorting the Daily Mail

Objective: Sort and distribute the medical office's daily mail.

Supplies: Office stamps (one with date and one with the name of the medical office), inkpad, paper clips, pencil

Affective Behaviors: Affective behaviors provide a professional approach to a skill that enhances the patient encounter. These behaviors may also display sensitivity to a patient's rights and enhance communication. Pay close attention to these skills, which will be in ***bold, italicized*** font.

Notes to the Student

____

____

____

____

____

____

Skills Assessment Requirements

Read and familiarize yourself with the procedure; complete the minimum practice requirements. Document each MPR using proper charting technique. Complete each procedure within a reasonable amount of time, with a minimum of 85% accuracy.

Name: ______________________

Date: ______________________

POINT VALUE
✦ = 3–6 points
✶ = 7–9 points

		PRACTICE TRIAL	GRADED TRIAL # 1	GRADED TRIAL # 2	NOTES
1. ✦	Have all supplies in place when processing the mail.				
2. ✦	Before opening it, sort the mail into first class, personal/ confidential, second class, third class, and fourth class.				
3. ✦	Discard and recycle all third-class mail, unless instructed otherwise.				
4. ✶	Place the current date and time of arrival on each piece of mail.				
5. ✦	Stamp the name of the medical office on all periodicals and newspapers.				
6. ✦	Lay all envelopes flat to reduce the motions involved in opening a large amount of mail.				
7. ✶	Do not open mail marked "personal/confidential." Place it in the physician's box unopened, unless instructed otherwise.				
8. ✦	Attach all enclosures in each envelope with a paper clip.				
9. ✦	Open all mail and clip together the inside contents before handling the individual correspondence.				
10. ✦	Annotate the mail.				
11. ✶	Route the mail immediately.				

Name: ______________________________

Date: ______________________________

Document: Enter the appropriate information in the chart below.

Grading

Points Earned	_______		
Points Possible	_______	75	75
Percent Grade (Points Earned/Points Possible)	_______		
PASS:	_______	❑ YES ❑ NO ❑ N/A	❑ YES ❑ NO ❑ N/A

Instructor Sign-Off

Instructor: ______________________________ **Date:** ______________

Name: ______________________________

Date: ______________________________

Procedure 13-1:

Adding or Changing Items on a Patient's Record

Objective: Add an item to a patient's record and correctly change an error in documentation.

Supplies: Medical record to be added to or changed; black pen; correct information or documentation to be added or changed

Affective Behaviors: Affective behaviors provide a professional approach to a skill that enhances the patient encounter. These behaviors may also display sensitivity to a patient's rights and enhance communication. Pay close attention to these skills, which will be in ***bold, italicized*** font.

Notes to the Student

____

____

____

____

____

____

Skills Assessment Requirements

Read and familiarize yourself with the procedure; complete the minimum practice requirements. Document each MPR using proper charting technique. Complete each procedure within a reasonable amount of time, with a minimum of 85% accuracy.

Name: ____________________

Date: ____________________

POINT VALUE
✦ = 3–6 points
✶ = 7–9 points

		PRACTICE TRIAL	GRADED TRIAL # 1	GRADED TRIAL # 2	NOTES
	Adding items to a record				
1. ✦	Locate the last entry in the medical record.				
2. ✦	Using a pen with black ink, place the current date on the next line of the record immediately after the last entry.				
3. ✶	On the same line, after the date, place the statement "late entry."				
4. ✦	Note the date on which the information to be added was gathered.				
5. ✦	Enter the information that was originally omitted.				
6. ✶	Sign the entry with your full name and credentials.				
	Changing items in the record				
1. ✦	Locate the incorrect information.				
2. ✶	Using a pen with black ink, draw a single line through the incorrect information so that the information is not obscured and can still be read.				
3. ✶	Place the date of the correction, your initials, and the letters "m.e." above the correct information.				
4. ✦	Enter the correct information.				

Name: ______________________________

Date: ______________________________

Document: Enter the appropriate information in the chart below.

Grading

Points Earned	_______		
Points Possible	_______	42 30	42 30
Percent Grade (Points Earned/Points Possible)	_______		
PASS:	_______	❑ YES ❑ NO ❑ N/A	❑ YES ❑ NO ❑ N/A

Instructor Sign-Off

Instructor: ______________________________ **Date:** ____________________

Name: ______________________________

Date: ______________________________

Procedure 13-2:

Organizing a Patient's Medical Record

Objective: Update a patient's medical record, verifying the right record and putting the information in the correct place in the record.

Supplies: Patient medical record, assorted documents for filing in record

Affective Behaviors: Affective behaviors provide a professional approach to a skill that enhances the patient encounter. These behaviors may also display sensitivity to a patient's rights and enhance communication. Pay close attention to these skills, which will be in ***bold, italicized*** font.

Notes to the Student

____

____

____

____

____

____

Skills Assessment Requirements

Read and familiarize yourself with the procedure; complete the minimum practice requirements. Document each MPR using proper charting technique. Complete each procedure within a reasonable amount of time, with a minimum of 85% accuracy.

Name: ______________________________

Date: ______________________________

POINT VALUE
✦ = 3–6 points
✶ = 7–9 points

		PRACTICE TRIAL	GRADED TRIAL # 1	GRADED TRIAL # 2	NOTES
1. ✶	Verify that you have the right records for the patient record you have been given.				
2. ✦	File documents given to you in the correct areas of the file, according to your facility policy, for consistency. For example, file laboratory reports with other laboratory reports.				
3. ✦	Return medical record to correct place in alphabetical order with other files.				

Name: ______________________

Date: ______________________

Document: Enter the appropriate information in the chart below.

Grading

Points Earned	_____		
Points Possible	_____	21	21
Percent Grade (Points Earned/Points Possible)	_____		
PASS:	_____	❑ YES ❑ NO ❑ N/A	❑ YES ❑ NO ❑ N/A

Instructor Sign-Off

Instructor: ______________________ **Date:** ______________________

Name: ______________________________

Date: ______________________________

Procedure 13-3:

Filing a Record Alphabetically

Objective: File a patient record in the correct order using the alphabetical filing method.

Supplies: Patient record, alphabetic files

Affective Behaviors: Affective behaviors provide a professional approach to a skill that enhances the patient encounter. These behaviors may also display sensitivity to a patient's rights and enhance communication. Pay close attention to these skills, which will be in ***bold, italicized*** font.

Notes to the Student

____

____

____

____

____

____

Skills Assessment Requirements

Read and familiarize yourself with the procedure; complete the minimum practice requirements. Document each MPR using proper charting technique. Complete each procedure within a reasonable amount of time, with a minimum of 85% accuracy.

Name: ______________________________

Date: ______________________________

POINT VALUE
✦ = 3–6 points
∗ = 7–9 points

		PRACTICE TRIAL	GRADED TRIAL # 1	GRADED TRIAL # 2	NOTES
1. ✦	Locate the medical record files.				
2. ✦	Observe the name on the medical record to be filed.				
3. ✦	Locate the two medical record files between which the record to be filed belongs.				
4. ✦	Within the set of records containing the same last name as the record to be filed, locate the records with the same-letter first name as the record to be filed.				
5. ✦	Using the alphabet as a guide, place the record to be filed after the record that comes before it in the alphabet but before the record that comes after it.				
6. ✦	If there is a marker in place for the "out" record, remove the marker.				
7. ✦	Document on the office record that the chart was filed.				

Name: ______________________

Date: ______________________

Document: Enter the appropriate information in the chart below.

Grading

Points Earned	______		
Points Possible	______	48	48
Percent Grade (Points Earned/Points Possible)	______		
PASS:	______	❑ YES ❑ NO ❑ N/A	❑ YES ❑ NO ❑ N/A

Instructor Sign-Off

Instructor: ______________________ **Date:** ______________________

Name: ______________________________

Date: ______________________________

Procedure 13-4:

Filing a Record Numerically Using the Terminal-Digit Filing System

Objective: File a patient record in the correct order using the terminal-digit filing system.

Supplies: Patient record, numeric file

Affective Behaviors: Affective behaviors provide a professional approach to a skill that enhances the patient encounter. These behaviors may also display sensitivity to a patient's rights and enhance communication. Pay close attention to these skills, which will be in ***bold, italicized*** font.

Notes to the Student

____

____

____

____

____

____

Skills Assessment Requirements

Read and familiarize yourself with the procedure; complete the minimum practice requirements. Document each MPR using proper charting technique. Complete each procedure within a reasonable amount of time, with a minimum of 85% accuracy.

Name: ______________________

Date: ______________________

POINT VALUE
✦ = 3–6 points
✶ = 7–9 points

		PRACTICE TRIAL	GRADED TRIAL # 1	GRADED TRIAL # 2	NOTES
1. ✦	Locate the medical record file.				
2. ✦	Observe the numbers on the record to be filed.				
3. ✦	Locate the two medical record files between which the record to be filed belongs.				
4. ✦	If there is a marker in place for the "out" record, remove the marker.				
5. ✦	Document on the office record that the chart was filed.				

Name: ______________________

Date: ______________________

Document: Enter the appropriate information in the chart below.

Grading

Points Earned	______		
Points Possible	______	30	30
Percent Grade (Points Earned/Points Possible)	______		
PASS:	______	❑ YES ❑ NO ❑ N/A	❑ YES ❑ NO ❑ N/A

Instructor Sign-Off

Instructor: ______________________ **Date:** ______________________

Name: ______________________________

Date: ______________________________

Procedure 13-5:

Locating Missing Files

Objective: Locate misfiled records.

Supplies: Patient record, numeric file

Affective Behaviors: Affective behaviors provide a professional approach to a skill that enhances the patient encounter. These behaviors may also display sensitivity to a patient's rights and enhance communication. Pay close attention to these skills, which will be in ***bold, italicized*** font.

Notes to the Student

____

____

____

____

____

____

Skills Assessment Requirements

Read and familiarize yourself with the procedure; complete the minimum practice requirements. Document each MPR using proper charting technique. Complete each procedure within a reasonable amount of time, with a minimum of 85% accuracy.

Name: ______________________

Date: ______________________

POINT VALUE
✦ = 3–6 points
✶ = 7–9 points

		PRACTICE TRIAL	GRADED TRIAL # 1	GRADED TRIAL # 2	NOTES
1. ✦	Look for a file with a sound-alike or look-alike name.				
2. ✦	If the patient has a first name that might also be considered a last name, look under the section it would be if it were misfiled under the first name.				
3. ✦	If using a color-coded system, look for a folder that is out of place based on the color-coded label.				
4. ✦	If using a numeric system, look for a transposition of numbers.				
5. ✦	Look for a transposition of letters, alternate letters, or files that were filed before and after the missing record.				
6. ✦	Look on the physician's and billing clerk's desk and through in and out baskets.				
7. ✦	Ask others in the office to assist you.				

Name: ___________________________

Date: ___________________________

Document: Enter the appropriate information in the chart below.

Grading

Points Earned	______		
Points Possible	______	42	42
Percent Grade (Points Earned/Points Possible)	______		
PASS:	______	❏ YES ❏ NO ❏ N/A	❏ YES ❏ NO ❏ N/A

Instructor Sign-Off

Instructor: ___________________________ **Date:** ___________________________

Name: ______________________________

Date: ______________________________

Procedure 14-1:

Correcting an Entry in the Electronic Medical Record

Objective: Correct an entry in the electronic medical record.

Supplies: Computer with electronic patient medical record software

Affective Behaviors: Affective behaviors provide a professional approach to a skill that enhances the patient encounter. These behaviors may also display sensitivity to a patient's rights and enhance communication. Pay close attention to these skills, which will be in ***bold, italicized*** font.

Notes to the Student

____

____

____

____

____

____

Skills Assessment Requirements

Read and familiarize yourself with the procedure; complete the minimum practice requirements. Document each MPR using proper charting technique. Complete each procedure within a reasonable amount of time, with a minimum of 85% accuracy.

Name: ______________________________

Date: ______________________________

POINT VALUE
✦ = 3–6 points
✶ = 7–9 points

		PRACTICE TRIAL	GRADED TRIAL # 1	GRADED TRIAL # 2	NOTES
1. ✦	Identify the correct patient electronic medical record where the error was made.				
2. ✦	Locate the error within the record.				
3. ✶	Using the rules associated with the software you are using, make the appropriate correction within the medical record.				
4. ✶	Sign off on the changes as necessary, according to the steps required within the software program.				
5. ✦	Verify the change made is correct.				
6. ✶	Save the changes made to the medical record before closing the patient's electronic medical record.				

Name: ______________________________

Date: ______________________________

Document: Enter the appropriate information in the chart below.

Grading

Points Earned	______		
Points Possible	______	45	45
Percent Grade (Points Earned/Points Possible)	______		
PASS:	______	❑ YES ❑ NO ❑ N/A	❑ YES ❑ NO ❑ N/A

Instructor Sign-Off

Instructor: ______________________________ **Date:** ____________________

Name: ______________________________

Date: ______________________________

Procedure 15-1:

Preparing a Patient Ledger Card

Objective: Prepare a patient ledger card with all pertinent information.

Supplies: Blank patient ledger card; black ink pen; completed patient demographic form; computer or typewriter

Affective Behaviors: Affective behaviors provide a professional approach to a skill that enhances the patient encounter. These behaviors may also display sensitivity to a patient's rights and enhance communication. Pay close attention to these skills, which will be in ***bold, italicized*** font.

Notes to the Student

____

____

____

____

____

____

Skills Assessment Requirements

Read and familiarize yourself with the procedure; complete the minimum practice requirements. Document each MPR using proper charting technique. Complete each procedure within a reasonable amount of time, with a minimum of 85% accuracy.

Name: ______________________________

Date: ______________________________

POINT VALUE
✦ = 3–6 points
✶ = 7–9 points

		PRACTICE TRIAL	GRADED TRIAL # 1	GRADED TRIAL # 2	NOTES
	Method: If you are not using a computerized system and instead use paper ledger cards, the steps are followed as listed below; however, you will fill in the appropriate areas of the ledger card using a black ink pen instead of typing or keying into the computer.				
1. ✦	Type or key into the computer the patient's name in the correct format: last name, first name, middle initial.				
2. ✦	Type or key into the computer the patient's address, including zip code.				
3. ✦	Type or key into the computer the patient's telephone number, including area code. If applicable, document the patient's home, work, and cell phone numbers.				
4. ✦	Type or key into the computer the patient's insurance information, including name, address, and telephone number of the insurance company; subscriber name and ID; group number; and effective date.				

Name: ______________________________

Date: ______________________________

Document: Enter the appropriate information in the chart below.

Grading

Points Earned	_______		
Points Possible	_______	24	24
Percent Grade (Points Earned/Points Possible)	_______		
PASS:	_______	❑ YES ❑ NO ❑ N/A	❑ YES ❑ NO ❑ N/A

Instructor Sign-Off

Instructor: ______________________________ **Date:** ____________________

Name: ______________________________

Date: ______________________________

Procedure 15-2:

Making Collection Calls

Objective: Place a call requesting payment from a patient.

Supplies: Patient's ledger card and/or financial record; demographic information; telephone; black ink pen

Affective Behaviors: Affective behaviors provide a professional approach to a skill that enhances the patient encounter. These behaviors may also display sensitivity to a patient's rights and enhance communication. Pay close attention to these skills, which will be in ***bold, italicized*** font.

Notes to the Student

____

____

____

____

____

____

Skills Assessment Requirements

Read and familiarize yourself with the procedure; complete the minimum practice requirements. Document each MPR using proper charting technique. Complete each procedure within a reasonable amount of time, with a minimum of 85% accuracy.

Name: ______________________

Date: ______________________

POINT VALUE
✦ = 3–6 points
∗ = 7–9 points

		PRACTICE TRIAL	GRADED TRIAL # 1	GRADED TRIAL # 2	NOTES
1. ✦	Based on the collection policy of the office, determine how many days overdue the bill must be before the first call is made.				
2. ✦	Review the account activity prior to placing the call.				
3. ✦	Find a quiet area of office in which to work while placing collection calls.				
4. ✦	Make collection calls only Monday through Saturday from 8 A.M. to 9 P.M.				
5. ✦	Locate the patient's telephone number and place the call.				
6. ✦	Once the call is answered, confidently ask to speak with the patient.				
7. ✦	If the patient is unavailable, you may leave a message; however, the message should simply state the caller's name, who the message is for, and the telephone number where the caller may be reached.				
8. ∗	***When speaking with the patient, politely introduce yourself and ask if this is a good time to talk.*** If the patient tells you it is not a good time, ask what time would be better and make a note of that in the chart. Call the patient back at the stated time.				

Name: ______________________

Date: ______________________

POINT VALUE
✦ = 3–6 points
✶ = 7–9 points

		PRACTICE TRIAL	GRADED TRIAL # 1	GRADED TRIAL # 2	NOTES
9. ✶	***When speaking with the patient, be polite, project confidence, and state the facts and purpose of the call.***				
10. ✦	Ask the patient if there is a reason for nonpayment. If the patient is able to provide a reason, document the response.				
11. ✦	Ask the patient when you might expect payment and document that response as well.				
12. ✦	***Politely thank the patient for his or her time, and repeat the terms agreed upon.***				
13. ✦	Document the interaction in the patient's financial record.				

Name: ______________________________

Date: ______________________________

Document: Enter the appropriate information in the chart below.

Grading

Points Earned	______		
Points Possible	______	94	94
Percent Grade (Points Earned/Points Possible)	______		
PASS:	______	❏ YES ❏ NO ❏ N/A	❏ YES ❏ NO ❏ N/A

Instructor Sign-Off

Instructor: ______________________________ **Date:** ____________________

Name: ______________________

Date: ______________________

Procedure 15-3:

Writing a Collection Letter

Objective: Compose a collection letter requesting payment.

Supplies: Patient's ledger card and/or financial record; demographic information; computer; black ink pen

Affective Behaviors: Affective behaviors provide a professional approach to a skill that enhances the patient encounter. These behaviors may also display sensitivity to a patient's rights and enhance communication. Pay close attention to these skills, which will be in ***bold, italicized*** font.

Notes to the Student

____

____

____

____

____

____

Skills Assessment Requirements

Read and familiarize yourself with the procedure; complete the minimum practice requirements. Document each MPR using proper charting technique. Complete each procedure within a reasonable amount of time, with a minimum of 85% accuracy.

Name: ______________________

Date: ______________________

POINT VALUE
✦ = 3–6 points
✶ = 7–9 points

		PRACTICE TRIAL	GRADED TRIAL # 1	GRADED TRIAL # 2	NOTES
1. ✦	Based on the collection policy of the office, determine at what point the first letter is sent.				
2. ✦	Review the account activity prior to drafting the letter.				
3. ✦	Locate the patient's demographic information, including his or her address.				
4. ✦	Using the computer, compose a rough draft of the letter, ensuring that proper formatting, grammar, and punctuation are used.				
5. ✦	The first paragraph should summarize the reason for the letter and any payments the patient has made on the account.				
6. ✦	The second paragraph should state the desired action of the patient.				
7. ✦	Ensure that the letter is in a polite tone without any threats for lack of compliance.				
8. ✦	The third paragraph or closing paragraph should thank the patient in advance for his or her prompt attention to the matter and should encourage the patient to contact the office.				
9. ✶	Once the rough draft is complete, read through the document again, checking for spelling, grammar, and formatting errors.				
10. ✶	Correct any errors, and then print and sign the document.				

Name: ________________________________

Date: ________________________________

POINT VALUE
✦ = 3–6 points
✶ = 7–9 points

		PRACTICE TRIAL	GRADED TRIAL # 1	GRADED TRIAL # 2	NOTES
11. ✦	Make a copy of the letter and place it in the patient's record.				
12. ✦	Place the letter in an addressed envelope and mail it to the patient. In the patient's record, note the day the letter was mailed.				

Name: ______________________________

Date: ______________________________

Document: Enter the appropriate information in the chart below.

Grading

Points Earned	______		
Points Possible	______	78	78
Percent Grade (Points Earned/Points Possible)	______		
PASS:	______	❑ YES ❑ NO ❑ N/A	❑ YES ❑ NO ❑ N/A

Instructor Sign-Off

Instructor: ______________________________ **Date:** ______________

Name: ______________________________

Date: ______________________________

Procedure 15-4:

Posting a Payment from a Collection Agency

Objective: Post a payment from a collection agency.

Supplies: *Manual Posting System:* day sheet, ledger card, pegboard, calculator, pen, collection agency payment; *Computerized Posting System:* calculator, computer, collection agency payment

Affective Behaviors: Affective behaviors provide a professional approach to a skill that enhances the patient encounter. These behaviors may also display sensitivity to a patient's rights and enhance communication. Pay close attention to these skills, which will be in ***bold, italicized*** font.

Notes to the Student

____

____

____

____

____

____

Skills Assessment Requirements

Read and familiarize yourself with the procedure; complete the minimum practice requirements. Document each MPR using proper charting technique. Complete each procedure within a reasonable amount of time, with a minimum of 85% accuracy.

Name: ____________________

Date: ____________________

POINT VALUE
✦ = 3–6 points
✶ = 7–9 points

		PRACTICE TRIAL	GRADED TRIAL # 1	GRADED TRIAL # 2	NOTES
	Steps for a manual system				
1. ✦	After verifying the correct patient account to apply the payment to, align the patient's ledger card to the next line on the day sheet.				
2. ✶	Enter the patient's name and previous balance into the appropriate column.				
3. ✦	Enter the date of the payment, the name of the collection agency, and the amount of the payment in the appropriate columns.				
4. ✦	Enter the amount of the payment on the deposit portion of the day sheet in the checks column.				
5. ✶	Subtract the payment from the previous patient balance and record the new balance on the patent's ledger card.				
6. ✦	If an adjustment is to be made to the account due to the collection agency fee, record the amount in brackets in the adjustment column of the ledger card. Enter it with the description "Collection agency fee."				
7. ✦	Subtract the amount of the adjustment from the previous patient balance and record the new balance on the patient's ledger card.				

Name: ______________________________

Date: ______________________________

POINT VALUE
✦ = 3–6 points
✶ = 7–9 points

		PRACTICE TRIAL	GRADED TRIAL # 1	GRADED TRIAL # 2	NOTES
	Steps for a computerized system				
1. ✦	Locate the patient's account in the computer.				
2. ✶	Verify that the patient's account is correct and follow the steps appropriate for your software program to post the payment.				
3. ✦	Choose "Collection Payment" to indicate the source of the payment.				
4. ✦	Following the instructions and training you received for the software program, enter the amount of any fee due to the collection agency, if applicable.				
5. ✶	Verify that the amount of payment and the fee are correct, and save the changes in the program according to software specifications.				

Name: ________________________________

Date: ________________________________

Document: Enter the appropriate information in the chart below.

Grading

Points Earned	______		
Points Possible	______	48 36	48 36
Percent Grade (Points Earned/Points Possible)	______		
PASS:	______	❑ YES ❑ NO ❑ N/A	❑ YES ❑ NO ❑ N/A

Instructor Sign-Off

Instructor:________________________________ **Date:**____________________

Name: ___________________________

Date: ___________________________

Procedure 15-5:

Perform Accounts Receivable

Objective: Demonstrate skills to ensure that patient accounts are in balance and financial obligations are met in a timely manner.

Supplies: Data; computer or ledger; telephone

Affective Behaviors: Affective behaviors provide a professional approach to a skill that enhances the patient encounter. These behaviors may also display sensitivity to a patient's rights and enhance communication. Pay close attention to these skills, which will be in ***bold, italicized*** font.

Notes to the Student

Skills Assessment Requirements

Read and familiarize yourself with the procedure; complete the minimum practice requirements. Document each MPR using proper charting technique. Complete each procedure within a reasonable amount of time, with a minimum of 85% accuracy.

Name: ______________________

Date: ______________________

POINT VALUE
✦ = 3–6 points
∗ = 7–9 points

		PRACTICE TRIAL	GRADED TRIAL # 1	GRADED TRIAL # 2	NOTES
1. ✦	Review the accounts receivable account aging.				
2. ✦	Determine if third-party (insurance) payments have been received and posted to the patient accounts being reviewed.				
3. ✦	Contact insurance carriers to resolve any outstanding payments, according to the facility policies.				
4. ✦	Update the patient accounts with appropriate notes.				

Name: ______________________

Date: ______________________

Document: Enter the appropriate information in the chart below.

Grading

Points Earned	______		
Points Possible	______	24	24
Percent Grade (Points Earned/Points Possible)	______		
PASS:	______	❑ YES ❑ NO ❑ N/A	❑ YES ❑ NO ❑ N/A

Instructor Sign-Off

Instructor: ______________________ **Date:** ______________________

Name: ______________________________

Date: ______________________________

Procedure 15-6:

Using a Pegboard System

Objective: Process patient accounts using the write-it-once system without error in posting of mathematics.

Supplies: Pegboard, superbills, new day sheet, ledger cards for each patient scheduled during the day, calculator

Affective Behaviors: Affective behaviors provide a professional approach to a skill that enhances the patient encounter. These behaviors may also display sensitivity to a patient's rights and enhance communication. Pay close attention to these skills, which will be in ***bold, italicized*** font.

Notes to the Student

____

____

____

____

____

____

Skills Assessment Requirements

Read and familiarize yourself with the procedure; complete the minimum practice requirements. Document each MPR using proper charting technique. Complete each procedure within a reasonable amount of time, with a minimum of 85% accuracy.

Name: ______________________________

Date: ______________________________

POINT VALUE
✦ = 3–6 points
✶ = 7–9 points

		PRACTICE TRIAL	GRADED TRIAL # 1	GRADED TRIAL # 2	NOTES
1. ✦	Place a new day sheet and strip of superbills on the pegboard, fastened securely into the pegs.				
2. ✦	Complete all the information required at the top of the day sheet.				
3. ✦	Carry balances forward from the previous day sheet and enter them in Section 4.				
4. ✦	Remove the superbill from the pegboard and clip it to the front of the patient's chart for the physician to enter the procedures performed that day on the appropriate line of the superbill, fill in the diagnosis, and sign the form after the physician sees the patient.				
5. ✦	*To record charges*, place the ledger card under the next superbill and turn back the top two pages of the superbill. Write the amount of the charges, pressing firmly and evenly to press through to the forms and day sheet.				
6. ✦	*To record payment*, the medical assistant or receptionist will enter the correct charge next to every procedure or service and place this total on the front of the superbill. Place the superbill back on the pegboard with the ledger card under the last page of the charge slip. Finish recording this transaction by filling in all the information that the office requires in the far right-hand columns.				

Name: ____________________

Date: ____________________

POINT VALUE ✦ = 3–6 points ✶ = 7–9 points		PRACTICE TRIAL	GRADED TRIAL # 1	GRADED TRIAL # 2	NOTES
7. ✦	*To post adjustments*, when an adjustment is made (e.g., a discount given to another health professional), the medical assistant or receptionist will enter the correct discounted amount into the computer system or subtract it from the balance due from the insurance company. If the adjustment is for nonsufficient funds, add the check amount and service fee charged by the bank to the patient balance.				
8. ✦	*To post collection agency payments*, if the patient pays a collection agency and the collection agency forwards the money, credit that payment to the patient account and write "Collection agency payment of $X" (the amount received) next to it.				
9. ✦	If a credit balance exists and the physician or office manager approves, issue a refund check to the patient.				

Name: ______________________________

Date: ______________________________

Document: Enter the appropriate information in the chart below.

Grading

Points Earned	_______		
Points Possible	_______	54	54
Percent Grade (Points Earned/Points Possible)	_______		
PASS:	_______	❑ YES ❑ NO ❑ N/A	❑ YES ❑ NO ❑ N/A

Instructor Sign-Off

Instructor: ______________________________ **Date:** ____________________

Name: ______________________________

Date: ______________________________

Procedure 16-1:

Prepare a Check

Objective: Correctly prepare a check.

Supplies: Blank checks with stub or record; black ink pen

Affective Behaviors: Affective behaviors provide a professional approach to a skill that enhances the patient encounter. These behaviors may also display sensitivity to a patient's rights and enhance communication. Pay close attention to these skills, which will be in ***bold, italicized*** font.

Notes to the Student

____

____

____

____

____

____

Skills Assessment Requirements

Read and familiarize yourself with the procedure; complete the minimum practice requirements. Document each MPR using proper charting technique. Complete each procedure within a reasonable amount of time, with a minimum of 85% accuracy.

Name: ______________________________

Date: ______________________________

POINT VALUE
✦ = 3–6 points
✶ = 7–9 points

		PRACTICE TRIAL	GRADED TRIAL # 1	GRADED TRIAL # 2	NOTES
1. ✦	Move all checks in the pad to the left so that the lowest-numbered check will be laid across the check register.				
2. ✦	Fill in the check stub or check record *before* writing the check.				
3. ✦	Use ink or a typewriter to complete the check and stub.				
4. ✦	Write the name of the payee on the "Pay to the Order of" line.				
5. ✦	Write the full amount of the check on the "Pay" line.				
6. ✦	Write the full date and check number in the designated boxes.				
7. ✶	Write the amount of the check using numbers in the designated area. Fill in all blank spaces and leave no room for anyone to add anything. Always begin writing or entering figures at the extreme left side.				
8. ✦	Date the check on the date it is written.				
9. ✦	Make sure that the dollar amount written on the second line agrees with the numerical dollar amount entered in the space on the first line.				
10. ✶	Subtract the amount of this check from the "Balance Forward" line. Write the amount as the new balance forward.				

Name: ______________________________

Date: ______________________________

Document: Enter the appropriate information in the chart below.

Grading

Points Earned	______		
Points Possible	______	66	66
Percent Grade (Points Earned/Points Possible)	______		
PASS:	______	❑ YES ❑ NO ❑ N/A	❑ YES ❑ NO ❑ N/A

Instructor Sign-Off

Instructor: ______________________________ **Date:** ______________

Name: ______________________________

Date: ______________________________

Procedure 16-2:

Post Nonsufficient Funds (NSF) Checks

Objective: Demonstrate the process for posting nonsufficient funds (NSF) checks.

Supplies: Data; computer or ledger card; pen

Affective Behaviors: Affective behaviors provide a professional approach to a skill that enhances the patient encounter. These behaviors may also display sensitivity to a patient's rights and enhance communication. Pay close attention to these skills, which will be in ***bold, italicized*** font.

Notes to the Student

____

____

____

____

____

____

Skills Assessment Requirements

Read and familiarize yourself with the procedure; complete the minimum practice requirements. Document each MPR using proper charting technique. Complete each procedure within a reasonable amount of time, with a minimum of 85% accuracy.

Name: ____________________

Date: ____________________

POINT VALUE
✦ = 3–6 points
✶ = 7–9 points

		PRACTICE TRIAL	GRADED TRIAL # 1	GRADED TRIAL # 2	NOTES
1. ✦	Record the amount of the NSF check and service fee in the adjustment column on the day sheet and ledger card.				
2. ✶	Accurately record the NSF check to show that the amount has been added to the balance instead of subtracted from it in the patient's account.				
3. ✦	Note the reason for the adjustment in the patient's account.				

Name: ____________________

Date: ____________________

Document: Enter the appropriate information in the chart below.

Grading

Points Earned	_______		
Points Possible	_______	21	21
Percent Grade (Points Earned/Points Possible)	_______		
PASS:	_______	❑ YES ❑ NO ❑ N/A	❑ YES ❑ NO ❑ N/A

Instructor Sign-Off

Instructor: ____________________ **Date:** ____________________

Name: ______________________________

Date: ______________________________

Procedure 16-3:

Prepare a Deposit Slip

Objective: Correctly complete a deposit slip.

Supplies: Pen; deposit slip; checks and currency to be deposited; endorsing stamp; calculator

Affective Behaviors: Affective behaviors provide a professional approach to a skill that enhances the patient encounter. These behaviors may also display sensitivity to a patient's rights and enhance communication. Pay close attention to these skills, which will be in ***bold, italicized*** font.

Notes to the Student

____

____

____

____

____

____

Skills Assessment Requirements

Read and familiarize yourself with the procedure; complete the minimum practice requirements. Document each MPR using proper charting technique. Complete each procedure within a reasonable amount of time, with a minimum of 85% accuracy.

Name: ______________________

Date: ______________________

POINT VALUE
✦ = 3–6 points
✶ = 7–9 points

		PRACTICE TRIAL	GRADED TRIAL # 1	GRADED TRIAL # 2	NOTES
1. ✦	Using the endorsing stamp, endorse all the checks to be deposited.				
2. ✦	Complete the information on the front of the deposit slip.				
3. ✶	If there is cash to be deposited, enter the amount in the upper-right box on the deposit slip beside the "Cash" indicator. In the boxes that list "Currency," list the total amount of all cash paper money to be deposited. In the "Coin" boxes, list the total amount of all coin money to be deposited.				
4. ✦	List each check to be deposited on a different line. If you have more checks than will fit on the front, list each additional check on the reverse side of the deposit slip.				
5. ✦	Beside the numbers, list the name of the person who wrote the check. In the box beside the numbered box, list the amount of the check.				
6. ✦	List each check in a different numbered box.				
7. ✶	Use a calculator to add all the checks and enter the total of all checks in the space labeled "Total" at the bottom of the reverse side of the deposit slip. Place this amount on the front of the deposit slip in the space labeled "Total from Side."				

Name: ______________________________

Date: ______________________________

POINT VALUE
✦ = 3–6 points
✶ = 7–9 points

		PRACTICE TRIAL	GRADED TRIAL # 1	GRADED TRIAL # 2	NOTES
8. ✶	Use the calculator to add the total amount of the cash and checks being deposited. List this amount in the space labeled "Total" and the space labeled "Net Deposit" on the front of the deposit slip.				
9. ✦	Place the deposit slip along with the cash and checks listed on the slip in an envelope for deposit at the bank.				

Name: ______________________

Date: ______________________

Document: Enter the appropriate information in the chart below.

Grading

Points Earned	_______		
Points Possible	_______	72	72
Percent Grade (Points Earned/Points Possible)	_______		
PASS:	_______	❏ YES ❏ NO ❏ N/A	❏ YES ❏ NO ❏ N/A

Instructor Sign-Off

Instructor: ______________________ **Date:** ______________________

Name: ______________________________

Date: ______________________________

Procedure 16-4:

Reconciling a Bank Statement

Objective: Reconcile a bank statement.

Supplies: Current and previous bank statements; cancelled checks (if returned by the bank); checkbook stubs

Affective Behaviors: Affective behaviors provide a professional approach to a skill that enhances the patient encounter. These behaviors may also display sensitivity to a patient's rights and enhance communication. Pay close attention to these skills, which will be in ***bold, italicized*** font.

Notes to the Student

____

____

____

____

____

____

Skills Assessment Requirements

Read and familiarize yourself with the procedure; complete the minimum practice requirements. Document each MPR using proper charting technique. Complete each procedure within a reasonable amount of time, with a minimum of 85% accuracy.

Name: ______________________________

Date: ______________________________

POINT VALUE
✦ = 3–6 points
✶ = 7–9 points

		PRACTICE TRIAL	GRADED TRIAL # 1	GRADED TRIAL # 2	NOTES
1. ✦	Compare the beginning balance of the current statement with the ending balance of the previous month's statement. They should be the same.				
2. ✦	Write the current ending balance in the appropriate space on the reverse side of the bank statement.				
3. ✦	Compare the deposits noted on the statement against your records or receipts by making a check mark next to each correct number.				
4. ✶	List separately all outstanding deposits. Add these together and place the total on the reverse side of the statement in the space provided.				
5. ✦	Add the ending balance to the total of deposits not already included, and write this amount on the "Total" line.				
6. ✦	Compare the value of the checks listed on the statement with the value listed in the checkbook or check stubs.				
7. ✶	Note all numbers missing from the sequential list of check numbers. List all outstanding checks. Add the total for outstanding checks and place that figure on the line indicated on the back of the statement.				
8. ✦	Subtract the total figure for checks outstanding from the previous total on the back of the statement to determine the current balance. This amount should agree with the amount in your checking account.				

Name: ______________________________

Date: ______________________________

Document: Enter the appropriate information in the chart below.

Grading

Points Earned	_______		
Points Possible	_______	54	54
Percent Grade (Points Earned/Points Possible)	_______		
PASS:	_______	❑ YES ❑ NO ❑ N/A	❑ YES ❑ NO ❑ N/A

Instructor Sign-Off

Instructor: ______________________________ **Date:** ______________

Name: ______________________________

Date: ______________________________

Procedure 16-5:

Generating Payroll in a Medical Office

Objective: Manually generate payroll.

Supplies: Pen, calculator, checkbook, employee time card, employee payroll record, payroll register, tax tables

Affective Behaviors: Affective behaviors provide a professional approach to a skill that enhances the patient encounter. These behaviors may also display sensitivity to a patient's rights and enhance communication. Pay close attention to these skills, which will be in ***bold, italicized*** font.

Notes to the Student

Skills Assessment Requirements

Read and familiarize yourself with the procedure; complete the minimum practice requirements. Document each MPR using proper charting technique. Complete each procedure within a reasonable amount of time, with a minimum of 85% accuracy.

Name: ______________________________

Date: ______________________________

POINT VALUE
✦ = 3–6 points
✶ = 7–9 points

		PRACTICE TRIAL	GRADED TRIAL # 1	GRADED TRIAL # 2	NOTES
1. ✦	Gather all necessary equipment.				
2. ✦	Using the employee's time card, calculate the total number of regular hours worked and the total number of overtime hours worked. Enter the totals on the payroll register.				
3. ✶	In the employee payroll record, obtain the employee's pay rate. Multiply the pay rate by the total number of regular hours worked. Next, calculate (multiply) the overtime pay rate and the total number of overtime hours. Enter the totals for each on the payroll register. Add the regular hours earned and overtime hours earned, and place this amount on the payroll register under the heading "Total Gross."				
4. ✶	Gather the employee payroll record and tax tables. Decide how much to withhold for federal income tax. Next, calculate the total FICA tax to be withheld for Medicare and Social Security. Enter these amounts on the payroll register in the appropriate places.				
5. ✶	Determine how much to withhold for local and state taxes. Enter these amounts on the payroll register in the appropriate places.				
6. ✦	Compute the employer's contributions to the unemployment fund of the state the employee currently resides in and FUTA. Document these calculations on the employer's account.				

Name: ______________________________

Date: ______________________________

POINT VALUE
✦ = 3–6 points
✶ = 7–9 points

		PRACTICE TRIAL	GRADED TRIAL # 1	GRADED TRIAL # 2	NOTES
7. ✦	Determine if there are any other deductions (insurance, retirement, 401K plan, etc.).				
8. ✦	To calculate the net earnings, subtract the total amount of deductions from the gross earnings.				
9. ✦	Complete the check stub and check with required information.				

Name: ______________________________

Date: ______________________________

Document: Enter the appropriate information in the chart below.

Grading

Points Earned	________		
Points Possible	________	72	72
Percent Grade (Points Earned/Points Possible)	________		
PASS:	________	❑ YES ❑ NO ❑ N/A	❑ YES ❑ NO ❑ N/A

Instructor Sign-Off

Instructor: ______________________________ **Date:** ______________

Name: ______________________

Date: ______________________

Procedure 17-1:

Performing Billing and Collection Procedures

Objective: Demonstrate the ability to record payments received from the patient, to record patient information using a patient ledger card and day sheet, and to generate an insurance bill using a charge slip. Demonstrate the ability to then record a payment and provide a receipt to the patient.

Supplies: Day sheet, ledger card, co-payment check, receipt book, pen, calculator

Affective Behaviors: Affective behaviors provide a professional approach to a skill that enhances the patient encounter. These behaviors may also display sensitivity to a patient's rights and enhance communication. Pay close attention to these skills, which will be in ***bold, italicized*** font.

Notes to the Student

____

____

____

____

____

____

Skills Assessment Requirements

Read and familiarize yourself with the procedure; complete the minimum practice requirements. Document each MPR using proper charting technique. Complete each procedure within a reasonable amount of time, with a minimum of 85% accuracy.

Name: ______________________________

Date: ______________________________

POINT VALUE
✦ = 3–6 points
✶ = 7–9 points

		PRACTICE TRIAL	GRADED TRIAL # 1	GRADED TRIAL # 2	NOTES
1. ✦	Pull the appropriate ledger card and place it directly on the day sheet.				
2. ✦	Temporarily remove the strip of charge slips from the pegboard.				
3. ✦	Enter the patient's previous balance on the day sheet. The ledger card does not extend to this column.				
4. ✦	Post the date, patient's name, descriptions, and co-payment amount.				
5. ✶	Calculate the new balance by subtracting the payment from the previous balance.				
6. ✦	Generate an insurance bill for the remaining balance.				
7. ✦	Create a receipt for the patient.				

Name: ____________________

Date: ____________________

Document: Enter the appropriate information in the chart below.

Grading

Points Earned	______		
Points Possible	______	45	45
Percent Grade (Points Earned/Points Possible)	______		
PASS:	______	❑ YES ❑ NO ❑ N/A	❑ YES ❑ NO ❑ N/A

Instructor Sign-Off

Instructor: ____________________ **Date:** ____________________

Name: ______________________________

Date: ______________________________

Procedure 17-2:

Applying Third-Party Guidelines

Objective: Apply knowledge of third-party guidelines to obtain preauthorization for a procedure.

Supplies: Insurance card, telephone, patient record

Affective Behaviors: Affective behaviors provide a professional approach to a skill that enhances the patient encounter. These behaviors may also display sensitivity to a patient's rights and enhance communication. Pay close attention to these skills, which will be in ***bold, italicized*** font.

Notes to the Student

____

____

____

____

____

____

Skills Assessment Requirements

Read and familiarize yourself with the procedure; complete the minimum practice requirements. Document each MPR using proper charting technique. Complete each procedure within a reasonable amount of time, with a minimum of 85% accuracy.

Name: ______________________________

Date: ______________________________

POINT VALUE
✦ = 3–6 points
∗ = 7–9 points

		PRACTICE TRIAL	GRADED TRIAL # 1	GRADED TRIAL # 2	NOTES
1. ✦	Gather information about the patient.				
2. ✦	Locate the insurance carrier's telephone number.				
3. ✦	Call the insurance carrier and introduce yourself, giving the name of the office.				
4. ✦	Instruct the insurance carrier that the physician recommends the procedure and that the third-party carrier requires preauthorization.				
5. ✦	Give the insurance carrier the necessary information as requested.				
6. ∗	Document in the patient's chart the preauthorization number for the procedure.				

Name: ________________________________

Date: ________________________________

Document: Enter the appropriate information in the chart below.

Grading

Points Earned	_______		
Points Possible	_______	39	39
Percent Grade (Points Earned/Points Possible)	_______		
PASS:	_______	❑ YES ❑ NO ❑ N/A	❑ YES ❑ NO ❑ N/A

Instructor Sign-Off

Instructor: ________________________________ **Date:** ____________________

Name: ______________________________

Date: ______________________________

Procedure 17-3:

Applying Managed Care Policies and Procedures

Objective: Demonstrate knowledge of managed care policies.

Supplies: Insurance card, copier

Affective Behaviors: Affective behaviors provide a professional approach to a skill that enhances the patient encounter. These behaviors may also display sensitivity to a patient's rights and enhance communication. Pay close attention to these skills, which will be in ***bold, italicized*** font.

Notes to the Student

____

____

____

____

____

____

Skills Assessment Requirements

Read and familiarize yourself with the procedure; complete the minimum practice requirements. Document each MPR using proper charting technique. Complete each procedure within a reasonable amount of time, with a minimum of 85% accuracy.

Name: ______________________________

Date: ______________________________

POINT VALUE
✦ = 3–6 points
✶ = 7–9 points

		PRACTICE TRIAL	GRADED TRIAL # 1	GRADED TRIAL # 2	NOTES
1. ✦	***Greet the patient*** and request the insurance card.				
2. ✶	Check the patient's insurance card to see if coverage is current.				
3. ✶	Correctly enter the insurance information from the card into the database.				
4. ✦	Photocopy the insurance card.				
5. ✦	Return the card to the patient.				

Name: ______________________

Date: ______________________

Document: Enter the appropriate information in the chart below.

Grading

Points Earned	________		
Points Possible	________	36	36
Percent Grade (Points Earned/Points Possible)	________		
PASS:	________	❑ YES ❑ NO ❑ N/A	❑ YES ❑ NO ❑ N/A

Instructor Sign-Off

Instructor: ______________________ **Date:** ______________________

Name: ______________________

Date: ______________________

Procedure 18-1:

Completing the CMS-1500 Form

Objective: Correctly complete the CMS-1500 form.

Supplies: Patient's medical record; patient's insurance information; patient's ledger card; superbill; CMS-1500 form; black ink pen; computer and printer (or typewriter)

Affective Behaviors: Affective behaviors provide a professional approach to a skill that enhances the patient encounter. These behaviors may also display sensitivity to a patient's rights and enhance communication. Pay close attention to these skills, which will be in ***bold, italicized*** font.

Notes to the Student

____

____

____

____

____

____

Skills Assessment Requirements

Read and familiarize yourself with the procedure; complete the minimum practice requirements. Document each MPR using proper charting technique. Complete each procedure within a reasonable amount of time, with a minimum of 85% accuracy.

Name: ______________________________

Date: ______________________________

POINT VALUE
✦ = 3–6 points
✶ = 7–9 points

		PRACTICE TRIAL	GRADED TRIAL # 1	GRADED TRIAL # 2	NOTES
1. ✦	Gather information about the patient.				
2. ✦	Gather all necessary materials.				
3. ✶	Using Figure 18-3 in your textbook, fill in all necessary sections of the CMS-1500 form using a computer or typewriter.				
4. ✶	Double-check all the boxes on the form for accuracy.				

Name: ______________________

Date: ______________________

Document: Enter the appropriate information in the chart below.

Grading

Points Earned	_____		
Points Possible	_____	30	30
Percent Grade (Points Earned/Points Possible)	_____		
PASS:	_____	❑ YES ❑ NO ❑ N/A	❑ YES ❑ NO ❑ N/A

Instructor Sign-Off

Instructor: ______________________ **Date:** ______________________

Name: ______________________________

Date: ______________________________

Procedure 19-1:

ICD-9-CM Coding

Objective: Accurately assign an ICD-9-CM code.

Supplies: Patient's medical record; patient's insurance card; computer with printer or typewriter; medical reference material; superbill with the doctor's diagnosis

Affective Behaviors: Affective behaviors provide a professional approach to a skill that enhances the patient encounter. These behaviors may also display sensitivity to a patient's rights and enhance communication. Pay close attention to these skills, which will be in ***bold, italicized*** font.

Notes to the Student

____

____

____

____

____

____

Skills Assessment Requirements

Read and familiarize yourself with the procedure; complete the minimum practice requirements. Document each MPR using proper charting technique. Complete each procedure within a reasonable amount of time, with a minimum of 85% accuracy.

Name: ______________________

Date: ______________________

POINT VALUE
✦ = 3–6 points
✶ = 7–9 points

		PRACTICE TRIAL	GRADED TRIAL # 1	GRADED TRIAL # 2	NOTES
1. ✦	Locate the condition or diagnosis on the superbill or in the patient's medical record.				
2. ✦	In *Volume II: Alphabetic Index* of the ICD-9-CM, locate the condition or diagnosis.				
3. ✦	Examine the diagnostic statements to determine if the main term specifically describes that disease. If it does not, look at the modifiers listed under that main term to find a more specific code.				
4. ✦	Locate the code in *Volume I: Tabular Index*.				
5. ✦	Match the code description in the *Tabular Index* with the diagnosis in the patient's medical record.				
6. ✦	Use the codes from 0021.0 through V82.9 in the ICD-9-CM to describe the main reason for the patient's office visit.				
7. ✦	First, list the ICD-9-CM code for the condition, problem, or diagnosis that is the main reason for the visit. Then, list coexisting conditions under additional codes.				
8. ✦	Use codes at their highest level of specificity—fifth-digit codes first, followed by fourth-digit codes, then third-digit codes, and so on.				
9. ✦	Do not code questionable, probable, or ruled-out diagnoses.				

Name: ______________________________

Date: ______________________________

POINT VALUE
✦ = 3–6 points
✶ = 7–9 points

		PRACTICE TRIAL	GRADED TRIAL # 1	GRADED TRIAL # 2	NOTES
10. ✦	V codes describe factors that influence the health status of the patient, such as pregnancy test or vaccination, and are not used to code current illnesses.				
11. ✦	E codes are used for identifying external environmental events or conditions such as the course of injury, some adverse effect, or poisoning. E codes (E930–E949) are mandatory when coding the use of drugs.				
12. ✦	M codes, in Appendix A of *Volume I*, relate to the morphology of neoplasm. Morphology codes are used only by tumor registries for reporting proposes.				
13. ✶	List all diagnosis codes (up to four) on the insurance claim form, with the primary diagnosis listed first.				
14. ✶	Always double-check your coding and ensure proper use of abbreviations and symbols prior to assigning the final code.				

Name: ______________________________

Date: ______________________________

Document: Enter the appropriate information in the chart below.

Grading

Points Earned	______		
Points Possible	______	90	90
Percent Grade (Points Earned/Points Possible)	______		
PASS:	______	❑ YES ❑ NO ❑ N/A	❑ YES ❑ NO ❑ N/A

Instructor Sign-Off

Instructor: ______________________________ **Date:** ______________

Name: ______________________________

Date: ______________________________

Procedure 19-2:

Assigning a CPT Code

Objective: Accurately assign a CPT code.

Supplies: Patient's medical record, computer, medical billing software, current CPT coding book, suberbill with procedure marked

Affective Behaviors: Affective behaviors provide a professional approach to a skill that enhances the patient encounter. These behaviors may also display sensitivity to a patient's rights and enhance communication. Pay close attention to these skills, which will be in ***bold, italicized*** font.

Notes to the Student

____

____

____

____

____

____

Skills Assessment Requirements

Read and familiarize yourself with the procedure; complete the minimum practice requirements. Document each MPR using proper charting technique. Complete each procedure within a reasonable amount of time, with a minimum of 85% accuracy.

Name: ____________________

Date: ____________________

POINT VALUE
✦ = 3–6 points
✶ = 7–9 points

		PRACTICE TRIAL	GRADED TRIAL # 1	GRADED TRIAL # 2	NOTES
1. ✦	Locate the complete procedure on the superbill.				
2. ✦	If the only procedure done was a physician visit, locate the CPT E/M codes section of the CPT book.				
3. ✦	Determine by the patient's medical record whether this office visit was a first-time or follow-up visit.				
4. ✦	Also determine by the patient's medical record whether this visit involved the patient's attending physician or a consulting physician.				
5. ✦	Note where the visit took place.				
6. ✶	Locate the level of visit within the place of service codes.				
7. ✦	If there was a surgical procedure, locate the code for it.				
8. ✦	Locate the code for any necessary equipment used in surgery.				
9. ✦	Code any radiologic procedures.				
10. ✶	Locate the procedure done in Sections 7000 to 7999.				
11. ✶	Locate, in the appropriate section, the part of the body on which the procedure was done.				
12. ✦	Locate the correct procedure, being careful to note if the test was bilateral, unilateral, etc.				
13. ✦	Code a laboratory test if done in Sections 80000 to 89999.				
14. ✦	Code any injected medication(s).				
15. ✶	Compare the CPT codes with the ICD codes before finalizing the bill.				

Name: ______________________________

Date: ______________________________

Document: Enter the appropriate information in the chart below.

Grading

Points Earned	______		
Points Possible	______	102	102
Percent Grade (Points Earned/Points Possible)	______		
PASS:	______	❑ YES ❑ NO ❑ N/A	❑ YES ❑ NO ❑ N/A

Instructor Sign-Off

Instructor: ______________________________ **Date:** ______________________________

Name: ______________________________

Date: ______________________________

Procedure 20-1:

Staff Meeting Procedures

Objective: Explain and present the steps in preparing for and conducting a staff meeting.

Supplies: Agenda items received from staff; meeting agenda; means of keeping time (watch, clock, stopwatch, etc.); room for the meeting; any audio or video equipment that may be needed

Affective Behaviors: Affective behaviors provide a professional approach to a skill that enhances the patient encounter. These behaviors may also display sensitivity to a patient's rights and enhance communication. Pay close attention to these skills, which will be in ***bold, italicized*** font.

Notes to the Student

____

____

____

____

____

____

Skills Assessment Requirements

Read and familiarize yourself with the procedure; complete the minimum practice requirements. Document each MPR using proper charting technique. Complete each procedure within a reasonable amount of time, with a minimum of 85% accuracy.

Name: ______________________________

Date: ______________________________

POINT VALUE
✦ = 3–6 points
∗ = 7–9 points

		PRACTICE TRIAL	GRADED TRIAL # 1	GRADED TRIAL # 2	NOTES
1. ✦	One week before the meeting, request agenda items from the staff.				
2. ✦	Before the meeting, create a meeting agenda with all topics to be discussed. Include the date, time, and place of the meeting. List who will be running (facilitating) the meeting. Assign a length of time to each topic and a person who will be responsible for that topic.				
3. ✦	Start the meeting on time.				
4. ✦	BegIn by briefly covering the previous meeting.				
5. ✦	Try to stay on schedule as much as possible.				
6. ✦	Allow for time at the end of the meeting to have open discussion of any new business.				
7. ✦	Adjourn the meeting.				
8. ✦	After the meeting, have the minutes of the meeting typed and distributed to all involved.				

Name: ______________________________

Date: ______________________________

Document: Enter the appropriate information in the chart below.

Grading

Points Earned	_______		
Points Possible	_______	48	48
Percent Grade (Points Earned/Points Possible)	_______		
PASS:	_______	❑ YES ❑ NO ❑ N/A	❑ YES ❑ NO ❑ N/A

Instructor Sign-Off

Instructor: ______________________________ **Date:** ____________________

Name: ______________________________

Date: ______________________________

Procedure 20-2:

Developing a Patient Information Booklet

Objective: Develop a booklet to inform patients about the services provided by your medical office.

Supplies: Computer, design software (if including images), high-quality paper, printer (or an independent printing service)

Affective Behaviors: Affective behaviors provide a professional approach to a skill that enhances the patient encounter. These behaviors may also display sensitivity to a patient's rights and enhance communication. Pay close attention to these skills, which will be in ***bold, italicized*** font.

Notes to the Student

____

____

____

____

____

____

Skills Assessment Requirements

Read and familiarize yourself with the procedure; complete the minimum practice requirements. Document each MPR using proper charting technique. Complete each procedure within a reasonable amount of time, with a minimum of 85% accuracy.

Name: ______________________________

Date: ______________________________

POINT VALUE
✦ = 3–6 points
✶ = 7–9 points

		PRACTICE TRIAL	GRADED TRIAL # 1	GRADED TRIAL # 2	NOTES
1. ✦	Make the booklet as appealing as possible. Leave a white border around all page edges. Use large print for the elderly reader's benefit. The booklet should be small enough that it will fit easily into a pocket or purse.				
2. ✦	Write the booklet with the reader in mind and at a reading level appropriate for the target audience.				
3. ✦	Avoid long paragraphs of explanation. Keep the sentences short and concise, and use as many bulleted points as possible.				
4. ✶	Proofread the booklet for grammatical and content errors.				
5. ✦	Provide a list of the regular office hours.				
6. ✦	List any special services offered by the practice or clinic, such as patient education classes or blood pressure testing programs.				
7. ✦	Explain the procedure for having a prescription refilled.				
8. ✦	Explain the procedure for processing medical insurance forms.				
9. ✦	Include a general statement about payment of fees, especially if payment is expected at the time of delivery of services. Do not discuss specific fees in patient brochures.				

Name: ______________________________

Date: ______________________________

POINT VALUE
✦ = 3–6 points
✶ = 7–9 points

		PRACTICE TRIAL	GRADED TRIAL # 1	GRADED TRIAL # 2	NOTES
10. ✦	Provide information about the physician and the staff. Include the name and telephone number of the office manager, the personnel responsible for insurance processing, and the patient educator.				
11. ✦	State what procedure to follow in case of an emergency. Ask the patient to keep this number near his or her telephone.				
12. ✦	Include a telephone number at the end of the brochure to use when additional information is needed.				
13. ✦	***End the brochure by thanking the patient for taking the time to read the literature.***				

Name: ______________________________

Date: ______________________________

Document: Enter the appropriate information in the chart below.

Grading

Points Earned	_______		
Points Possible	_______	81	81
Percent Grade (Points Earned/Points Possible)	_______		
PASS:	_______	❑ YES ❑ NO ❑ N/A	❑ YES ❑ NO ❑ N/A

Instructor Sign-Off

Instructor: ______________________________ **Date:** ____________________

Name: ______________________________

Date: ______________________________

Procedure 34-1:

Disposal of Infectious Wastes and Substances

Objective: Demonstrate proficiency in the safe handling and disposal of infectious waste and substances.

Supplies: Biohazard container, red plastic bag, hazardous waste

Affective Behaviors: Affective behaviors provide a professional approach to a skill that enhances the patient encounter. These behaviors may also display sensitivity to a patient's rights and enhance communication. Pay close attention to these skills, which will be in ***bold, italicized*** font.

Notes to the Student

____

____

____

____

____

____

Skills Assessment Requirements

Read and familiarize yourself with the procedure; complete the minimum practice requirements. Document each MPR using proper charting technique. Complete each procedure within a reasonable amount of time, with a minimum of 85% accuracy.

Name: ______________________________

Date: ______________________________

POINT VALUE
✦ = 3–6 points
✶ = 7–9 points

		PRACTICE TRIAL	GRADED TRIAL # 1	GRADED TRIAL # 2	NOTES
1. ✦	Line an infectious waste container (red biohazard container) with a red plastic bag if this has not already been done.				
2. ✶	Discard *only* infectious waste in the infectious waste container.				
3. ✶	Contain liquid in a non-permeable bag before depositing it in the infectious waste container.				
4. ✦	Do not discard contaminated glass in the biohazard container.				
5. ✶	Close the red bag correctly, tying it securely closed.				
6. ✦	Transport the closed red bag from the site to the dirty utility area and store it in the designated biohazard trash-holding area.				

Name: ______________________________

Date: ______________________________

Document: Enter the appropriate information in the chart below.

Grading

Points Earned	_______		
Points Possible	_______	45	45
Percent Grade (Points Earned/Points Possible)	_______		
PASS:	_______	❑ YES ❑ NO ❑ N/A	❑ YES ❑ NO ❑ N/A

Instructor Sign-Off

Instructor: ______________________________ **Date:** ______________________

Name: ______________________________

Date: ______________________________

Procedure 34-2:

Performing Hand Washing

Objective: Demonstrate proper aseptic hand-washing technique without error.

Supplies: Sink; water; soap; nail brush and/or an orange cuticle stick; disposable towel and waste container

Affective Behaviors: Affective behaviors provide a professional approach to a skill that enhances the patient encounter. These behaviors may also display sensitivity to a patient's rights and enhance communication. Pay close attention to these skills, which will be in ***bold, italicized*** font.

Notes to the Student

____

____

____

____

____

____

Skills Assessment Requirements

Read and familiarize yourself with the procedure; complete the minimum practice requirements. Document each MPR using proper charting technique. Complete each procedure within a reasonable amount of time, with a minimum of 85% accuracy.

Name: ______________________________

Date: ______________________________

POINT VALUE
✦ = 3–6 points
✶ = 7–9 points

		PRACTICE TRIAL	GRADED TRIAL # 1	GRADED TRIAL # 2	NOTES
1. ✶	Remove all jewelry (only exception is a wedding band) and artificial nails.				
2. ✦	Stand at the sink without allowing your clothing to touch the sink.				
3. ✦	Adjust running water to the correct lukewarm temperature.				
4. ✦	Wet your hands under the running water.				
5. ✦	Place liquid soap in the palm of one hand, beginning to rub your hands together to form a lather.				
6. ✶	Work soap into lather by moving it over the entire surface of the hands, including the palms and sides and backs of both hands, for 15–30 seconds.				
7. ✦	Use a circular motion and friction.				
8. ✦	Interlace the fingers, and move soapy water between them.				
9. ✶	Keep the hands pointed down. Hands and forearms should be at elbow level or below during procedure.				
10. ✦	Use nail brush and/or an orange cuticle stick to clean under the fingernails.				
11. ✶	Rinse the hands under running water with the fingers pointed down, taking care not to touch the sink or faucet.				

Name: ___________________________

Date: ___________________________

POINT VALUE
✦ = 3–6 points
✶ = 7–9 points

		PRACTICE TRIAL	GRADED TRIAL # 1	GRADED TRIAL # 2	NOTES
12. ✦	Reapply soap and wash the wrists and forearms for 15–30 seconds using a circular motion.				
13. ✦	Rinse the hands thoroughly under running water. Let the water continue to run.				
14. ✦	Dry the hands with a paper towel. Discard the paper towel used to dry the hands.				
15. ✶	Turn the faucet off with a dry paper towel and discard the towel.				

Name: ______________________________

Date: ______________________________

Document: Enter the appropriate information in the chart below.

Grading

Points Earned	________		
Points Possible	________	105	105
Percent Grade (Points Earned/Points Possible)	________		
PASS:	________	❏ YES ❏ NO ❏ N/A	❏ YES ❏ NO ❏ N/A

Instructor Sign-Off

Instructor: ______________________________ **Date:** ____________________

Name: ______________________________

Date: ______________________________

Procedure 34-3:

Applying and Removing Nonsterile Gloves

Objective: Demonstrate the proper technique for applying and removing nonsterile gloves.

Supplies: Nonsterile gloves, biohazard waste container

Affective Behaviors: Affective behaviors provide a professional approach to a skill that enhances the patient encounter. These behaviors may also display sensitivity to a patient's rights and enhance communication. Pay close attention to these skills, which will be in ***bold, italicized*** font.

Notes to the Student

____

____

____

____

____

____

Skills Assessment Requirements

Read and familiarize yourself with the procedure; complete the minimum practice requirements. Document each MPR using proper charting technique. Complete each procedure within a reasonable amount of time, with a minimum of 85% accuracy.

Name: ____________________

Date: ____________________

POINT VALUE
✦ = 3–6 points
✶ = 7–9 points

		PRACTICE TRIAL	GRADED TRIAL # 1	GRADED TRIAL # 2	NOTES
1. ✦	Perform proper hand hygiene.				
2. ✦	Choose appropriate glove size.				
3. ✦	Hold a glove at the wrist opening, insert fingers, and pull the glove up to the wrist. Repeat for second glove.				
4. ✶	Check gloves for holes or flaws. Discard gloves and repeat if necessary.				
5. ✶	To remove the gloves, use the fingers of one gloved hand to grasp the other glove at the wrist, palm side. Pull the glove over the hand while turning it inside out. Hold it in the palm of the gloved hand. Slide the fingers of the ungloved hand under the cuff of the remaining glove, grasp the inside, and pull it down over the glove and off the hand.				
6. ✦	Dispose of the gloves in the appropriate biohazard waste container.				
7. ✦	Perform proper hand hygiene.				

Name: ______________________________

Date: ______________________________

Document: Enter the appropriate information in the chart below.

Grading

Points Earned	______		
Points Possible	______	48	48
Percent Grade (Points Earned/Points Possible)	______		
PASS:	______	❑ YES ❑ NO ❑ N/A	❑ YES ❑ NO ❑ N/A

Instructor Sign-Off

Instructor: ______________________________ **Date:** ______________

Name: ______________________________

Date: ______________________________

Procedure 34-4:

Performing Transmission-Based Precaution: Isolation Techniques

Objective: Demonstrate the proper use of barrier protection to prevent the spread of infectious disease.

Supplies: Disposable gowns, masks, caps, nonsterile gloves, sterile gloves, sink with running water, paper towels

Affective Behaviors: Affective behaviors provide a professional approach to a skill that enhances the patient encounter. These behaviors may also display sensitivity to a patient's rights and enhance communication. Pay close attention to these skills, which will be in ***bold, italicized*** font.

Notes to the Student

____

____

____

____

____

____

Skills Assessment Requirements

Read and familiarize yourself with the procedure; complete the minimum practice requirements. Document each MPR using proper charting technique. Complete each procedure within a reasonable amount of time, with a minimum of 85% accuracy.

Name: ______________________________

Date: ______________________________

POINT VALUE
✦ = 3–6 points
✶ = 7–9 points

		PRACTICE TRIAL	GRADED TRIAL # 1	GRADED TRIAL # 2	NOTES
1. ✶	Review and be familiar with orders and agency protocols specific to your organization regarding the use of personal protective equipment (PPE). Examples of PPE: • Disposable gloves • Mask • Gown • Facemask				
2. ✦	Assemble appropriate equipment based upon the type of protection required for the procedure.				
3. ✦	Remove lab coat and jewelry.				
4. ✦	Perform proper hand hygiene.				
5. ✶	Apply the appropriate disposable apparel. When applying a cap, be sure hair and ears are covered completely. When applying a gown over clothes, first hold the gown in front of the body and place arms through the sleeves. Pull the sleeves on, covering the wrists. Tie the gown securely at the neck and back. When applying a mask, place the mask over the bridge of the nose. Ensure a snug fit by pinching the metal strip or by tying the mask. Apply protective eyewear.				
6. ✦	Apply nonsterile gloves and pull up over cuffs of gown, covering wrists completely.				

Name: ______________________

Date: ______________________

POINT VALUE
✦ = 3–6 points
✶ = 7–9 points

		PRACTICE TRIAL	GRADED TRIAL # 1	GRADED TRIAL # 2	NOTES
7. ✶	Remove barrier protection in following order: Untie the waist of the gown. Remove gloves. Perform hand hygiene. Untie the neck of the gown. Remove the gown by pulling it down from the shoulders. Turn the gown inside out and remove arms from sleeves.				
8. ✶	Hold the gown away from your body with the contaminated area on the inside. Fold and discard gown in biohazard container.				
9. ✦	Remove mask and discard.				
10. ✦	Perform proper hand hygiene.				

Name: ______________________________

Date: ______________________________

Document: Enter the appropriate information in the chart below.

Grading

Points Earned	________		
Points Possible	________	72	72
Percent Grade (Points Earned/Points Possible)	________		
PASS:	________	❑ YES ❑ NO ❑ N/A	❑ YES ❑ NO ❑ N/A

Instructor Sign-Off

Instructor: ______________________________ **Date:** ____________________

Name: ______________________________

Date: ______________________________

Procedure 34-5:

Sanitizing Instruments

Objective: Demonstrate the proper cleaning and sanitizing of instruments.

Supplies: Instruments; basin; disposable gloves; rubber gloves; cleaning brush; germicidal agent or low pH detergent; water; towel

Affective Behaviors: Affective behaviors provide a professional approach to a skill that enhances the patient encounter. These behaviors may also display sensitivity to a patient's rights and enhance communication. Pay close attention to these skills, which will be in ***bold, italicized*** font.

Notes to the Student

____

____

____

____

____

____

Skills Assessment Requirements

Read and familiarize yourself with the procedure; complete the minimum practice requirements. Document each MPR using proper charting technique. Complete each procedure within a reasonable amount of time, with a minimum of 85% accuracy.

Name: ______________________________

Date: ______________________________

POINT VALUE
✦ = 3–6 points
✶ = 7–9 points

		PRACTICE TRIAL	GRADED TRIAL # 1	GRADED TRIAL # 2	NOTES
1. ✶	Apply rubber gloves over disposable gloves.				
2. ✦	Fill basin approximately halfway with a low-sudsing detergent or germicidal agent (sanitizing solution).				
3. ✦	Rinse all instruments and place them in the sanitizing solution.				
4. ✶	Scrub each instrument individually with a brush and detergent under running water. Open the instruments and scrub all serrated edges and hinged areas.				
5. ✦	Thoroughly rinse instruments again under hot water.				
6. ✦	After thoroughly rinsing instruments, roll them in a clean, dry towel to finish drying.				
7. ✶	Check the condition of the instruments for defects or remaining soil.				
8. ✦	Wrap instruments for sterilization when dry.				

Name: ______________________________

Date: ______________________________

Document: Enter the appropriate information in the chart below.

Grading

Points Earned	______		
Points Possible	______	57	57
Percent Grade (Points Earned/Points Possible)	______		
PASS:	______	❑ YES ❑ NO ❑ N/A	❑ YES ❑ NO ❑ N/A

Instructor Sign-Off

Instructor: ______________________________ **Date:** ______________

Name: ______________________________

Date: ______________________________

Procedure 34-6:

Wrapping and Labeling Instruments for Autoclaving

Objective: Demonstrate the proper procedure for wrapping, packaging, and labeling instruments for autoclaving (sterilization).

Supplies: Instruments, wrapping material, sterilization indicator strip, indelible pen, tape

Affective Behaviors: Affective behaviors provide a professional approach to a skill that enhances the patient encounter. These behaviors may also display sensitivity to a patient's rights and enhance communication. Pay close attention to these skills, which will be in ***bold, italicized*** font.

Notes to the Student

____

____

____

____

____

____

Skills Assessment Requirements

Read and familiarize yourself with the procedure; complete the minimum practice requirements. Document each MPR using proper charting technique. Complete each procedure within a reasonable amount of time, with a minimum of 85% accuracy.

Name: ______________________________

Date: ______________________________

POINT VALUE
✦ = 3–6 points
✶ = 7–9 points

		PRACTICE TRIAL	GRADED TRIAL # 1	GRADED TRIAL # 2	NOTES
1. ✦	Perform proper hand hygiene.				
2. ✦	Place a square of wrapping material on the table so that it appears in a diamond shape when you are facing it. Ensure the wrapping material is large enough to completely cover the entire article you are wrapping for autoclaving.				
3. ✶	Place the item in the center of the wrapping material. If the instrument is hinged, open it so that the hinge is in the open position. If the instrument has a sharp point/tip, cover it with gauze to prevent a puncture through the wrapping material.				
4. ✦	Place the indicator strip in the center of the package.				
5. ✶	Fold the bottom point of the "diamond" up and over the instruments. Fold a small portion of the point back over so that it can be used to pick up the wrapping when it is opened for use.				
6. ✶	Fold right side of the "diamond" up and over the instruments. Again, fold a small portion back, as described above.				
7. ✶	Fold the left side of the "diamond" over until it covers the instruments. Again, fold a small portion back.				
8. ✶	Fold the bottom of the point of the "diamond" up until it reaches the top point.				
9. ✦	Make sure the pack is folded securely.				

Name: ____________________

Date: ____________________

POINT VALUE ✦ = 3–6 points ∗ = 7–9 points		PRACTICE TRIAL	GRADED TRIAL # 1	GRADED TRIAL # 2	NOTES
10. ✦	Using a piece of autoclave tape, securely tape the pack closed.				
11. ∗	Label the package with the contents (instruments or items inside), your initials, and the date.				
12. ✦	If you are using bags for autoclaving, place the item and indicator strip inside the bag. Seal the bag and label as described above.				

Name: ______________________________

Date: ______________________________

Document: Enter the appropriate information in the chart below.

Grading

Points Earned	_____		
Points Possible	_____	90	90
Percent Grade (Points Earned/Points Possible)	_____		
PASS:	_____	❑ YES ❑ NO ❑ N/A	❑ YES ❑ NO ❑ N/A

Instructor Sign-Off

Instructor: ______________________________ **Date:** ______________

Name: ______________________________

Date: ______________________________

Procedure 34-7:

Sterilizing Instruments in an Autoclave

Objective: Load and operate an autoclave correctly to prevent the spread of pathogens.

Supplies: Autoclave; instruments sanitized and wrapped for autoclaving; distilled water

Affective Behaviors: Affective behaviors provide a professional approach to a skill that enhances the patient encounter. These behaviors may also display sensitivity to a patient's rights and enhance communication. Pay close attention to these skills, which will be in ***bold, italicized*** font.

Notes to the Student

____

____

____

____

____

____

Skills Assessment Requirements

Read and familiarize yourself with the procedure; complete the minimum practice requirements. Document each MPR using proper charting technique. Complete each procedure within a reasonable amount of time, with a minimum of 85% accuracy.

Name: ___________________________

Date: ___________________________

POINT VALUE
✦ = 3–6 points
✶ = 7–9 points

		PRACTICE TRIAL	GRADED TRIAL # 1	GRADED TRIAL # 2	NOTES
1. ✦	Perform proper hand hygiene and assemble materials.				
2. ✦	Check the level of distilled water in the autoclave reservoir and fill as necessary to the fill line.				
3. ✶	Load the autoclave, paying close attention to the following: • Trays and packs should be loaded on their sides. • Containers should be loaded on their sides with lids off or ajar. • Mixed loads are loaded with hard objects on bottom racks and softer items on top racks. • Large packs are to be placed 2 to 4 inches apart; small packets 1 to 2 inches apart.				
4. ✶	Read the manufacturer's instructions and follow them exactly. (Most autoclaves follow similar protocols.)				
5. ✦	With the door open, turn the control knob to "Fill" and observe the water reaching the fill line.				
6. ✦	Turn the knob to the autoclave position (this shuts off the water).				
7. ✦	When pressure reaches 15 to 17 pounds per square inch and temperature reaches 250°F to 270°F, set the timer for the required time according to the manufacture's protocol.				

Name: ______________________________

Date: ______________________________

POINT VALUE
✦ = 3–6 points
✶ = 7–9 points

		PRACTICE TRIAL	GRADED TRIAL # 1	GRADED TRIAL # 2	NOTES
8. ✦	When timing is complete, turn autoclave knob to "Vent."				
9. ✶	When the pressure reaches zero, open the chamber door about 1 inch and allow items to dry completely before removing them. (This takes approximately 30–45 minutes.)				
10. ✦	Remove wrapped items and check the autoclave tape for color change. Store in dry, closed cabinet for use.				
11. ✦	Record date, time, and types of items autoclaved into log and initial.				

Name: ______________________

Date: ______________________

Document: Enter the appropriate information in the chart below.

Grading

Points Earned	______		
Points Possible	______	75	75
Percent Grade (Points Earned/Points Possible)	______		
PASS:	______	❑ YES ❑ NO ❑ N/A	❑ YES ❑ NO ❑ N/A

Instructor Sign-Off

Instructor: ______________________ **Date:** ______________________

Name: ____________________

Date: ____________________

Procedure 34-8:

Chemically Sterilizing Instruments

Objective: Demonstrate chemical sterilization of heat-sensitive instruments to prevent the spread of pathogens.

Supplies: Chemical disinfectant; goggles; utility gloves; sink; glass or stainless steel container with cover; sterile towels; sterile transfer forceps; sterile basin; sanitized instrument

Affective Behaviors: Affective behaviors provide a professional approach to a skill that enhances the patient encounter. These behaviors may also display sensitivity to a patient's rights and enhance communication. Pay close attention to these skills, which will be in ***bold, italicized*** font.

Notes to the Student

Skills Assessment Requirements

Read and familiarize yourself with the procedure; complete the minimum practice requirements. Document each MPR using proper charting technique. Complete each procedure within a reasonable amount of time, with a minimum of 85% accuracy.

Name: ______________________________

Date: ______________________________

POINT VALUE
✦ = 3–6 points
✶ = 7–9 points

		PRACTICE TRIAL	GRADED TRIAL # 1	GRADED TRIAL # 2	NOTES
1. ✦	Sanitize instruments appropriately.				
2. ✶	Select appropriate chemical needed for instruments to be sterilized.				
3. ✶	Follow directions on original germicidal label. If opening for the first time, write the date on the container and follow instructions to prepare the chemical agent. Change chemical agent every 7 to 14 days or as recommended by manufacturer or facility protocol.				
4. ✦	Use enough of the chemical agent to completely submerge instruments in appropriate container.				
5. ✦	Cover tightly. Record date, time, and initials.				
6. ✶	Do not open during the sterilization process.				
7. ✦	When timing is complete, remove the instruments using sterile gloves or sterile transfer forceps. Rinse with sterile water over sterile basin.				
8. ✦	Thoroughly dry instruments with sterile towel and place on sterile field.				
9. ✦	Remove gloves and perform proper hand hygiene.				

Name: ____________________

Date: ____________________

Document: Enter the appropriate information in the chart below.

Grading

Points Earned	_______		
Points Possible	_______	63	63
Percent Grade (Points Earned/Points Possible)	_______		
PASS:	_______	❑ YES ❑ NO ❑ N/A	❑ YES ❑ NO ❑ N/A

Instructor Sign-Off

Instructor: ______________________________ **Date:** ______________

Name: ______________________________

Date: ______________________________

Procedure 35-1:

Measuring Adult Weight and Height

Objective: Obtain height and weight measurements and perform adequate math conversions.

Supplies: Balance scale with bar to measure height; paper towel; pen; patient record

Affective Behaviors: Affective behaviors provide a professional approach to a skill that enhances the patient encounter. These behaviors may also display sensitivity to a patient's rights and enhance communication. Pay close attention to these skills, which will be in ***bold, italicized*** font.

Notes to the Student

____

____

____

____

____

____

Skills Assessment Requirements

Read and familiarize yourself with the procedure; complete the minimum practice requirements. Document each MPR using proper charting technique. Complete each procedure within a reasonable amount of time, with a minimum of 85% accuracy.

Name: ______________________

Date: ______________________

POINT VALUE
✦ = 3–6 points
✶ = 7–9 points

		PRACTICE TRIAL	GRADED TRIAL # 1	GRADED TRIAL # 2	NOTES
1. ✦	Perform proper hand hygiene.				
2. ✶	Identify the patient and ***explain the procedure***.				
3. ✦	***If patient removes shoes, place a paper towel on the scale. Heavy objects such as keys or purses should be set aside.***				
4. ✶	Set all weights to zero. Adjust balance as needed.				
5. ✦	***Assist the patient onto the scale, and ask the patient to stand still.***				
6. ✦	Move the large weight into the groove closest to the weight you estimate for the patient. If the balance bar pointer touches the bottom of the frame, move the large weight back one notch. Move the small weight by tapping it gently until it reaches a point at which the pointer floats in the center of the frame.				
7. ✶	Leave the weight in place.				
8. ✦	***Ask the patient to place his or her back to the scale, stand erect, and look straight ahead.***				
9. ✶	Raise the height bar in a collapsed position, making sure that the tip is over the patient's head.				
10. ✦	Open the bar to the horizontal position and bring it down gently to touch the top of the patient's head. Leave the setting in place.				

Name: ______________________________

Date: ______________________________

POINT VALUE
✦ = 3–6 points
✶ = 7–9 points

		PRACTICE TRIAL	GRADED TRIAL # 1	GRADED TRIAL # 2	NOTES
11. ✦	***Assist the patient in stepping off the scale.***				
12. ✶	Read the weight by adding the number at the large weight to the number behind the small weight to the nearest quarter pound. Record this measurement in the patient's record.				
13. ✶	Read the height as marked behind the movable level of lthe ruled bar. Record the measurement to the nearest quarter inch on the patient's record.				
14. ✶	Return the weights to zero and the height bar to the normal position.				
15. ✦	Discard the paper towel if used.				
16. ✦	Perform proper hand hygiene.				

Name: ______________________________

Date: ______________________________

Document: Enter the appropriate information in the chart below.

Grading

Points Earned	______		
Points Possible	______	117	117
Percent Grade (Points Earned/Points Possible)	______		
PASS:	______	❑ YES ❑ NO ❑ N/A	❑ YES ❑ NO ❑ N/A

Instructor Sign-Off

Instructor: ______________________________ **Date:** ______________

Name: ______________________________

Date: ______________________________

Procedure 35-2:

Measuring Oral Temperature Using an Electronic or Digital Thermometer

Objective: Provide an accurate temperature reading and document it properly.

Supplies: Electronic or digital thermometer (rechargeable); probe cover; waste container; pen; patient record

Affective Behaviors: Affective behaviors provide a professional approach to a skill that enhances the patient encounter. These behaviors may also display sensitivity to a patient's rights and enhance communication. Pay close attention to these skills, which will be in ***bold, italicized*** font.

Notes to the Student

____

____

____

____

____

____

Skills Assessment Requirements

Read and familiarize yourself with the procedure; complete the minimum practice requirements. Document each MPR using proper charting technique. Complete each procedure within a reasonable amount of time, with a minimum of 85% accuracy.

Name: ______________________________

Date: ______________________________

POINT VALUE
✦ = 3–6 points
✶ = 7–9 points

		PRACTICE TRIAL	GRADED TRIAL # 1	GRADED TRIAL # 2	NOTES
1. ✦	Perform proper hand hygiene.				
2. ✦	Assemble equipment.				
3. ✶	***Identify the patient and explain the procedure.***				
4. ✦	Remove the thermometer unit from the base and attach the probe (blue for oral).				
5. ✦	Remove the thermometer probe from the holder.				
6. ✶	Insert the thermometer probe into the disposable tip box to secure the tip.				
7. ✶	Insert into the patient's mouth on either side of the lingual frenulum and ***instruct the patient to close his or her mouth.***				
8. ✶	When temperature signal is seen or heard, remove the thermometer from the patient's mouth and read the result in the LED window.				
9. ✶	Dispose of the thermometer tip in the waste container.				
10. ✦	Return the thermometer probe to the storage place.				
11. ✦	Replace the unit on the rechargeable base.				
12. ✦	Perform proper hand hygiene.				
13. ✶	Document the results.				

Name: ____________________

Date: ____________________

Document: Enter the appropriate information in the chart below.

Grading

Points Earned	_____		
Points Possible	_____	96	96
Percent Grade (Points Earned/Points Possible)	_____		
PASS:	_____	❑ YES ❑ NO ❑ N/A	❑ YES ❑ NO ❑ N/A

Instructor Sign-Off

Instructor: ____________________ **Date:** ____________________

Name: ______________________________

Date: ______________________________

Procedure 35-3:

Measuring Rectal Temperature Using an Electronic Thermometer

Objective: Provide an accurate temperature reading and document it properly.

Supplies: Electronic thermometer; red (rectal) probe; disposable thermometer sheathe; disposable gloves; patient's records; pen/pencil; tissue; watch with second hand; water-soluble lubricant; biohazard waste container

Affective Behaviors: Affective behaviors provide a professional approach to a skill that enhances the patient encounter. These behaviors may also display sensitivity to a patient's rights and enhance communication. Pay close attention to these skills, which will be in ***bold, italicized*** font.

Notes to the Student

____

____

____

____

____

____

Skills Assessment Requirements

Read and familiarize yourself with the procedure; complete the minimum practice requirements. Document each MPR using proper charting technique. Complete each procedure within a reasonable amount of time, with a minimum of 85% accuracy.

Name: ______________________________

Date: ______________________________

POINT VALUE
✦ = 3–6 points
✶ = 7–9 points

		PRACTICE TRIAL	GRADED TRIAL # 1	GRADED TRIAL # 2	NOTES
1. ✦	Perform proper hand hygiene.				
2. ✦	Apply gloves.				
3. ✶	Identify the patient and ***explain the procedure***.				
4. ✦	***Instruct the patient to remove appropriate clothing so that the rectal area can be accessed. Provide privacy for the patient.***				
5. ✦	***Assist the patient onto the examining table and cover the patient with a sheet or drape.***				
6. ✦	***Instruct the patient to lie on his or her left side with top leg bent (Sims' position).***				
7. ✦	Remove the electronic thermometer from the base and place a cover on the probe.				
8. ✦	Place a small amount of lubricant on a tissue. Dip the probe in the lubricant.				
9. ✶	With one hand, raise the upper buttock to expose the anus or anal opening. ***If you are unable to see the anal opening, ask the patient to bear down slightly.***				
10. ✶	With the other hand, gently insert the lubricated end of the thermometer approximately 1½ inches into the anal canal. Do not force the thermometer into the anal canal. Rotating the thermometer may make insertion easier.				
11. ✦	Hold the thermometer in place until the result is signaled.				
12. ✦	Read the thermometer.				

Name: ______________________________

Date: ______________________________

POINT VALUE
✦ = 3–6 points
✶ = 7–9 points

		PRACTICE TRIAL	GRADED TRIAL # 1	GRADED TRIAL # 2	NOTES
13. ✦	Withdraw the thermometer and dispose of the plastic sheath in the biohazard container.				
14. ✦	Wipe the anus from front to back, removing any excess lubricant.				
15. ✦	***Assist the patient from the examination table. Instruct the patient to dress and assist if needed.***				
16. ✦	Remove your gloves and place in a biohazard waste container. Perform proper hand hygiene.				
17. ✶	Reread the thermometer and document the temperature in the patient's record using "R" to indicate a rectal reading.				

Name: ______________________

Date: ______________________

Document: Enter the appropriate information in the chart below.

Grading

Points Earned	______		
Points Possible	______	114	114
Percent Grade (Points Earned/Points Possible)	______		
PASS:	______	❑ YES ❑ NO ❑ N/A	❑ YES ❑ NO ❑ N/A

Instructor Sign-Off

Instructor: ______________________ **Date:** ______________

Name: ______________________________

Date: ______________________________

Procedure 35-4:

Measuring Axillary Temperature

Objective: Provide an accurate temperature reading and document it properly.

Supplies: Electronic thermometer and probe; paper and pen; patient's record; tissue; watch with second hand; biohazard waste container

Affective Behaviors: Affective behaviors provide a professional approach to a skill that enhances the patient encounter. These behaviors may also display sensitivity to a patient's rights and enhance communication. Pay close attention to these skills, which will be in ***bold, italicized*** font.

Notes to the Student

____

____

____

____

____

____

Skills Assessment Requirements

Read and familiarize yourself with the procedure; complete the minimum practice requirements. Document each MPR using proper charting technique. Complete each procedure within a reasonable amount of time, with a minimum of 85% accuracy.

Name: ____________________

Date: ____________________

POINT VALUE
✦ = 3–6 points
✶ = 7–9 points

		PRACTICE TRIAL	GRADED TRIAL # 1	GRADED TRIAL # 2	NOTES
1. ✦	Perform proper hand hygiene.				
2. ✶	Identify the patient and ***explain the procedure***.				
3. ✦	Remove the thermometer from its base and place cover on probe.				
4. ✦	Ask the patient to expose the axilla.				
5. ✦	Using a tissue, pat the axilla dry of perspiration.				
6. ✦	Place the probe with cover into the axillary space.				
7. ✶	Ask the patient to remain still and hold his or her arm tightly against the body while the temperature registers. *Note:* This is when the MA can take pulse and respirations.				
8. ✦	When the thermometer beeps, read the thermometer, then remove and discard the probe in the waste container.				
9. ✦	Return the thermometer to the storage base.				
10. ✶	Reread the thermometer and record the temperature in the patient's record. Document results in the patient's record using "AX" to indicate an axillary temperature.				
11. ✦	Perform proper hand hygiene.				

Name: ______________________________

Date: ______________________________

Document: Enter the appropriate information in the chart below.

Grading

Points Earned	_______		
Points Possible	_______	75	75
Percent Grade (Points Earned/Points Possible)	_______		
PASS:	_______	❑ YES ❑ NO ❑ N/A	❑ YES ❑ NO ❑ N/A

Instructor Sign-Off

Instructor: ______________________________ **Date:** ______________

Name: ______________________________

Date: ______________________________

Procedure 35-5:

Measuring Temperature Using an Aural (Tympanic Membrane) Thermometer

Objective: Provide an accurate temperature reading and document it properly.

Supplies: Tympanic membrane thermometer; disposable protective probe cover; paper and pen; patient record; biohazard waste container

Affective Behaviors: Affective behaviors provide a professional approach to a skill that enhances the patient encounter. These behaviors may also display sensitivity to a patient's rights and enhance communication. Pay close attention to these skills, which will be in ***bold, italicized*** font.

Notes to the Student

____

____

____

____

____

____

Skills Assessment Requirements

Read and familiarize yourself with the procedure; complete the minimum practice requirements. Document each MPR using proper charting technique. Complete each procedure within a reasonable amount of time, with a minimum of 85% accuracy.

Name: ______________________________

Date: ______________________________

POINT VALUE ✦ = 3–6 points ✶ = 7–9 points		PRACTICE TRIAL	GRADED TRIAL # 1	GRADED TRIAL # 2	NOTES
1. ✦	Perform proper hand hygiene.				
2. ✶	***Identify the patient and explain the procedure.*** *Note:* To avoid error, call the patient by name and check against the name on the patient's record.				
3. ✦	Remove the thermometer unit from its base. The display will read "Ready."				
4. ✦	Attach the disposable cover to the earpiece probe.				
5. ✶	With one hand, gently pull upward on thc adult patient's ear or pull back and downward if the patient is a child or infant.				
6. ✦	Gently insert the plastic-covered tip of the probe into the ear canal.				
7. ✦	Press the button that activates the thermometer.				
8. ✦	Observe the temperature reading on the display window.				
9. ✦	Gently withdraw the thermometer.				
10. ✦	Eject the used probe cover into a biohazard waste container.				
11. ✶	Document the results in the patient's record using "T" to indicate tympanic temperature.				
12. ✦	Replace the unit on the rechargeable base.				
13. ✦	Perform proper hand hygiene.				

Name: ___________________________

Date: ___________________________

Document: Enter the appropriate information in the chart below.

Grading

Points Earned	______		
Points Possible	______	87	87
Percent Grade (Points Earned/Points Possible)	______		
PASS:	______	❑ YES ❑ NO ❑ N/A	❑ YES ❑ NO ❑ N/A

Instructor Sign-Off

Instructor: ___________________________ **Date:** ___________________________

Name: ______________________________

Date: ______________________________

Procedure 35-6:

Measuring Temperature Using a Heat-Sensitive Wearable Thermometer

Objective: Accurately measure a dermal temperature with a disposable thermometer.

Supplies: Wearable heat-sensitive thermometer (chemical strip, liquid crystal); paper and pen; patient's record; tissue; watch with second hand; biohazard waste container

Affective Behaviors: Affective behaviors provide a professional approach to a skill that enhances the patient encounter. These behaviors may also display sensitivity to a patient's rights and enhance communication. Pay close attention to these skills, which will be in ***bold, italicized*** font.

Notes to the Student

____

____

____

____

____

____

Skills Assessment Requirements

Read and familiarize yourself with the procedure; complete the minimum practice requirements. Document each MPR using proper charting technique. Complete each procedure within a reasonable amount of time, with a minimum of 85% accuracy.

Name: ______________________________

Date: ______________________________

POINT VALUE
✦ = 3–6 points
✶ = 7–9 points

		PRACTICE TRIAL	GRADED TRIAL # 1	GRADED TRIAL # 2	NOTES
1. ✦	Perform proper hand hygiene.				
2. ✦	Gather equipment and assemble supplies.				
3. ✦	***Identify the patient and explain the procedure.***				
4. ✦	Dry the patient's forehead.				
5. ✦	Place the thermometer strip on the patient's forehead.				
6. ✦	Read the correct temperature by reading color changes.				
7. ✦	Record the temperature in the patient's record.				
8. ✦	Discard strip.				
9. ✦	Perform proper hand hygiene.				

Name: ______________________________

Date: ______________________________

Document: Enter the appropriate information in the chart below.

Grading

Points Earned	________		
Points Possible	________	54	54
Percent Grade (Points Earned/Points Possible)	________		
PASS:	________	❑ YES ❑ NO ❑ N/A	❑ YES ❑ NO ❑ N/A

Instructor Sign-Off

Instructor: ______________________________ **Date:** ____________________

Name: ______________________________

Date: ______________________________

Procedure 35-7:

Measuring Temperature Using a Temporal Artery Thermometer

Objective: Accurately measure body temperature using a temporal thermometer.

Supplies: Temporal artery thermometer; paper and pen; patient record

Affective Behaviors: Affective behaviors provide a professional approach to a skill that enhances the patient encounter. These behaviors may also display sensitivity to a patient's rights and enhance communication. Pay close attention to these skills, which will be in ***bold, italicized*** font.

Notes to the Student

____

____

____

____

____

____

Skills Assessment Requirements

Read and familiarize yourself with the procedure; complete the minimum practice requirements. Document each MPR using proper charting technique. Complete each procedure within a reasonable amount of time, with a minimum of 85% accuracy.

Name: ______________________

Date: ______________________

POINT VALUE
✦ = 3–6 points
✶ = 7–9 points

		PRACTICE TRIAL	GRADED TRIAL # 1	GRADED TRIAL # 2	NOTES
1. ✦	Perform proper hand hygiene.				
2. ✦	Assemble the equipment. Clean the probe.				
3. ✶	Identify the patient and ***explain the procedure***. *Note:* To avoid error, call the patient by name and check against the name on the patient's record.				
4. ✦	***Brush aside the patient's hair.***				
5. ✦	***Place the probe flush on the center of the patient's forehead and depress the red button.***				
6. ✶	***Keep the button depressed and slowly slide the probe on the midline across the forehead to the hairline.***				
7. ✦	***Lift the probe from the forehead and touch it on the neck just behind the earlobe.***				
8. ✦	Release the button and read the temperature.				
9. ✦	Record the results in the patient's record.				
10. ✦	Perform proper hand hygiene.				

Name: ______________________

Date: ______________________

Document: Enter the appropriate information in the chart below.

Grading

Points Earned	_______		
Points Possible	_______	66	66
Percent Grade (Points Earned/Points Possible)	_______		
PASS:	_______	❑ YES ❑ NO ❑ N/A	❑ YES ❑ NO ❑ N/A

Instructor Sign-Off

Instructor: ______________________ **Date:** ______________________

Name: ______________________________

Date: ______________________________

Procedure 35-8:

Measuring Radial Pulse

Objective: Provide an accurate radial pulse reading and document it properly.

Supplies: Paper and pen; patient's record; watch with second hand

Affective Behaviors: Affective behaviors provide a professional approach to a skill that enhances the patient encounter. These behaviors may also display sensitivity to a patient's rights and enhance communication. Pay close attention to these skills, which will be in ***bold, italicized*** font.

Notes to the Student

____

____

____

____

____

____

Skills Assessment Requirements

Read and familiarize yourself with the procedure; complete the minimum practice requirements. Document each MPR using proper charting technique. Complete each procedure within a reasonable amount of time, with a minimum of 85% accuracy.

Name: ______________________

Date: ______________________

POINT VALUE
✦ = 3–6 points
✶ = 7–9 points

		PRACTICE TRIAL	GRADED TRIAL # 1	GRADED TRIAL # 2	NOTES
1. ✦	Perform proper hand hygiene.				
2. ✶	Identify the patient and ***explain the procedure***.				
3. ✦	Ask the patient about any recent physical activity or smoking.				
4. ✦	Ask the patient to sit down and place his or her arm in a comfortable, supported position. *Note:* The hand should be at chest level with the palm down.				
5. ✶	Place your finger tips on the radial artery on the thumb side of the wrist.				
6. ✦	Check the quality of the pulse.				
7. ✦	Start counting pulse beats when the second hand on your watch is at 3, 6, 9, or 12.				
8. ✶	Count the pulse for one full minute.				
9. ✦	Immediately write the number of pulse beats per minute on a piece of paper.				
10. ✦	Perform proper hand hygiene.				
11. ✶	Correctly document the results in the patient's record, describing any abnormalities in pulse rate.				

Name: ______________________________

Date: ______________________________

Document: Enter the appropriate information in the chart below.

Grading

Points Earned	______		
Points Possible	______	78	78
Percent Grade (Points Earned/Points Possible)	______		
PASS:	______	❑ YES ❑ NO ❑ N/A	❑ YES ❑ NO ❑ N/A

Instructor Sign-Off

Instructor: ______________________________ **Date:** ______________

Name: ____________________

Date: ____________________

Procedure 35-9:

Measuring Apical–Radial Pulse (Two Persons)

Objective: Provide an accurate apical–radial pulse reading and document it properly.

Supplies: Stethoscope; alcohol wipe/cotton ball with 70 percent isopropyl alcohol; paper and pencil; patient record; watch with second hand

Affective Behaviors: Affective behaviors provide a professional approach to a skill that enhances the patient encounter. These behaviors may also display sensitivity to a patient's rights and enhance communication. Pay close attention to these skills, which will be in ***bold, italicized*** font.

Notes to the Student

____

____

____

____

____

____

Skills Assessment Requirements

Read and familiarize yourself with the procedure; complete the minimum practice requirements. Document each MPR using proper charting technique. Complete each procedure within a reasonable amount of time, with a minimum of 85% accuracy.

Name: ______________________________

Date: ______________________________

POINT VALUE
✦ = 3–6 points
✶ = 7–9 points

		PRACTICE TRIAL	GRADED TRIAL # 1	GRADED TRIAL # 2	NOTES
1. ✦	Perform proper hand hygiene.				
2. ✶	Prepare stethoscope using alcohol wipes or cotton balls with alcohol on earpieces and diaphragm of scope.				
3. ✦	Identify the patient and ***explain the procedure***.				
4. ✦	***The first person will uncover the left side of the patient's chest and provide a drape if necessary.*** Warm chest piece of the stethoscope, with opening of earpiece tips forward.				
5. ✶	Locate the apex of the heart by palpating the fifth intercostal space (between fifth and sixth ribs) at the midclavicular line. *Note:* This is found just below the nipple.				
6. ✶	The second person locates the radial pulse in the thumb side of the wrist 1 inch below the base of the thumb.				
7. ✦	When the heart beat is heard by the first person, a nod is made to the second person and counting begins. Ideally, the count should begin when the second hand is at 3, 6, 9, or 12. *Note:* Both systole and diastole (or lub/dub) count as one beat.				
8. ✶	Both should begin timing for one full minute.				

Name: ______________________________

Date: ______________________________

POINT VALUE
✦ = 3–6 points
✶ = 7–9 points

		PRACTICE TRIAL	GRADED TRIAL # 1	GRADED TRIAL # 2	NOTES
9. ✦	Remove the stethoscope and earpieces.				
10. ✦	Record the rate and quality of heartbeats. Include both apical and radial rates using the designation "AP." Calculate the deficit by subtracting the radial pulse rate from the apical pulse rate. *Note:* A pulse deficit may indicate that the heart contractions are not strong enough to produce a palpable radial pulse.				
11. ✦	***Assist patient with dressing if necessary.*** ***Assist the patient from the examining table.***				
12. ✦	Disinfect stethoscope and perform proper hand hygiene.				

Name: ______________________________

Date: ______________________________

Document: Enter the appropriate information in the chart below.

Grading

Points Earned	______		
Points Possible	______	84	84
Percent Grade (Points Earned/Points Possible)	______		
PASS:	______	❑ YES ❑ NO ❑ N/A	❑ YES ❑ NO ❑ N/A

Instructor Sign-Off

Instructor: ______________________________ **Date:** ______________

Name: ______________________________

Date: ______________________________

Procedure 35-10:

Measuring Respirations

Objective: Accurately measure respiration and document it properly.

Supplies: Watch with sweep second hand

Affective Behaviors: Affective behaviors provide a professional approach to a skill that enhances the patient encounter. These behaviors may also display sensitivity to a patient's rights and enhance communication. Pay close attention to these skills, which will be in ***bold, italicized*** font.

Notes to the Student

____

____

____

____

____

____

Skills Assessment Requirements

Read and familiarize yourself with the procedure; complete the minimum practice requirements. Document each MPR using proper charting technique. Complete each procedure within a reasonable amount of time, with a minimum of 85% accuracy.

Name: ______________________________

Date: ______________________________

POINT VALUE
✦ = 3–6 points
✶ = 7–9 points

		PRACTICE TRIAL	GRADED TRIAL # 1	GRADED TRIAL # 2	NOTES
1. ✦	Perform proper hand hygiene.				
2. ✶	Identify the patient and ***explain the procedure***.				
3. ✦	Assist the patient into a comfortable position.				
4. ✦	Place your hand on the patient's wrist in position to take the pulse, or place your hand on the patient's chest.				
5. ✶	Count each breathing cycle by observing and/or feeling the rise and fall of the patient's chest or upper abdomen.				
6. ✶	Count for one full minute using a watch with a sweep second hand. If the rate is atypical or unusual in any way, take it for another minute.				
7. ✶	Document the respiratory rate in the patient's record, noting the date, time, and any abnormality in rate, rhythm, and depth. Be sure to include your signature.				

Name: ______________________________

Date: ______________________________

Document: Enter the appropriate information in the chart below.

Grading

Points Earned	______		
Points Possible	______	54	54
Percent Grade (Points Earned/Points Possible)	______		
PASS:	______	❑ YES ❑ NO ❑ N/A	❑ YES ❑ NO ❑ N/A

Instructor Sign-Off

Instructor: ______________________________ **Date:** ______________________________

Name: ______________________________

Date: ______________________________

Procedure 35-11:

Measuring Blood Pressure

Objective: Obtain an accurate systolic and diastolic reading.

Supplies: Sphygmomanometer; stethoscope; 70 percent isopropyl alcohol; alcohol sponges or cotton balls; paper and pen; patient's record

Affective Behaviors: Affective behaviors provide a professional approach to a skill that enhances the patient encounter. These behaviors may also display sensitivity to a patient's rights and enhance communication. Pay close attention to these skills, which will be in ***bold, italicized*** font.

Notes to the Student

____

____

____

____

____

____

Skills Assessment Requirements

Read and familiarize yourself with the procedure; complete the minimum practice requirements. Document each MPR using proper charting technique. Complete each procedure within a reasonable amount of time, with a minimum of 85% accuracy.

Name: ______________________________

Date: ______________________________

POINT VALUE
✦ = 3–6 points
✶ = 7–9 points

		PRACTICE TRIAL	GRADED TRIAL # 1	GRADED TRIAL # 2	NOTES
1. ✦	Perform proper hand hygiene.				
2. ✶	Assemble the equipment. Use a sponge or cotton ball with alcohol to thoroughly cleanse the earpieces, bell, and diaphragm pieces of the stethoscope. Allow the alcohol to dry.				
3. ✦	***Identify the patient and explain the procedure.***				
4. ✦	***Assist the patient into a comfortable position. BP may be taken with the patient in a sitting or lying position. The patient's arm should be at heart level. Ask the patient not to cross his or her legs or talk during the procedure.*** *Note:* If the patient's arm is below heart level, the BP reading will be higher than normal; if the arm is higher than heart level, the BP will be lower than normal.				
5. ✦	Place the sphygmomanometer on a solid surface with the gauge within 3 feet for easy viewing.				
6. ✶	***Uncover the patient's arm by asking the patient to roll back his or her sleeve 5 inches above the elbow. If the sleeve becomes constricting when rolled back, ask the patient to slip his or her arm out of the sleeve.*** *Note:* Never take a BP reading through clothing.				

Name: ____________________

Date: ____________________

POINT VALUE
✦ = 3–6 points
✶ = 7–9 points

		PRACTICE TRIAL	GRADED TRIAL # 1	GRADED TRIAL # 2	NOTES
7. ✦	Have the patient straighten his or her arm with palms up. Apply a proper-size cuff over the brachial artery 1 to 2 inches above the antecubital space (bend in the elbow). Many cuffs are marked with arrows or circles to be placed over the artery. Hold the edge of the cuff in place as you wrap the remainder of the cuff tightly around the arm securing the Velcro closure.				
8. ✦	Palpate with your fingertips to locate the brachial artery in the antecubital space.				
9. ✶	Pump air into the cuff quickly and evenly until the level of mercury is 20 to 30 mmHg above the point at which the radial pulse is no longer palpable. Note the level, rapidly deflate, and wait 60 seconds.				
10. ✦	Place the earpieces in your ears and the diaphragm (or bell) of the stethoscope over the area where you feel the brachial artery pulsing. Hold the diaphragm in place with one hand on the chest piece without placing your thumb over the diaphragm. The stethoscope tubing should hang freely and not touch any object or the patient during the reading.				

Name: ______________________

Date: ______________________

POINT VALUE
✦ = 3–6 points
✶ = 7–9 points

		PRACTICE TRIAL	GRADED TRIAL # 1	GRADED TRIAL # 2	NOTES
11. ✦	Close the thumbscrew on the hand bulb by turning clockwise with your dominant hand. Close the thumbscrew just enough so that no air can leak out. Do not close so tightly that you will have difficulty reopening it with one hand.				
12. ✶	Slowly turn the thumbscrew counterclockwise with your dominant hand. Allow the pressure reading to fall only 2 to 3 mmHg at a time.				
13. ✦	Listen for the point at which the first clear sound is heard. Note where this occurred on the manometer. This is the systolic pressure.				
14. ✶	Slowly continue to allow the cuff to deflate. The sounds will change from loud to murmur and then fade away. Read the mercury column (or spring gauge scale) at the point where the sound is no longer heard. This is the diastolic pressure.				
15. ✦	Quickly open the thumbscrew all the way to release the air and deflate the cuff completely.				
16. ✦	If you are unsure about the BP reading, wait at least a minute or two before taking a second reading. *Note:* Never take more than two readings in one arm.				

Name: ____________________

Date: ____________________

POINT VALUE
✦ = 3–6 points
✶ = 7–9 points

		PRACTICE TRIAL	GRADED TRIAL # 1	GRADED TRIAL # 2	NOTES
17. ✶	Immediately write the BP as a fraction on paper. You may inform the patient of the reading if this is the policy in your office.				
18. ✦	Remove the cuff.				
19. ✦	Clean the earpieces of the stethoscope with an alcohol sponge.				
20. ✦	Perform proper hand hygiene.				
21. ✶	Document results, including the date, time, BP reading, and your name, in the patient's record.				

Name: ______________________

Date: ______________________

Document: Enter the appropriate information in the chart below.

Grading

Points Earned	_______		
Points Possible	_______	141	141
Percent Grade (Points Earned/Points Possible)	_______		
PASS:	_______	❏ YES ❏ NO ❏ N/A	❏ YES ❏ NO ❏ N/A

Instructor Sign-Off

Instructor: ______________________ **Date:** ______________________

Name: ______________________________

Date: ______________________________

Procedure 35-12:

Measuring Systolic Blood Pressure Using the Palpatory Method

Objective: Obtain an accurate systolic reading.

Supplies: Sphygmomanometer; stethoscope; 70 percent isopropyl alcohol; alcohol sponges or cotton balls; paper and pen; patient's record

Affective Behaviors: Affective behaviors provide a professional approach to a skill that enhances the patient encounter. These behaviors may also display sensitivity to a patient's rights and enhance communication. Pay close attention to these skills, which will be in ***bold, italicized*** font.

Notes to the Student

The American Heart Association recommends that approximate systolic BP be determined first by palpating radial pulse, then pumping up the cuff until the pulse is no longer felt. This is standard procedure in many cases.

Skills Assessment Requirements

Read and familiarize yourself with the procedure; complete the minimum practice requirements. Document each MPR using proper charting technique. Complete each procedure within a reasonable amount of time, with a minimum of 85% accuracy.

Name: ______________________________

Date: ______________________________

POINT VALUE ✦ = 3–6 points ✶ = 7–9 points		PRACTICE TRIAL	GRADED TRIAL # 1	GRADED TRIAL # 2	NOTES
1. ✦	Assemble the equipment.				
2. ✦	Perform proper hand hygiene.				
3. ✦	***Have the patient sit in a comfortable position with the hand at heart level.*** Place the correct-size blood pressure cuff on the arm about 1 inch over the inside elbow area.				
4. ✦	Locate the radial pulse on the thumb side of the wrist.				
5. ✶	Inflate the blood pressure cuff until the pulse disappears, being sure to note the reading. Continue to inflate about 30 mmHg above the point at which the radial artery pulse disappeared.				
6. ✶	Slowly deflate the cuff 2 to 3 mmHg per second while keeping the fingers on the pulse. The point at which the pulse is felt is the systolic blood pressure.				
7. ✦	Remove the cuff and perform proper hand hygiene.				
8. ✶	Record the systolic pressure as "palpated systolic pressure."				

Name: ______________________________

Date: ______________________________

Document: Enter the appropriate information in the chart below.

Grading

Points Earned	______		
Points Possible	______	57	57
Percent Grade (Points Earned/Points Possible)	______		
PASS:	______	❑ YES ❑ NO ❑ N/A	❑ YES ❑ NO ❑ N/A

Instructor Sign-Off

Instructor: ______________________________ **Date:** ______________

Name: ______________________________

Date: ______________________________

Procedure 35-13:

Determining the Fat-Fold Measurement in an Adult

Objective: Accurately determine and record body fat measurement.

Supplies: Fat-fold body calipers; patient's record; pen and paper

Affective Behaviors: Affective behaviors provide a professional approach to a skill that enhances the patient encounter. These behaviors may also display sensitivity to a patient's rights and enhance communication. Pay close attention to these skills, which will be in ***bold, italicized*** font.

Notes to the Student

____

____

____

____

____

____

Skills Assessment Requirements

Read and familiarize yourself with the procedure; complete the minimum practice requirements. Document each MPR using proper charting technique. Complete each procedure within a reasonable amount of time, with a minimum of 85% accuracy.

Name: ______________________________

Date: ______________________________

POINT VALUE
✦ = 3–6 points
✶ = 7–9 points

		PRACTICE TRIAL	GRADED TRIAL # 1	GRADED TRIAL # 2	NOTES
1. ✦	Gather equipment and supplies.				
2. ✦	Perform proper hand hygiene.				
3. ✶	Read caliper directions.				
4. ✦	Identify the patient and ***explain the procedure***. *Note:* To avoid error, call the patient by name and check against the name on the patient's record.				
5. ✦	***Grasp the triceps in the upper arm with the thumb and index finger.*** Do not pinch too hard.				
6. ✦	Place the calipers over the fold and measure.				
7. ✶	Record the measurement.				
8. ✦	***Grasp the subscapular region beneath the shoulder blade, obtain the caliper reading, and record it.***				
9. ✦	***At the suprailiac area (located posterior and immediately superior to the fanning of the hip bone), obtain the caliper reading and record it.***				
10. ✶	Determine the total percentage of body fat, using a table provided by the manufacturer or the calipers.				
11. ✦	Perform proper hand hygiene.				
12. ✦	Document the result in the patient's record.				

Name: ______________________________

Date: ______________________________

Document: Enter the appropriate information in the chart below.

Grading

Points Earned	_______		
Points Possible	_______	81	81
Percent Grade (Points Earned/Points Possible)	_______		
PASS:	_______	❏ YES ❏ NO ❏ N/A	❏ YES ❏ NO ❏ N/A

Instructor Sign-Off

Instructor: ______________________________ **Date:** ______________

Name: ______________________________

Date: ______________________________

Procedure 35-14:

Calculating Adult Body Mass Index

Objective: Accurately calculate adult body mass index.

Supplies: Patient's record; pen and paper; scale for height and weight; BMI formula or nomogram, or chart for BMI

Affective Behaviors: Affective behaviors provide a professional approach to a skill that enhances the patient encounter. These behaviors may also display sensitivity to a patient's rights and enhance communication. Pay close attention to these skills, which will be in ***bold, italicized*** font.

Notes to the Student

____

____

____

____

____

____

Skills Assessment Requirements

Read and familiarize yourself with the procedure; complete the minimum practice requirements. Document each MPR using proper charting technique. Complete each procedure within a reasonable amount of time, with a minimum of 85% accuracy.

Name: ______________________

Date: ______________________

POINT VALUE
✦ = 3–6 points
✶ = 7–9 points

		PRACTICE TRIAL	GRADED TRIAL # 1	GRADED TRIAL # 2	NOTES
1. ✦	Perform proper hand hygiene.				
2. ✦	If recent height and weight measurements are not available, follow the steps in Procedure 35-1 for measuring adult height and weight.				
3. ✦	Insert the patient's height and weight into the formula, using pounds and inches or kilograms and meters, according to facility policy.				
4. ✦	Formula for pounds and inches: BMI = Weight in pounds ÷ (Height in inches × Height in inches) × 703				
5. ✶	*Example:* Weight of 175 lbs; Height of 64 inches 175 ÷ (64 × 64) = 0.0427 0.0427 × 703 = 30.0 BMI A BMI between 19 and 25 is considered a healthy weight, 25–30 is considered overweight, and over 30 is considered obese.				
6. ✶	Record the results in the patient's record.				

Name: ______________________

Date: ______________________

Document: Enter the appropriate information in the chart below.

Grading

Points Earned	______		
Points Possible	______	42	42
Percent Grade (Points Earned/Points Possible)	______		
PASS:	______	❑ YES ❑ NO ❑ N/A	❑ YES ❑ NO ❑ N/A

Instructor Sign-Off

Instructor: ______________________ **Date:** ______________________

Name: ______________________________

Date: ______________________________

Procedure 36-1:

Cleaning the Examination Room

Objective: Prepare and clean the examination room.

Supplies: Disinfectant, paper towels, disposable gloves, examination table, pillow, gown

Affective Behaviors: Affective behaviors provide a professional approach to a skill that enhances the patient encounter. These behaviors may also display sensitivity to patient's rights and enhance communication. Pay close attention to these skills, which will be in ***bold, italicized*** font.

Notes to the Student

____

____

____

____

____

____

Skills Assessment Requirements

Read and familiarize yourself with the procedure; complete the minimum practice requirements. Document each MPR using proper charting technique. Complete each procedure within a reasonable amount of time, with a minimum of 85% accuracy.

Name: ______________________

Date: ______________________

POINT VALUE
✦ = 3–6 points
✶ = 7–9 points

		PRACTICE TRIAL	GRADED TRIAL # 1	GRADED TRIAL # 2	NOTES
1. ✦	Perform proper hand hygiene.				
2. ✶	Put on a clean pair of gloves.				
3. ✦	Roll the soiled disposable gown up and dispose of it in the appropriate waste container.				
4. ✦	Roll the soiled examination table paper covering into a ball and dispose of it in the appropriate waste container.				
5. ✦	Remove the soiled pillow case and place it in the appropriate container.				
6. ✦	Remove any other soiled items or equipment from the examination room.				
7. ✶	Clean the examination table and counter surfaces with disinfectant and paper towels.				
8. ✦	Dispose of cleaning materials in the appropriate container.				
9. ✦	Remove soiled gloves and dispose of them in the proper container.				
10. ✦	Perform proper hand hygiene.				
11. ✦	Put a clean paper covering on the examination table.				
12. ✦	Put a new pillow covering on the pillow.				
13. ✶	Be sure that the examination room is clean, clutter-free, and odor-free.				

Name: ______________________________

Date: ______________________________

Document: Enter the appropriate information in the chart below.

Grading

Points Earned	_______		
Points Possible	_______	87	87
Percent Grade (Points Earned/Points Possible)	_______		
PASS:	_______	❑ YES ❑ NO ❑ N/A	❑ YES ❑ NO ❑ N/A

Instructor Sign-Off

Instructor: ______________________________ **Date:** ______________

Name: ______________________________

Date: ______________________________

Procedure 36-2:

Documenting a Chief Complaint During a Patient Interview

Objective: Accurately document the chief complaint during a patient interview using correct charting format and abbreviations.

Supplies: Patient record; narrative or progress note form; black or blue ink pen

Affective Behaviors: Affective behaviors provide a professional approach to a skill that enhances the patient encounter. These behaviors may also display sensitivity to a patient's rights and enhance communication. Pay close attention to these skills, which will be in ***bold, italicized*** font.

Notes to the Student

____

____

____

____

____

____

Skills Assessment Requirements

Read and familiarize yourself with the procedure; complete the minimum practice requirements. Document each MPR using proper charting technique. Complete each procedure within a reasonable amount of time, with a minimum of 85% accuracy.

Name: ______________________

Date: ______________________

POINT VALUE
✦ = 3–6 points
✶ = 7–9 points

		PRACTICE TRIAL	GRADED TRIAL # 1	GRADED TRIAL # 2	NOTES
1. ✦	Gather supplies, including the medical record with problem list or progress notes form.				
2. ✦	Briefly review the patient's medical history before greeting the patient.				
3. ✦	Greet and identify the patient, and escort him or her to the examination room.				
4. ✶	***Ask open-ended questions to gather information about why the patient is being seen today. Maintain eye contact and actively listen to the patient's responses.***				
5. ✦	Gather information about PI by asking questions such as: • What makes the problem better or worse? • When did it start? • Where does it hurt? • Rate the pain on a pain scale of 0 to 10.				
6. ✶	Document the CC and PI on the correct form in the patient's record using the patient's own words when appropriate.				
7. ✦	Thank the patient and state that the doctor will be in shortly.				
8. ✦	***Before leaving the room, make sure the patient is comfortable.***				

Name: ______________________________

Date: ______________________________

Document: Enter the appropriate information in the chart below.

Grading

Points Earned	_______		
Points Possible	_______	54	54
Percent Grade (Points Earned/Points Possible)	_______		
PASS:	_______	❑ YES ❑ NO ❑ N/A	❑ YES ❑ NO ❑ N/A

Instructor Sign-Off

Instructor: ______________________________ **Date:** ____________________

Name: ______________________________

Date: ______________________________

Procedure 36-3:

Interviewing a New Patient to Obtain Medical History Information and Preparing for a Physical Examination

Objective: Obtain pertinent patient information for the medical history to assist the physician in establishing the cause and treatment of the present illness (PI) by interview. Include the chief complaint (CC), past history (PH), social or personal history (SH), and family history (FH).

Supplies: Medical history form; clipboard; pen; scale; equipment for vital signs; urine container; gown and drape

Affective Behaviors: Affective behaviors provide a professional approach to a skill that enhances the patient encounter. These behaviors may also display sensitivity to a patient's rights and enhance communication. Pay close attention to these skills, which will be in ***bold, italicized*** font.

Notes to the Student

____

____

____

____

____

____

Skills Assessment Requirements

Read and familiarize yourself with the procedure; complete the minimum practice requirements. Document each MPR using proper charting technique. Complete each procedure within a reasonable amount of time, with a minimum of 85% accuracy.

Name: ______________________________

Date: ______________________________

POINT VALUE
✦ = 3–6 points
✶ = 7–9 points

		PRACTICE TRIAL	GRADED TRIAL # 1	GRADED TRIAL # 2	NOTES
1. ✶	***Identify the patient, greet the patient warmly, and identify yourself.***				
2. ✦	Explain the procedure.				
3. ✦	Provide a private area to conduct the interview.				
4. ✦	If not already complete, ask the patient to fill out the required demographic information on the registration form. ***Assist the patient in completing the form if necessary.***				
5. ✶	Review the patient data portion; ***ask for any additional information necessary***.				
6. ✦	***Ask why the patient is being seen by the physician today (CC).***				
7. ✶	Record the CC in the patient's own words (as appropriate).				
8. ✦	***Using observations skills, ask the patient other open-ended questions to gather necessary information about the CC. Record this information under PI.***				
9. ✦	Gather other information about PH, FH, and SH; document in patient's record.				
10. ✶	***Ask the patient if he or she has any allergies.*** Document according to facility protocol (red ink/specific area for recording allergy information).				
11. ✦	Document any other relevant observations or information.				
12. ✦	Record all information using correct charting guidelines.				

Name: ______________________________

Date: ______________________________

POINT VALUE
✦ = 3–6 points
✶ = 7–9 points

		PRACTICE TRIAL	GRADED TRIAL # 1	GRADED TRIAL # 2	NOTES
13. ✶	Correct any charting errors, drawing one line through error and adding the date and your initials. Record the correct information.				
14. ✦	If required or appropriate, ask patient to provide urine specimen or to empty his or her bladder.				
15. ✶	Obtain a complete set of vital signs (temperature, pulse, respirations, blood pressure, height, and weight). Immediately document this data in the patient's record.				
16. ✦	***Explain what clothes the patient needs to remove, proper donning of the exam gown, and where the patient should sit and wait.***				
17. ✦	***Explain what procedures will follow;*** tell the patient that the physician will be in shortly.				
18. ✦	Place the patient's record with the history and complaint in the designated place for the physician.				

Name: ______________________________

Date: ______________________________

Document: Enter the appropriate information in the chart below.

Grading

Points Earned	______		
Points Possible	______	126	126
Percent Grade (Points Earned/Points Possible)	______		
PASS:	______	❑ YES ❑ NO ❑ N/A	❑ YES ❑ NO ❑ N/A

Instructor Sign-Off

Instructor: ______________________________ **Date:** ____________________

Name: ______________________

Date: ______________________

Procedure 36-4:

Positioning the Patient in the Supine Position

Objective: Assist the patient into the supine position.

Supplies: Patient gown and drape; examination table

Affective Behaviors: Affective behaviors provide a professional approach to a skill that enhances the patient encounter. These behaviors may also display sensitivity to a patient's rights and enhance communication. Pay close attention to these skills, which will be in ***bold, italicized*** font.

Notes to the Student

____

____

____

____

____

____

Skills Assessment Requirements

Read and familiarize yourself with the procedure; complete the minimum practice requirements. Document each MPR using proper charting technique. Complete each procedure within a reasonable amount of time, with a minimum of 85% accuracy.

Name: ______________________________

Date: ______________________________

POINT VALUE
✦ = 3–6 points
✶ = 7–9 points

		PRACTICE TRIAL	GRADED TRIAL # 1	GRADED TRIAL # 2	NOTES
1. ✶	***Greet and identify the patient. Introduce yourself, and escort him or her to the examination room.***				
2. ✦	Perform proper hand hygiene.				
3. ✦	***Explain the procedure to the patient.*** Provide a gown and ask the patient to completely undress and put on the gown. Assist the patient if necessary. For a breast examination, instruct the patient to tie the gown in the front.				
4. ✦	***Ask the patient to sit on the examination table. Assist the patient onto the table.*** If a separate step stool is used, stabilize it with your feet as the patient steps up to prevent the stool from sliding.				
5. ✦	Pull out the foot extension. Ask the patient to lie back on the table. ***Assist the patient by supporting the patient's back.***				
6. ✦	Place a pillow under the patient's head.				
7. ✦	***Cover the patient with the drape from his or her chest to ankles.***				
8. ✦	After the examination, ***assist the patient to a sitting position***. Allow the patient to remain seated to prevent dizziness.				
9. ✦	Push the foot extension into place while supporting the patient's feet.				

Name: ______________________________

Date: ______________________________

POINT VALUE
✦ = 3–6 points
✶ = 7–9 points

		PRACTICE TRIAL	GRADED TRIAL # 1	GRADED TRIAL # 2	NOTES
10. ✦	When the patient is stable and the examination is complete, ***assist the patient to a standing position and hold the patient's arm while he or she steps down***. Stabilize the step stool with your feet again. Give further instructions as needed. ***Prior to leaving the examination room, ask the patient if he or she has any questions.***				
11. ✦	Clean the examination room.				
12. ✦	Perform proper hand hygiene.				

Name: ______________________

Date: ______________________

Document: Enter the appropriate information in the chart below.

Grading

Points Earned	______		
Points Possible	______	75	75
Percent Grade (Points Earned/Points Possible)	______		
PASS:	______	❑ YES ❑ NO ❑ N/A	❑ YES ❑ NO ❑ N/A

Instructor Sign-Off

Instructor: ______________________ **Date:** ______________________

Name: ______________________________

Date: ______________________________

Procedure 36-5:

Positioning the Patient in the Dorsal Recumbent Position

Objective: Assist the patient into the dorsal recumbent position.

Supplies: Patient gown and drape; examination table

Affective Behaviors: Affective behaviors provide a professional approach to a skill that enhances the patient encounter. These behaviors may also display sensitivity to a patient's rights and enhance communication. Pay close attention to these skills, which will be in ***bold, italicized*** font.

Notes to the Student

____

____

____

____

____

____

Skills Assessment Requirements

Read and familiarize yourself with the procedure; complete the minimum practice requirements. Document each MPR using proper charting technique. Complete each procedure within a reasonable amount of time, with a minimum of 85% accuracy.

Name: ______________________________

Date: ______________________________

POINT VALUE ✦ = 3–6 points ✶ = 7–9 points		PRACTICE TRIAL	GRADED TRIAL # 1	GRADED TRIAL # 2	NOTES
1. ✶	***Greet and identify the patient. Introduce yourself, and escort him or her to the examination room.***				
2. ✦	Perform proper hand hygiene.				
3. ✦	***Explain the procedure to the patient.*** Provide a gown and ask the patient to completely undress and to put on the gown. Assist the patient if necessary.				
4. ✦	Instruct the patient to sit on the end of the examination table. ***Assist the patient onto the table.*** If a separate step stool is used, stabilize it with your feet as the patient steps up to prevent the stool from sliding.				
5. ✦	Pull out the foot extension. Ask the patient to lie back on the table. ***Assist the patient by supporting the patient's back.***				
6. ✦	***Ask the patient to bend his or her knees and place the feet flat on the table.*** Push in the foot extension.				
7. ✦	***Cover the patient with the drape from the patient's chest to ankles.***				
8. ✦	Place a pillow under the patient's head.				
9. ✦	Place the light source and rolling stool in place for the examiner.				
10. ✦	After the examination, ***assist the patient to a sitting position***. Allow the patient to remain seated to prevent dizziness.				

Name: ____________________

Date: ____________________

POINT VALUE
✦ = 3–6 points
✶ = 7–9 points

		PRACTICE TRIAL	GRADED TRIAL # 1	GRADED TRIAL # 2	NOTES
11. ✦	When the patient is stable and the examination is complete, ***assist the patient to a standing position and hold the patient's arm while he or she steps down***. Stabilize the step stool with your feet again. Give further instructions as needed. ***Prior to leaving the examination room, ask the patient if he or she has any questions.***				
12. ✦	Clean the examination room.				
13. ✦	Perform proper hand hygiene.				

Name: ______________________________

Date: ______________________________

Document: Enter the appropriate information in the chart below.

Grading

Points Earned	______		
Points Possible	______	81	81
Percent Grade (Points Earned/Points Possible)	______		
PASS:	______	❑ YES ❑ NO ❑ N/A	❑ YES ❑ NO ❑ N/A

Instructor Sign-Off

Instructor: ______________________________ **Date:** ______________

Name: ______________________________

Date: ______________________________

Procedure 36-6:

Positioning the Patient in the Lithotomy Position

Objective: Assist the patient into the lithotomy position.

Supplies: Patient gown and drape; examination table with stirrups

Affective Behaviors: Affective behaviors provide a professional approach to a skill that enhances the patient encounter. These behaviors may also display sensitivity to a patient's rights and enhance communication. Pay close attention to these skills, which will be in ***bold, italicized*** font.

Notes to the Student

____

____

____

____

____

____

Skills Assessment Requirements

Read and familiarize yourself with the procedure; complete the minimum practice requirements. Document each MPR using proper charting technique. Complete each procedure within a reasonable amount of time, with a minimum of 85% accuracy.

Name: ______________________

Date: ______________________

POINT VALUE
✦ = 3–6 points
✶ = 7–9 points

		PRACTICE TRIAL	GRADED TRIAL # 1	GRADED TRIAL # 2	NOTES
1. ✶	***Greet and identify the patient. Introduce yourself, and escort him or her to the examination room.***				
2. ✦	Perform proper hand hygiene.				
3. ✦	***Explain the procedure to the patient.*** Provide a gown and ask the patient to completely undress and put on the gown. Assist the patient if necessary.				
4. ✦	Instruct the patient to sit on the end of the examination table. ***Assist the patient onto the table.*** If a separate step stool is used, stabilize it with your feet as the patient steps up to prevent the stool from sliding.				
5. ✦	***Cover the patient's legs with a drape.***				
6. ✦	Pull out the foot extension. Ask the patient to lie back on the table. ***Assist the patient by supporting the patient's back.***				
7. ✦	Position the stirrups level with the height of the table, about 1 foot from the side of the table, and lock them in place.				
8. ✦	***Ask the patient to slide down on the table until the buttocks is on the edge of the table end.***				
9. ✦	***Ask the patient to bend his or her knees and place his or her feet in the stirrups.*** Position the drape for privacy with a point between the legs. Push in the foot extension.				
10. ✦	Place the light source and rolling stool in place for the examiner.				

Name: ____________________

Date: ____________________

POINT VALUE
✦ = 3–6 points
∗ = 7–9 points

		PRACTICE TRIAL	GRADED TRIAL # 1	GRADED TRIAL # 2	NOTES
11. ✦	***Place a pillow under the patient's head.***				
12. ✦	When the examination is complete, pull out the foot extension and help the patient remove his or her feet from the stirrups and place them on the foot extension.				
13. ✦	***Ask the patient to slide up on the table, assisting as necessary. Keep the drape in place to ensure privacy.***				
14. ✦	***Assist the patient to a sitting position and push in the foot extension.*** Allow the patient to remain seated to prevent dizziness.				
15. ✦	When the patient is stable and the examination is complete, ***assist the patient to a standing position and hold the patient's arm while he or she steps down***. Stabilize the step stool with your feet again. Give further instructions as needed. ***Prior to leaving the examination room, ask the patient if he or she has any questions.***				
16. ✦	Clean the examination room.				
17. ✦	Perform proper hand hygiene.				

Name: ______________________________

Date: ______________________________

Document: Enter the appropriate information in the chart below.

Grading

Points Earned	______		
Points Possible	______	105	105
Percent Grade (Points Earned/Points Possible)	______		
PASS:	______	❑ YES ❑ NO ❑ N/A	❑ YES ❑ NO ❑ N/A

Instructor Sign-Off

Instructor: ______________________________ **Date:** ______________

Name: ______________________________

Date: ______________________________

Procedure 36-7:

Positioning the Patient in the Fowler's Position

Objective: Assist the patient into the Fowler's position.

Supplies: Patient gown and drape; examination table with stirrups

Affective Behaviors: Affective behaviors provide a professional approach to a skill that enhances the patient encounter. These behaviors may also display sensitivity to a patient's rights and enhance communication. Pay close attention to these skills, which will be in ***bold, italicized*** font.

Notes to the Student

____

____

____

____

____

____

Skills Assessment Requirements

Read and familiarize yourself with the procedure; complete the minimum practice requirements. Document each MPR using proper charting technique. Complete each procedure within a reasonable amount of time, with a minimum of 85% accuracy.

Name: ______________________________

Date: ______________________________

POINT VALUE
✦ = 3–6 points
✶ = 7–9 points

		PRACTICE TRIAL	GRADED TRIAL # 1	GRADED TRIAL # 2	NOTES
1. ✶	***Greet and identify the patient. Introduce yourself, and escort him or her to the examination room.***				
2. ✦	Perform proper hand hygiene.				
3. ✦	***Explain the procedure to the patient.*** Provide a gown and ask the patient to completely undress and put on the gown. Assist the patient if necessary.				
4. ✦	Instruct the patient to sit on the end of the examination table. ***Assist the patient onto the table.*** If a separate step stool is used, stabilize it with your feet as the patient steps up to prevent the stool from sliding.				
5. ✦	***Cover the patient's legs with a drape.***				
6. ✦	***Assist the patient to slide back and lean on the raised end of the table.***				
7. ✦	Pull out the foot extension while supporting the patient's feet.				
8. ✦	Raise the head of the table to a 90-degree angle for Fowler's position and to a 45-degree angle for the Semi-Fowler's position.				
9. ✦	***Place a pillow under the patient's knees to relieve strain on the lower back. Adjust the drape as needed.***				

Name: ______________________________

Date: ______________________________

POINT VALUE
✦ = 3–6 points
✶ = 7–9 points

		PRACTICE TRIAL	GRADED TRIAL # 1	GRADED TRIAL # 2	NOTES
10. ✦	When the examination is complete, push in the foot extension. ***Ask the patient to remain seated at the end of the table to prevent dizziness.*** ***Note: Inform the patient before lowering the table. Ask the patient to lean forward while you support the patient's back and lower the table.***				
11. ✦	When the patient is stable and the examination is complete, ***assist the patient to a standing position and hold the patient's arm while he or she steps down***. Stabilize the step stool with your feet again. Give further instructions as needed. ***Prior to leaving the examination room, ask the patient if he or she has any questions.***				
12. ✦	Clean the examination room.				
13. ✦	Perform proper hand hygiene.				

Name: ______________________________

Date: ______________________________

Document: Enter the appropriate information in the chart below.

Grading

Points Earned	______		
Points Possible	______	87	87
Percent Grade (Points Earned/Points Possible)	______		
PASS:	______	❑ YES ❑ NO ❑ N/A	❑ YES ❑ NO ❑ N/A

Instructor Sign-Off

Instructor: ______________________________ **Date:** ______________

Name: ______________________________

Date: ______________________________

Procedure 36-8:

Positioning the Patient in the Prone Position

Objective: Assist the patient into the Prone position.

Supplies: Patient gown and drape; examination table

Affective Behaviors: Affective behaviors provide a professional approach to a skill that enhances the patient encounter. These behaviors may also display sensitivity to a patient's rights and enhance communication. Pay close attention to these skills, which will be in ***bold, italicized*** font.

Notes to the Student

____

____

____

____

____

____

Skills Assessment Requirements

Read and familiarize yourself with the procedure; complete the minimum practice requirements. Document each MPR using proper charting technique. Complete each procedure within a reasonable amount of time, with a minimum of 85% accuracy.

Name: ______________________

Date: ______________________

POINT VALUE
✦ = 3–6 points
✶ = 7–9 points

		PRACTICE TRIAL	GRADED TRIAL # 1	GRADED TRIAL # 2	NOTES
1. ✶	***Greet and identify the patient. Introduce yourself, and escort him or her to the examination room.***				
2. ✦	Perform proper hand hygiene.				
3. ✦	***Explain the procedure to the patient.*** Provide a gown and ask the patient to undress and put on the gown. ***Assist the patient if necessary.***				
4. ✦	Instruct the patient to sit on the examination table. ***Assist the patient onto the table.*** If a separate step stool is used, stabilize it with your feet as the patient steps up to prevent the stool from sliding.				
5. ✦	Pull out the foot extension. Ask the patient to lie back on the table. ***Assist the patient by supporting the patient's back.***				
6. ✦	***Ask the patient to turn toward you onto his or her side, then onto the abdomen. Position yourself close to the middle of the table to prevent the patient from falling.***				
7. ✦	***Place a pillow under the patient's head and feet as needed for comfort. Cover with a drape from the patient's shoulders to ankles.***				
8. ✦	***Cover the patient with the drape from the patient's chest to ankles.***				

Name: ______________________________

Date: ______________________________

POINT VALUE
✦ = 3–6 points
✶ = 7–9 points

		PRACTICE TRIAL	GRADED TRIAL # 1	GRADED TRIAL # 2	NOTES
9. ✦	When the examination is complete, ask the patient to turn toward you and ***assist the patient to a sitting position***. Allow the patient to remain seated to prevent dizziness.				
10. ✦	Push the foot extension into place while supporting the patient's feet.				
11. ✦	When the patient is stable and the examination is complete, ***assist the patient to a standing position and hold the patient's arm while he or she steps down***. Stabilize the step stool with your feet again. Give further instructions as needed. ***Prior to leaving the examination room, ask the patient if he or she has any questions.***				
12. ✦	Clean the examination room.				
13. ✦	Perform proper hand hygiene.				

Name: ______________________________

Date: ______________________________

Document: Enter the appropriate information in the chart below.

Grading

Points Earned	______		
Points Possible	______	81	81
Percent Grade (Points Earned/Points Possible)	______		
PASS:	______	❏ YES ❏ NO ❏ N/A	❏ YES ❏ NO ❏ N/A

Instructor Sign-Off

Instructor: ______________________________ **Date:** ______________

Name: ______________________________

Date: ______________________________

Procedure 36-9:

Positioning the Patient in the Sims' Position

Objective: Assist the patient into the Sims' position.

Supplies: Patient gown and drape; examination table

Affective Behaviors: Affective behaviors provide a professional approach to a skill that enhances the patient encounter. These behaviors may also display sensitivity to a patient's rights and enhance communication. Pay close attention to these skills, which will be in ***bold, italicized*** font.

Notes to the Student

____

____

____

____

____

____

Skills Assessment Requirements

Read and familiarize yourself with the procedure; complete the minimum practice requirements. Document each MPR using proper charting technique. Complete each procedure within a reasonable amount of time, with a minimum of 85% accuracy.

Name: ____________________

Date: ____________________

POINT VALUE
✦ = 3–6 points
✶ = 7–9 points

		PRACTICE TRIAL	GRADED TRIAL # 1	GRADED TRIAL # 2	NOTES
1. ✶	***Greet and identify the patient. Introduce yourself, and escort him or her to the examination room.***				
2. ✦	Perform proper hand hygiene.				
3. ✦	***Explain the procedure to the patient.*** Provide a gown and ask the patient to undress and put on the gown. ***Assist the patient if necessary.***				
4. ✦	Instruct the patient to sit on the examination table. ***Assist the patient onto the table.*** If a separate step stool is used, stabilize it with your feet as the patient steps up to prevent the stool from sliding.				
5. ✦	Pull out the foot extension. Ask the patient to lie back on the table. ***Assist the patient by supporting the patient's back.***				
6. ✦	***Ask the patient to turn toward you*** onto his or her left side, placing the body weight on the chest with the left knee flexed slightly. Position yourself close to the middle of the table to prevent the patient from falling.				
7. ✦	Ask the patient to flex the right knee to a 90-degree angle. Bend the patient's right arm at the elbow with his or her hand toward the head. Place a pillow under the patient's head for comfort.				
8. ✦	***Cover the patient with the drape from the patient's shoulders to ankles.***				

Name: ______________________________

Date: ______________________________

POINT VALUE
✦ = 3–6 points
✶ = 7–9 points

		PRACTICE TRIAL	GRADED TRIAL # 1	GRADED TRIAL # 2	NOTES
9. ✦	When the examination or procedure is complete, ask the patient to turn toward you and onto his or her back. ***Assist the patient to a sitting position.*** Ask the patient to remain seated to prevent dizziness.				
10. ✦	Push the foot extension into place while supporting the patient's feet.				
11. ✦	When the patient is stable and the examination is complete, ***assist the patient to a standing position and hold the patient's arm while he or she steps down***. Stabilize the step stool with your feet again. Give further instructions as needed. ***Prior to leaving the examination room, ask the patient if he or she has any questions.***				
12. ✦	Clean the examination room.				
13. ✦	Perform proper hand hygiene.				

Name: ____________________

Date: ____________________

Document: Enter the appropriate information in the chart below.

Grading

Points Earned	______		
Points Possible	______	81	81
Percent Grade (Points Earned/Points Possible)	______		
PASS:	______	❏ YES ❏ NO ❏ N/A	❏ YES ❏ NO ❏ N/A

Instructor Sign-Off

Instructor: ____________________ **Date:** ____________________

Name: ______________________________

Date: ______________________________

Procedure 36-10:

Positioning the Patient in the Knee-Chest Position

Objective: Assist the patient into the Knee-Chest position.

Supplies: Patient gown and drape; examination table

Affective Behaviors: Affective behaviors provide a professional approach to a skill that enhances the patient encounter. These behaviors may also display sensitivity to a patient's rights and enhance communication. Pay close attention to these skills, which will be in ***bold, italicized*** font.

Notes to the Student

____

____

____

____

____

____

Skills Assessment Requirements

Read and familiarize yourself with the procedure; complete the minimum practice requirements. Document each MPR using proper charting technique. Complete each procedure within a reasonable amount of time, with a minimum of 85% accuracy.

Name: ______________________________

Date: ______________________________

POINT VALUE
✦ = 3–6 points
✶ = 7–9 points

		PRACTICE TRIAL	GRADED TRIAL # 1	GRADED TRIAL # 2	NOTES
1. ✶	***Greet and identify the patient. Introduce yourself, and escort him or her to the examination room.***				
2. ✦	Perform proper hand hygiene.				
3. ✦	***Explain the procedure to the patient.*** Provide a gown and ask the patient to undress and put on the gown. ***Assist the patient if necessary.***				
4. ✦	Instruct the patient to sit on the examination table. ***Assist the patient onto the table.*** If a separate step stool is used, stabilize it with your feet as the patient steps up to prevent the stool from sliding.				
5. ✦	***Cover the legs with a drape.***				
6. ✦	Pull out the foot extension. Ask the patient to lie back on the table. ***Assist the patient by supporting the patient's back.***				
7. ✦	***Ask the patient*** to turn toward you onto his or her abdomen, providing assistance as needed. Position yourself close to the middle of the table to prevent the patient from falling.				
8. ✦	***Assist the patient*** onto his or her knees, with hips bent and keeping the chest on the table. Buttocks will be raised in the air, arms bent, head turned to the side, and hands next to the head. The patient may rest his or her weight on the elbows if it is more comfortable. Place a pillow under the patient's head for comfort.				

Name: ______________________________

Date: ______________________________

POINT VALUE
✦ = 3–6 points
∗ = 7–9 points

		PRACTICE TRIAL	GRADED TRIAL # 1	GRADED TRIAL # 2	NOTES
9. ✦	***Adjust the drape so the point of the drape is between the patient's legs.***				
10. ✦	When the examination or procedure is complete, help the patient to lie flat on the abdomen. When the patient is ready, ask him or her to turn toward you and onto his or her back. ***Assist the patient to a sitting position.*** Ask the patient to remain seated to prevent dizziness.				
11. ✦	Push the foot extension into place while supporting the patient's feet.				
12. ✦	When the patient is stable and the examination is complete, ***assist the patient to a standing position and hold the patient's arm while he or she steps down***. Stabilize the step stool with your feet again. Give further instructions as needed. ***Prior to leaving the examination room, ask the patient if he or she has any questions.***				
13. ✦	Clean the examination room.				
14. ✦	Perform proper hand hygiene.				

Name: ______________________

Date: ______________________

Document: Enter the appropriate information in the chart below.

Grading

Points Earned	______		
Points Possible	______	87	87
Percent Grade (Points Earned/Points Possible)	______		
PASS:	______	❑ YES ❑ NO ❑ N/A	❑ YES ❑ NO ❑ N/A

Instructor Sign-Off

Instructor: ______________________ **Date:** ______________________

Name: ______________________________

Date: ______________________________

Procedure 36-11:

Assisting with a Complete Physical Examination

Objective: Assist with the physical examination by preparing the room and the necessary equipment, while observing proper sequencing and ensuring patient safety with limited direction.

Supplies: Examination equipment (varies depending on type and purpose of examination and personal preference of the physician); examination table with clean sheet; pillow with clean cover; Snellen chart; urine specimen container; sphygmomanometer; stethoscope; tape measure; thermometer; probe cover; gown and drape; gloves; waste container; pencil or pen

Affective Behaviors: Affective behaviors provide a professional approach to a skill that enhances the patient encounter. These behaviors may also display sensitivity to a patient's rights and enhance communication. Pay close attention to these skills, which will be in ***bold, italicized*** font.

Notes to the Student

____

____

____

____

____

____

Skills Assessment Requirements

Read and familiarize yourself with the procedure; complete the minimum practice requirements. Document each MPR using proper charting technique. Complete each procedure within a reasonable amount of time, with a minimum of 85% accuracy.

Name: ______________________

Date: ______________________

POINT VALUE
✦ = 3–6 points
✶ = 7–9 points

		PRACTICE TRIAL	GRADED TRIAL #1	GRADED TRIAL #2	NOTES
1. ✦	Perform proper hand hygiene.				
2. ✦	Assemble all equipment in the examination room.				
3. ✶	***Identify the patient, escort him or her to the examination room, and explain the procedure.***				
4. ✦	If a urine specimen is needed for testing, provide the patient with a urine specimen container and give instructions at this time. If no specimen is needed, offer the patient an opportunity to use the restroom before the examination begins.				
5. ✶	Take vital signs and measurements. Properly document this data in the patient's record immediately.				
6. ✦	***Provide the patient with a gown and drape, and give instructions on undressing. Allow the patient to undress in privacy.***				
7. ✶	Have the patient sit on the examination table with his or her legs hanging over; ***place a drape sheet over the patient's legs***.				
8. ✦	Tell the physician that the patient is ready.				
9. ✦	Assist the physician as needed.				
10. ✦	Apply gloves when handling soiled equipment that may contain biohazardous materials, such as body secretions (e.g., laryngeal mirror).				

Name: ______________________

Date: ______________________

POINT VALUE
✦ = 3–6 points
✶ = 7–9 points

		PRACTICE TRIAL	GRADED TRIAL # 1	GRADED TRIAL # 2	NOTES
11. ✦	As the physician progresses from one section of the body to the next, ***reposition the drape to expose only the portion of the patient being examined at that time***.				
12. ✦	Use gloves when handling specimens.				
13. ✶	Label all specimens as soon as possible.				
14. ✦	When the examination is complete, ***assist the patient in slowly sitting up***.				
15. ✦	***Assist the patient off the examination table.***				
16. ✦	***Ask the patient if he or she requires help dressing. If no help is needed, allow the patient to dress in privacy.***				
17. ✦	***Instruct the patient where to go after dressing.***				
18. ✦	After the patient leaves the examination room, discard all disposable materials in the appropriate sharps/waste containers.				
19. ✦	Replace supplies in the examination room.				
20. ✶	Clean the examination table, and replace linens and gowns.				
21. ✦	Ensure all documentation of the examination is complete in the patient's record.				

Name: ______________________________

Date: ______________________________

Document: Enter the appropriate information in the chart below.

Grading

Points Earned	______		
Points Possible	______	141	141
Percent Grade (Points Earned/Points Possible)	______		
PASS:	______	❑ YES ❑ NO ❑ N/A	❑ YES ❑ NO ❑ N/A

Instructor Sign-Off

Instructor: ______________________________ **Date:** ______________

Name: ______________________________

Date: ______________________________

Procedure 37-1:

Performing a Scratch Test

Objective: Determine specific substances that cause an allergic reaction in the patient.

Supplies: Allergen extracts; control solution; cotton balls; alcohol; disposable sterile needles and lancets; timer; tape; ruler; cold pack or ice bag; patient's record; disposable gloves; biohazard waste containers, including sharps container

Affective Behaviors: Affective behaviors provide a professional approach to a skill that enhances the patient encounter. These behaviors may also display sensitivity to a patient's rights and enhance communication. Pay close attention to these skills, which will be in ***bold, italicized*** font.

Notes to the Student

____

____

____

____

____

____

Skills Assessment Requirements

Read and familiarize yourself with the procedure; complete the minimum practice requirements. Document each MPR using proper charting technique. Complete each procedure within a reasonable amount of time, with a minimum of 85% accuracy.

Name: ______________________________

Date: ______________________________

POINT VALUE
✦ = 3–6 points
✶ = 7–9 points

		PRACTICE TRIAL	GRADED TRIAL # 1	GRADED TRIAL # 2	NOTES
1. ✦	Assemble all necessary equipment and supplies and perform proper hand hygiene.				
2. ✦	***Identify the patient, introduce yourself, and explain the procedure.***				
3. ✦	***Assist the patient onto the examination table if necessary.***				
4. ✦	Apply gloves, swab the test site (either upper arm or back) with alcohol, and allow it to air dry.				
5. ✦	Label the skin surface with adhesive tape in rows about 1½ to 2 inches apart.				
6. ✶	Place a drop of allergen above or below the correct label. Be consistent.				
7. ✶	Using a separate sterile lancet or needle for each extract, make a small scratch (no more than 1/8 inch deep) on the skin below each drop.				
8. ✦	Set the timer for the specified reaction time. Time is usually 10 to 30 minutes.				
9. ✦	After the specified time period elapses, clean each site with alcohol and cotton ball, taking care not to remove labels.				
10. ✶	Examine and measure each site, and record the results in the patient's record.				
11. ✦	Have the physician check each site.				

Name: ______________________________

Date: ______________________________

POINT VALUE
✦ = 3–6 points
✶ = 7–9 points

		PRACTICE TRIAL	GRADED TRIAL # 1	GRADED TRIAL # 2	NOTES
12. ✶	Apply cold packs or ice bag to relieve itching if necessary.				
13. ✦	Dispose of used material properly.				
14. ✦	***Assist the patient off the examination table, and allow time and privacy for the patient to dress, offering aid as needed.***				
15. ✦	Clean the examination room. Record any further data in the patient's record.				
16. ✦	Perform proper hand hygiene.				

Name: ______________________________

Date: ______________________________

Document: Enter the appropriate information in the chart below.

Grading

Points Earned	______		
Points Possible	______	108	108
Percent Grade (Points Earned/Points Possible)	______		
PASS:	______	❑ YES ❑ NO ❑ N/A	❑ YES ❑ NO ❑ N/A

Instructor Sign-Off

Instructor: ______________________________ **Date:** ______________

Name: ______________________________

Date: ______________________________

Procedure 37-2:

Taking a Wound Culture

Objective: Obtain a sample from a wound by using a swab technique without error.

Supplies: Gloves; culture tube with sterile swab and transport media; tape for dressing; sterile water for cleansing wound; sterile 4 × 4 gauze dressing; hazardous waste container; bag for soiled dressing; prepared label culture tube or pen for labeling tube

Affective Behaviors: Affective behaviors provide a professional approach to a skill that enhances the patient encounter. These behaviors may also display sensitivity to a patient's rights and enhance communication. Pay close attention to these skills, which will be in **bold, italicized** font.

Notes to the Student

____

____

____

____

____

____

Skills Assessment Requirements

Read and familiarize yourself with the procedure; complete the minimum practice requirements. Document each MPR using proper charting technique. Complete each procedure within a reasonable amount of time, with a minimum of 85% accuracy.

Name: ______________________________

Date: ______________________________

POINT VALUE
✦ = 3–6 points
✶ = 7–9 points

		PRACTICE TRIAL	GRADED TRIAL # 1	GRADED TRIAL # 2	NOTES
1. ✦	Perform proper hand hygiene.				
2. ✦	Assemble all necessary equipment and supplies.				
3. ✶	**Identify the patient and explain the procedure.**				
4. ✦	Apply gloves.				
5. ✶	Remove any dressing from the wound, if applicable, noting amount and type of exudates. Place in bag.				
6. ✦	Observe the wound for redness, crusting, swelling, and odor.				
7. ✶	Place a sterile swab in the wound and rotate the swab back and forth. Place the swab in the sterile culture tube. Crush the ampoule of preservative that is in the culture tube and seal the tube. Label the culture tube with the patient's name, the identification number, the source of the specimen, and the date.				
8. ✦	Remove gloves, perform proper hand hygiene, and don sterile gloves.				
9. ✶	Clean the wound using sterile water and 4 × 4 gauze squares.				
10. ✦	Apply sterile dressing over the wound.				

Name: ______________________________

Date: ______________________________

POINT VALUE
✦ = 3–6 points
✶ = 7–9 points

		PRACTICE TRIAL	GRADED TRIAL # 1	GRADED TRIAL # 2	NOTES
11. ✶	***Instruct the patient in wound care.***				
12. ✦	Remove the gloves and dispose of them in a hazardous waste container.				
13. ✶	Document the procedure in the patient's record.				

Name: ______________________________

Date: ______________________________

Document: Enter the appropriate information in the chart below.

Grading

Points Earned	______		
Points Possible	______	96	96
Percent Grade (Points Earned/Points Possible)	______		
PASS:	______	❑ YES ❑ NO ❑ N/A	❑ YES ❑ NO ❑ N/A

Instructor Sign-Off

Instructor: ______________________________ **Date:** ____________________

Name: ______________________________

Date: ______________________________

Procedure 37-3:

Assisting with a Sigmoidoscopy

Objective: Assist the physician during a sigmoidoscopy examination; provide comfort and support for the patient during the exam.

Supplies: Sigmoidoscope with obturator; flexible or inflexible (metal or plastic) anoscope; rectal speculum; insufflator; suction equipment; sterile specimen container with preservative; sterile biopsy forceps; long cotton tip applications; lubricating jelly; basin of warm water; patient drape; gloves; patient gown; examination table pad; tissue; biohazard waste container

Affective Behaviors: Affective behaviors provide a professional approach to a skill that enhances the patient encounter. These behaviors may also display sensitivity to a patient's rights and enhance communication. Pay close attention to these skills, which will be in ***bold, italicized*** font.

Notes to the Student

____

____

____

____

____

____

Skills Assessment Requirements

Read and familiarize yourself with the procedure; complete the minimum practice requirements. Document each MPR using proper charting technique. Complete each procedure within a reasonable amount of time, with a minimum of 85% accuracy.

Name: ______________________________

Date: ______________________________

POINT VALUE
✦ = 3–6 points
✶ = 7–9 points

		PRACTICE TRIAL	GRADED TRIAL # 1	GRADED TRIAL # 2	NOTES
1. ✦	Perform proper hand hygiene.				
2. ✶	Assemble equipment and supplies, check light bulbs on all equipment, and prepare basin of warm water to receive used instruments. Test suction equipment; place obturator within the sigmoidoscope.				
3. ✦	***Identify patient and explain procedure. Verify that the patient has followed the enema and diet instructions. Check to make sure the consent form has been signed.***				
4. ✦	***Ask the patient to undress, put on a gown, and empty the bladder.***				
5. ✦	***Assist patient into the Sims', lateral, or knee-chest position, or onto the proctology table.***				
6. ✦	***Drape patient, and place a towel or disposable examination pad under the perineal area.***				
7. ✦	Apply gloves.				
8. ✦	Place lubricant on the physician's gloved fingers for a digital examination.				
9. ✶	Place metal scope in a basin of warm water to warm it before insertion into patient.				
10. ✦	Lubricate the tip of the scope.				
11. ✦	Attach both the inflation bulb (for air inflation during the procedure) and the light source. Turn on scope immediately before physician use.				

Name: ______________________

Date: ______________________

POINT VALUE
✦ = 3–6 points
✶ = 7–9 points

		PRACTICE TRIAL	GRADED TRIAL # 1	GRADED TRIAL # 2	NOTES
12. ✦	***Remind the patient to take deep breaths and relax abdominal muscles. Observe patient for undue reactions.***				
13. ✦	Assist the physician by handing instruments and equipment, such as suction and cotton-tipped applicators, as they are needed. Place used equipment, including suction tubing, into the basin of water.				
14. ✦	Assist with biopsy by holding open specimen container to receive specimen while maintaining sterility of container.				
15. ✦	Clean around the patient's anal opening with tissue. Discard the tissue in biohazard waste container.				
16. ✦	Remove gloves and perform proper hand hygiene.				
17. ✦	***Assist the patient to slowly sit up.***				
18. ✦	***Ask patient to dress, and provide assistance as needed.***				
19. ✶	Label specimen container with patient's name, address, date, time, source of the specimen, and ID number.				
20. ✶	Apply gloves and clean the equipment. Sterilize and sanitize equipment as needed, and clean the examination room.				
21. ✶	Remove gloves and document the procedure. The physician will document the results of the procedure.				

Name: ______________________________

Date: ______________________________

Document: Enter the appropriate information in the chart below.

Grading

Points Earned	________		
Points Possible	________	141	141
Percent Grade (Points Earned/Points Possible)	________		
PASS:	________	❑ YES ❑ NO ❑ N/A	❑ YES ❑ NO ❑ N/A

Instructor Sign-Off

Instructor: ______________________________ **Date:** ____________________

Name: ______________________________

Date: ______________________________

Procedure 37-4:

Administering a Disposable Enema

Objective: Assist in cleansing fecal material from bowel in preparation for a diagnostic examination.

Supplies: Examination table, disposable enema, lubricant, Mayo tray, towel, gloves, tissues drape, pen, patient's record

Affective Behaviors: Affective behaviors provide a professional approach to a skill that enhances the patient encounter. These behaviors may also display sensitivity to a patient's rights and enhance communication. Pay close attention to these skills, which will be in ***bold, italicized*** font.

Notes to the Student

____

____

____

____

____

____

Skills Assessment Requirements

Read and familiarize yourself with the procedure; complete the minimum practice requirements. Document each MPR using proper charting technique. Complete each procedure within a reasonable amount of time, with a minimum of 85% accuracy.

Name: ______________________________

Date: ______________________________

POINT VALUE
✦ = 3–6 points
✶ = 7–9 points

		PRACTICE TRIAL	GRADED TRIAL # 1	GRADED TRIAL # 2	NOTES
1. ✦	Assemble equipment. Warm the disposable enema container prior to using it to avoid causing abdominal cramping.				
2. ✦	***Identify patient and explain procedure.***				
3. ✦	Perform proper hand hygiene.				
4. ✦	***Instruct the patient to disrobe from the waist down. Assist the patient onto the examination table as needed.***				
5. ✦	***Ask the patient to assume the Sims' position (left side with right knee at 90-degree angle).*** Drape the patient for comfort and privacy.				
6. ✦	Apply gloves.				
7. ✦	Remove the tip from the enema container. Apply a small amount of lubricant.				
8. ✶	Separate the buttocks to expose the anus and gently insert the lubricant tip about 2 inches into the anus, with the tip pointing toward the patient's navel.				
9. ✶	***Instruct the patient to take deep breaths while you slowly empty the contents of the container.***				
10. ✦	***Ask the patient to retain the liquid as long as possible to ensure good results: 5 to 10 minutes should help the enema to work.***				
11. ✦	After withdrawing the tip, gently wipe the anal area with a tissue to remove excess lubricant.				

Name: ______________________________

Date: ______________________________

POINT VALUE
✦ = 3–6 points
✶ = 7–9 points

		PRACTICE TRIAL	GRADED TRIAL # 1	GRADED TRIAL # 2	NOTES
12. ✶	***Provide a bedpan or direct the patient to the rest room, instructing the patient not to flush the toilet until you have checked the results.***				
13. ✦	***Review instructions with the patient, as necessary, for the next test procedure.***				
14. ✦	Clean the room; discard disposable enema equipment in appropriate waste containers.				
15. ✦	Remove gloves and perform proper hand hygiene.				
16. ✶	Document the patient's record.				

Name: ______________________________

Date: ______________________________

Document: Enter the appropriate information in the chart below.

Grading

Points Earned	_______		
Points Possible	_______	108	108
Percent Grade (Points Earned/Points Possible)	_______		
PASS:	_______	❑ YES ❑ NO ❑ N/A	❑ YES ❑ NO ❑ N/A

Instructor Sign-Off

Instructor: ______________________________ **Date:** ______________________________

Name: ______________________________

Date: ______________________________

Procedure 37-5:

Instructing the Patient in Collecting a Stool Specimen

Objective: Instruct patients on how to obtain an adequate stool specimen for laboratory testing.

Supplies: Sterile specimen container with lid (for culture or ova and parasite testing); three occult blood slides with envelope and applicator sticks (for testing for occult blood); lab request form; pen; patient's record; label; printed instructions; tongue depressor; biohazard transport bag; note pad; bedpan or other container for the collection of stool

Affective Behaviors: Affective behaviors provide a professional approach to a skill that enhances the patient encounter. These behaviors may also display sensitivity to a patient's rights and enhance communication. Pay close attention to these skills, which will be in ***bold, italicized*** font.

Notes to the Student

Check the physician's orders for the type of test to be performed prior to collecting the specimen.

____

____

____

____

____

____

Skills Assessment Requirements

Read and familiarize yourself with the procedure; complete the minimum practice requirements. Document each MPR using proper charting technique. Complete each procedure within a reasonable amount of time, with a minimum of 85% accuracy.

Name: ______________________________

Date: ______________________________

POINT VALUE
✦ = 3–6 points
✶ = 7–9 points

		PRACTICE TRIAL	GRADED TRIAL # 1	GRADED TRIAL # 2	NOTES
1. ✦	Assemble needed items next to the patient.				
2. ✦	Label the specimen container or the occult blood slides and fill in the lab request form.				
3. ✦	Identify patient ***and explain the physician orders. Give the patient a copy of the printed instructions and review them together.***				
4. ✶	***Instruct the patient on how to obtain a small amount of stool.*** *Note:* 3–4 tablespoons for culture, ova, and parasites; small amount on the applicator stick for occult blood. For the culture, ova, and parasites, nothing else may be placed in the container (no toilet paper, tissues, urine, or menses), and to maintain sterility, patients are not to touch the inside of the cup or cover. The patient may use a sterile tongue depressor to obtain larger samples of stool from the bedpan or speci-pan. Patient compliance is difficult, and it is up to you to put the patient at ease as much as possible.				
5. ✶	***Instruct the patient to write the date and time of the specimen, place it in a biohazard transport bag, and bring it as soon as possible with the laboratory request form to the laboratory or office.*** Storage and time of delivery directions depend on the test performed and are specified in the testing facility manual.				
6. ✦	***Have the patient or family member repeat instructions to you to verify comprehension.***				
7. ✶	Document that the instructions were given to the patient.				

Name: ______________________________

Date: ______________________________

Document: Enter the appropriate information in the chart below.

Grading

Points Earned	_______		
Points Possible	_______	51	51
Percent Grade (Points Earned/Points Possible)	_______		
PASS:	_______	❏ YES ❏ NO ❏ N/A	❏ YES ❏ NO ❏ N/A

Instructor Sign-Off

Instructor: ______________________________ **Date:** ____________________

Name: ______________________

Date: ______________________

Procedure 37-6:

Testing for Occult Blood

Objective: Test feces for occult blood.

Supplies: 3 occult blood slides, applications, envelope, timer, patient's record, pen, gloves, color developer

Affective Behaviors: Affective behaviors provide a professional approach to a skill that enhances the patient encounter. These behaviors may also display sensitivity to a patient's rights and enhance communication. Pay close attention to these skills, which will be in ***bold, italicized*** font.

Notes to the Student

Note: Many test kits are available on the market. Each one has its own set of directions, color developer, slides, and control monitors. The test kit directions should be followed exactly.

Skills Assessment Requirements

Read and familiarize yourself with the procedure; complete the minimum practice requirements. Document each MPR using proper charting technique. Complete each procedure within a reasonable amount of time, with a minimum of 85% accuracy.

Name: ______________________________

Date: ______________________________

POINT VALUE
✦ = 3–6 points
✶ = 7–9 points

		PRACTICE TRIAL	GRADED TRIAL # 1	GRADED TRIAL # 2	NOTES
1. ✦	Perform proper hand hygiene.				
2. ✦	Apply gloves. Place a paper towel on the area to hold the slides.				
3. ✶	Check the name and date on the occult blood slides.				
4. ✶	Check the expiration date on the color developer.				
5. ✦	Open the window flap on the back of slide and apply 2 drops of the developer to Box A and Box B.				
6. ✶	Interpret the results in 30 to 60 seconds or according to the manufacturer's directions. A positive result will exhibit the color blue around the edge of the specimen; a negative result will not change color. Any amount of blue color is positive.				
7. ✶	For quality control purposes, perform a test on positive and negative controls as required by the manufacturer.				
8. ✦	Test the remaining slides in the same manner.				
9. ✦	Dispose of all materials in a biohazard waste container. Clean the work area.				
10. ✦	Remove gloves.				
11. ✦	Perform proper hand hygiene.				
12. ✶	Document the results in the patient's record.				

Name: ____________________

Date: ____________________

Document: Enter the appropriate information in the chart below.

Grading

Points Earned	_______		
Points Possible	_______	87	87
Percent Grade (Points Earned/Points Possible)	_______		
PASS:	_______	❑ YES ❑ NO ❑ N/A	❑ YES ❑ NO ❑ N/A

Instructor Sign-Off

Instructor: ____________________ **Date:** ____________________

Name: ______________________________

Date: ______________________________

Procedure 37-7:

Performing a Pupil Check on a Patient

Objective: Correctly check patient's pupils for size, dilation, constriction accommodation, and equal reaction to light.

Supplies: Pen light; patient's record; pen

Affective Behaviors: Affective behaviors provide a professional approach to a skill that enhances the patient encounter. These behaviors may also display sensitivity to a patient's rights and enhance communication. Pay close attention to these skills, which will be in ***bold, italicized*** font.

Notes to the Student

____

____

____

____

____

____

Skills Assessment Requirements

Read and familiarize yourself with the procedure; complete the minimum practice requirements. Document each MPR using proper charting technique. Complete each procedure within a reasonable amount of time, with a minimum of 85% accuracy.

Name: ______________________________

Date: ______________________________

POINT VALUE
✦ = 3–6 points
✶ = 7–9 points

		PRACTICE TRIAL	GRADED TRIAL # 1	GRADED TRIAL # 2	NOTES
1. ✦	***Identify patient and introduce yourself.***				
2. ✦	***Observe the patient for responsiveness to your introduction.***				
3. ✦	***Explain the procedure. (It may help to partially darken the room.)***				
4. ✦	***Ask the patient to look straight ahead.***				
5. ✶	Using a penlight or flashlight, approach from the side and shine the light on one pupil at a time. Observe for constriction of the pupil.				
6. ✦	Shine the light on the pupil again and observe the other pupil for constriction.				
7. ✦	Hold the eyes open and observe the size of the pupils. They should be equal in size.				
8. ✶	Hold an object, penlight, or pen about 10 cm. (4 in.) from the bridge of the patient's nose. ***Ask the patient to look at the top of the object and then at an object on the wall across the room.*** Observe for pupil response. (Pupil should constrict when looking at close objects and dilate when looking across the room.)				
9. ✦	Move the pen toward the patient's nose. Pupils should converge toward the patient's nose.				

Name: ______________________________

Date: ______________________________

POINT VALUE
✦ = 3–6 points
✶ = 7–9 points

		PRACTICE TRIAL	GRADED TRIAL # 1	GRADED TRIAL # 2	NOTES
10. ✦	Observe the shape of the pupils. They should be equal or similar in shape.				
11. ✦	***Explain to the patient what other tests will be performed.***				
12. ✶	Document in the patient's record either using the abbreviation for Pupils Equal, Round, Reactive to Light and Accommodation (PERRLA), or with the details of whatever result was obtained.				

Name: ______________________________

Date: ______________________________

Document: Enter the appropriate information in the chart below.

Grading

Points Earned	______		
Points Possible	______	81	81
Percent Grade (Points Earned/Points Possible)	______		
PASS:	______	❑ YES ❑ NO ❑ N/A	❑ YES ❑ NO ❑ N/A

Instructor Sign-Off

Instructor: ______________________________ **Date:** ______________________

Name: ______________________________

Date: ______________________________

Procedure 37-8:

Assisting with a Neurologic Examination

Objective: Assist the physician with a neurologic screening examination.

Supplies: Percussion hammer; safety pin; tongue depressor; mayo tray; penlight; cotton ball; tuning fork; neurological wheel; ophthalmoscope; otoscope; hot and cold water; materials with different odors

Affective Behaviors: Affective behaviors provide a professional approach to a skill that enhances the patient encounter. These behaviors may also display sensitivity to a patient's rights and enhance communication. Pay close attention to these skills, which will be in ***bold, italicized*** font.

Notes to the Student

____

____

____

____

____

____

Skills Assessment Requirements

Read and familiarize yourself with the procedure; complete the minimum practice requirements. Document each MPR using proper charting technique. Complete each procedure within a reasonable amount of time, with a minimum of 85% accuracy.

Name: ______________________________

Date: ______________________________

POINT VALUE
✦ = 3–6 points
✶ = 7–9 points

		PRACTICE TRIAL	GRADED TRIAL # 1	GRADED TRIAL # 2	NOTES
1. ✦	Perform proper hand hygiene.				
2. ✦	Assemble equipment on the tray and cover the tray.				
3. ✦	Identify patient and ***explain procedure***.				
4. ✶	***Evaluate the patient's mental status while taking a medical history, paying attention to responses, memory, and coherence of thought, overall mood, and awareness.***				
5. ✦	If ordered, perform a visual acuity test.				
6. ✦	***Assist the patient onto the examination table*** and drape as needed for comfort.				
7. ✦	The physician will test reflexes with the percussion hammer.				
8. ✶	Sensory ability and skin sensations are tested using a safety pin, neurological wheel, and cotton ball, and the patient's recognition of simple objects are tested by touch (key, pen, coin).				
9. ✦	The physician will check the cranial nerves by having the patient touch the finger to the nose, touch the heel to the shin, and mover the heel down the opposite shin.				
10. ✦	Assist the physician as needed during the remainder of the examination by handing equipment.				

Name: ______________________________

Date: ______________________________

POINT VALUE ✦ = 3–6 points ✶ = 7–9 points		PRACTICE TRIAL	GRADED TRIAL # 1	GRADED TRIAL # 2	NOTES
11. ✦	***Assist the patient off the table*** if the physician wants to evaluate gait or to have the patient perform the Romberg test successfully (patient closes eyes and stands with feet together without swaying).				
12. ✦	***Assist the patient off the table and instruct him or her to dress. Assist and provide privacy as needed.***				
13. ✦	Clean the examination room.				
14. ✦	Perform proper hand hygiene.				
15. ✶	Document the patient's record.				

Name: ______________________________

Date: ______________________________

Document: Enter the appropriate information in the chart below.

Grading

Points Earned	_______		
Points Possible	_______	99	99
Percent Grade (Points Earned/Points Possible)	_______		
PASS:	_______	❑ YES ❑ NO ❑ N/A	❑ YES ❑ NO ❑ N/A

Instructor Sign-Off

Instructor: ______________________________ **Date:** ____________________

Name: ________________________________

Date: ________________________________

Procedure 38-1:

Instructing a Patient on Breast Self-Examination

Objective: Instruct a patient on performing a breast self-examination.

Supplies: Breast model, if available; pamphlets; patient record

Affective Behaviors: Affective behaviors provide a professional approach to a skill that enhances the patient encounter. These behaviors may also display sensitivity to a patient's rights and enhance communication. Pay close attention to these skills, which will be in ***bold, italicized*** font.

Notes to the Student

____

____

____

____

____

____

Skills Assessment Requirements

Read and familiarize yourself with the procedure; complete the minimum practice requirements. Document each MPR using proper charting technique. Complete each procedure within a reasonable amount of time, with a minimum of 85% accuracy.

Name: ______________________________

Date: ______________________________

POINT VALUE
✦ = 3–6 points
✶ = 7–9 points

		PRACTICE TRIAL	GRADED TRIAL # 1	GRADED TRIAL # 2	NOTES
1. ✶	Assemble equipment and supplies. Perform proper hand hygiene.				
2. ✶	Identify the patient and explain the importance of breast self-examinations. ***Introduce yourself to the patient if you haven't already done so.***				
3. ✦	In shower: • Raise right arm and use left hand to examine the right breast, then raise left arm and use right hand to examine left breast. • Using the flat portions of the fingertips, check breast and underarm tissue, feeling for any lump or thickening. • Touch every part of the breast when skin is wet.				
4. ✦	Before a mirror: • Inspect the breast for any irregularity in shape while arms are at the side of the body. • Look for swelling, dimpling, or puckering of the skin, as well as lumps or changes in the nipples, such as retracting. • Gently squeeze both nipples and check for discharge. • Raise the arms overhead and look for size, shape, and contour changes in each breast. • With palms resting on hips, flex chest muscles to check for obvious differences in breasts.				

Name: ______________________________

Date: ______________________________

POINT VALUE
✦ = 3–6 points
∗ = 7–9 points

		PRACTICE TRIAL	GRADED TRIAL # 1	GRADED TRIAL # 2	NOTES
5. ✦	While laying down: • To examine the right breast, place a pillow or folded towel behind the right shoulder and place the right hand behind the head. • Examine the right breast with the left hand and the left breast with the right hand. • Using your hand, with fingers flat, gently press the breast tissue using small circular motions, starting at the outermost top of the breast in the 12 o'clock position and spiraling toward the nipple. Cover all breast tissue, feeling for lumps or abnormal changes in breast tissue. • Gently squeeze the nipple of each breast to check for lumps or discharge. • Repeat for the left breast.				
6. ✦	With arm resting on a firm surface, use the same circular motion to examine the underarm area. (This is also breast tissue.) Repeat the procedure for both underarm areas.				

Name: ______________________________

Date: ______________________________

POINT VALUE
✦ = 3–6 points
✶ = 7–9 points

		PRACTICE TRIAL	GRADED TRIAL # 1	GRADED TRIAL # 2	NOTES
7. ✦	Report any abnormalities to the physician. This self-exam is not a substitute for periodic examinations by the physician. ***Recognize that this instruction may be embarrassing for some patients, and remain sensitive to their feelings and needs. Prior to leaving the examination room, ask the patient if she has any questions.***				
8. ✶	Document patient education in the patient's chart, and note any concerns or questions. ***Sign the entry with your name and credentials.***				

Name: ______________________________

Date: ______________________________

Document: Enter the appropriate information in the chart below.

Grading

Points Earned	______		
Points Possible	______	57	57
Percent Grade (Points Earned/Points Possible)	______		
PASS:	______	❑ YES ❑ NO ❑ N/A	❑ YES ❑ NO ❑ N/A

Instructor Sign-Off

Instructor: ______________________________ **Date:** ______________

Name: ______________________________

Date: ______________________________

Procedure 38-2:

Assisting with a Pelvic Examination and Pap Test

Objective: Set up and assist with a gynecologic examination, including collection without error of "dry" or "liquid" prep-method Pap smear.

Supplies: Vaginal speculum; water-soluble lubricant; cotton-tipped applicator; patient drape; Pap smear materials—*Dry-prep*: cervical spatula brush; glass slides; fixative spray or liquid slide holder; identification label; *Liquid-based prep*: plastic cervical spatula, broom, or brush; cytology medium transport vial; identification label; laboratory request form; cleansing tissue; gloves; container for contaminated vaginal speculum; gooseneck lam; biohazard waste container

Affective Behaviors: Affective behaviors provide a professional approach to a skill that enhances the patient encounter. These behaviors may also display sensitivity to a patient's rights and enhance communication. Pay close attention to these skills, which will be in ***bold, italicized*** font.

Notes to the Student

The physician will chart the procedure. ______________________________

Skills Assessment Requirements

Read and familiarize yourself with the procedure; complete the minimum practice requirements. Document each MPR using proper charting technique. Complete each procedure within a reasonable amount of time, with a minimum of 85% accuracy.

Name: ______________________________

Date: ______________________________

POINT VALUE ✦ = 3–6 points ✶ = 7–9 points		PRACTICE TRIAL	GRADED TRIAL # 1	GRADED TRIAL # 2	NOTES
	For "dry prep" collection				
1. ✦	Assemble equipment.				
2. ✦	Perform proper hand hygiene.				
3. ✦	Label the slides and complete the laboratory form.				
4. ✶	Identify the patient and ***explain the procedure***.				
5. ✶	***Direct the patient to the restroom to empty her bladder.***				
6. ✶	***Ask the patient to remover her clothing and put on the gown with the opening in front.***				
7. ✶	***Drape the patient appropriately, and assist her into the supine position for breast and abdominal examination.***				
8. ✶	When the physician is ready to collect the Pap specimen, ***assist and instruct the patient to assume the dorsal lithotomy position with her buttocks at the edge of the table and her feet in the stirrups. Knees should be relaxed and rotated outward. Expose the genitalia by moving the drape away from this area while it still covers the legs.***				
9. ✦	Adjust the gooseneck lamp and place the physician's stool in the proper position at the end of examination table.				

Name: ______________________________

Date: ______________________________

POINT VALUE ✦ = 3–6 points ✶ = 7–9 points		PRACTICE TRIAL	GRADED TRIAL # 1	GRADED TRIAL # 2	NOTES
10. ✶	Assist the physician with the procedure: • Apply gloves. • Hand gloves and equipment to the physician as needed. Place lubricant onto the speculum as the physician holds it. • Hold the microscopic slides as the physician smears the slides. Mark the slides *C* for cervical, *V* for vaginal, and *E* for endocervical. • Spray fixative from about 6 inches away from the slide. • Place the slide into a container with the appropriate label.				
11. ✦	Hold the receptacle as the physician places the contaminated speculum into it. Set the container into the sink for later cleaning.				
12. ✦	Apply lubricant to the physician's gloved fingers in preparation for the manual examination.				
13. ✦	Properly dispose of gloves in a biohazard waste container and perform proper hygiene.				
14. ✶	Assist the patient to sit up by (a) helping her move back on the table, (b) taking her feet out of the stirrups, and (c) helping her to a sitting position.				
15. ✶	Sanitize and sterilize equipment as needed.				
16. ✶	Perform proper hand hygiene.				

Name: ______________________________

Date: ______________________________

POINT VALUE
✦ = 3–6 points
✶ = 7–9 points

		PRACTICE TRIAL	GRADED TRIAL # 1	GRADED TRIAL # 2	NOTES
17. ✶	Prepare the Pap specimen to be sent to the laboratory.				
	For "liquid-based prep" collection				
18. ✶	Proceed through steps 1–9 above.				
19. ✶	Open the vial of liquid transport medium and hold it so the physician can place both the plastic spatula and either the brush or the broom containing the specimen into the vial.				
20. ✶	Rinse the broom vigorously by pushing it to the bottom of the vial 10 times.				
21. ✶	Use the spatula to scrape cells from the brush, and swirl both the spatula and brush in the vial to mix before removing.				
22. ✶	Label the vial and dispose of hazardous waste appropriately.				
23. ✶	Proceed through steps 1–17 above.				

Name: ______________________________

Date: ______________________________

Document: Enter the correct information in the chart below.

Grading

Points Earned	______		
Points Possible	______	186	186
Percent Grade (Points Earned/Points Possible)	______		
PASS:	______	❑ YES ❑ NO ❑ N/A	❑ YES ❑ NO ❑ N/A

Instructor Sign-Off

Instructor: ______________________________ **Date:** ______________

Name: ________________________

Date: ________________________

Procedure 38-3:

Instructing a Male Patient How to Perform a Testicular Self-Examination

Objective: Instruct a patient on performing a testicular self-examination.

Supplies: Instruction sheet; testicular examination model or illustration

Affective Behaviors: Affective behaviors provide a professional approach to a skill that enhances the patient encounter. These behaviors may also display sensitivity to a patient's rights and enhance communication. Pay close attention to these skills, which will be in ***bold, italicized*** font.

Notes to the Student

____

____

____

____

____

____

Skills Assessment Requirements

Read and familiarize yourself with the procedure; complete the minimum practice requirements. Document each MPR using proper charting technique. Complete each procedure within a reasonable amount of time, with a minimum of 85% accuracy.

Name: ____________________

Date: ____________________

POINT VALUE
✦ = 3–6 points
✶ = 7–9 points

		PRACTICE TRIAL	GRADED TRIAL # 1	GRADED TRIAL # 2	NOTES
1. ✶	Identify the patient and ***introduce yourself***.				
2. ✶	***Explain to the patient that he should perform the examination in the shower or right after a warm shower, which causes the scrotal tissue to relax.***				
3. ✶	***Using the testicular model or illustration, explain that he should place his middle and index fingers underneath the scrotum and thumb on top and use a gentle motion to roll the testes between the fingers.*** ***Indicate on the model or illustration the location of the epididymis, the soft tubular cord behind the testis that stores and carries sperm. The patient should know what the epididymis feels like so he does not confuse it with a lump.***				
4. ✶	Explain that the entire procedure should be repeated on the second testicle.				
5. ✶	***Encourage the patient to immediately report to his physician any lumps or thickening found during an examination, since early testicular cancer cases have a high cure rate.***				
6. ✶	Document the instruction in the patient's record.				

Name: ____________________

Date: ____________________

Document: Enter the appropriate information in the chart below.

Grading

Points Earned	_______		
Points Possible	_______	54	54
Percent Grade (Points Earned/Points Possible)	_______		
PASS:	_______	❑ YES ❑ NO ❑ N/A	❑ YES ❑ NO ❑ N/A

Instructor Sign-Off

Instructor: ____________________ **Date:** ____________________

Name: ______________________

Date: ______________________

Procedure 39-1:

Testing Visual Acuity Using a Snellen Eye Chart

Objective: Screen a patient for distance acuity using a Snellen eye chart.

Supplies: Snellen eye chart; eye shield or occluder; pointer; pen; patient document; alcohol and gauze

Affective Behaviors: Affective behaviors provide a professional approach to a skill that enhances the patient encounter. These behaviors may also display sensitivity to a patient's rights and enhance communication. Pay close attention to these skills, which will be in ***bold, italicized*** font.

Notes to the Student

____

____

____

____

____

____

Skills Assessment Requirements

Read and familiarize yourself with the procedure; complete the minimum practice requirements. Document each MPR using proper charting technique. Complete each procedure within a reasonable amount of time, with a minimum of 85% accuracy.

Name: ______________________________

Date: ______________________________

POINT VALUE ✦ = 3–6 points ✶ = 7–9 points		PRACTICE TRIAL	GRADED TRIAL # 1	GRADED TRIAL # 2	NOTES
1. ✦	Assemble equipment.				
2. ✦	Review the physician's order.				
3. ✦	Perform proper hand hygiene and ***identify the patient***.				
4. ✦	***Explain the procedure.***				
5. ✶	***Determine patient's ability to recognize letters.*** *Note:* If the patient is unable to read letters, use an alternate chart to accommodate patient's abilities.				
6. ✦	Use pointer, and point to letters or appropriate symbols in random order.				
7. ✶	Place the patient 20 feet from the chart, either seated or standing, with Snellen chart at eye level.				
8. ✦	Follow office policy regarding testing with or without corrective lenses.				
9. ✦	Have patient read the lines with both eyes first at a distance of 20 feet.				
10. ✦	Follow office policies regarding which eye to test first. Have patient cover the other eye with a cup or occluder. *Note:* The occluder should be positioned in such a way that it does not interfere with the position of the patient's glasses.				

Name: ____________________

Date: ____________________

POINT VALUE
✦ = 3–6 points
✶ = 7–9 points

		PRACTICE TRIAL	GRADED TRIAL # 1	GRADED TRIAL # 2	NOTES
11. ✶	Starting with the 20/70 line, ***ask the patient to identify*** each line and proceed down the chart to the last line the patient can read without error. ***Note: Be sure to check for any squinting or tilting of the head, which would indicate difficulty in identifying letters.***				
12. ✶	Record the ratio numbers adjacent to the line the patient can read without error. If there is an error, note it.				
13. ✶	Repeat the procedure with the other eye and record result. *Note:* Follow office policy for charting abbreviations.				
14. ✦	Clean the occluder with gauze and alcohol.				
15. ✦	Remove and dispose of gloves. Perform proper hand hygiene.				
16. ✶	Document results accurately in the patient's chart.				

Name: ______________________________

Date: ______________________________

Document: Enter the appropriate information in the chart below.

Grading

Points Earned	______		
Points Possible	______	114	114
Percent Grade (Points Earned/Points Possible)	______		
PASS:	______	❑ YES ❑ NO ❑ N/A	❑ YES ❑ NO ❑ N/A

Instructor Sign-Off

Instructor: ______________________________ **Date:** ______________________

Name: ______________________________

Date: ______________________________

Procedure 39-2:

Screening for Near Vision Acuity

Objective: Screen near vision acuity using the Jaeger system.

Supplies: Jaeger card, pen, patient record

Affective Behaviors: Affective behaviors provide a professional approach to a skill that enhances the patient encounter. These behaviors may also display sensitivity to a patient's rights and enhance communication. Pay close attention to these skills, which will be in ***bold, italicized*** font.

Notes to the Student

____

____

____

____

____

____

Skills Assessment Requirements

Read and familiarize yourself with the procedure; complete the minimum practice requirements. Document each MPR using proper charting technique. Complete each procedure within a reasonable amount of time, with a minimum of 85% accuracy.

Name: ______________________________

Date: ______________________________

POINT VALUE
✦ = 3–6 points
✶ = 7–9 points

		PRACTICE TRIAL	GRADED TRIAL # 1	GRADED TRIAL # 2	NOTES
1. ✦	Perform proper hand hygiene.				
2. ✦	Review the physician's order.				
3. ✦	Assemble equipment.				
4. ✦	***Identify patient and introduce yourself.***				
5. ✦	***Explain the procedure.***				
6. ✦	In a well-lit room, have the patient hold the Jaeger card at a distance of 14 to 16 inches.				
7. ✦	***Ask the patient*** to read aloud with both eyes open the smallest paragraph or line possible without error.				
8. ✶	Document the results accurately in the patient's record, noting any unusual symptoms such as squinting.				

Name: ______________________________

Date: ______________________________

Document: Enter the appropriate information in the chart below.

Grading

Points Earned	_______		
Points Possible	_______	51	51
Percent Grade (Points Earned/Points Possible)	_______		
PASS:	_______	❑ YES ❑ NO ❑ N/A	❑ YES ❑ NO ❑ N/A

Instructor Sign-Off

Instructor: ______________________________ **Date:** ____________________

Name: ______________________

Date: ______________________

Procedure 39-3:

Screening for Color Vision Acuity

Objective: Screen a patient for color vision defects.

Supplies: Ishihara screening book/cards, pen, patient record

Affective Behaviors: Affective behaviors provide a professional approach to a skill that enhances the patient encounter. These behaviors may also display sensitivity to a patient's rights and enhance communication. Pay close attention to these skills, which will be in ***bold, italicized*** font.

Notes to the Student

____

____

____

____

____

____

Skills Assessment Requirements

Read and familiarize yourself with the procedure; complete the minimum practice requirements. Document each MPR using proper charting technique. Complete each procedure within a reasonable amount of time, with a minimum of 85% accuracy.

Name: ____________________

Date: ____________________

POINT VALUE
✦ = 3–6 points
✶ = 7–9 points

		PRACTICE TRIAL	GRADED TRIAL # 1	GRADED TRIAL # 2	NOTES
1. ✦	Perform proper hand hygiene.				
2. ✦	Review the physician's order.				
3. ✦	Assemble equipment.				
4. ✦	***Identify the patient and introduce yourself.***				
5. ✦	***Explain the procedure.***				
6. ✦	Have the patient assume a comfortable position and ask the patient to keep both eyes open.				
7. ✶	In a well-lit room at a distance of 30 inches, ***ask the patient to identify*** the number that is formed by the colored dots on each card or page within 3 seconds per page or card.				
8. ✦	***If the patient is unable to identify the numbers, have the patient trace the numbers with his or her finger.***				
9. ✦	Score each plate as it is read. If the patient is able to identify a number, record the number seen after the plate number. If the patient is unable to identify a number on the plate, record the plate number and mark an X next to it.				
10. ✶	Note any unusual symptoms.				
11. ✦	Document the results accurately in the patient's record.				

Name: ______________________

Date: ______________________

Document: Enter the appropriate information in the chart below.

Grading

Points Earned	_______		
Points Possible	_______	72	72
Percent Grade (Points Earned/Points Possible)	_______		
PASS:	_______	❑ YES ❑ NO ❑ N/A	❑ YES ❑ NO ❑ N/A

Instructor Sign-Off

Instructor: ______________________ **Date:** ______________

Name: ______________________________

Date: ______________________________

Procedure 39-4:

Irrigation of the Eye

Objective: Cleanse or irrigate the eye.

Supplies: Gloves, sterile basin, emesis basin, sterile solution, towel, sterile irrigating syringe, sterile gauze, towel, tissues, pen, patient record

Affective Behaviors: Affective behaviors provide a professional approach to a skill that enhances the patient encounter. These behaviors may also display sensitivity to a patient's rights and enhance communication. Pay close attention to these skills, which will be in ***bold, italicized*** font.

Notes to the Student

____

____

____

____

____

____

Skills Assessment Requirements

Read and familiarize yourself with the procedure; complete the minimum practice requirements. Document each MPR using proper charting technique. Complete each procedure within a reasonable amount of time, with a minimum of 85% accuracy.

Name: ____________________

Date: ____________________

POINT VALUE
✦ = 3–6 points
∗ = 7–9 points

		PRACTICE TRIAL	GRADED TRIAL # 1	GRADED TRIAL # 2	NOTES
1. ✦	***Identify the patient and explain the procedure.***				
2. ✦	Review the physician's order.				
3. ✦	Assemble all equipment and supplies.				
4. ∗	Check the name, expiration date, and concentration of the solution. Bring the solution to room temperature. *Note:* Be sure to check medicine 3 times!				
5. ✦	***Place the patient in a comfortable position, either sitting or lying down.***				
6. ✦	***Place a towel over the patient's shoulder.***				
7. ✦	Perform proper hand hygiene.				
8. ✦	Open the irrigating solution and fill the syringe.				
9. ✦	***Ask the patient to tilt his or her head to the affected side, if seated, and hold the basin.***				
10. ✦	***Open the patient's eye using the index finger and thumb of your nondominant hand.***				
11. ✦	Hold a tissue on the patient's cheekbone below the lower lid, and pull down and expose the conjunctiva.				
12. ∗	Hold the syringe one-half-inch from the eye.				
13. ∗	Gently irrigate from inner to outer canthus, or corner of the eye, aiming at the lower conjunctiva.				

Name: ______________________________

Date: ______________________________

POINT VALUE
✦ = 3–6 points
✶ = 7–9 points

		PRACTICE TRIAL	GRADED TRIAL # 1	GRADED TRIAL # 2	NOTES
14. ✦	Continue irrigating until all of the solution is used.				
15. ✦	Dry the area around the eye with sterile gauze.				
16. ✦	Dispose of equipment properly.				
17. ✦	Perform proper hand hygiene.				
18. ✶	Document the information, including the name and expiration date of the irrigation solutions, in the patient's record.				

Name: ______________________

Date: ______________________

Document: Enter the appropriate information in the chart below.

Grading

Points Earned	_______		
Points Possible	_______	120	120
Percent Grade (Points Earned/Points Possible)	_______		
PASS:	_______	❑ YES ❑ NO ❑ N/A	❑ YES ❑ NO ❑ N/A

Instructor Sign-Off

Instructor: ______________________ **Date:** ______________________

Name: ____________________

Date: ____________________

Procedure 39-5:

Instilling Eye Medication

Objective: Instill eye medication as ordered by the physician.

Supplies: Sterile medication; sterile eyedropper; tissues; sterile gauze squares; gloves; drape or towel

Affective Behaviors: Affective behaviors provide a professional approach to a skill that enhances the patient encounter. These behaviors may also display sensitivity to a patient's rights and enhance communication. Pay close attention to these skills, which will be in ***bold, italicized*** font.

Notes to the Student

____

____

____

____

____

____

Skills Assessment Requirements

Read and familiarize yourself with the procedure; complete the minimum practice requirements. Document each MPR using proper charting technique. Complete each procedure within a reasonable amount of time, with a minimum of 85% accuracy.

Name: ______________________

Date: ______________________

POINT VALUE
✦ = 3–6 points
✶ = 7–9 points

		PRACTICE TRIAL	GRADED TRIAL # 1	GRADED TRIAL # 2	NOTES
1. ✦	Perform proper hand hygiene.				
2. ✦	Review the physician's order.				
3. ✦	***Properly identify the patient and explain the procedure.***				
4. ✶	Check the name, expiration date, and concentration of the solution. *Note:* Be sure to check medicine 3 times!				
5. ✦	Ask the patient if he or she has any allergies to the medication.				
6. ✦	***Hand the patient a tissue to blot the cheeks.***				
7. ✦	Put on gloves.				
8. ✦	Position the patient with the head tilted back and looking upward.				
9. ✦	Pull down the lower eyelid, exposing the conjunctiva.				
10. ✶	Place the dropper about one-half-inch above the eyeball with your dominant hand. Insert the proper number of drops in the center of the conjunctiva or, if ointment is used, apply a thin strip from the inner to the outer canthus.				
11. ✶	Do not touch the dropper or ointment tube to eye.				
12. ✦	Ask the patient to gently close eye and rotate the eyeball.				
13. ✶	Remove excess medication from the inner canthus to the outer canthus using sterile gauze.				
14. ✦	***Explain to the patient that his or her vision may be blurry.***				

Name: ______________________________

Date: ______________________________

POINT VALUE
✦ = 3–6 points
✶ = 7–9 points

		PRACTICE TRIAL	GRADED TRIAL # 1	GRADED TRIAL # 2	NOTES
15. ✦	Cleanse the area and dispose of unused medication.				
16. ✦	Remove gloves and perform proper hand hygiene.				
17. ✶	Document procedure in the patient's record.				

Name: ___________________________

Date: ___________________________

Document: Enter the appropriate information in the chart below.

Grading

Points Earned	_______		
Points Possible	_______	117	117
Percent Grade (Points Earned/Points Possible)	_______		
PASS:	_______	❏ YES ❏ NO ❏ N/A	❏ YES ❏ NO ❏ N/A

Instructor Sign-Off

Instructor: ___________________________ **Date:** _______________

Name: ______________________________

Date: ______________________________

Procedure 39-6:

Irrigation of the Ear

Objective: Irrigate ear as ordered by the physician.

Supplies: Gloves, ear syringe, sterile basin, emesis basin, warm irrigation solution, towels, cotton balls

Affective Behaviors: Affective behaviors provide a professional approach to a skill that enhances the patient encounter. These behaviors may also display sensitivity to a patient's rights and enhance communication. Pay close attention to these skills, which will be in ***bold, italicized*** font.

Notes to the Student

____

____

____

____

____

____

Skills Assessment Requirements

Read and familiarize yourself with the procedure; complete the minimum practice requirements. Document each MPR using proper charting technique. Complete each procedure within a reasonable amount of time, with a minimum of 85% accuracy.

Name: ______________________

Date: ______________________

POINT VALUE
✦ = 3–6 points
✶ = 7–9 points

		PRACTICE TRIAL	GRADED TRIAL # 1	GRADED TRIAL # 2	NOTES
1. ✦	Review the physician's order.				
2. ✦	Perform proper hand hygiene.				
3. ✦	Assemble the equipment.				
4. ✶	Check the name, concentration, and expiration date of solution. *Note:* Be sure to check solution 3 times!				
5. ✶	***Properly identify the patient and explain the procedure.***				
6. ✦	Apply gloves.				
7. ✦	Have the patient sit with the affected ear tilted slightly downward.				
8. ✦	Place a towel over the patient's shoulder and ask the patient to hold the emesis basin.				
9. ✦	Clean the external ear canal with a moistened cotton ball, if necessary.				
10. ✶	Pour warmed solution into a sterile basin and fill the syringe with 50 cc of solution.				
11. ✶	For adults, pull the auricle up and out to straighten the ear canal. *Note:* For children younger than age three, pull earlobe down and back to straighten ear canal.				
12. ✦	Expel air from the syringe and insert the tip into the ear canal. Aim the stream of flow toward the roof of the canal.				
13. ✶	Repeat until the return from the ear canal is clear or no cerumen is visible upon otoscope examination.				

Name: ______________________________

Date: ______________________________

POINT VALUE
✦ = 3–6 points
✶ = 7–9 points

		PRACTICE TRIAL	GRADED TRIAL # 1	GRADED TRIAL # 2	NOTES
14. ✦	Remove basin, dry outer ear, and remove towel.				
15. ✦	Give the patient cotton balls to wipe any further external drainage from the ear.				
16. ✦	***Instruct the patient about home care, if needed. Ask patient if he or she has any questions.***				
17. ✦	Dispose of waste material properly and clean all equipment used.				
18. ✦	Perform proper hand hygiene.				
19. ✶	Document the procedure and the patient's reaction. Note any drainage, cerumen impaction, or patient symptoms such as vertigo or pain.				

Name: ______________________________

Date: ______________________________

Document: Enter the appropriate information in the chart below.

Grading

Points Earned	_______		
Points Possible	_______	132	132
Percent Grade (Points Earned/Points Possible)	_______		
PASS:	_______	❑ YES ❑ NO ❑ N/A	❑ YES ❑ NO ❑ N/A

Instructor Sign-Off

Instructor: ______________________________ **Date:** ______________________________

Name: ______________________

Date: ______________________

Procedure 39-7:

Instilling Ear Medication

Objective: Instill ear medication as ordered by physician.

Supplies: Otic drops in dropper bottle, cotton balls, gloves

Affective Behaviors: Affective behaviors provide a professional approach to a skill that enhances the patient encounter. These behaviors may also display sensitivity to a patient's rights and enhance communication. Pay close attention to these skills, which will be in ***bold, italicized*** font.

Notes to the Student

Skills Assessment Requirements

Read and familiarize yourself with the procedure; complete the minimum practice requirements. Document each MPR using proper charting technique. Complete each procedure within a reasonable amount of time, with a minimum of 85% accuracy.

Name: ______________________

Date: ______________________

POINT VALUE
✦ = 3–6 points
✶ = 7–9 points

		PRACTICE TRIAL	GRADED TRIAL # 1	GRADED TRIAL # 2	NOTES
1. ✦	Review the physician's order.				
2. ✦	Perform proper hand hygiene.				
3. ✦	Assemble the equipment.				
4. ✦	***Identify the patient.***				
5. ✶	Check the medication label for the name, concentration, and expiration date. *Note:* Be sure to check the label 3 times!				
6. ✦	If the medication is cold, warm it by rolling the bottle between the palms.				
7. ✶	***Have the patient sit or lie down with the affected ear tilted facing up.***				
8. ✦	Pull the earlobe down and back for a child, and pull the auricle up and out for an adult, to straighten the ear canal.				
9. ✶	Place the dropper in the ear canal; avoid touching the sides of the ear canal.				
10. ✶	Instill the appropriate number of drops along the sides of the ear canal.				
11. ✦	Instruct the patient to remain in the same position for 3–5 minutes.				
12. ✦	***Give instructions for home care if needed. Ask the patient if he or she has any questions.***				

Name: ______________________________

Date: ______________________________

POINT VALUE
✦ = 3–6 points
∗ = 7–9 points

		PRACTICE TRIAL	GRADED TRIAL # 1	GRADED TRIAL # 2	NOTES
13. ✦	Dispose of equipment and clean the area.				
14. ✦	Perform proper hand hygiene.				
15. ∗	Document the procedure, medication information, and patient reaction in the patient's record.				

Name: ______________________

Date: ______________________

Document: Enter the appropriate information in the chart below.

Grading

Points Earned	______		
Points Possible	______	105	105
Percent Grade (Points Earned/Points Possible)	______		
PASS:	______	❑ YES ❑ NO ❑ N/A	❑ YES ❑ NO ❑ N/A

Instructor Sign-Off

Instructor: ______________________ **Date:** ______________________

Name: ______________________________

Date: ______________________________

Procedure 39-8:

Assisting with Audiometry

Objective: Perform audiometric testing without error.

Supplies: Audiometer with headphones; quiet room or small, enclosed cubicle; patient record; pen

Affective Behaviors: Affective behaviors provide a professional approach to a skill that enhances the patient encounter. These behaviors may also display sensitivity to a patient's rights and enhance communication. Pay close attention to these skills, which will be in ***bold, italicized*** font.

Notes to the Student

____

____

____

____

____

____

Skills Assessment Requirements

Read and familiarize yourself with the procedure; complete the minimum practice requirements. Document each MPR using proper charting technique. Complete each procedure within a reasonable amount of time, with a minimum of 85% accuracy.

Name: ______________________________

Date: ______________________________

POINT VALUE
✦ = 3–6 points
✶ = 7–9 points

		PRACTICE TRIAL	GRADED TRIAL # 1	GRADED TRIAL # 2	NOTES
1. ✦	Check physician's orders.				
2. ✦	Perform proper hand hygiene.				
3. ✦	Assemble all equipment and supplies, and prepare the room.				
4. ✶	Test equipment and be sure that power is on.				
5. ✦	***Identify the patient and explain the procedure.***				
6. ✦	Establish the signal response the patient will give if no automatic button is available. (Nodding the head or holding up a hand are common signals.)				
7. ✦	***Have the patient sit in a comfortable position.***				
8. ✦	Place headphones over the patient's ears.				
9. ✶	Begin with low frequency and high decibel levels and watch the patient to record if the machine does not automatically record.				
10. ✶	Gradually increase frequency until the test is completed in the first ear.				
11. ✦	Proceed to the other ear and repeat the testing procedure.				
12. ✦	Remove the headphones.				
13. ✦	Clean the equipment and work area.				
14. ✦	Perform proper hand hygiene.				
15. ✶	Document the procedure in the patient's record.				

Name: ____________________

Date: ____________________

Document: Enter the appropriate information in the chart below.

Grading

Points Earned	______		
Points Possible	______	102	102
Percent Grade (Points Earned/Points Possible)	______		
PASS:	______	❑ YES ❑ NO ❑ N/A	❑ YES ❑ NO ❑ N/A

Instructor Sign-Off

Instructor: ____________________ **Date:** ____________________

Name: ______________________________

Date: ______________________________

Procedure 39-9:

Instilling Nasal Medications

Objective: Instill nasal medication as ordered by the physician.

Supplies: Physician's order, patient record, nasal medication, sterile medicine dropper, tissues, gloves

Affective Behaviors: Affective behaviors provide a professional approach to a skill that enhances the patient encounter. These behaviors may also display sensitivity to a patient's rights and enhance communication. Pay close attention to these skills, which will be in ***bold, italicized*** font.

Notes to the Student

____

____

____

____

____

____

Skills Assessment Requirements

Read and familiarize yourself with the procedure; complete the minimum practice requirements. Document each MPR using proper charting technique. Complete each procedure within a reasonable amount of time, with a minimum of 85% accuracy.

Name: ______________________

Date: ______________________

POINT VALUE
✦ = 3–6 points
✶ = 7–9 points

		PRACTICE TRIAL	GRADED TRIAL # 1	GRADED TRIAL # 2	NOTES
1. ✦	Check physician's orders.				
2. ✦	Perform proper hand hygiene.				
3. ✦	Assemble all equipment and supplies.				
4. ✦	***Identify the patient and explain the procedure.***				
5. ✦	Place patient in supine position with a pillow under the neck. ***Make the patient as comfortable as possible.*** Position the patient with head lower than the shoulders to instill medication into the ethmoid and sphenoid sinuses. To instill medication into the maxillary and frontal sinuses, have the patient assume the same back-lying position, with the head turned toward the side to be treated.				
6. ✶	Check the medication name, dosage and expiration date. *Note:* Be sure to check the medication 3 times!				
7. ✶	Draw the medication into a dropper and hold it over the center of the affected nostril. *Note:* Take care not to touch the dropper to the inside of the nostril.				
8. ✦	Administer the medication. Repeat in the other nostril if ordered.				
9. ✦	Tell the patient to stay in that position for 5 minutes to prevent medication from running out of the nostril.				

Name: ____________________

Date: ____________________

POINT VALUE
✦ = 3–6 points
✶ = 7–9 points

		PRACTICE TRIAL	GRADED TRIAL # 1	GRADED TRIAL # 2	NOTES
10. ✦	***Provide tissues for the patient to use to wipe excess from the skin.***				
11. ✦	Discard the dropper in proper waste container. Recap medication and store appropriately.				
12. ✦	Clean the area and remove gloves.				
13. ✦	***Provide home instruction, if needed. Ask the patient if he or she has any questions.***				
14. ✦	Perform proper hand hygiene.				
15. ✶	Document the procedure in the patient's record.				

Name: ______________________

Date: ______________________

Document: Enter the appropriate information in the chart below.

Grading

Points Earned	______		
Points Possible	______	99	99
Percent Grade (Points Earned/Points Possible)	______		
PASS:	______	❏ YES ❏ NO ❏ N/A	❏ YES ❏ NO ❏ N/A

Instructor Sign-Off

Instructor: ______________________ **Date:** ______________

Name: ______________________________

Date: ______________________________

Procedure 40-1:

Wrapping an Infant or Small Child

Objective: Wrap an infant or small child securely to restrain movement.

Supplies: Small sheet or receiving blanket; examination table; patient record; pen

Affective Behaviors: Affective behaviors provide a professional approach to a skill that enhances the patient encounter. These behaviors may also display sensitivity to a patient's rights and enhance communication. Pay close attention to these skills, which will be in ***bold, italicized*** font.

Notes to the Student

Size of sheet or blanket depends on age and size of child. Be sure to choose the appropriate size.

Skills Assessment Requirements

Read and familiarize yourself with the procedure; complete the minimum practice requirements. Document each MPR using proper charting technique. Complete each procedure within a reasonable amount of time, with a minimum of 85% accuracy.

Name: ______________________________

Date: ______________________________

POINT VALUE
✦ = 3–6 points
✶ = 7–9 points

		PRACTICE TRIAL	GRADED TRIAL # 1	GRADED TRIAL # 2	NOTES
1. ✦	***Introduce yourself to the parent and child.***				
2. ✶	***Speak to the child in soft, soothing tones, and explain to the parent or child what you are going to do.***				
3. ✦	Perform proper hand hygiene.				
4. ✦	***Place the child on the table. Have the parent undress the child or undress, as needed.***				
5. ✦	Place a receiving blanket or small sheet on the table and fold the top corner down. Fold the bottom corner up.				
6. ✶	***Place the child diagonally on the blanket, keeping one hand on the abdomen to ensure safety.***				
7. ✦	Wrap the right corner across the torso, covering the right arm, and tuck snugly under the left arm.				
8. ✦	Wrap the left corner across the torso, covering the left arm, and tuck snugly under the torso.				
9. ✶	To restrain the head, place yourself at the end of the table where the infant's head is located and ***place one hand on either side of the head. Avoid sealing the ears or touching the fontanels.***				
10. ✶	***Speak soothingly to comfort the child and ease fears as much as possible.***				

Name: ______________________________

Date: ______________________________

POINT VALUE
✦ = 3–6 points
✶ = 7–9 points

		PRACTICE TRIAL	GRADED TRIAL # 1	GRADED TRIAL # 2	NOTES
11. ✦	When the procedure is completed, ***pick up and comfort the child for a few moments***. Then proceed to redress or continue with examination as directed.				
12. ✦	Clean the examination room.				
13. ✦	Perform proper hand hygiene.				

Name: ________________________________

Date: ________________________________

Document: Enter the appropriate information in the chart below.

Grading

Points Earned	______		
Points Possible	______	90	90
Percent Grade (Points Earned/Points Possible)	______		
PASS:	______	❑ YES ❑ NO ❑ N/A	❑ YES ❑ NO ❑ N/A

Instructor Sign-Off

Instructor: ________________________________ **Date:** ________________

Name: ______________________________

Date: ______________________________

Procedure 40-2:

Measuring Pediatric Vital Signs

Objective: Perform all steps of the procedures and provide readings with accuracy according to instructor guidelines.

Supplies: Gloves, tympanic thermometer, glass thermometer, electronic thermometer, watch with second hand, pediatric stethoscope, pediatric blood pressure cuff

Affective Behaviors: Affective behaviors provide a professional approach to a skill that enhances the patient encounter. These behaviors may also display sensitivity to a patient's rights and enhance communication. Pay close attention to these skills, which will be in ***bold, italicized*** font.

Notes to the Student

____

____

____

____

____

____

Skills Assessment Requirements

Read and familiarize yourself with the procedure; complete the minimum practice requirements. Document each MPR using proper charting technique. Complete each procedure within a reasonable amount of time, with a minimum of 85% accuracy.

Name: ______________________

Date: ______________________

POINT VALUE
✦ = 3–6 points
✶ = 7–9 points

		PRACTICE TRIAL	GRADED TRIAL # 1	GRADED TRIAL # 2	NOTES
1. ✦	Gather necessary equipment and supplies.				
2. ✦	***Identify the patient, introduce yourself, and explain the procedures to the parent.***				
3. ✶	***Speak reassuringly to the child to win his or her trust.***				
4. ✦	Perform proper hand hygiene.				
5. ✦	***Explain to the parent how he or she can assist you by holding the infant, if necessary.***				
	Obtain temperature using tympanic thermometer				
1. ✦	Remove the thermometer from its base and check that it is ready.				
2. ✦	Attach the disposable probe cover to the earpiece.				
3. ✶	Gently pull down and back on the earlobe to straighten the canal.				
4. ✦	Insert the probe into the ear canal.				
5. ✦	Press the “scan” button.				
6. ✦	Remove the thermometer from the ear and read the temperature reading.				
7. ✦	Eject the probe cover into the appropriate waste container.				
8. ✶	Record the temperature reading. (Remember to use a “T” for tympanic reading.)				
9. ✦	Return the thermometer to its base.				

Name: ____________________

Date: ____________________

POINT VALUE
✦ = 3–6 points
✶ = 7–9 points

		PRACTICE TRIAL	GRADED TRIAL # 1	GRADED TRIAL # 2	NOTES
	Obtain axillary temperature				
1. ✦	Remove the thermometer from its container, rinse it with cool water, and inspect it for defects.				
2. ✦	Shake down the thermometer to 95° F/35° C.				
3. ✦	Place the thermometer in the infant's armpit and hold arm across chest for the required 10 minutes.				
4. ✶	Read the thermometer and record the temperature, using "AX" to indicate the axillary method.				
5. ✦	Clean and disinfect the thermometer when you are finished with the patient.				
	Obtain rectal temperature using a digital thermometer with red probe				
1. ✦	Put on gloves.				
2. ✦	Attach the red disposable tip to the top of the probe.				
3. ✶	***Lubricate the thermometer to provide easy insertion.***				
4. ✦	Place the child on the bed in a supine or prone position.				
5. ✶	Insert the thermometer one-half-inch into the rectum, and hold it in place with your hand to prevent expelling or breakage.				
6. ✶	Hold the child securely to restrict movement.				
7. ✦	Leave the thermometer in for the required time.				
8. ✦	Remove the thermometer, wipe off the lubricant, and take a reading.				

Name: ______________________________

Date: ______________________________

POINT VALUE
✦ = 3–6 points
✶ = 7–9 points

		PRACTICE TRIAL	GRADED TRIAL # 1	GRADED TRIAL # 2	NOTES
9. ✶	Record the reading in the patient record, using "R" to indicate that the rectal method was used.				
	Measure apical pulse/heart rate				
1. ✶	Place the stethoscope on the child's chest at the midpoint between the sternum and the left nipple.				
2. ✦	Listen for the heartbeat.				
3. ✦	Count the apical pulse for 1 full minute.				
4. ✶	Record the apical pulse using the "Ap" before the pulse to indicate an apical pulse reading.				
	Measure infant respirations for one full minute				
1. ✦	Place your hand on the infant's chest, and count the rise and fall of the chest for one respiration.				
2. ✶	Document results in the patient's record.				
	Measure the infant's blood pressure using a pediatric cuff and stethoscope				
1.✦	Wrap the cuff securely around the upper arm.				
2. ✦	Feel for the brachial pulse.				
3. ✦	Place the stethoscope ear-pieces in your ears and place the diaphragm near the pulse point.				
4. ✦	Pump the cuff up until the pulse is no longer heard.				

Name: ______________________________

Date: ______________________________

POINT VALUE
✦ = 3–6 points
✶ = 7–9 points

		PRACTICE TRIAL	GRADED TRIAL # 1	GRADED TRIAL # 2	NOTES
5. ✶	Release the valve slowly while listening for systolic and diastolic sounds.				
6. ✶	Document the results in the patient's record.				

Name: ______________________

Date: ______________________

Document: Enter the appropriate information in the chart below.

Grading

Points Earned	______		
Points Possible	______	279	279
Percent Grade (Points Earned/Points Possible)	______		
PASS:	______	❑ YES ❑ NO ❑ N/A	❑ YES ❑ NO ❑ N/A

Instructor Sign-Off

Instructor: ______________________ **Date:** ______________________

Name: ______________________________

Date: ______________________________

Procedure 40-3:

Measuring the Weight and Height of an Infant

Objective: Obtain the weight and height of an infant.

Supplies: Baby scale; patient record; pen; small towel or protector for scale; tape measure

Affective Behaviors: Affective behaviors provide a professional approach to a skill that enhances the patient encounter. These behaviors may also display sensitivity to a patient's rights and enhance communication. Pay close attention to these skills, which will be in ***bold, italicized*** font.

Notes to the Student

____

____

____

____

____

____

Skills Assessment Requirements

Read and familiarize yourself with the procedure; complete the minimum practice requirements. Document each MPR using proper charting technique. Complete each procedure within a reasonable amount of time, with a minimum of 85% accuracy.

Name: ______________________________

Date: ______________________________

POINT VALUE
✦ = 3–6 points
✶ = 7–9 points

		PRACTICE TRIAL	GRADED TRIAL # 1	GRADED TRIAL # 2	NOTES
	Measure weight				
1. ✶	***Introduce yourself and identify the infant by stating infant's name to the parent. Have the infant remain with the parent or caregiver while you prepare the equipment. Explain the procedure.***				
2. ✦	Place a towel or paper protector on the baby scale.				
3. ✦	Perform proper hand hygiene.				
4. ✶	Balance the scale by placing all weights to the left side and turning the adjustment bolt until the balance bar pointer is in the middle.				
5. ✦	***Undress the infant. Gently lay the infant on the scale. Remember to always keep one hand on the infant until the weights are adjusted. Do not leave the infant unattended at any time.***				
6. ✶	***Keeping one hand over the infant's body as a safety precaution,*** move the large pound weight into the groove closest to the weight estimated for the baby. Then move the smaller ounce weight by tapping it gently until the pointer floats in the center of the frame.				
7. ✶	Keep the weights in place while moving the infant to the examination table for height measurement under the caregiver's care while you record the weight.				

Name: ______________________________

Date: ______________________________

POINT VALUE
✦ = 3–6 points
✶ = 7–9 points

		PRACTICE TRIAL	GRADED TRIAL # 1	GRADED TRIAL # 2	NOTES
	Measure height				
1. ✶	Holding the tape measure with one hand, place the tape at the top of the side of the infant's head. Stretch the infant out full-length as you pull the tape measure down to the bottom of the feet. If you are using a table with a measure bar, place the infant's head on one end of the table with the soles of the feet touching the footboard. *Note:* It is best to have two people measure the length of an infant. The parent can assist by keeping the infant's head still. If the child is active, make pencil marks on the examination table paper at the top of the head and at the heel. Remove child and measure area between the marks.				
2. ✦	Note the height in inches and fractions of an inch, and write the measurement on the exam table paper.				
3. ✶	***Ask the parent to hold the infant while the height and weight are charted in the infant record.***				
4. ✦	Tell the measurements to the parent.				
5. ✦	Discard the scale cover or place it in the laundry bin.				
6. ✦	Perform proper hand hygiene.				

Name: ____________________

Date: ____________________

Document: Enter the appropriate information in the chart below.

Grading

Points Earned	______		
Points Possible	______	96	96
Percent Grade (Points Earned/Points Possible)	______		
PASS:	______	❑ YES ❑ NO ❑ N/A	❑ YES ❑ NO ❑ N/A

Instructor Sign-Off

Instructor: ______________________________ **Date:** ____________________

Name: ___________________________

Date: ___________________________

Procedure 40-4:

Measuring the Head Circumference of an Infant or Small Child

Objective: Obtain an accurate measurement of the head circumference of an infant or small child.

Supplies: Flexible tape measure, growth chart

Affective Behaviors: Affective behaviors provide a professional approach to a skill that enhances the patient encounter. These behaviors may also display sensitivity to a patient's rights and enhance communication. Pay close attention to these skills, which will be in ***bold, italicized*** font.

Notes to the Student

____

____

____

____

____

____

Skills Assessment Requirements

Read and familiarize yourself with the procedure; complete the minimum practice requirements. Document each MPR using proper charting technique. Complete each procedure within a reasonable amount of time, with a minimum of 85% accuracy.

Name: ____________________

Date: ____________________

POINT VALUE
✦ = 3–6 points
✶ = 7–9 points

		PRACTICE TRIAL	GRADED TRIAL # 1	GRADED TRIAL # 2	NOTES
1. ✦	***Identify the patient.***				
2. ✶	***Talk to the infant to gain trust.***				
3. ✦	***Explain the procedure to the patient's parent or caregiver.***				
4. ✦	Perform proper hand hygiene.				
5. ✦	Position the patient on the examination table or have the caregiver hold the infant.				
6. ✶	Hold the end of the tape (0) on the forehead, over the patient's eyebrows.				
7. ✦	Bring the tape around the head and over the ears to meet in the front.				
8. ✦	Take the measurement with accuracy to a fraction of an inch or centimeter.				
9. ✦	Repeat procedure if in any doubt about measurements.				
10. ✦	Perform proper hand hygiene.				
11. ✶	Document results in patient's record and on growth chart.				

Name: ______________________

Date: ______________________

Document: Enter the appropriate information in the chart below.

Grading

Points Earned	_______		
Points Possible	_______	75	75
Percent Grade (Points Earned/Points Possible)	_______		
PASS:	_______	❑ YES ❑ NO ❑ N/A	❑ YES ❑ NO ❑ N/A

Instructor Sign-Off

Instructor: ______________________ **Date:** ______________________

Name: ___________________________

Date: ___________________________

Procedure 40-5:

Measuring the Chest Circumference of a Child

Objective: Accurately measure the circumference of a child's chest.

Supplies: Tape measurer, examination table, patient record, pen

Affective Behaviors: Affective behaviors provide a professional approach to a skill that enhances the patient encounter. These behaviors may also display sensitivity to a patient's rights and enhance communication. Pay close attention to these skills, which will be in ***bold, italicized*** font.

Notes to the Student

____

____

____

____

____

____

Skills Assessment Requirements

Read and familiarize yourself with the procedure; complete the minimum practice requirements. Document each MPR using proper charting technique. Complete each procedure within a reasonable amount of time, with a minimum of 85% accuracy.

Name: ______________________________

Date: ______________________________

POINT VALUE ✦ = 3–6 points ✶ = 7–9 points		PRACTICE TRIAL	GRADED TRIAL # 1	GRADED TRIAL # 2	NOTES
1. ✦	***Introduce yourself, identify the patient, and explain the procedure.***				
2. ✶	***Talk to the patient soothingly to gain trust.***				
3. ✦	Perform proper hand hygiene.				
4. ✦	Position the child on the table in the supine position. *Note:* If the patient is older than age 2, he or she may sit on the table.				
5. ✶	Place the end of the tape (0) in the center of the child's chest in line with the child's nipples. Slip the tape under the child's body and bring it to meet the other end of the tape. Take a measurement in centimeters to the nearest 0.01 or in inches to the nearest one-half-inch.				
6. ✶	***Place the child in the caregiver's care before recording the results.***				
7. ✦	Perform proper hand hygiene.				

Name: ____________________

Date: ____________________

Document: Enter the appropriate information in the chart below.

Grading

Points Earned	______		
Points Possible	______	51	51
Percent Grade (Points Earned/Points Possible)	______		
PASS:	______	❑ YES ❑ NO ❑ N/A	❑ YES ❑ NO ❑ N/A

Instructor Sign-Off

Instructor: ____________________ **Date:** ____________________

Name: ______________________________

Date: ______________________________

Procedure 40-6:

Calculating Growth Percentiles

Objective: Plot the age, weight, and height of a patient, and obtain correct percentiles.

Supplies: Patient's record with weight and height values; pen; growth chart; patient record

Affective Behaviors: Affective behaviors provide a professional approach to a skill that enhances the patient encounter. These behaviors may also display sensitivity to a patient's rights and enhance communication. Pay close attention to these skills, which will be in ***bold, italicized*** font.

Notes to the Student

____

____

____

____

____

____

Skills Assessment Requirements

Read and familiarize yourself with the procedure; complete the minimum practice requirements. Document each MPR using proper charting technique. Complete each procedure within a reasonable amount of time, with a minimum of 85% accuracy.

Name: ____________________

Date: ____________________

POINT VALUE
✦ = 3–6 points
✶ = 7–9 points

		PRACTICE TRIAL	GRADED TRIAL # 1	GRADED TRIAL # 2	NOTES
1. ✦	Select the proper growth chart for the patient.				
2. ✶	Locate the child's age in the horizontal axis at the bottom of the chart. Draw an imaginary vertical line on the chart.				
3. ✶	Locate the proper growth value and draw an imaginary horizontal line on the chart.				
4. ✶	Find the point at which the two imaginary lines intersect on the graph and place a dot there.				
5. ✶	Follow the curved line closest to the dot upward, then read the percentile located on the right side of the chart.				
6. ✶	If the dot you placed falls between two curved lines, estimate the percentile that falls between the two closest percentile lines.				
7. ✶	Record the results in the patient's record.				

Name: ______________________

Date: ______________________

Document: Enter the appropriate information in the chart below.

Grading

Points Earned	_______		
Points Possible	_______	60	60
Percent Grade (Points Earned/Points Possible)	_______		
PASS:	_______	❑ YES ❑ NO ❑ N/A	❑ YES ❑ NO ❑ N/A

Instructor Sign-Off

Instructor: ______________________ **Date:** ______________

Name: ______________________________

Date: ______________________________

Procedure 40-7:

Perform a Snellen Eye Exam on a Child

Objective: Perform a Snellen eye exam for distance visual acuity on a child.

Supplies: Snellen eye chart; occulator; pen and paper; 20-foot distance mark on floor

Affective Behaviors: Affective behaviors provide a professional approach to a skill that enhances the patient encounter. These behaviors may also display sensitivity to a patient's rights and enhance communication. Pay close attention to these skills, which will be in ***bold, italicized*** font.

Notes to the Student

____

____

____

____

____

____

Skills Assessment Requirements

Read and familiarize yourself with the procedure; complete the minimum practice requirements. Document each MPR using proper charting technique. Complete each procedure within a reasonable amount of time, with a minimum of 85% accuracy.

Name: ______________________________

Date: ______________________________

POINT VALUE
✦ = 3–6 points
✶ = 7–9 points

		PRACTICE TRIAL	GRADED TRIAL # 1	GRADED TRIAL # 2	NOTES
1. ✦	Assemble the equipment.				
2. ✦	***Identify the patient and introduce yourself.***				
3. ✶	***Explain the procedure to the patient and parent.***				
4. ✦	Perform proper hand hygiene.				
5. ✶	***Ask the child to indicate which way the legs on the E are pointing to make sure the child understands the directions.***				
6. ✦	If the child understands, position him or her in front of the Snellen E chart at a distance of 20 feet.				
7. ✦	***Make sure the child is comfortable.***				
8. ✦	***Ask the child to hold the occulator over his or her first eye and remind the child to keep both eyes open.***				
9. ✶	***Point to the Es on the chart and make sure the child is pointing his or her fingers in the same direction as the E on the chart. Proceed until you have results from the first eye.***				
10. ✶	Repeat with the other eye.				
11. ✶	Document results in the patient's record using written words. *Note:* Write out the words fully. (Do not use the abbreviations OS, OD, and OU.)				

Name: ______________________________

Date: ______________________________

POINT VALUE
✦ = 3–6 points
✶ = 7–9 points

		PRACTICE TRIAL	GRADED TRIAL # 1	GRADED TRIAL # 2	NOTES
12. ✦	***Compliment the child and parent on how well the child performed.***				
13. ✦	Perform proper hand hygiene.				
14. ✦	Sanitize and replace the equipment.				

Name: ______________________________

Date: ______________________________

Document: Enter the appropriate information in the chart below.

Grading

Points Earned	_____		
Points Possible	_____	99	99
Percent Grade (Points Earned/Points Possible)	_____		
PASS:	_____	❑ YES ❑ NO ❑ N/A	❑ YES ❑ NO ❑ N/A

Instructor Sign-Off

Instructor: ______________________________ **Date:** ______________

Name: ______________________________

Date: ______________________________

Procedure 40-8:

Applying a Pediatric Urine Collection Device

Objective: Properly apply a urinary collection device.

Supplies: Pediatric urine collection bag, laboratory specimen container with label, antiseptic wipes, gloves, biohazard waste container

Affective Behaviors: Affective behaviors provide a professional approach to a skill that enhances the patient encounter. These behaviors may also display sensitivity to a patient's rights and enhance communication. Pay close attention to these skills, which will be in ***bold, italicized*** font.

Notes to the Student

____

____

____

____

____

____

Skills Assessment Requirements

Read and familiarize yourself with the procedure; complete the minimum practice requirements. Document each MPR using proper charting technique. Complete each procedure within a reasonable amount of time, with a minimum of 85% accuracy.

Name: ______________________________

Date: ______________________________

POINT VALUE
✦ = 3–6 points
✶ = 7–9 points

		PRACTICE TRIAL	GRADED TRIAL # 1	GRADED TRIAL # 2	NOTES
1. ✦	Assemble all equipment and supplies.				
2. ✦	***Introduce yourself, identify the patient, and explain the procedure to the parent.***				
3. ✦	Perform proper hand hygiene and put on gloves.				
4. ✦	***Ask the parent to place the child on the examination table in a supine position and remove the diaper.***				
5. ✶	Cleanse the genitalia with antiseptic wipes. *Male:* Cleanse the urinary meatus using a circular motion. Repeat with a clean wipe if the infant is uncircumcised, retracting the foreskin to clean the meatus. When finished cleaning, replace the foreskin to the normal position. *Female:* Hold the labia open with your nondominant hand and cleanse from superior to inferior (front to back). Discard the wipe and repeat with a new wipe.				
6. ✶	Make sure the area is dry. Unfold the collection device and remove the upper portion of the paper, protecting the adhesive surface. Apply the device to the mons pubis and press it securely into place. Continue removing the paper and applying the device to the perineum, securing it and ***making sure that it does not stick to the patient's leg.***				

Name: ______________________

Date: ______________________

POINT VALUE
✦ = 3–6 points
✶ = 7–9 points

		PRACTICE TRIAL	GRADED TRIAL # 1	GRADED TRIAL # 2	NOTES
7. ✦	***Offer water and suggest that the parent try to coax the child to increase fluid intake to help obtain the urine specimen.***				
8. ✦	When sufficient urine sample is collected, remove the bag, ***wipe down the area that the bag was attached to, and rediaper the infant***.				
9. ✶	Pour the sample into a labeled laboratory container and handle it according to the routine practice in your facility.				
10. ✦	Dispose of all equipment in the biohazard waste container.				
11. ✦	Remove gloves and perform proper hand hygiene.				
12. ✶	Record the procedure in the patient's record.				

Name: ______________________________

Date: ______________________________

Document: Enter the appropriate information in the chart below.

Grading

Points Earned	_______		
Points Possible	_______	84	84
Percent Grade (Points Earned/Points Possible)	_______		
PASS:	_______	❑ YES ❑ NO ❑ N/A	❑ YES ❑ NO ❑ N/A

Instructor Sign-Off

Instructor: ______________________________ **Date:** ______________________________

Name: ______________________

Date: ______________________

Procedure 41-1:

Communicating Effectively with the Elderly

Objective: Communicate effectively with a new elderly patient preparing for a physical examination.

Supplies: Pen and paper; patient history form; examination table; gown and drape; other physical examination equipment, as needed

Affective Behaviors: Affective behaviors provide a professional approach to a skill that enhances the patient encounter. These behaviors may also display sensitivity to a patient's rights and enhance communication. Pay close attention to these skills, which will be in ***bold, italicized*** font.

Notes to the Student

____

____

____

____

____

____

Skills Assessment Requirements

Read and familiarize yourself with the procedure; complete the minimum practice requirements. Document each MPR using proper charting technique. Complete each procedure within a reasonable amount of time, with a minimum of 85% accuracy.

Name: ______________________________

Date: ______________________________

POINT VALUE
✦ = 3–6 points
✶ = 7–9 points

		PRACTICE TRIAL	GRADED TRIAL # 1	GRADED TRIAL # 2	NOTES
1. ✦	***Welcome the patient in the front office warmly and with a smile.***				
2. ✦	***Face the patient, and speak clearly and directly to him or her.***				
3. ✶	***Introduce yourself. Be sincere and polite.***				
4. ✦	***Address the patient as "Mr.," "Mrs.," or "Ms." unless otherwise instructed by the patient.***				
5. ✶	***Observe the patient for cues to indicate comprehension of your remarks.***				
6. ✦	***If the patient does not appear to comprehend, paraphrase using other words or simple gestures.***				
7. ✦	***Escort the patient to the exam room. If the patient has a walker or cane, walk closely to them and assist as needed.***				
8. ✦	***Allow sufficient time for the patient to process information.***				
9. ✦	***Observe the patient's overall physical ability to comply with your requests.***				
10. ✦	***Offer assistance as needed. Allow the patient to do as much for him or herself as possible.***				
11. ✦	***Ask the patient to be seated while you being to gather information for the patient history.***				

Name: ______________________________

Date: ______________________________

POINT VALUE
✦ = 3–6 points
✶ = 7–9 points

		PRACTICE TRIAL	GRADED TRIAL # 1	GRADED TRIAL # 2	NOTES
12. ✶	***Speak respectfully, and convey a feeling of warmth and empathy. If the patient's reply to questions becomes too lengthy, gently interrupt and bring the patient back to the subject.***				
13. ✦	***Never assume that the patient is incapable of understanding because of his or her age.***				
14. ✦	***If some answers appear to be inappropriate, do not correct the patient. Gently distract the patient and proceed with the patient history.***				
15. ✦	***Set aside questions that received inappropriate answers, and ask them of the caregiver or family member at a later time.***				
16. ✦	***Do not leave the patient unattended if he or she is confused.***				
17. ✶	***Do not argue with the patient's view of reality! Always use relaxed body language, calm facial expressions, and a caring touch when caring for confused patients.***				
18. ✶	Document all findings in the patient's record.				

Name: ______________________

Date: ______________________

Document: Enter the appropriate information in the chart below.

Grading

Points Earned	______		
Points Possible	______	123	123
Percent Grade (Points Earned/Points Possible)	______		
PASS:	______	❑ YES ❑ NO ❑ N/A	❑ YES ❑ NO ❑ N/A

Instructor Sign-Off

Instructor: ______________________ **Date:** ______________________

Name: ______________________________

Date: ______________________________

Procedure 41-2:

Instructing Stroke Patients According to Their Needs

Objective: Provide patient instruction on the lifestyle changes required after the patient has suffered a stroke.

Supplies: Pen and paper; patient history form

Affective Behaviors: Affective behaviors provide a professional approach to a skill that enhances the patient encounter. These behaviors may also display sensitivity to a patient's rights and enhance communication. Pay close attention to these skills, which will be in ***bold, italicized*** font.

Notes to the Student

Some stroke patients will suffer irreversible loss of function on one side of their body (hemiplegia).

____

____

____

____

____

Skills Assessment Requirements

Read and familiarize yourself with the procedure; complete the minimum practice requirements. Document each MPR using proper charting technique. Complete each procedure within a reasonable amount of time, with a minimum of 85% accuracy.

Name: ______________________________

Date: ______________________________

POINT VALUE
✦ = 3–6 points
✶ = 7–9 points

		PRACTICE TRIAL	GRADED TRIAL # 1	GRADED TRIAL # 2	NOTES
1. ✦	***Welcome the patient in the front office warmly and with a smile.***				
2. ✦	***Face the patient, and speak clearly and directly to him or her.***				
3. ✶	***Introduce yourself. Be sincere and polite.***				
4. ✦	***Address the patient as "Mr.," "Mrs.," or "Ms." unless otherwise instructed by the patient.***				
5. ✶	***If the patient does not appear to comprehend, paraphrase using other words or simple gestures.***				
6. ✦	***Escort the patient to the exam room. If the patient has a walker or cane, walk closely to them and assist as needed.***				
7. ✦	***Observe the patient's overall physical ability to comply with your requests.***				
8. ✦	***Offer assistance as needed. Allow the patient to do as much for him or herself as possible.***				
9. ✦	***Ask the patient to be seated while you being to gather information for the patient history.***				

Name: ______________________

Date: ______________________

POINT VALUE
✦ = 3–6 points
✶ = 7–9 points

		PRACTICE TRIAL	GRADED TRIAL # 1	GRADED TRIAL # 2	NOTES
10. ✶	***Instruct the patient regarding the physician's recommendations for regular blood pressure screenings, such as obtaining an automatic BP machine from the drug store or having readings performed in the office.***				
11. ✦	***Explain how other medical conditions (including heart disease, atrial fibrillation, high cholesterol, and diabetes) will be closely monitored, along with any change or adjustments made to medication.***				
12. ✶	***Make the patient aware of the warning signs of depression and offer coping strategies for stressors, such as physical limitations, potential loss of income, and financial concerns.***				
13. ✶	***Discuss with the patient factors that he or she is unable to control against recurring stroke, including family history, age, gender, and race.***				
14. ✶	***Discuss with the patient factors that he or she is able to control against recurring stroke, including smoking, drinking, diet modifications, and exercise. Encourage the patient to become proactive in lifestyle changes.***				
15. ✶	Document all findings and impressions in the patient's record.				

Name: ______________________________

Date: ______________________________

Document: Enter the appropriate information in the chart below.

Grading

Points Earned	________		
Points Possible	________	111	111
Percent Grade (Points Earned/Points Possible)	________		
PASS:	________	❏ YES ❏ NO ❏ N/A	❏ YES ❏ NO ❏ N/A

Instructor Sign-Off

Instructor: ______________________________ **Date:** ______________________

Name: ______________________________

Date: ______________________________

Procedure 42-1:

Surgical Hand Hygiene/Surgical Scrub

Objective: Perform a surgical scrub on hands and arms using the correct technique for the appropriate length of time.

Supplies: Nail file, germicidal dispenser soap, sterile scrub brush, sterile towel pack, packaged sterile gloves, running water

Affective Behaviors: Affective behaviors provide a professional approach to a skill that enhances the patient encounter. These behaviors may also display sensitivity to a patient's rights and enhance communication. Pay close attention to these skills, which will be in ***bold, italicized*** font.

Notes to the Student

____

____

____

____

____

____

Skills Assessment Requirements

Read and familiarize yourself with the procedure; complete the minimum practice requirements. Document each MPR using proper charting technique. Complete each procedure within a reasonable amount of time, with a minimum of 85% accuracy.

Name: ______________________________

Date: ______________________________

POINT VALUE
✦ = 3–6 points
✶ = 7–9 points

		PRACTICE TRIAL	GRADED TRIAL # 1	GRADED TRIAL # 2	NOTES
1. ✦	Assemble all equipment.				
2. ✶	Remove all jewelry. Use the nail file to remove any visible dirt from beneath fingernails before scrubbing. *Note:* Microorganisms can accumulate in crevices of rings or watches and under fingernails.				
3. ✦	Stand at the sink without allowing your body to touch it.				
4. ✦	Remove your lab coat. Roll or pull up your sleeves above the elbows. Keep your hands and arms above waist level at all times.				
5. ✦	Turn on the water and regulate the temperature to warm, not hot.				
6. ✶	Place your hands under the running water, keeping them pointed up, allowing water to run from fingertips to elbows.				
7. ✦	Apply soap and lather well.				
8. ✶	Vigorously scrub your hands and wrists with a scrub brush. Wash thoroughly between the fingers. Scrub under the fingernails. Scrub toward the elbows. Scrub for 5 minutes on each hand.				
9. ✦	Raise your hands, bending your arm at the elbow, and place your hands under running water to rinse off the soap. Continue letting water flow from fingertips to elbows.				
10. ✦	Perform a second lather and scrub each hand for 3 minutes, if this is the policy of your facility.				

Name: ______________________________

Date: ______________________________

POINT VALUE
✦ = 3–6 points
✶ = 7–9 points

		PRACTICE TRIAL	GRADED TRIAL # 1	GRADED TRIAL # 2	NOTES
11. ✶	Using a sterile towel, pat your hands dry, moving from fingertips to wrists, and then on to the elbows. Continue holding the hands above the elbows.				
12. ✦	Turn off the faucet using a fresh towel if a foot lever is not available.				
13. ✦	Glove immediately after completing the scrub. Keep your hands folded together and above your waist until the procedure begins.				

Name: ____________________

Date: ____________________

Document: Enter the appropriate information in the chart below.

Grading

Points Earned	______		
Points Possible	______	90	90
Percent Grade (Points Earned/Points Possible)	______		
PASS:	______	❑ YES ❑ NO ❑ N/A	❑ YES ❑ NO ❑ N/A

Instructor Sign-Off

Instructor: ____________________ **Date:** ____________________

Name: ______________________________

Date: ______________________________

Procedure 42-2:

Surgical Gloving

Objective: Apply sterile gloves without a break in sterile technique.

Supplies: Double-wrapped sterile glove pack

Affective Behaviors: Affective behaviors provide a professional approach to a skill that enhances the patient encounter. These behaviors may also display sensitivity to a patient's rights and enhance communication. Pay close attention to these skills, which will be in ***bold, italicized*** font.

Notes to the Student

This procedure follows a surgical hand scrub.

Skills Assessment Requirements

Read and familiarize yourself with the procedure; complete the minimum practice requirements. Document each MPR using proper charting technique. Complete each procedure within a reasonable amount of time, with a minimum of 85% accuracy.

Name: ____________________

Date: ____________________

POINT VALUE
✦ = 3–6 points
✶ = 7–9 points

		PRACTICE TRIAL	GRADED TRIAL # 1	GRADED TRIAL # 2	NOTES
1. ✦	Assemble all equipment. Check the tape or seal for expiration date and condition of pack.				
2. ✦	Place the pack on a flat surface at waist height with the cuffed end of the gloves toward you.				
3. ✶	Open the outside wrapper by touching only the outside of the pack. Leave the opened wrapper in place to provide a sterile work field.				
4. ✶	Open the inner wrapper without reaching over the pack or touching the inside of the wrapper. Pull inner wrapper edges to each side without touching the inside of the pack.				
5. ✦	Using the thumb and fingers of your left hand, pick up the glove on the right side of the pack by grasping the folded inside edge of the cuff. The glove can be dangled slightly off the sterile packing material for easier insertion.				
6. ✶	Pull the glove onto the right hand using only the thumb and fingers of the left hand. Do not allow your fingers to touch the rest of the glove.				
7. ✦	Place the fingers of the right-gloved hand under the cuff of the left hand and up over the left wrist.				
8. ✦	With the gloved right hand, place your fingers under the cuff of the left glove and pull up over the left wrist. The thumb should not touch the cuff.				

Name: ______________________________

Date: ______________________________

POINT VALUE
✦ = 3–6 points
✶ = 7–9 points

		PRACTICE TRIAL	GRADED TRIAL # 1	GRADED TRIAL # 2	NOTES
9. ✦	After the gloves are in place, the fingers can be adjusted, if necessary, by using the gloved hands.				
10. ✶	Remove gloves by grasping the edge of the first glove and pull over the hand, turning it inside out. Discard the first glove into the proper waste container. Remove the other glove by grasping the edge of the cuff with your fingers, pulling this second glove down over your hand and turning it inside out. Discard appropriately.				
11. ✦	Perform proper hand hygiene.				

Name: ______________________________

Date: ______________________________

Document: Enter the appropriate information in the chart below.

Grading

Points Earned	_______		
Points Possible	_______	78	78
Percent Grade (Points Earned/Points Possible)	_______		
PASS:	_______	❑ YES ❑ NO ❑ N/A	❑ YES ❑ NO ❑ N/A

Instructor Sign-Off

Instructor: ______________________________ **Date:** ________________

Name: ______________________________

Date: ______________________________

Procedure 42-3:

Opening a Sterile Packet

Objective: Open a sterile packet and use it to set up a sterile field without a break in the sterile technique.

Supplies: Sterile packet, Mayo stand, waste container, sterile forceps

Affective Behaviors: Affective behaviors provide a professional approach to a skill that enhances the patient encounter. These behaviors may also display sensitivity to a patient's rights and enhance communication. Pay close attention to these skills, which will be in ***bold, italicized*** font.

Notes to the Student

____

____

____

____

____

____

Skills Assessment Requirements

Read and familiarize yourself with the procedure; complete the minimum practice requirements. Document each MPR using proper charting technique. Complete each procedure within a reasonable amount of time, with a minimum of 85% accuracy.

Name: ______________________________

Date: ______________________________

POINT VALUE
✦ = 3–6 points
✶ = 7–9 points

		PRACTICE TRIAL	GRADED TRIAL # 1	GRADED TRIAL # 2	NOTES
1. ✦	Assemble all equipment. Adjust the Mayo stand to the correct working height.				
2. ✦	Perform proper hand hygiene.				
3. ✦	Place the sterile packet on the Mayo stand with the folded edge on top. Position the packet on the stand so that the top flap will fold away from you.				
4. ✦	Remove the tape or fastener and check the sterilization indicator and date. Discard waste in the proper container.				
5. ✶	Pull the corner of the pack that is tucked under and lay this flap away from you. It will hang down over the edge of the Mayo stand.				
6. ✶	With both hands, pull the next two flaps to each side. The packet will still be covered with the last layer of the outer wrapper.				
7. ✶	Grasp the corner of the last flap without reaching over the sterile field and open the flap toward your body without touching it.				
8. ✦	The inside of the outer wrapper is now your sterile field. If you need to arrange items within this field, use sterile forceps. If an inner packet needs to be opened with an instrument setup, someone wearing sterile gloves must open it.				

Name: ______________________________

Date: ______________________________

Document: Enter the appropriate information in the chart below.

Grading

Points Earned	_______		
Points Possible	_______	57	57
Percent Grade (Points Earned/Points Possible)	_______		
PASS:	_______	❑ YES ❑ NO ❑ N/A	❑ YES ❑ NO ❑ N/A

Instructor Sign-Off

Instructor: ______________________________ **Date:** ____________________

Name: ______________________________

Date: ______________________________

Procedure 42-4:

Dropping a Sterile Packet onto a Sterile Field

Objective: Place (drop) a sterile item onto a sterile field or into a sterile gloved hand without contaminating the item or the field.

Supplies: Sterile pack

Affective Behaviors: Affective behaviors provide a professional approach to a skill that enhances the patient encounter. These behaviors may also display sensitivity to a patient's rights and enhance communication. Pay close attention to these skills, which will be in ***bold, italicized*** font.

Notes to the Student

____

____

____

____

____

____

Skills Assessment Requirements

Read and familiarize yourself with the procedure; complete the minimum practice requirements. Document each MPR using proper charting technique. Complete each procedure within a reasonable amount of time, with a minimum of 85% accuracy.

Name: ______________________________

Date: ______________________________

POINT VALUE
✦ = 3–6 points
✶ = 7–9 points

		PRACTICE TRIAL	GRADED TRIAL # 1	GRADED TRIAL # 2	NOTES
1. ✦	Assemble all necessary equipment, check the expiration date on all items, and be sure that all items are in sealed condition.				
2. ✦	Locate the "pull-apart" edge on the sterile package and pull it apart, using the thumb and forefinger of each hand. Be careful not to let your fingers touch the inside of the package.				
3. ✶	Pull the sterile package apart by securely placing the remaining three fingers of each hand against the outside of the package on each side. The wrapper edges will be pulled back away from the sterile item to allow it to drop easily onto the sterile field.				
4. ✶	Hold the package securely about 8–10 inches above the sterile field and drop the contents of the package on it, allowing at least 1 inch from each side. The physician may choose to take the item directly from you using his or her gloved hand.				
5. ✦	Discard the wrapper in the proper waste container or set it aside, away from the sterile field, until after the procedure.				

Name: ______________________________

Date: ______________________________

Document: Enter the appropriate information in the chart below.

Grading

Points Earned	______		
Points Possible	______	36	36
Percent Grade (Points Earned/Points Possible)	______		
PASS:	______	❑ YES ❑ NO ❑ N/A	❑ YES ❑ NO ❑ N/A

Instructor Sign-Off

Instructor: ______________________________ **Date:** ______________

Name: ______________________________

Date: ______________________________

Procedure 42-5:

Transferring Sterile Objects Using Transfer Forceps

Objective: Move sterile objects within or onto a sterile field or gloved hand without contaminating the item or the field.

Supplies: Sterile transfer forceps in container with sterilant solution, Mayo stand with sterile field setup, sterile 4 × 4 gauze package

Affective Behaviors: Affective behaviors provide a professional approach to a skill that enhances the patient encounter. These behaviors may also display sensitivity to a patient's rights and enhance communication. Pay close attention to these skills, which will be in ***bold, italicized*** font.

Notes to the Student

____

____

____

____

____

____

Skills Assessment Requirements

Read and familiarize yourself with the procedure; complete the minimum practice requirements. Document each MPR using proper charting technique. Complete each procedure within a reasonable amount of time, with a minimum of 85% accuracy.

Name: ______________________________

Date: ______________________________

POINT VALUE ✦ = 3–6 points ✶ = 7–9 points		PRACTICE TRIAL	GRADED TRIAL # 1	GRADED TRIAL # 2	NOTES
1. ✶	Grasp forceps handles firmly without separating the tips and remove vertically from the container. (Remove vertically to avoid dripping solution onto exposed contaminated portion of forceps.)				
2. ✦	Dry the tips of the forceps by holding forceps vertically with tips down and gently tapping the tips together to drop excess solution onto dry, sterile 4 × 4 gauze.				
3. ✶	Hold the forceps vertically with the tip down. Do not touch the sterile field. Grasp the item to be transferred firmly at its midsection.				
4. ✦	Place the sterile item within the sterile field.				
5. ✦	Place the forceps back into the container without touching the sides of the container.				
6. ✶	Clean and sterilize the forceps and container in the autoclave. Change the solution.				

Name: ______________________________

Date: ______________________________

Document: Enter the appropriate information in the chart below.

Grading

Points Earned	_______		
Points Possible	_______	45	45
Percent Grade (Points Earned/Points Possible)	_______		
PASS:	_______	❑ YES ❑ NO ❑ N/A	❑ YES ❑ NO ❑ N/A

Instructor Sign-Off

Instructor: ______________________________ **Date:** ____________________

Name: ______________________________

Date: ______________________________

Procedure 42-6:

Transferring Sterile Solutions onto a Sterile Field

Objective: Pour sterile fluid into a sterile basin on a sterile field without spilling the solution or contaminating the field.

Supplies: Sterile saline or other solution, as ordered; sterile basin; Mayo stand or side tray; waste container

Affective Behaviors: Affective behaviors provide a professional approach to a skill that enhances the patient encounter. These behaviors may also display sensitivity to a patient's rights and enhance communication. Pay close attention to these skills, which will be in ***bold, italicized*** font.

Notes to the Student

____

____

____

____

____

____

Skills Assessment Requirements

Read and familiarize yourself with the procedure; complete the minimum practice requirements. Document each MPR using proper charting technique. Complete each procedure within a reasonable amount of time, with a minimum of 85% accuracy.

Name: ______________________

Date: ______________________

POINT VALUE
✦ = 3–6 points
✶ = 7–9 points

		PRACTICE TRIAL	GRADED TRIAL # 1	GRADED TRIAL # 2	NOTES
1. ✦	Perform proper hand hygiene.				
2. ✦	Assemble all supplies and equipment. Check all expiration dates on the solution and sterile basin pack.				
3. ✦	Sep up a sterile basin or cup on the Mayo stand tray using the inside wrapper to create a sterile field.				
4. ✶	Remove the cap of the solution and place it on a clean surface with the outer edge down (inside facing up). Avoid touching the inner surface of the cap.				
5. ✦	Double-check the label on the bottle before pouring the solution.				
6. ✦	Pour a small amount of the liquid into a waste container for discarding.				
7. ✶	Pour the solution from the bottle with the label held against the palm of your hand.				
8. ✶	Hold the bottle about 6 inches above the basin and pour slowly to avoid splashing the solution.				
9. ✦	Replace the lid immediately after pouring is complete.				

Name: ______________________

Date: ______________________

Document: Enter the appropriate information in the chart below.

Grading

Points Earned	______		
Points Possible	______	63	63
Percent Grade (Points Earned/Points Possible)	______		
PASS:	______	❑ YES ❑ NO ❑ N/A	❑ YES ❑ NO ❑ N/A

Instructor Sign-Off

Instructor: ______________________ **Date:** ______________________

Name: ______________________________

Date: ______________________________

Procedure 42-7:

Assisting with Minor Surgery

Objective: Prepare all materials and equipment for immediate use in a surgical procedure using sterile techniques.

Supplies: Mayo stand; side stand; transfer forceps and container; sharps container; waste container/plastic bag; biohazard waste container; anesthetic; alcohol swab; sterile specimen container (depending on procedure); sterile pack

Affective Behaviors: Affective behaviors provide a professional approach to a skill that enhances the patient encounter. These behaviors may also display sensitivity to a patient's rights and enhance communication. Pay close attention to these skills, which will be in ***bold, italicized*** font.

Notes to the Student

____

____

____

____

____

____

Skills Assessment Requirements

Read and familiarize yourself with the procedure; complete the minimum practice requirements. Document each MPR using proper charting technique. Complete each procedure within a reasonable amount of time, with a minimum of 85% accuracy.

Name: ______________________________

Date: ______________________________

POINT VALUE
✦ = 3–6 points
✶ = 7–9 points

		PRACTICE TRIAL	GRADED TRIAL # 1	GRADED TRIAL # 2	NOTES
1. ✦	Perform proper hand hygiene.				
2. ✦	Open sterile tray packs onto the Mayo stand tray and side stand. Use sterile wrapper to create a sterile field. The wrapper will hang over the edges of the tray.				
3. ✦	Use sterile transfer forceps to move instruments to the tray or place equipment from inside packets. Materials in a peel-away package should be flipped or dropped onto the tray.				
4. ✦	Open the sterile needle and syringe unit, and drop them gently onto the sterile field. *Note:* Do not reach over the sterile field.				
5. ✦	Open sterile drape packs, sterile towels, and towel clamp packs; drop these gently onto the tray.				
6. ✦	Open a set of sterile gloves for the physician.				
7. ✶	After the tray is ready with all equipment open and arranged, place a sterile towel or sterile drape over the tray, touching only the corners of the sterile towel. Do not leave the room once the tray is set up.				
8. ✶	When the physician has donned the sterile gloves, remove the sterile towel covering the tray of instruments.				

Name: ______________________________

Date: ______________________________

POINT VALUE
✦ = 3–6 points
✶ = 7–9 points

		PRACTICE TRIAL	GRADED TRIAL # 1	GRADED TRIAL # 2	NOTES
9. ✦	Remove the sterile towel from the tray by standing to one side and grasping the two distal corners. Lift the towel toward you so that you do not reach over the unprotected sterile field.				
10. ✶	Cleanse the vial of anesthetic with a sterile alcohol swab and hold it upside down in the palm of your hand with the label facing toward the physician. Hold it steady while the physician draws up the anesthetic.				
11. ✦	Stand to one side of the patient and assist the physician as requested. Provide additional supplies as needed. *Note:* If you assist by handing instruments to the physician, you must perform a surgical scrub and wear a sterile gown and gloves.				
12. ✦	Hold all containers for specimens, drainage, or contaminated 4 × 4's. Wear nonsterile gloves to protect yourself from drainage.				
13. ✦	Collect and place all soiled instruments in a basin out of the patient's view.				
14. ✦	Place all soiled gauze, sponges, and dressings in a plastic bag. Do not allow wet items to remain on the sterile field.				

Name: ______________________________

Date: ______________________________

POINT VALUE ✦ = 3–6 points ✶ = 7–9 points		PRACTICE TRIAL	GRADED TRIAL # 1	GRADED TRIAL # 2	NOTES
15. ✶	Immediately label all specimens as they are obtained. Close the specimen container tightly.				
16. ✦	***Periodically reassure the patient by quietly asking how he or she is feeling. Do not touch the patient with soiled gloves.***				
17. ✦	When the procedure is complete, wash your hands before assisting the patient. ***Assist in moving the patient to a recovery area (if that is facility policy) before cleaning the area.*** To dispose of soiled dressing, use the following steps: • Remove gloves. • Place one hand into the empty plastic bag. • Using the hand covered with the plastic bag, pick up all soiled materials. With the other hand, pull the outside of the bag over the soiled dressings. • Dispose of the bag in a biohazard waste container. • Perform proper hand hygiene and document the procedure.				
18. ✦	***Allow the patient to rest and recover from the anesthetic. Periodically check the patient's vital signs according to facility policy.***				

Name: ______________________

Date: ______________________

POINT VALUE ✦ = 3–6 points ✶ = 7–9 points		PRACTICE TRIAL	GRADED TRIAL # 1	GRADED TRIAL # 2	NOTES
19. ✦	***Provide clear verbal and written postoperative instructions to the patient. Make sure that the patient is stable before he or she leaves the office.***				
20. ✶	Prepare the requisition slip and send the specimen to the laboratory.				
21. ✶	Clean, sanitize, and sterilize the instruments. Clean and sanitize the procedure room in preparation for the next patient.				
22. ✦	Perform proper hand hygiene.				

Name: ______________________________

Date: ______________________________

Document: Enter the appropriate information in the chart below.

Grading

Points Earned	______		
Points Possible	______	150	150
Percent Grade (Points Earned/Points Possible)	______		
PASS:	______	❏ YES ❏ NO ❏ N/A	❏ YES ❏ NO ❏ N/A

Instructor Sign-Off

Instructor: ______________________________ **Date:** ______________

Name: ____________________

Date: ____________________

Procedure 42-8:

Preparing the Patient's Skin for Surgical Procedures

Objective: Prepare the patient's skin at the surgical site using a sterile scrub and shaving (if required).

Supplies: Sink; sterile gloves; Mayo stand; packs; gown and drape; sterile towels; sterile gauze and syringe; sterile saline; biohazard waste container; pencil or pen; paper

Affective Behaviors: Affective behaviors provide a professional approach to a skill that enhances the patient encounter. These behaviors may also display sensitivity to a patient's rights and enhance communication. Pay close attention to these skills, which will be in ***bold, italicized*** font.

Notes to the Student

____

____

____

____

____

____

Skills Assessment Requirements

Read and familiarize yourself with the procedure; complete the minimum practice requirements. Document each MPR using proper charting technique. Complete each procedure within a reasonable amount of time, with a minimum of 85% accuracy.

Name: ______________________________

Date: ______________________________

POINT VALUE
✦ = 3–6 points
✶ = 7–9 points

		PRACTICE TRIAL	GRADED TRIAL # 1	GRADED TRIAL # 2	NOTES
1. ✦	Assemble equipment by placing packs on Mayo stand or side tray and opening outer wraps from all packs.				
2. ✦	Perform proper hand hygiene.				
3. ✶	***Identify the patient and explain the procedure.***				
4. ✦	***Have the patient remove any necessary clothing and jewelry and put on a gown. Ask the patient to void if necessary.***				
5. ✦	***Position and drape the patient to expose the operative site.***				
6. ✦	Unwrap the basin pack. Pour germicidal soap solution into the first basin, sterile saline into the second basin, and antiseptic into the third.				
7. ✦	Wash your hands using sterile scrub and apply sterile gloves.				
8. ✦	Drape the skin with two sterile towels placed 3 to 5 inches above and below the surgical site.				
9. ✶	With a sterile gauze or sponge, apply soapy solution from the first basin to the patient's skin. Use a circular motion, starting at the site of the proposed incision and move outward. Pass over each skin area only once. Place each used sponge into the waste receptacle immediately.				
10. ✶	Use the following techniques appropriate for the type of shaving the physician orders.				

Name: ______________________________

Date: ______________________________

POINT VALUE ✦ = 3–6 points ✶ = 7–9 points		PRACTICE TRIAL	GRADED TRIAL # 1	GRADED TRIAL # 2	NOTES
	Instructions for a dry shave: 1. Clip the hair as short as possible with scissors. 2. Apply firm traction to the skin with the nondominant hand. 3. Using either hair clippers or a razor, remove hair in the direction of hair growth. *Note:* Never shave against the grain, as this will cause unnecessary irritation to the skin and increase the likelihood of nicks. 4. Take a fresh sterile gauze or sponge for each cleansing wipe. Repeat this process until the area is completely washed. The last area cleansed will be the outer edges. 5. Rinse using sterile saline on a clean gauze or sponge. Pat dry with a dry gauze only on the area that has been washed. Avoid touching any other skin area.				

Name: ______________________________

Date: ______________________________

POINT VALUE
✦ = 3–6 points
✶ = 7–9 points

		PRACTICE TRIAL	GRADED TRIAL # 1	GRADED TRIAL # 2	NOTES
	If shaving is ordered and a dry shave is not specified, proceed with the following steps: 1. Apply soap solution to the site area. Remove the razor from shave preparation pack. Pull the skin taut and shave the surgical site in the same direction as the hair is growing. Rinse with a saline solution, using the single-pass, circular motion as before, and pat dry. 2. Reapply soap solution to the area and repeat the preceding process according to your office policy (around 5 minutes). 3. Pat the entire area dry with the third sterile towel. 4. Apply the antiseptic solution using two cotton applicators together in the same single-pass, circular motion.				
11. ✶	Cover the prepared surgical site with the remaining sterile towel.				
12. ✦	Properly dispose of gloves and soiled materials in a biohazard waste container.				
13. ✦	Perform proper hand hygiene.				
14. ✶	Document the procedure completely in the patient record.				

Name: ______________________________

Date: ______________________________

Document: Enter the appropriate information in the chart below.

Grading

Points Earned	_______		
Points Possible	_______	99	99
Percent Grade (Points Earned/Points Possible)	_______		
PASS:	_______	❑ YES ❑ NO ❑ N/A	❑ YES ❑ NO ❑ N/A

Instructor Sign-Off

Instructor: ______________________________ **Date:** ______________________________

Name: ______________________________

Date: ______________________________

Procedure 42-9:

Assisting with Suturing

Objective: Assist with suture repair of an incision or laceration using sterile technique.

Supplies: Mayo stand; side stand; anesthetic; sterile transfer forceps; sterile saline; waste container/plastic bag; biohazard waste container; sharps container; sterile gloves (2 pairs); sterile pack; scalpel blades pack; needle and syringe pack; suture and needle pack; 2 sterile basins; suture pack

Affective Behaviors: Affective behaviors provide a professional approach to a skill that enhances the patient encounter. These behaviors may also display sensitivity to a patient's rights and enhance communication. Pay close attention to these skills, which will be in ***bold, italicized*** font.

Notes to the Student

____

____

____

____

____

____

Skills Assessment Requirements

Read and familiarize yourself with the procedure; complete the minimum practice requirements. Document each MPR using proper charting technique. Complete each procedure within a reasonable amount of time, with a minimum of 85% accuracy.

Name: ______________________________

Date: ______________________________

POINT VALUE
✦ = 3–6 points
✶ = 7–9 points

		PRACTICE TRIAL	GRADED TRIAL # 1	GRADED TRIAL # 2	NOTES
1. ✦	Use a sterile hand scrub and gloving procedure.				
2. ✦	Stand across from the physician.				
3. ✦	Place 2 gauze sponges, ready for the physician, near the wound site.				
4. ✦	Assist by using additional sponges to keep the wound dry.				
5. ✶	Pass instruments, such as scissors, to the physician with a firm snap of the handle into his or her hand without letting go until the physician has a firm grasp.				
6. ✦	Place the blade into the scalpel using a hemostat.				
7. ✶	Hand the scalpel to the physician with the blade edge down to avoid cutting the physician.				
8. ✦	Continue to use sponges to keep the wound clear and free of drainage and blood.				
9. ✦	Pass all instruments to the physician as requested. Try to anticipate the next instrument that the physician will need, such as another hemostat or scissors for cutting the suture.				
10. ✦	Pass the toothed forceps to the physician if laceration edges need to be grasped.				

Name: ______________________

Date: ______________________

POINT VALUE
✦ = 3–6 points
✶ = 7–9 points

		PRACTICE TRIAL	GRADED TRIAL # 1	GRADED TRIAL # 2	NOTES
11. ✶	Mount the needle in the needle holder and pass the needle and needle holder as one unit to the physician, being careful to keep the suture within the sterile field. Pass the needle holder with the needle pointing outward. Hold the suture with the other hand and do not let go until the physician sees it.				
12. ✦	Using the suture scissors, prepare to cut the suture as directed by the physician (usually one-half to one-quarter inch from the knot).				
13. ✶	Sponge the closed wound once with a sponge and discard it.				
14. ✦	Repeat the above step with each suture.				
15. ✶	Apply a layer of sterile dressing (i.e., sterile gauze) over the wound. Sterile dressing should extend a minimum of 2 inches past all edges of the wound. *Note:* Forceps can be used to apply the dressing.				
16. ✦	Apply a second layer of gauze over the wound site.				
17. ✦	Apply a third layer of wound dressing, such as a SurgiPad.				
18. ✦	Secure the edges of the dressing with paper tape or waterproof membrane, depending on physician's preference.				

Name: ____________________

Date: ____________________

POINT VALUE
✦ = 3–6 points
✶ = 7–9 points

		PRACTICE TRIAL	GRADED TRIAL # 1	GRADED TRIAL # 2	NOTES
19. ✶	Place all soiled instruments after they are used onto the sterile field if they will be used again; discard others in the instrument basin if the physician is finished with them.				
20. ✦	When the procedure is complete, remove your gloves and use proper hand hygiene before assisting the patient.				
21. ✦	***Allow the patient to rest and recover from the anesthetic.*** Periodically check the patient's vital signs and document them.				
22. ✶	***Provide clear verbal and written after-care instructions for the patient. Make sure that the patient is stable before allowing him or her to leave the office.***				
23. ✶	Clean, sanitize, and sterilize all instruments. Clean and sanitize the procedure room and prepare it for the next patient.				
24. ✦	Perform proper hand hygiene.				
25. ✶	Document the procedure, the patient response, and the postoperative instructions given to the patient.				

Name: ______________________

Date: ______________________

Document: Enter the appropriate information in the chart below.

Grading

Points Earned	______		
Points Possible	______	177	177
Percent Grade (Points Earned/Points Possible)	______		
PASS:	______	❑ YES ❑ NO ❑ N/A	❑ YES ❑ NO ❑ N/A

Instructor Sign-Off

Instructor: ______________________ **Date:** ______________

Name: ______________________________

Date: ______________________________

Procedure 42-10:

Removing Sutures

Objective: Remove sutures using proper sterile technique as ordered by the physician.

Supplies: Suture removal pack

Affective Behaviors: Affective behaviors provide a professional approach to a skill that enhances the patient encounter. These behaviors may also display sensitivity to a patient's rights and enhance communication. Pay close attention to these skills, which will be in ***bold, italicized*** font.

Notes to the Student

____

____

____

____

____

____

Skills Assessment Requirements

Read and familiarize yourself with the procedure; complete the minimum practice requirements. Document each MPR using proper charting technique. Complete each procedure within a reasonable amount of time, with a minimum of 85% accuracy.

Name: ______________________

Date: ______________________

POINT VALUE
✦ = 3–6 points
✶ = 7–9 points

		PRACTICE TRIAL	GRADED TRIAL # 1	GRADED TRIAL # 2	NOTES
	Removal of sutures				
1. ✦	Assemble all equipment and supplies needed; check expiration dates on all packs.				
2. ✦	Perform proper hand hygiene.				
3. ✦	***Identify the patient.***				
4. ✶	***Explain the procedure to the patient and place him or her in a comfortable position.***				
5. ✦	Perform proper hand hygiene.				
6. ✦	Remove the dressing from the site using proper technique and dispose of it in the appropriate waste container.				
7. ✦	Perform proper hand hygiene.				
8. ✶	Open the suture removal pack using proper sterile technique.				
9. ✶	Apply sterile gloves using proper sterile technique.				
10. ✦	Cleanse the wound as needed.				
11. ✦	Place a gauze sponge next to the wound to hold the removed sutures.				
12. ✦	Grasp the knot of the suture with forceps and lift it gently.				
13. ✦	Insert the suture scissors and cut the suture at skin level. Pull out the suture.				
14. ✶	Place the cut suture on the gauze pad and check to see that all the pieces of the suture have been removed.				

Name: ____________________

Date: ____________________

POINT VALUE
✦ = 3–6 points
✶ = 7–9 points

		PRACTICE TRIAL	GRADED TRIAL # 1	GRADED TRIAL # 2	NOTES
15. ✦	Repeat these steps until all sutures have been removed.				
16. ✶	Count the removed sutures, making sure that all sutures have been removed.				
	Removal of staples				
1. ✦	Follow steps 1–10 of suture removal.				
2. ✦	Place the lower tips of a sterile staple remover under the staple.				
3. ✶	Squeeze the handles together until they are completely closed, thus bending the staple and removing the staple edges from the skin. *Note:* Do not lift the staple remover when squeezing the handles.				
4. ✦	When both ends of the staple are visible, gently move the staple away from the incision site.				
5. ✦	Hold the staple remover over a disposable container, release the handles, and release the staple.				
6. ✶	Repeat these steps until all staples are removed. Count the number of staples to ensure all been removed.				

Name: ____________________

Date: ____________________

POINT VALUE
✦ = 3–6 points
✶ = 7–9 points

		PRACTICE TRIAL	GRADED TRIAL # 1	GRADED TRIAL # 2	NOTES
	Closing steps for either suture or staple removal				
1. ✶	Clean the wound with antiseptic and allow it to dry.				
2. ✦	Dress wound as ordered.				
3. ✦	Properly dispose of equipment and supplies.				
4. ✦	Remove and dispose of gloves. Perform proper hand hygiene.				
5. ✦	***Instruct patient on wound care.***				
6. ✶	Document the procedure, including condition of the wound, number of staples/sutures removed, and patient wound care instructions, in the patient's record.				

Name: ____________________

Date: ____________________

Document: Enter the appropriate information in the chart below.

Grading

Points Earned	_______		
Points Possible	_______	195	195
Percent Grade (Points Earned/Points Possible)	_______		
PASS:	_______	❏ YES ❏ NO ❏ N/A	❏ YES ❏ NO ❏ N/A

Instructor Sign-Off

Instructor: ____________________ **Date:** ____________________

Name: ______________________________

Date: ______________________________

Procedure 42-11:

Changing a Sterile Dressing

Objective: Change a wound dressing using sterile technique.

Supplies: Gloves; antiseptic solution; solution container; prepackaged dressing pack; thumb forceps; sterile cotton balls; sterile gloves; sterile dressing; adhesive tape; scissors (for tape); waste container/plastic bag; biohazard waste container; Mayo stand or side tray

Affective Behaviors: Affective behaviors provide a professional approach to a skill that enhances the patient encounter. These behaviors may also display sensitivity to a patient's rights and enhance communication. Pay close attention to these skills, which will be in ***bold, italicized*** font.

Notes to the Student

____

____

____

____

____

____

Skills Assessment Requirements

Read and familiarize yourself with the procedure; complete the minimum practice requirements. Document each MPR using proper charting technique. Complete each procedure within a reasonable amount of time, with a minimum of 85% accuracy.

Name: ______________________

Date: ______________________

POINT VALUE
✦ = 3–6 points
✶ = 7–9 points

		PRACTICE TRIAL	GRADED TRIAL # 1	GRADED TRIAL # 2	NOTES
1. ✦	Assemble all equipment and supplies needed using the Mayo stand.				
2. ✦	Perform proper hand hygiene.				
3. ✦	Prepare the sterile field using aseptic technique with prepackaged dressing packet. Employ sterile transfer forceps to place additional needed sterile items onto the sterile field.				
4. ✶	***Identify the patient and explain the procedure.***				
5. ✦	***Assist the patient into a comfortable position with the area to be dressed resting on a support, such as an examination table.***				
6. ✦	Apply nonsterile gloves.				
7. ✶	Remove the soiled dressing from the wound by loosening the tape with gloved hands and/or forceps and pulling it from both sides toward the wound. Without passing the soiled dressing over the sterile field, place it in the soiled waste bag. Do not allow the dressing to touch the outside or edges of the bag.				
8. ✶	Inspect the wound for signs of infection and inflammation, and for signs of healing. Note any discharge by type, amount, color, and odor.				

Name: ____________________

Date: ____________________

POINT VALUE
✦ = 3–6 points
✶ = 7–9 points

		PRACTICE TRIAL	GRADED TRIAL # 1	GRADED TRIAL # 2	NOTES
9. ✦	Remove and discard gloves and forceps properly. Disposable gloves and forceps are placed in the biohazard waste container. Reusable forceps are placed in the basin for later cleaning.				
10. ✦	Drop antiseptic on several gauze sponges until they are moist but not saturated.				
11. ✦	Open sterile gloves and apply them properly, maintaining sterile technique.				
12. ✶	Clean the wound using sterile forceps to hold the sponges. Cleanse the wound by moving from top to bottom once. Use a new sponge with antiseptic for each wipe. Next, cleanse from the inside of the wound to the outside edges, moving in concentric circles.				
13. ✦	Pick up the sterile dressing with gloved hands and place it over the wound.				
14. ✦	Discard your gloves and forceps properly.				

Name: ______________________________

Date: ______________________________

POINT VALUE
✦ = 3–6 points
✶ = 7–9 points

		PRACTICE TRIAL	GRADED TRIAL # 1	GRADED TRIAL # 2	NOTES
15. ✶	Apply tape or other material as ordered to hold the dressing in place. Do not apply it too tightly, as this will restrict circulation. The strips of tape should be long enough to hold the dressing in place. Do not wrap the tape entirely around an extremity or completely cover a dressing. *Note:* Some facilities require that you add your initials and the date of the dressing. Follow office policy.				
16. ✦	***Instruct the patient on dressing care and schedule a followup appointment to see the physician.***				
17. ✶	Document the procedure, including date, time, location, condition of the wound, and instructions given to the patient.				

Name: ______________________

Date: ______________________

Document: Enter the appropriate information in the chart below.

Grading

Points Earned	_______		
Points Possible	_______	120	120
Percent Grade (Points Earned/Points Possible)	_______		
PASS:	_______	❑ YES ❑ NO ❑ N/A	❑ YES ❑ NO ❑ N/A

Instructor Sign-Off

Instructor: ______________________ **Date:** ______________________

Name: ______________________________

Date: ______________________________

Procedure 42-12:

Applying a Bandage Over a Sterile Dressing

Objective: Apply a bandage to the forearm.

Supplies: Gloves; bandage material prescribed by physician or office procedures; bandage scissors; tape

Affective Behaviors: Affective behaviors provide a professional approach to a skill that enhances the patient encounter. These behaviors may also display sensitivity to a patient's rights and enhance communication. Pay close attention to these skills, which will be in ***bold, italicized*** font.

Notes to the Student

____

____

____

____

____

____

Skills Assessment Requirements

Read and familiarize yourself with the procedure; complete the minimum practice requirements. Document each MPR using proper charting technique. Complete each procedure within a reasonable amount of time, with a minimum of 85% accuracy.

Name: ______________________

Date: ______________________

POINT VALUE
✦ = 3–6 points
✶ = 7–9 points

		PRACTICE TRIAL	GRADED TRIAL # 1	GRADED TRIAL # 2	NOTES
1. ✦	Assemble all equipment and supplies needed.				
2. ✦	Perform proper hand hygiene.				
3.✦	***Identify the patient.***				
4. ✦	Apply nonsterile gloves.				
5. ✦	***Explain the procedure.***				
6. ✦	Hold the bandage against the skin with the nondominant hand 1 inch below the sterile dressing.				
7. ✶	Wrap the bandage around the wrist two or three times to secure it. Wrap from distal to proximal.				
8. ✶	Check to see that the bandage has not restricted the blood flow.				
9. ✦	Continue wrapping to at least 1 inch above the dressing.				
10. ✦	Wrap two more times to secure the bandage, and then cut the bandage.				
11. ✦	Tape the cut end to the bandage. ***Do not tape the end to the patient's skin.***				
12. ✶	Check again for any blood flow restriction.				
13. ✦	Remove and dispose of gloves.				
14. ✦	Perform proper hand hygiene.				
15. ✦	***Explain home care to the patient.***				
16. ✶	Document the procedure in the patient's record.				

Name: ______________________________

Date: ______________________________

Document: Enter the appropriate information in the chart below.

Grading

Points Earned	________		
Points Possible	________	108	108
Percent Grade (Points Earned/Points Possible)	________		
PASS:	________	❑ YES ❑ NO ❑ N/A	❑ YES ❑ NO ❑ N/A

Instructor Sign-Off

Instructor: ______________________________ **Date:** ______________________

Name: ____________________

Date: ____________________

Procedure 43-1:

Perform Adult Rescue Breathing and One-Rescuer CPR

Objective: Correctly administer rescue breathing for an adult and one-rescuer CPR for an adult, within the designated time frame.

Supplies: Approved mannequin, gloves, ventilator mask, mouth guard

Affective Behaviors: Affective behaviors provide a professional approach to a skill that enhances the patient encounter. These behaviors may also display sensitivity to a patient's rights and enhance communication. Pay close attention to these skills, which will be in ***bold, italicized*** font.

Notes to the Student

____

____

____

____

____

____

Skills Assessment Requirements

Read and familiarize yourself with the procedure; complete the minimum practice requirements. Document each MPR using proper charting technique. Complete each procedure within a reasonable amount of time, with a minimum of 85% accuracy.

Name: ____________________

Date: ____________________

POINT VALUE
✦ = 3–6 points
✶ = 7–9 points

		PRACTICE TRIAL	GRADED TRIAL # 1	GRADED TRIAL # 2	NOTES
1. ✦	***Asses the patient and determine if help is needed. Shout, "Are you okay?" while gently shaking the patient's shoulders.***				
2. ✦	If the adult patient is unresponsive, activate EMS immediately by calling 911, and then get an AED, if available.				
3. ✶	Assess the ABCs. To check the airway, perform a head-tilt, chin-lift maneuver or, if a neck injury is suspected, a jaw thrust. Look and feel for breath and chest movement. Attempt to get another person to call 911. If you are alone, begin the rescue sequence for 1 minute, and then attempt to call 911 yourself. If gloves are available, put them on. If you have a ventilator mask, place it on the patient.				
4. ✦	If breathing is absent, put on a mouth guard and administer 2 rescue breaths. If your breaths do not cause the chest to rise, look in the patient's mouth and remove an object if you see one. If you see no obstructions, make a second attempt to administer a rescue breath.				

Name: ____________________

Date: ____________________

POINT VALUE
✦ = 3–6 points
✶ = 7–9 points

		PRACTICE TRIAL	GRADED TRIAL # 1	GRADED TRIAL # 2	NOTES
5. ✶	If the breaths cause the chest to rise, assess the patient's circulation by feeling for a pulse at the carotid artery (find the Adam's apple with two fingers and slide the fingers to the side of the neck). If you feel a pulse, begin rescue breathing. Administer 1 breath every 5 seconds or 10 to 12 breaths every minute. After 1 minute, reassess the patient for breathing and pulse.				
6. ✦	If you do not feel a pulse, begin chest compressions. Kneel at the patient's side. Place your hand in the center of the chest between the nipples.				
7. ✦	Place your other hand on top of the first hand, making sure to lift your fingers off the chest, using only the heels of your hands to administer compressions.				
8. ✦	Keeping your shoulders directly over your hand, compress the chest 1-and-one-half to 2 inches, and then allow the sternum to relax. Do not lift your hands off the chest.				
9. ✶	Continue to compress the chest a total of 30 times, and then administer 2 breaths.				
10. ✶	Repeat this sequence for 4 total cycles. Reassess the patient.				

Name: ______________________________

Date: ______________________________

POINT VALUE
✦ = 3–6 points
✶ = 7–9 points

		PRACTICE TRIAL	GRADED TRIAL # 1	GRADED TRIAL # 2	NOTES
11. ✶	If necessary, continue CPR until pulse and breathing return or you are relieved by more advanced medial personnel, or the person is pronounced dead by the physician.				
12. ✦	Wash your hands and document the incident in the patient's chart.				

Name: ______________________________

Date: ______________________________

Document: Enter the appropriate information in the chart below.

Grading

Points Earned	______		
Points Possible	______	87	87
Percent Grade (Points Earned/Points Possible)	______		
PASS:	______	❑ YES ❑ NO ❑ N/A	❑ YES ❑ NO ❑ N/A

Instructor Sign-Off

Instructor: ______________________________ **Date:** ______________

Name: ______________________________

Date: ______________________________

Procedure 43-2:

Perform Infant or Young Child Rescue Breathing and One-Rescuer CPR

Objective: Correctly administer rescue breathing for a child and one-rescuer CPR for a child, within the designated time frame.

Supplies: Approved mannequin, gloves, ventilator mask, mouth guard

Affective Behaviors: Affective behaviors provide a professional approach to a skill that enhances the patient encounter. These behaviors may also display sensitivity to a patient's rights and enhance communication. Pay close attention to these skills, which will be in ***bold, italicized*** font.

Notes to the Student

____

____

____

____

____

____

Skills Assessment Requirements

Read and familiarize yourself with the procedure; complete the minimum practice requirements. Document each MPR using proper charting technique. Complete each procedure within a reasonable amount of time, with a minimum of 85% accuracy.

Name: ______________________________

Date: ______________________________

POINT VALUE ✦ = 3–6 points ✶ = 7–9 points		PRACTICE TRIAL	GRADED TRIAL # 1	GRADED TRIAL # 2	NOTES
1. ✦	***Asses the patient and determine if help is needed. Shout the name of the infant or child, and sharply poke at the feet. Never shake an infant.***				
2. ✦	If the infant is unresponsive, perform CPR for 2 minutes prior to activating EMS by calling 911, and then get an AED, if available.				
3. ✶	***Carefully place the patient on the back, being cautious not to move the head or allow the neck to twist, especially if a spinal cord injury is suspected.***				
4. ✦	Gently, with two fingers, tilt the patient's head and open the airway.				
5. ✶	Place your ear close to the patient's mouth to listen for breathing sounds; watch to see if the chest rises or falls, indicating breathing; and feel for any breathing from the patient's nose or mouth.				
6. ✦	If breathing is absent, secure a mouth guard over the patient's mouth and nose. Administer 2 rescue breaths. If your breaths do not cause the chest to rise, look in the patient's mouth and remove any object seen. If no object is seen, make a second attempt to administer a rescue breath.				

Name: ______________________________

Date: ______________________________

POINT VALUE
✦ = 3–6 points
✶ = 7–9 points

		PRACTICE TRIAL	GRADED TRIAL # 1	GRADED TRIAL # 2	NOTES
7. ✦	If the breaths cause the chest to rise, check the patient's pulse at the brachial artery. If you feel a pulse, begin rescue breathing by administering 1 breath every 5 seconds or 10 to 12 breaths every minute.				
8. ✦	If you do not feel a pulse, begin chest compressions. Place two fingers in the center of the chest just below the nipple line. Compressions should be made one-third to one-half the depth of the chest. Perform 30 quick compressions.				
9. ✶	Give 2 more rescue breaths followed by 30 more compressions. Continue the 30:2 ratio of compressions and breaths.				
10. ✶	After 2 minutes, leave the infant and call if you are *still alone*. Continue compressions and breaths until the infant recovers or EMS arrives.				
11. ✦	Wash your hands and document the incident in the patient's chart.				

Name: ______________________________

Date: ______________________________

Document: Enter the appropriate information in the chart below.

Grading

Points Earned	______		
Points Possible	______	78	78
Percent Grade (Points Earned/Points Possible)	______		
PASS:	______	❑ YES ❑ NO ❑ N/A	❑ YES ❑ NO ❑ N/A

Instructor Sign-Off

Instructor: ______________________________ **Date:** ______________________

Name: ______________________

Date: ______________________

Procedure 43-3:

Use an Automated External Defibrillator

Objective: Correctly use an automated external defibrillator (AED) within the time frame designated by the instructor.

Supplies: AED machine; patient chart

Affective Behaviors: Affective behaviors provide a professional approach to a skill that enhances the patient encounter. These behaviors may also display sensitivity to a patient's rights and enhance communication. Pay close attention to these skills, which will be in ***bold, italicized*** font.

Notes to the Student

____

____

____

____

____

____

Skills Assessment Requirements

Read and familiarize yourself with the procedure; complete the minimum practice requirements. Document each MPR using proper charting technique. Complete each procedure within a reasonable amount of time, with a minimum of 85% accuracy.

Name: ______________________

Date: ______________________

POINT VALUE
✦ = 3–6 points
✶ = 7–9 points

		PRACTICE TRIAL	GRADED TRIAL # 1	GRADED TRIAL # 2	NOTES
1. ✶	Place the AED next to the patient's left ear. This position allows the rescuers clear access to the chest and airway for continued rescue measures.				
2. ✶	Turn the AED on and follow the voice prompts.				
3. ✶	You will be prompted to attach the electrode pads to the patient's chest on the sternum and at the apex of the heart, following the diagram for correct placement. Use adult-size electrode pads on patients 8 years of age and older. Child-size electrode pads are used for patients between the ages of 1 and 8 years or who weigh less than 55 pounds.				
4. ✶	Next, you will be directed to allow the machine to analyze the heart rhythm to determine if it is a shockable rhythm. CPR should cease while the machine is analyzing.				
5. ✶	The machine will begin a charging sequence prior to shocking and warn rescuers to stand back. The voice prompt will then tell you to press the SHOCK button to administer the electrical current to the patient.				
6. ✶	If the machine indicates "No Shock Advised," assess the patient's breathing and circulation. Continue CPR as needed until advanced medical personnel arrive.				

Name: ____________________

Date: ____________________

Document: Enter the appropriate information in the chart below.

Grading

Points Earned	_______		
Points Possible	_______	54	54
Percent Grade (Points Earned/Points Possible)	_______		
PASS:	_______	❏ YES ❏ NO ❏ N/A	❏ YES ❏ NO ❏ N/A

Instructor Sign-Off

Instructor: ____________________ **Date:** ____________________

Name: ______________________

Date: ______________________

Procedure 43-4:

Respond to an Adult with an Obstructed Airway

Objective: Correctly administer the Heimlich maneuver to an adult, within the designated time frame.

Supplies: Approved mannequin; gloves; ventilation mask with one-way valve for unconscious patient

Affective Behaviors: Affective behaviors provide a professional approach to a skill that enhances the patient encounter. These behaviors may also display sensitivity to a patient's rights and enhance communication. Pay close attention to these skills, which will be in ***bold, italicized*** font.

Notes to the Student

____

____

____

____

____

____

Skills Assessment Requirements

Read and familiarize yourself with the procedure; complete the minimum practice requirements. Document each MPR using proper charting technique. Complete each procedure within a reasonable amount of time, with a minimum of 85% accuracy.

Name: ___________________________

Date: ___________________________

POINT VALUE
✦ = 3–6 points
✶ = 7–9 points

		PRACTICE TRIAL	GRADED TRIAL # 1	GRADED TRIAL # 2	NOTES
1. ✦	Once it has been established that the patient is choking, with no air exchanged, direct someone to call 911 ***and shout, "Are you choking?" or "Can you speak?" If the answer is no—as indicated by a head shake—tell the patient you are going to begin emergency treatment***.				
2. ✶	***Stand behind the patient with your feet slightly apart, placing one foot between the patient's feet and one to the outside.*** This stance will give you greater stability, and if the patient should pass out, you can safely guide him or her down your thigh.				
3. ✶	***Place the index finger of one hand at the person's navel or belt buckle to mark that spot. If the patient is a pregnant woman, place your finger above the enlarged uterus.***				
4. ✶	***Make a fist with your other hand and place it, thumb side to patient, above your other hand. If the person is very large or far along in pregnancy, you may have to do chest compressions.***				
5. ✦	Place your marking hand over your curled fist and begin to give *quick inward and upward thrusts.*				

Name: ______________________________

Date: ______________________________

POINT VALUE ✦ = 3–6 points ✶ = 7–9 points		PRACTICE TRIAL	GRADED TRIAL # 1	GRADED TRIAL # 2	NOTES
6. ✶	There is no set number of thrusts to give to an adult who remains conscious. ***Continue to give quick and forceful thrusts until the object is expelled from the patient's mouth or the patient becomes unconscious.***				
7. ✦	***If the patient becomes unconscious, gently lower him or her to the ground.***				
8. ✶	Activate EMS and put on gloves.				
9. ✶	Immediately begin CPR with 30 chest compressions and 2 rescue breaths.				
10. ✶	***Before administering the rescue breaths, open the airway with the head-tilt, chin-lift maneuver. Look for a foreign body in the patient's mouth and remove any that is visible.*** *Note:* Blind finger sweeps are no longer recommended and should NOT be performed.				
11. ✦	Continue with cycles of 30 compressions and 2 rescue breaths until the foreign body is expelled or advanced medical personal arrive to relieve you.				
12. ✦	Wash your hands and document the event in the patient's chart.				

Name: ______________________________

Date: ______________________________

Document: Enter the appropriate information in the chart below.

Grading

Points Earned	______		
Points Possible	______	93	93
Percent Grade (Points Earned/Points Possible)	______		
PASS:	______	❑ YES ❑ NO ❑ N/A	❑ YES ❑ NO ❑ N/A

Instructor Sign-Off

Instructor: ______________________________ **Date:** ______________

Name: ______________________________

Date: ______________________________

Procedure 43-5:

Administer Oxygen

Objective: Correctly administer oxygen therapy to an adult within the time frame designated by the instructor.

Supplies: Portable oxygen tank; pressure regulator; oxygen flow meter; sterile, prepackaged, disposable nasal cannula with tubing; gloves; oximeter; patient's record

Affective Behaviors: Affective behaviors provide a professional approach to a skill that enhances the patient encounter. These behaviors may also display sensitivity to a patient's rights and enhance communication. Pay close attention to these skills, which will be in ***bold, italicized*** font.

Notes to the Student

____

____

____

____

____

____

Skills Assessment Requirements

Read and familiarize yourself with the procedure; complete the minimum practice requirements. Document each MPR using proper charting technique. Complete each procedure within a reasonable amount of time, with a minimum of 85% accuracy.

Name: ______________________________

Date: ______________________________

POINT VALUE
✦ = 3–6 points
✶ = 7–9 points

		PRACTICE TRIAL	GRADED TRIAL # 1	GRADED TRIAL # 2	NOTES
1. ✦	Gather all needed equipment.				
2. ✦	Perform proper hand hygiene.				
3. ✶	***Identify the patient and warmly greet him or her. State your name and confirm the physician's order for oxygen therapy.***				
4. ✦	Check the pressure reading on the oxygen tank to make sure the tank has enough oxygen in it.				
5. ✦	Start the flow of oxygen by opening the cylinder.				
6. ✦	Attach the cannula tubing to the flow meter. Adjust the oxygen flow to the physician's order.				
7. ✦	Hold the cannula tips over the inside of your wrist, without touching the skin, to determine if the oxygen is flowing.				
8. ✦	Apply gloves.				
9. ✦	Place the tips of the nasal cannula into the patient's nostrils. Wrap the tubing behind the patient's ears.				
10. ✦	Instruct the patient to breathe normally through the mouth and nose. (Some patients instinctively hold their breath or avoid breathing through the nose when an object is placed in the nostrils.)				

Name: ______________________________

Date: ______________________________

POINT VALUE
✦ = 3–6 points
✶ = 7–9 points

		PRACTICE TRIAL	GRADED TRIAL # 1	GRADED TRIAL # 2	NOTES
11. ✦	Check the patient's oxygen level with an oximeter. Place the probe over the index finger and record the reading. If necessary, have the patient take a short walk to verify that the oxygen flow rate is sufficient for activity.				
12. ✶	***Ask the patient if he or she has any questions, thank the patient and bid him or her a good day,*** and document the procedure in the patient's chart.				

Name: ______________________________

Date: ______________________________

Document: Enter the correct information in the chart below.

Grading

Points Earned	______		
Points Possible	______	78	78
Percent Grade (Points Earned/Points Possible)	______		
PASS:	______	❑ YES ❑ NO ❑ N/A	❑ YES ❑ NO ❑ N/A

Instructor Sign-Off

Instructor: ______________________________ **Date:** ______________

Name: ______________________________

Date: ______________________________

Procedure 43-6:

Demonstrate the Application of a Pressure Bandage

Objective: Correctly demonstrate the application of a pressure dressing.

Supplies: Dressing supplies or makeshift materials; gloves and other PPE; biohazard waste container

Affective Behaviors: Affective behaviors provide a professional approach to a skill that enhances the patient encounter. These behaviors may also display sensitivity to a patient's rights and enhance communication. Pay close attention to these skills, which will be in ***bold, italicized*** font.

Notes to the Student

____

____

____

____

____

____

Skills Assessment Requirements

Read and familiarize yourself with the procedure; complete the minimum practice requirements. Document each MPR using proper charting technique. Complete each procedure within a reasonable amount of time, with a minimum of 85% accuracy.

Name: ______________________________

Date: ______________________________

POINT VALUE
✦ = 3–6 points
✶ = 7–9 points

		PRACTICE TRIAL	GRADED TRIAL # 1	GRADED TRIAL # 2	NOTES
1. ✦	***Immediately escort the patient to an examination room.***				
2. ✦	Perform proper hand hygiene. Gather all necessary supplies.				
3. ✶	Apply gloves and other appropriate PPE.				
4. ✶	Under the physician's supervision, ***apply direct pressure with a dressing placed on the open wound***. ***If possible, elevate the affected part.***				
5. ✦	After assessment, the physician will decide if EMS should be contacted.				
6. ✦	Apply additional dressings as needed. Do not remove the original dressing.				
7. ✶	Apply pressure to pressure points as necessary and with the physician's supervision.				
8. ✶	If bleeding is controlled, anchor the dressing to maintain pressure.				
9. ✦	***If the physician orders, prepare the patient for transport to an emergency care facility.***				
10. ✶	Dispose of waste in a biohazard waste container.				
11. ✦	Remove and discard gloves.				
12. ✶	Perform proper hand hygiene and document the procedure in the patient's chart.				

Name: ____________________

Date: ____________________

Document: Enter the appropriate information in the chart below.

Grading

Points Earned	_______		
Points Possible	_______	90	90
Percent Grade (Points Earned/Points Possible)	_______		
PASS:	_______	❏ YES ❏ NO ❏ N/A	❏ YES ❏ NO ❏ N/A

Instructor Sign-Off

Instructor: ____________________ **Date:** ____________________

Name: ______________________________

Date: ______________________________

Procedure 43-7:

Demonstrate the Application of Triangular, Figure-Eight, and Tubular Bandages

Objective: Correctly apply triangular, figure-eight, and tubular bandaging.

Supplies: Elastic bandage; roller bandage; Kling™ bandage; tubular gauze and applicator; triangular bandage; tape; scissors

Affective Behaviors: Affective behaviors provide a professional approach to a skill that enhances the patient encounter. These behaviors may also display sensitivity to a patient's rights and enhance communication. Pay close attention to these skills, which will be in ***bold, italicized*** font.

Notes to the Student

____

____

____

____

____

____

Skills Assessment Requirements

Read and familiarize yourself with the procedure; complete the minimum practice requirements. Document each MPR using proper charting technique. Complete each procedure within a reasonable amount of time, with a minimum of 85% accuracy.

Name: ______________________

Date: ______________________

POINT VALUE
✦ = 3–6 points
✶ = 7–9 points

		PRACTICE TRIAL	GRADED TRIAL # 1	GRADED TRIAL # 2	NOTES
1. ✦	***Immediately escort the patient to an examination room. Identify yourself to the patient.*** You may need to assist the patient, depending on the severity, location, and type of injury.				
2. ✦	***Explain the procedure to the patient.***				
3. ✦	Perform proper hand hygiene.				
4. ✦	Gather necessary supplies.				
5. ✶	**Triangular bandage:** • Keep the injured arm as immobile as possible. • Carefully slide the triangular bandage under the area to be held. The two shorter sides of the triangle should be pointing toward the elbow, and the remaining longer edge should be parallel to the opposite body side. • Bring the lowest side of the triangle up and over the arm. • Tie the ends of the bandage behind and slightly to the side of the neck. • Tuck the peak of the bandage in toward the elbow point of the bandage. • The triangular bandage may also be wrapped around the head as a turban to anchor dressings onto the head.				

Name: ______________________________

Date: ______________________________

POINT VALUE
✦ = 3–6 points
✶ = 7–9 points

		PRACTICE TRIAL	GRADED TRIAL # 1	GRADED TRIAL # 2	NOTES
6. ✶	**Figure 8 bandage:** • Place the thumb of one hand on one end of the bandage to hold it in place. • Anchor the bandage with your other hand, and then complete one circle around the extremity or body part. • Continue to alternate wrapping above and below the body joint or dressing and circling behind the joint or dressing area until the injured area is covered adequately.				
7. ✶	**Tubular bandage:** • Choose an applicator that is larger than the extremity to be bandaged. Anchor the bandage with your other hand, and then complete one circle around the extremity or body part. • Cut an approximate amount of tubular gauze bandage and slide the gathered bandage onto the applicator. • Slide the applicator over the extremity. • Hold the bandage against the proximal end of the extremity and pull the applicator approximately 1 inch past the distal end. • Twist the bandage gauze one complete turn. • Next, slide the applicator toward the proximal end of the injury. *(continued)*				

Name: ______________________

Date: ______________________

POINT VALUE
✦ = 3–6 points
✶ = 7–9 points

		PRACTICE TRIAL	GRADED TRIAL # 1	GRADED TRIAL # 2	NOTES
	Tubular bandage: *(continued)* • Hold the proximal end of the tubular bandage gauze in place, and pull the applicator toward the distal end. • After pulling past the distal end, complete one twist. • Slide back and forth and twist the distal end of the dressing until the injured area is adequately covered. • Cut excess dressing, but remember to anchor the bandage at the proximal end.				
8. ✶	***Instruct the patient to watch for signs of circulation impairment.***				
9. ✦	Perform proper hand hygiene.				
10. ✶	Document the procedure and patient teaching.				

Name: ____________________

Date: ____________________

Document: Enter the correct information in the chart below.

Grading

Points Earned	______		
Points Possible	______	75	75
Percent Grade (Points Earned/Points Possible)	______		
PASS:	______	❏ YES ❏ NO ❏ N/A	❏ YES ❏ NO ❏ N/A

Instructor Sign-Off

Instructor: ____________________ **Date:** ____________________

Name: ______________________________

Date: ______________________________

Procedure 43-8:

Respond to a Patient Who Has Fainted

Objective: Correctly care for a patient who has fainted, within the time limit set by the instructor.

Supplies: Blanket; footstool or box

Affective Behaviors: Affective behaviors provide a professional approach to a skill that enhances the patient encounter. These behaviors may also display sensitivity to a patient's rights and enhance communication. Pay close attention to these skills, which will be in ***bold, italicized*** font.

Notes to the Student

____

____

____

____

____

____

Skills Assessment Requirements

Read and familiarize yourself with the procedure; complete the minimum practice requirements. Document each MPR using proper charting technique. Complete each procedure within a reasonable amount of time, with a minimum of 85% accuracy.

Name: ______________________________

Date: ______________________________

POINT VALUE
✦ = 3–6 points
✶ = 7–9 points

		PRACTICE TRIAL	GRADED TRIAL # 1	GRADED TRIAL # 2	NOTES
1. ✦	***If the patient communicates a faint feeling, help the patient sit, bend forward, and place the head on the knees. If the patient collapses with no warning, do not move the patient.*** The patient may have sustained a neck or back injury.				
2. ✦	Remain calm and notify the physician.				
3. ✦	***Loosen any tight clothing and cover the patient with the blanket for warmth.***				
4. ✦	***If the physician directs, use the footstool to support the patient's legs in a raised position.***				
5. ✦	If the physician directs, call for EMS.				
6. ✶	Once the emergency passes, Obtain a full set of vital signs and document all activities in the patient's medical record.				

Name: ____________________

Date: ____________________

Document: Enter the appropriate information in the chart below.

Grading

Points Earned	_______		
Points Possible	_______	39	39
Percent Grade (Points Earned/Points Possible)	_______		
PASS:	_______	❑ YES ❑ NO ❑ N/A	❑ YES ❑ NO ❑ N/A

Instructor Sign-Off

Instructor: ____________________ **Date:** ____________________

Name: ______________________________

Date: ______________________________

Procedure 43-9:

Demonstrate the Application of a Splint

Objective: Correctly apply a splint with minimal movement to the affected extremity and without impairment to circulation or neurological status.

Supplies: Makeshift or sterile dressing supplies; stiff or solid materials to immobilize the extremity; bandages or strips of material to secure splint materials

Affective Behaviors: Affective behaviors provide a professional approach to a skill that enhances the patient encounter. These behaviors may also display sensitivity to a patient's rights and enhance communication. Pay close attention to these skills, which will be in ***bold, italicized*** font.

Notes to the Student

____

____

____

____

____

____

Skills Assessment Requirements

Read and familiarize yourself with the procedure; complete the minimum practice requirements. Document each MPR using proper charting technique. Complete each procedure within a reasonable amount of time, with a minimum of 85% accuracy.

Name: ____________________

Date: ____________________

POINT VALUE
✦ = 3–6 points
✶ = 7–9 points

		PRACTICE TRIAL	GRADED TRIAL # 1	GRADED TRIAL # 2	NOTES
1. ✦	***Identify the patient and introduce yourself.***				
2. ✦	Obtain vital signs.				
3. ✦	***Ask the patient, if conscious, to speak his or her name.***				
4. ✶	***Ask about medication allergies and any prescription or over-the-counter medications the patient may be taking. Also inquire about the patient's medical history.***				
5. ✦	Assess the area of suspected fracture for bruising, bleeding, and open areas or protruding bones.				
6. ✶	***Moving the limb as little as possible and with gentle traction on the distal side, place the splint with padding under the limb or alongside the limb. You may have to ask other clinical staff for help to ensure the least amount of discomfort for the least amount of time.***				
7. ✦	Gently place sterile dressings or clean makeshift dressings over open areas.				
8. ✶	***Secure the splint by wrapping bandages or strips of material around the splint and the limb. The ties must be above and below the joints on both sides of the suspected fracture.***				

Name: ______________________________

Date: ______________________________

POINT VALUE
✦ = 3–6 points
✶ = 7–9 points

		PRACTICE TRIAL	GRADED TRIAL # 1	GRADED TRIAL # 2	NOTES
9. ✦	Add additional ties as necessary along the length of the splint.				
10. ✦	If possible, leave an exposed area, such as toes or fingers, so that circulation can be monitored.				
11. ✶	The splint should be snug enough to immobilize the limb, but not tight.				
12. ✶	Document the procedure in the patient's chart.				

Name: ______________________________

Date: ______________________________

Document: Enter the correct information in the chart below.

Grading

Points Earned	_______		
Points Possible	_______	87	87
Percent Grade (Points Earned/Points Possible)	_______		
PASS:	_______	❑ YES ❑ NO ❑ N/A	❑ YES ❑ NO ❑ N/A

Instructor Sign-Off

Instructor: ______________________________ **Date:** ______________________

Name: ______________________________

Date: ______________________________

Procedure 43-10:

Develop an Environmental Exposure Plan

Objective: Develop an environmental exposure plan.

Supplies: Pen, paper, computer, copy machine, various emergency supplies, waterproof containers

Affective Behaviors: Affective behaviors provide a professional approach to a skill that enhances the patient encounter. These behaviors may also display sensitivity to a patient's rights and enhance communication. Pay close attention to these skills, which will be in ***bold, italicized*** font.

Notes to the Student

____

____

____

____

____

____

Skills Assessment Requirements

Read and familiarize yourself with the procedure; complete the minimum practice requirements. Document each MPR using proper charting technique. Complete each procedure within a reasonable amount of time, with a minimum of 85% accuracy.

Name: ____________________

Date: ____________________

POINT VALUE
✦ = 3–6 points
✶ = 7–9 points

		PRACTICE TRIAL	GRADED TRIAL # 1	GRADED TRIAL # 2	NOTES
1. ✦	Create an emergency kit that can be used by your office in the event of an environmental emergency. Supplies may include flashlights; batteries; bottles of water; nonperishable food; bandages; alcohol and hydrogen peroxide; blankets; vinyl or latex gloves; tweezers; scissors; a self-powered radio; and medications (ibuprofen, acetaminophen, antihistamines, antibiotic ointment, tetanus vaccines, etc.).				
2. ✦	Enclose the kit in a waterproof container.				
3. ✦	Place the kit is a safe area, such as the medicine closet or storage closet.				
4. ✦	Create evacuation plans and make sure that every room in the medical office has a detailed exit route posted.				
5. ✦	Create a delineation chart that outlines responsibilities of office staff members in the event of an emergency.				
6. ✦	Create a list of safety zones that can be used in the event of an emergency (e.g., a safety zone for use in the event of a tornado, an outdoor safety zone for use in the event of a fire, a safety zone for use in the event of a flood).				

Name: ______________________________

Date: ______________________________

POINT VALUE
✦ = 3–6 points
✶ = 7–9 points

		PRACTICE TRIAL	GRADED TRIAL # 1	GRADED TRIAL # 2	NOTES
7. ✦	Make photocopies of the safety zone list, evacuation plan, and delineation chart for everyone in the office. Laminate and hang copies in the employee break room.				
8. ✦	Train all office staff on the environmental exposure plan within 10 days of hire.				

Name: ______________________________

Date: ______________________________

Document: Enter the appropriate information in the chart below.

Grading

Points Earned	______		
Points Possible	______	48	48
Percent Grade (Points Earned/Points Possible)	______		
PASS:	______	❑ YES ❑ NO ❑ N/A	❑ YES ❑ NO ❑ N/A

Instructor Sign-Off

Instructor: ______________________________ **Date:** ______________

Name: ______________________________

Date: ______________________________

Procedure 44-1:

Using and Cleaning the Microscope

Objective: Properly observe a slide under the microscope using 10×, 40×, and 100× oil immersion, and correctly clean and store the microscope.

Supplies: Microscope, specimen slide, lens paper, lens cleaner, dust cover for microscope

Affective Behaviors: Affective behaviors provide a professional approach to a skill that enhances the patient encounter. These behaviors may also display sensitivity to a patient's rights and enhance communication. Pay close attention to these skills, which will be in ***bold, italicized*** font.

Notes to the Student

____

____

____

____

____

____

Skills Assessment Requirements

Read and familiarize yourself with the procedure; complete the minimum practice requirements. Document each MPR using proper charting technique. Complete each procedure within a reasonable amount of time, with a minimum of 85% accuracy.

Name: ______________________________

Date: ______________________________

POINT VALUE
✦ = 3–6 points
✶ = 7–9 points

		PRACTICE TRIAL	GRADED TRIAL # 1	GRADED TRIAL # 2	NOTES
1. ✶	Carry the microscope with on hand on the arm and one hand supporting the base.				
2. ✦	Check to see that the stage is in the down position before beginning.				
3. ✦	Clean objectives with lens paper starting with 10× and ending with oil immersion (100×).				
4. ✦	Turn on the light. Rotate the nosepiece to the 10× objective over the stage.				
5. ✦	Place the prepared slide on the stage.				
6. ✦	Use the coarse adjustment knob to raise the stage until the objective is close to the slide on the stage.				
7. ✦	Look through the eyepiece and adjust the coarse focus knob until the microscope field is seen.				
8. ✦	Use the fine adjustment knob for a clearer image.				
9. ✦	Open the diaphragm; adjust the rheostat to focus, if necessary.				
10. ✦	Raise or lower the condenser to alter light refraction.				
11. ✦	Observe the slide.				
12. ✦	Change the objective to 40× and readjust. Use oil on 100× oil immersion.				

Name: ______________________________

Date: ______________________________

POINT VALUE
✦ = 3–6 points
✶ = 7–9 points

		PRACTICE TRIAL	GRADED TRIAL # 1	GRADED TRIAL # 2	NOTES
13.✶	When you are finished, always lower the stage before removing the slide.				
14. ✦	Turn off the light.				
15. ✦	Clean the eyepieces and objectives with lens paper, and the oil immersion lens with lens cleaner.				
16. ✦	Unplug the electrical cord and wrap it around the base.				
17. ✶	Cover the microscope with the dust cover.				
18. ✦	Clean the slide, and store or discard it in the appropriate sharps container.				

Name: ______________________________

Date: ______________________________

Document: Enter the appropriate information in the chart below.

Grading

Points Earned	______		
Points Possible	______	117	117
Percent Grade (Points Earned/Points Possible)	______		
PASS:	______	❑ YES ❑ NO ❑ N/A	❑ YES ❑ NO ❑ N/A

Instructor Sign-Off

Instructor: ______________________________ **Date:** ______________

Name: ______________________________

Date: ______________________________

Procedure 44-2:

Completing a Laboratory Requisition and Preparing a Specimen for Transport to an Outside Laboratory

Objective: Accurately complete a laboratory requisition form for specimen testing. Obtain and prepare the specimen(s) for transport to an outside laboratory.

Supplies: Order for laboratory test, patient's record, pen, laboratory requisition form, gloves, specimen container, laboratory logbook, biohazard waste container

Affective Behaviors: Affective behaviors provide a professional approach to a skill that enhances the patient encounter. These behaviors may also display sensitivity to a patient's rights and enhance communication. Pay close attention to these skills, which will be in ***bold, italicized*** font.

Notes to the Student

____

____

____

____

____

____

Skills Assessment Requirements

Read and familiarize yourself with the procedure; complete the minimum practice requirements. Document each MPR using proper charting technique. Complete each procedure within a reasonable amount of time, with a minimum of 85% accuracy.

Name: ______________________________

Date: ______________________________

POINT VALUE ✦ = 3–6 points ✶ = 7–9 points		PRACTICE TRIAL	GRADED TRIAL # 1	GRADED TRIAL # 2	NOTES
1. ✦	Check the patient record for lab tests orders.				
2. ✦	Verify which lab will complete the testing and locate the correct requisition form.				
3. ✦	Complete the patient demographic section.				
4. ✦	Complete the section requiring the physician's name, address, phone number, and account number.				
5. ✦	Complete the patient's insurance and billing information (if applicable).				
6. ✶	Clearly mark each box to indicate each test ordered by the physician. If a test is ordered and is not listed on the requisition, clearly write the name of the test on the lines provided.				
7. ✦	Indicate the type and source of the specimen to be tested.				
8. ✦	Enter the patient's diagnosis on the requisition.				
9. ✦	Verify that the patient's authorization of release and assignment of benefits has been completed.				
10. ✦	Assemble equipment and supplies needed to obtain the specimen.				
11. ✦	Perform proper hand hygiene and apply gloves.				
12. ✦	***Explain the procedure to the patient, ask for questions***, and obtain the specimen.				

Name: ______________________________

Date: ______________________________

POINT VALUE
✦ = 3–6 points
✶ = 7–9 points

		PRACTICE TRIAL	GRADED TRIAL # 1	GRADED TRIAL # 2	NOTES
13. ✶	Label the specimen with the patient's name, date, physician's name, time of collection, and other required information per facility protocol.				
14. ✦	Record the date and time of specimen collection on the laboratory requisition form.				
15. ✦	Process the specimens as needed or store appropriately until sent out.				
16. ✶	Attach the requisition securely to the specimen.				
17. ✦	Remove gloves and discard in biohazard waste container. Perform proper hand hygiene.				
18. ✦	Document in patient's record.				
19. ✦	Record specimen in laboratory logbook; include date, time of collection, receiving laboratory, and date specimen was sent.				

Name: ______________________

Date: ______________________

Document: Enter the appropriate information in the chart below.

Grading

Points Earned	______		
Points Possible	______	123	123
Percent Grade (Points Earned/Points Possible)	______		
PASS:	______	❑ YES ❑ NO ❑ N/A	❑ YES ❑ NO ❑ N/A

Instructor Sign-Off

Instructor: ______________________ **Date:** ______________________

Name: ______________________________

Date: ______________________________

Procedure 44-3:

Monitoring and Following up on Laboratory Test Results

Objective: Accurately review laboratory results and follow up with patient per physician's orders.

Supplies: Patient's record, laboratory test results, pen, log of patient's laboratory results

Affective Behaviors: Affective behaviors provide a professional approach to a skill that enhances the patient encounter. These behaviors may also display sensitivity to a patient's rights and enhance communication. Pay close attention to these skills, which will be in ***bold, italicized*** font.

Notes to the Student

____

____

____

____

____

____

Skills Assessment Requirements

Read and familiarize yourself with the procedure; complete the minimum practice requirements. Document each MPR using proper charting technique. Complete each procedure within a reasonable amount of time, with a minimum of 85% accuracy.

Name: ______________________________

Date: ______________________________

POINT VALUE
✦ = 3–6 points
✶ = 7–9 points

		PRACTICE TRIAL	GRADED TRIAL # 1	GRADED TRIAL # 2	NOTES
1. ✦	Review incoming lab results and compare them with the reference values provided by the lab. Abnormally high or low levels will be indicated by an H or an L.				
2. ✶	Highlight any abnormal results per facility policy. *Note:* Follow facility policy on contacting patients when results are abnormal. Results are NOT to be released to patient unless authorized by the physician.				
3. ✦	Attach laboratory results to patient's record and submit for physician's review. *Note:* Accuracy is critical when entering data electronically.				
4. ✦	Follow physician's orders regarding scheduling appointments or repeat testing.				
5. ✦	Document in patient's record accordingly.				

Name: ____________________

Date: ____________________

Document: Enter the appropriate information in the chart below.

Grading

Points Earned	______		
Points Possible	______	33	33
Percent Grade (Points Earned/Points Possible)	______		
PASS:	______	❑ YES ❑ NO ❑ N/A	❑ YES ❑ NO ❑ N/A

Instructor Sign-Off

Instructor: ____________________ **Date:** ____________________

Name: ______________________________

Date: ______________________________

Procedure 45-1:

Preparing a Smear

Objective: Prepare a smear for microscopic examination without error.

Supplies: Slides; thumb forceps; specimen from Culturette applicator; loop or swab; Bunsen burner (or methanol); microscope; oil immersion; gloves; biohazard waste container

Affective Behaviors: Affective behaviors provide a professional approach to a skill that enhances the patient encounter. These behaviors may also display sensitivity to a patient's rights and enhance communication. Pay close attention to these skills, which will be in ***bold, italicized*** font.

Notes to the Student

____

____

____

____

____

____

Skills Assessment Requirements

Read and familiarize yourself with the procedure; complete the minimum practice requirements. Document each MPR using proper charting technique. Complete each procedure within a reasonable amount of time, with a minimum of 85% accuracy.

Name: ______________________

Date: ______________________

POINT VALUE
✦ = 3–6 points
✶ = 7–9 points

		PRACTICE TRIAL	GRADED TRIAL # 1	GRADED TRIAL # 2	NOTES
1. ✦	Perform proper hand hygiene and apply gloves.				
2. ✦	Assemble equipment.				
3. ✦	Label a clean slide with patient's name, date, and type of specimen.				
4. ✶	Inoculate the slide by transferring the specimen to the slide by rolling a swab over the slide, ensuring that all areas of the swab touch the slide, or placing a drop of sterile saline on the slide after flaming a needle or loop. Pick up material from one type of colony, place it on the saline, and spread it gently over two-thirds of the slide.				
5. ✦	Allow the slide to dry for 20–30 minutes.				
6. ✶	Hold the slide with thumb forceps and pass the slide over the Bunsen burner flame. Let the slide cool, or flood the dry smear with methanol and let it dry to fix the slide if an open flame is not available.				
7. ✦	The slide is then ready to be stained.				

Name: ______________________________

Date: ______________________________

Document: Enter the appropriate information in the chart below.

Grading

Points Earned	______		
Points Possible	______	48	48
Percent Grade (Points Earned/Points Possible)	______		
PASS:	______	❑ YES ❑ NO ❑ N/A	❑ YES ❑ NO ❑ N/A

Instructor Sign-Off

Instructor: ______________________________ **Date:** ______________

Name: ______________________________

Date: ______________________________

Procedure 45-2:

Preparing a Wet Mount Slide

Objective: Prepare a wet mount slide for microscopic examination without error.

Supplies: Slides; cover slip; saline; specimen from a Culturette applicator or swab; paper/pen; microscope; gloves

Affective Behaviors: Affective behaviors provide a professional approach to a skill that enhances the patient encounter. These behaviors may also display sensitivity to a patient's rights and enhance communication. Pay close attention to these skills, which will be in ***bold, italicized*** font.

Notes to the Student

Observation and staining of the slide will be performed by a physician or laboratory specialist.

____

____

____

____

____

Skills Assessment Requirements

Read and familiarize yourself with the procedure; complete the minimum practice requirements. Document each MPR using proper charting technique. Complete each procedure within a reasonable amount of time, with a minimum of 85% accuracy.

Name: ______________________________

Date: ______________________________

POINT VALUE
✦ = 3–6 points
✶ = 7–9 points

		PRACTICE TRIAL	GRADED TRIAL # 1	GRADED TRIAL # 2	NOTES
1. ✦	Assemble all equipment.				
2. ✦	Use proper hand hygiene and apply gloves.				
3. ✶	Label a dry slide with the patient's name and the date.				
4. ✦	Inoculate the dry slide by rolling a swab containing the specimen across the surface.				
5. ✦	Place a drop of saline solution on top of the specimen.				
6. ✦	Place a cover slip on top of the smeared slide.				
7. ✦	Remove your gloves and wash your hands.				
8. ✶	Document the findings in the patient's record.				

Name: ____________________

Date: ____________________

Document: Enter the appropriate information in the chart below.

Grading

Points Earned	_______		
Points Possible	_______	54	54
Percent Grade (Points Earned/Points Possible)	_______		
PASS:	_______	❑ YES ❑ NO ❑ N/A	❑ YES ❑ NO ❑ N/A

Instructor Sign-Off

Instructor: ____________________ **Date:** ____________________

Name: ______________________________

Date: ______________________________

Procedure 45-3:

Performing a Gram Stain

Objective: Prepare a slide for a Gram stain in order to differentiate a gram-positive organism from a gram-negative organism.

Supplies: Gram-stain kit with decolorization, culture specimen, slides, Bunsen burner (or methanol), staining rack, water wash bottle, sink with water, immersion oil, stopwatch, gloves, slide stand, paper towels, biohazard waste container

Affective Behaviors: Affective behaviors provide a professional approach to a skill that enhances the patient encounter. These behaviors may also display sensitivity to a patient's rights and enhance communication. Pay close attention to these skills, which will be in ***bold, italicized*** font.

Notes to the Student

Examination of a Gram stain slide is beyond the scope of practice of medical assisting. It must be performed by a physician or laboratory specialist.

____

____

____

____

____

Skills Assessment Requirements

Read and familiarize yourself with the procedure; complete the minimum practice requirements. Document each MPR using proper charting technique. Complete each procedure within a reasonable amount of time, with a minimum of 85% accuracy.

Name: ______________________________

Date: ______________________________

POINT VALUE
✦ = 3–6 points
✶ = 7–9 points

		PRACTICE TRIAL	GRADED TRIAL # 1	GRADED TRIAL # 2	NOTES
1. ✦	Assemble all equipment.				
2. ✦	Use proper hand hygiene and apply gloves.				
3. ✦	Make a smear, label it, and allow it to air dry. Methanol or heat-fix the slide.				
4. ✦	Place the slide on a staining rack, smear side up.				
5. ✶	Pour crystal violet solution all over the slide. Let it stand for 1 minute.				
6. ✦	Tilt the slide, drain excess solution, and rinse it with water.				
7. ✶	Pour Gram's iodine stain all over the slide. Let it stand for 1 minute.				
8. ✦	Tilt the slide, drain excess iodine, and rinse it with water.				
9. ✶	Gently pour decolorizer with alcohol-acetone all over the slide for 15 seconds or until the color blue stops running.				
10. ✦	Rinse the slide with water.				
11. ✶	Pour safranin stain all over the slide. Let it stand for 30 seconds.				
12. ✦	Tilt the slide to drain excess stain and rinse with water. Wipe the back of the slide.				
13. ✦	Stand the slide on end on a paper towel or in a slide drying rack. Allow it to air dry.				
14. ✦	Examine the slide under a microscope using an oil immersion lens and oil.				

Name: ______________________________

Date: ______________________________

Document: Enter the appropriate information in the chart below.

Grading

Points Earned	_____		
Points Possible	_____	96	96
Percent Grade (Points Earned/Points Possible)	_____		
PASS:	_____	❑ YES ❑ NO ❑ N/A	❑ YES ❑ NO ❑ N/A

Instructor Sign-Off

Instructor: ______________________________ **Date:** ____________________

Name: ______________________________

Date: ______________________________

Procedure 45-4:

Obtaining a Throat Culture

Objective: Collect a throat or nasopharyngeal culture without contaminating the specimen.

Supplies: Culturette system, laboratory requisition, tongue depressor, gloves, biohazard waste container

Affective Behaviors: Affective behaviors provide a professional approach to a skill that enhances the patient encounter. These behaviors may also display sensitivity to a patient's rights and enhance communication. Pay close attention to these skills, which will be in ***bold, italicized*** font.

Notes to the Student

____

____

____

____

____

____

Skills Assessment Requirements

Read and familiarize yourself with the procedure; complete the minimum practice requirements. Document each MPR using proper charting technique. Complete each procedure within a reasonable amount of time, with a minimum of 85% accuracy.

Name: ___________________________

Date: ___________________________

POINT VALUE
✦ = 3–6 points
✶ = 7–9 points

		PRACTICE TRIAL	GRADED TRIAL # 1	GRADED TRIAL # 2	NOTES
1. ✦	Assemble all equipment.				
2. ✦	***Identify the patient and explain the procedure.***				
3. ✦	Perform proper hand hygiene and apply gloves.				
4. ✶	Position the patient facing a light source and instruct the patient to open his or her mouth as wide as possible and say "Aaaaah" (to diminish the gag reflex).				
5. ✦	Remove sterile swab from the Culturette.				
6. ✶	Depress the tongue, insert the swab, and roll it firmly across the back of the patient's throat or nasopharyngeal area where infected. Avoid the uvula. *Note:* Be careful not to contaminate the swab on the teeth, lips, tongue, or cheeks.				
7. ✶	Insert the swab in a plastic vial. Crush an internal vial of transport medium; make sure that the swab is saturated.				
8. ✦ 9. ✦	Place the swab in a labeled mailing/transport envelope and seal it shut or immediately inoculate culture plate if specimen is to be analyzed on site. Remove and dispose of gloves. Perform proper hand hygiene.				
10. ✶	Document the procedure in the patient's record.				

Name: ______________________________

Date: ______________________________

Document: Enter the appropriate information in the chart below.

Grading

Points Earned	_______		
Points Possible	_______	72	72
Percent Grade (Points Earned/Points Possible)	_______		
PASS:	_______	❑ YES ❑ NO ❑ N/A	❑ YES ❑ NO ❑ N/A

Instructor Sign-Off

Instructor: ______________________________ **Date:** ______________________

Name: ______________________________

Date: ______________________________

Procedure 45-5:

Obtaining a Sputum Specimen for Culture

Objective: Obtain a sputum specimen without contamination.

Supplies: Sterile sputum container with lid, laboratory requisition form, gloves, biohazard waste container

Affective Behaviors: Affective behaviors provide a professional approach to a skill that enhances the patient encounter. These behaviors may also display sensitivity to a patient's rights and enhance communication. Pay close attention to these skills, which will be in ***bold, italicized*** font.

Notes to the Student

____

____

____

____

____

____

Skills Assessment Requirements

Read and familiarize yourself with the procedure; complete the minimum practice requirements. Document each MPR using proper charting technique. Complete each procedure within a reasonable amount of time, with a minimum of 85% accuracy.

Name: ______________________________

Date: ______________________________

POINT VALUE
✦ = 3–6 points
✶ = 7–9 points

		PRACTICE TRIAL	GRADED TRIAL # 1	GRADED TRIAL # 2	NOTES
1. ✦	Assemble all equipment.				
2. ✦	Perform proper hand hygiene.				
3. ✶	***Identify the patient and explain the procedure.*** Provide written instructions that the patient can take home if necessary.				
4. ✦	Don gloves.				
5. ✶	***Instruct the patient to breathe in or out 2 to 4 times and cough deeply to raise sputum.*** Instruct the patient to expel the fluid into the center of the specimen container. A morning specimen is preferable.				
6. ✦	Be sure that no other fluids enter the cup, such as tears, mucus, or saliva.				
7. ✦	Place the lid securely on the container, and write the time and date the specimen was obtained. *Note:* If the patient is collecting the specimen at home, he or she should bring the sample into the office as soon as possible. The sample should not be refrigerated for more than 2 hours.				
8. ✶	Label the envelope with information, seal it shut, and transport it immediately.				
9. ✦	Remove and dispose of gloves. Perform proper hand hygiene.				
10. ✶	Document the procedure in the patient's record.				

Name: ______________________________

Date: ______________________________

Document: Enter the appropriate information in the chart below.

Grading

Points Earned	_______		
Points Possible	_______	72	72
Percent Grade (Points Earned/Points Possible)	_______		
PASS:	_______	❑ YES ❑ NO ❑ N/A	❑ YES ❑ NO ❑ N/A

Instructor Sign-Off

Instructor: ______________________________ **Date:** ______________

Name: ______________________________

Date: ______________________________

Procedure 45-6:

Performing a Urine Culture

Objective: Inoculate a urine plate to aid in the identification of a urinary tract infection.

Supplies: Lab requisition form, urine specimen, incinerator (electric or Bunsen burner), inoculating loop, agar plates, gloves, biohazard waste container

Affective Behaviors: Affective behaviors provide a professional approach to a skill that enhances the patient encounter. These behaviors may also display sensitivity to a patient's rights and enhance communication. Pay close attention to these skills, which will be in ***bold, italicized*** font.

Notes to the Student

____

____

____

____

____

____

Skills Assessment Requirements

Read and familiarize yourself with the procedure; complete the minimum practice requirements. Document each MPR using proper charting technique. Complete each procedure within a reasonable amount of time, with a minimum of 85% accuracy.

Name: ______________________

Date: ______________________

POINT VALUE
✦ = 3–6 points
✶ = 7–9 points

		PRACTICE TRIAL	GRADED TRIAL # 1	GRADED TRIAL # 2	NOTES
1. ✦	Assemble all equipment.				
2. ✦	Perform proper hand hygiene.				
3. ✦	Apply gloves and face protection.				
4. ✶	Verify that the name on the laboratory requisition and the specimen are the same.				
5. ✦	Swirl the urine sample to mix it. (Be sure that the lid is on.)				
6. ✶	Sterilize the loop, remove the lid, and place it between the inoculating plates.				
7. ✶	Inoculate each media plate in a pattern to allow for isolated colonies.				
8. ✶	Label the bottom of the plates with patient name, date, and type of specimen.				
9. ✶	Place the media in an incubator with the agar side up for 24 hours.				
10. ✦	Clean the area. Remove and dispose of the gloves.				
11. ✦	Perform proper hand hygiene.				
12. ✶	Document the procedure in the patient's record.				

Name: ______________________

Date: ______________________

Document: Enter the appropriate information in the chart below.

Grading

Points Earned	______		
Points Possible	______	90	90
Percent Grade (Points Earned/Points Possible)	______		
PASS:	______	❑ YES ❑ NO ❑ N/A	❑ YES ❑ NO ❑ N/A

Instructor Sign-Off

Instructor: ______________________ **Date:** ______________________

Name: ______________________________

Date: ______________________________

Procedure 45-7:

Obtaining a Stool Specimen for Culture and Sensitivity

Objective: Clearly instruct a patient on how to collect a stool sample for culture and sensitivity in a sterile container using correct infection control procedures.

Supplies: Sterile stool collection container or bedpan; tongue depressor or sterile applicator sticks; transportation/mailing container; labels; rubber band; laboratory requisition form; gloves; biohazard waste container

Affective Behaviors: Affective behaviors provide a professional approach to a skill that enhances the patient encounter. These behaviors may also display sensitivity to a patient's rights and enhance communication. Pay close attention to these skills, which will be in ***bold, italicized*** font.

Notes to the Student

____

____

____

____

____

____

Skills Assessment Requirements

Read and familiarize yourself with the procedure; complete the minimum practice requirements. Document each MPR using proper charting technique. Complete each procedure within a reasonable amount of time, with a minimum of 85% accuracy.

Name: ____________________

Date: ____________________

POINT VALUE
✦ = 3–6 points
✶ = 7–9 points

		PRACTICE TRIAL	GRADED TRIAL # 1	GRADED TRIAL # 2	NOTES
1. ✦	Assemble all equipment.				
2. ✦	Use proper hand hygiene.				
3. ✶	***Identify the patient and clearly explain the procedure. Provide written instructions if necessary.***				
4. ✦	Instruct the patient to defecate into the container or bed pan.				
5. ✦	When the patient returns with the specimen, don gloves.				
6. ✶	Using a tongue depressor or applicator stick, remove a small amount of stool from different parts of the specimen and place it in the specimen container. *Note:* Be sure no other contaminants are included (toilet paper, urine, toilet water, etc.).				
7. ✦	Correctly fill out the laboratory requisition form.				
8. ✶	Wrap the form around the container, securing it with a rubber band. Place it in the proper container for delivery.				
9. ✦	Clean the area. Remove and dispose of the gloves, and perform proper hand hygiene.				
10. ✶	Document the procedure in the patient's record.				

Name: ______________________

Date: ______________________

Document: Enter the appropriate information in the chart below.

Grading

Points Earned	______		
Points Possible	______	72	72
Percent Grade (Points Earned/Points Possible)	______		
PASS:	______	❑ YES ❑ NO ❑ N/A	❑ YES ❑ NO ❑ N/A

Instructor Sign-Off

Instructor: ______________________ **Date:** ______________

Name: ______________________________

Date: ______________________________

Procedure 45-8:

Obtaining a Stool Specimen for Ova and Parasites

Objective: Clearly instruct a patient on how to collect a stool sample (fresh and preserved specimens) for ova and parasites and sensitivity in a sterile container using correct infection control procedures.

Supplies: Stool collection kit with containers for fresh and preserved specimens, or bedpan; tongue depressor or sterile applicator sticks; transportation/mailing container; labels; laboratory requisition form; rubber band; gloves; biohazard waste container

Affective Behaviors: Affective behaviors provide a professional approach to a skill that enhances the patient encounter. These behaviors may also display sensitivity to a patient's rights and enhance communication. Pay close attention to these skills, which will be in ***bold, italicized*** font.

Notes to the Student

____

____

____

____

____

____

Skills Assessment Requirements

Read and familiarize yourself with the procedure; complete the minimum practice requirements. Document each MPR using proper charting technique. Complete each procedure within a reasonable amount of time, with a minimum of 85% accuracy.

Name: ______________________

Date: ______________________

POINT VALUE ✦ = 3–6 points ✶ = 7–9 points		PRACTICE TRIAL	GRADED TRIAL # 1	GRADED TRIAL # 2	NOTES
1. ✦	Assemble all equipment.				
2. ✦	Use proper hand hygiene.				
3. ✶	***Identify the patient and clearly explain the procedure. Provide written instructions if necessary.***				
4. ✦	Instruct the patient to defecate into the container or bed pan.				
5. ✦	When the patient returns with the specimen, don gloves.				
6. ✶	Using a tongue depressor or applicator stick, remove a small amount of stool from different parts of the specimen and place it in each vial, using a different depressor for each vial. *Note:* Be sure no other contaminants are included (toilet paper, urine, toilet water, etc.).				
7. ✦	Correctly fill out laboratory requisition form.				
8. ✶	Wrap the form around the container, securing it with a rubber band. Place it in the proper container for delivery.				
9. ✦	Clean the area. Remove and dispose of the gloves, and perform proper hand hygiene.				
10. ✶	Document the procedure in the patient's record.				

Name: ____________________

Date: ____________________

Document: Enter the appropriate information in the chart below.

Grading

Points Earned	______		
Points Possible	______	72	72
Percent Grade (Points Earned/Points Possible)	______		
PASS:	______	❑ YES ❑ NO ❑ N/A	❑ YES ❑ NO ❑ N/A

Instructor Sign-Off

Instructor: ______________________________ **Date:** ____________________

Name: ______________________

Date: ______________________

Procedure 45-9:

Obtaining a Stool Specimen for Examination for Pinworms

Objective: Collect a rectal swab using cellulose tape for pinworm examination.

Supplies: Slide; tongue depressor or swab; gauze; microscope; cellulose tape; laboratory requisition form

Affective Behaviors: Affective behaviors provide a professional approach to a skill that enhances the patient encounter. These behaviors may also display sensitivity to a patient's rights and enhance communication. Pay close attention to these skills, which will be in ***bold, italicized*** font.

Notes to the Student

____

____

____

____

____

____

Skills Assessment Requirements

Read and familiarize yourself with the procedure; complete the minimum practice requirements. Document each MPR using proper charting technique. Complete each procedure within a reasonable amount of time, with a minimum of 85% accuracy.

Name: ______________________________

Date: ______________________________

POINT VALUE
✦ = 3–6 points
✶ = 7–9 points

		PRACTICE TRIAL	GRADED TRIAL # 1	GRADED TRIAL # 2	NOTES
1. ✦	Assemble all equipment and supplies.				
2. ✦	Attach the sticky side of a piece of cellulose tape to the slide surface and wrapping tape around one end. Leave room to attach a small square of paper for labeling at the other end. *Note:* Do not use double-sided sticky or Magic tape.				
3. ✦	Perform proper hand hygiene and apply gloves.				
4. ✦	***Identify the patient and clearly explain the procedure. Prepare the patient on exam table or parent's lap with anal area exposed.***				
5. ✶	Peel tape off slide by the labeled end and wrap around tongue depressor or swab with the sticky side out.				
6. ✶	Press the tape on both sides of the area around the anus.				
7. ✦	Replace the tape on the slide with the sticky side down. Smooth it with gauze.				
8. ✦	Label the slide with the patient's name and the date. Correctly fill out the laboratory requisition form.				
9. ✦	Clean the area and dispose of all waste.				
10. ✦	Remove and dispose of the gloves, and perform proper hand hygiene.				
11. ✶	Document the procedure in the patient's record.				

Name: ______________________________

Date: ______________________________

Document: Enter the appropriate information in the chart below.

Grading

Points Earned	_______		
Points Possible	_______	75	75
Percent Grade (Points Earned/Points Possible)	_______		
PASS:	_______	❑ YES ❑ NO ❑ N/A	❑ YES ❑ NO ❑ N/A

Instructor Sign-Off

Instructor: ______________________________ **Date:** ____________________

Name: ____________________

Date: ____________________

Procedure 46-1:

Collecting a 24-Hour Urine Specimen

Objective: Clearly instruct a patient on how to collect a 24-hour urine specimen.

Supplies: 24-hour specimen container (some patients may require 2 containers); smaller collection container or toilet insert; patient instruction sheet; collection label; patient record; requisition slip; preservation additive and hazardous indicator label (as required); 1 L graduated cylinder; gloves; pen

Affective Behaviors: Affective behaviors provide a professional approach to a skill that enhances the patient encounter. These behaviors may also display sensitivity to a patient's rights and enhance communication. Pay close attention to these skills, which will be in a ***bold, italicized*** font.

Notes to the Student

____

____

____

____

____

____

Skills Assessment Requirements

Read and familiarize yourself with the procedure; complete the minimum practice requirements. Document each MPR using proper charting technique. Complete each procedure within a reasonable amount of time, with a minimum of 85% accuracy.

Name: ______________________________

Date: ______________________________

POINT VALUE
✦ = 3–6 points
✶ = 7–9 points

		PRACTICE TRIAL	GRADED TRIAL # 1	GRADED TRIAL # 2	NOTES
1. ✦	Verify orders for specific test in patient record.				
2. ✦	Assemble equipment and supplies. *Note:* Be sure to check laboratory directory for specific instructions (dietary restrictions or preservatives) for tests ordered.				
3. ✦	Perform proper hand hygiene.				
4. ✦	Label container with patient's name, start and end dates, and times for collection. *Note:* If indicated by the lab directory, add preservative to the container and correct chemical hazard label.				
5. ✦	***Identify the patient and greet the patient. Introduce yourself and guide the patient to the treatment area.***				
6. ✦	***Clearly instruct the patient on the following procedure for urine collection:*** • Wash hands. • Void into the toilet upon arising. • Record the time and the date (i.e., 7 A.M., Thursday, XX/XX/XXXX). • Collect all voided urine *after this time* for the next 24 hours until the recorded time is reached the next day (i.e., 7 A.M., Friday, XX/XX/XXXX). • Note on the label the date and time of each urination. • All urine will go into the 24-hour collection container.				

Name: ______________________

Date: ______________________

POINT VALUE
✦ = 3–6 points
✶ = 7–9 points

		PRACTICE TRIAL	GRADED TRIAL # 1	GRADED TRIAL # 2	NOTES
7. ✶	• DO NOT void directly into the large 24-hour collection container. • Void all urine into the smaller collection container or toilet insert, and pour it into the larger container. • Each time wash, rinse, and air-dry the smaller container. • After each specimen is placed in the larger specimen container, screw the lid tightly. • Store the container in the refrigerator or portable cooler unless otherwise indicated by the lab directory for the specific test.				
8. ✦	• The first voided specimen of the second morning is the last specimen to be added to the container, ending the collecting period. • At the end of the 24-hour period, bring the large container in as soon as possible to ensure accurate results. • ***Ask the patient if he or she has any questions prior to leaving the office and beginning the specimen collection.***				
9. ✦	***Provide a written copy of these instructions to the patient, along with the prepared container(s).***				
10. ✦	Document the supplies and instructions given in the patient's record.				

Name: ______________________

Date: ______________________

POINT VALUE ✦ = 3–6 points ✶ = 7–9 points		PRACTICE TRIAL	GRADED TRIAL # 1	GRADED TRIAL # 2	NOTES
11. ✦	Upon return of the specimen, ***verify the collection dates and times with patient for accuracy***.				
12. ✦	Perform proper hand hygiene and apply gloves.				
13. ✶	Fill out a lab requisition slip for the specimen. Be sure to check if any other additives need to be included per the laboratory directory for the specific testing.				
14. ✦	Mix the urine sample by swirling carefully. Measure and record total volume of collected urine.				
15. ✶	Pour an aliquot (portion obtained by dividing whole amount into equal portions) of urine into the container for delivery. Record the total volume of urine collected and preservative added (if any). Dispose of the remainder of the urine per laboratory directions.				
16. ✦	Clean the area, disposing of urine containers in biohazard waste containers.				
17. ✦	Remove and dispose of gloves. Perform proper hand hygiene.				
18. ✦	Record the date, time, volume of urine, and where specimen was sent in the patient's record.				

Name: ______________________________

Date: ______________________________

Document: Enter the appropriate information in the chart below.

Grading

Points Earned	_______		
Points Possible	_______	117	117
Percent Grade (Points Earned/Points Possible)	_______		
PASS:	_______	❑ YES ❑ NO ❑ N/A	❑ YES ❑ NO ❑ N/A

Instructor Sign-Off

Instructor: ______________________________ **Date:** ______________

Name: ______________________________

Date: ______________________________

Procedure 46-2:

Collecting a Clean-Catch Midstream Urine Specimen

Objective: Instruct both male and female patients to correctly obtain a contaminant-free, clean-catch midstream urine specimen.

Supplies: Sterile urine container, antiseptic towelettes, written patient instructions

Affective Behaviors: Affective behaviors provide a professional approach to a skill that enhances the patient encounter. These behaviors may also display sensitivity to a patient's rights and enhance communication. Pay close attention to these skills, which will be in ***bold, italicized*** font.

Notes to the Student

____

____

____

____

____

____

Skills Assessment Requirements

Read and familiarize yourself with the procedure; complete the minimum practice requirements. Document each MPR using proper charting technique. Complete each procedure within a reasonable amount of time, with a minimum of 85% accuracy.

Name: ______________________________

Date: ______________________________

POINT VALUE ✦ = 3–6 points ✶ = 7–9 points		PRACTICE TRIAL	GRADED TRIAL # 1	GRADED TRIAL # 2	NOTES
1. ✦	Assemble equipment and supplies. Perform proper hand hygiene.				
2. ✦	***Identify and greet the patient.***				
3. ✶	***Explain procedure to a* male *patient as follows:*** • Perform proper hand hygiene. • Expose penis. Pull foreskin back if uncircumcised, and hold back until the specimen has been collected. • Cleanse each side of the urethral opening from top to bottom using a separate antiseptic wipe, wiping in one direction only. Cleanse across the top of the urethral opening with a third antiseptic wipe, wiping in one direction only. • Be certain to avoid having any body part touch the inside of the specimen container. • Void a small amount into the toilet. Then, void into the container, taking care not to touch the insides of the container. Remove the container. • Continue voiding the remainder of the urine into the toilet. • Re-cap container, taking care not to contaminate the inside of the lid. • Deliver the specimen as directed.				

Name: ______________________________

Date: ______________________________

POINT VALUE ✦ = 3–6 points ✶ = 7–9 points		PRACTICE TRIAL	GRADED TRIAL # 1	GRADED TRIAL # 2	NOTES
4. ✶	***Explain procedure to* female *patient as follows:*** • Perform proper hand hygiene and remove underwear. • Expose urinary meatus by pulling apart labia and hold open with nondominant hand. • Use dominant hand to cleanse around one side of the urinary meatus from front to back with one antiseptic wipe. Use a second wipe to cleanse the other side in the same manner. Using a third wipe, cleanse across the opening of the meatus itself. Continue holding the labia apart until the procedure is complete. • Begin voiding into the toilet. Place the container into position and void into the container without touching the inside of the container with fingers. • Remove container and continue voiding into the toilet. • Wipe in usual manner and cover container with lid, avoiding contaminating the inside of the lid. • Deliver the specimen as directed.				
5. ✦	Label specimen container appropriately and complete the lab requisition form.				
6. ✦	Perform proper hand hygiene.				
7. ✶	Document chart appropriately.				

Name: ______________________________

Date: ______________________________

Document: Enter the appropriate information in the chart below.

Grading

Points Earned	______		
Points Possible	______	51	51
Percent Grade (Points Earned/Points Possible)	______		
PASS:	______	❑ YES ❑ NO ❑ N/A	❑ YES ❑ NO ❑ N/A

Instructor Sign-Off

Instructor: ______________________________ **Date:** ______________

Name: ______________________________

Date: ______________________________

Procedure 46-3:

Evaluating the Physical Characteristics of Urine

Objective: Evaluate the physical characteristics of urine and properly record the results.

Supplies: Urine specimen, centrifuge tube, laboratory slip, personal protective equipment, as needed

Affective Behaviors: Affective behaviors provide a professional approach to a skill that enhances the patient encounter. These behaviors may also display sensitivity to a patient's rights and enhance communication. Pay close attention to these skills, which will be in ***bold, italicized*** font.

Notes to the Student

____

____

____

____

____

____

Skills Assessment Requirements

Read and familiarize yourself with the procedure; complete the minimum practice requirements. Document each MPR using proper charting technique. Complete each procedure within a reasonable amount of time, with a minimum of 85% accuracy.

Name: ____________________

Date: ____________________

POINT VALUE
✦ = 3–6 points
✶ = 7–9 points

		PRACTICE TRIAL	GRADED TRIAL # 1	GRADED TRIAL # 2	NOTES
1. ✦	Assemble all equipment and supplies.				
2. ✦	Perform proper hand hygiene and apply gloves.				
3. ✦	Label a centrifuge tube with the patient's name.				
4. ✦	Mix the urine by carefully swirling it, avoiding spillage.				
5. ✶	Assess the color of the specimen and record it using appropriate terminology.				
6. ✶	Assess the clarity of the urine and record it using proper terminology.				
7. ✦	Clean and sanitize the work area.				
8. ✦	Remove and dispose of gloves properly.				
9. ✦	Perform proper hand hygiene, unless proceeding with complete urinalysis.				
10. ✶	Document your observations in the patient's record using proper terminology.				

Name: ____________________

Date: ____________________

Document: Enter the appropriate information in the chart below.

Grading

Points Earned	______		
Points Possible	______	69	69
Percent Grade (Points Earned/Points Possible)	______		
PASS:	______	❑ YES ❑ NO ❑ N/A	❑ YES ❑ NO ❑ N/A

Instructor Sign-Off

Instructor: ____________________ **Date:** ____________________

Name: ______________________________

Date: ______________________________

Procedure 46-4:

Measuring the Specific Gravity of Urine with a Refractometer

Objective: Measure the specific gravity of urine using a refractometer without error.

Supplies: Antiseptic cleaner; biohazard waste container; personal protective equipment; gloves; distilled water; medicine dropper or pipette; pen and paper; paper towels; refractometer; urine specimen

Affective Behaviors: Affective behaviors provide a professional approach to a skill that enhances the patient encounter. These behaviors may also display sensitivity to a patient's rights and enhance communication. Pay close attention to these skills, which will be in ***bold, italicized*** font.

Notes to the Student

____

____

____

____

____

____

Skills Assessment Requirements

Read and familiarize yourself with the procedure; complete the minimum practice requirements. Document each MPR using proper charting technique. Complete each procedure within a reasonable amount of time, with a minimum of 85% accuracy.

Name: ______________________________

Date: ______________________________

POINT VALUE
✦ = 3–6 points
✶ = 7–9 points

		PRACTICE TRIAL	GRADED TRIAL # 1	GRADED TRIAL # 2	NOTES
1. ✦	Assemble all equipment and supplies.				
2. ✦	Perform proper hand hygiene. Apply gloves and personal protective equipment, as needed.				
3. ✦	Before using the refractometer, perform a quality control check by using a sample of distilled water. The value of distilled water is 1.000.				
4. ✦	Clean the prism and refractometer cover with distilled water; wipe it dry.				
5. ✶	Close the cover. Using a dropper or pipette, place a drop of distilled water on the notched area of the cover. If the refractometer does not have an attached cover, place the water directly on the prism and then place a cover plate on top of the prism.				
6. ✶	Tilt the refractometer to allow light to enter. Read the specific gravity of the distilled water by noting the division line between the light and dark areas. The reading should be 1.000. If it isn't, retest with fresh distilled water.				
7. ✦	To test the urine sample, swirl the urine gently in the specimen cup; avoid splashing. Using the dropper or pipette, remove a small sample of urine and place 1–2 drops on the notched area of the cover.				

Name: ______________________________

Date: ______________________________

POINT VALUE
✦ = 3–6 points
✶ = 7–9 points

		PRACTICE TRIAL	GRADED TRIAL # 1	GRADED TRIAL # 2	NOTES
8. ✦	Refer back to step 6 to read the specific gravity.				
9. ✶	Record the reading on a piece of paper.				
10. ✦	Discard the urine according to OSHA guidelines.				
11. ✦	Remove the gloves and PPE, and dispose of them properly.				
12. ✦	Perform proper hand hygiene.				
13. ✶	Document the findings in the patient's record.				
14. ✦	Clean and sanitize the work area and equipment according to OSHA guidelines.				

Name: ____________________

Date: ____________________

Document: Enter the appropriate information in the chart below.

Grading

Points Earned	______		
Points Possible	______	96	96
Percent Grade (Points Earned/Points Possible)	______		
PASS:	______	❑ YES ❑ NO ❑ N/A	❑ YES ❑ NO ❑ N/A

Instructor Sign-Off

Instructor: ____________________ **Date:** ____________________

Name: ______________________________

Date: ______________________________

Procedure 46-5:

Testing the Chemical Characteristics of Urine with Reagent Strips

Objective: Perform chemical testing on urine using chemical reagent strips.

Supplies: Urine specimen; reagent test strips; timer; paper towels; laboratory slip; pen/pencil; personal protective equipment, as needed

Affective Behaviors: Affective behaviors provide a professional approach to a skill that enhances the patient encounter. These behaviors may also display sensitivity to a patient's rights and enhance communication. Pay close attention to these skills, which will be in ***bold, italicized*** font.

Notes to the Student

____

____

____

____

____

____

Skills Assessment Requirements

Read and familiarize yourself with the procedure; complete the minimum practice requirements. Document each MPR using proper charting technique. Complete each procedure within a reasonable amount of time, with a minimum of 85% accuracy.

Name: ____________________

Date: ____________________

POINT VALUE
✦ = 3–6 points
✶ = 7–9 points

		PRACTICE TRIAL	GRADED TRIAL # 1	GRADED TRIAL # 2	NOTES
1. ✦	Assemble all equipment and supplies.				
2. ✦	Perform proper hand hygiene. Apply gloves and personal protective equipment, as needed.				
3. ✶	Check the specimen for the patient identity, date, and time of collection.				
4. ✦	Check the expiration date on reagent strips.				
5. ✦	Allow urine to reach room temperature and swirl gently to mix.				
6. ✶	Dip a chemical reagent strip in urine, making sure that all pads on the strips are moistened.				
7. ✶	Read each pad by comparing it to the chart on the side of the reagent strip container, appropriately timing each test. Ignore any color change after the time has elapsed.				
8. ✶	Record the results on the patient's laboratory slip.				
9. ✦	Clean and sanitize the work area.				
10. ✦	Remove gloves and PPE, and perform proper hand hygiene.				

Name: ____________________

Date: ____________________

Document: Enter the appropriate information in the chart below.

Grading

Points Earned	_______		
Points Possible	_______	72	72
Percent Grade (Points Earned/Points Possible)	_______		
PASS:	_______	❑ YES ❑ NO ❑ N/A	❑ YES ❑ NO ❑ N/A

Instructor Sign-Off

Instructor: ______________________________ **Date:** ____________________

Name: ______________________________

Date: ______________________________

Procedure 46-6:

Testing for Glucose in Urine Using the Tablet Method

Objective: Perform procedure to test for sugar in the urine without error.

Supplies: Antiseptic cleaner; biohazard waste container; personal protective equipment, as needed; gloves; test tube; Clinitest tables; distilled water; dropper/pipette; urine specimen

Affective Behaviors: Affective behaviors provide a professional approach to a skill that enhances the patient encounter. These behaviors may also display sensitivity to a patient's rights and enhance communication. Pay close attention to these skills, which will be in ***bold, italicized*** font.

Notes to the Student

____

____

____

____

____

____

Skills Assessment Requirements

Read and familiarize yourself with the procedure; complete the minimum practice requirements. Document each MPR using proper charting technique. Complete each procedure within a reasonable amount of time, with a minimum of 85% accuracy.

Name: ______________________________

Date: ______________________________

POINT VALUE
✦ = 3–6 points
✶ = 7–9 points

		PRACTICE TRIAL	GRADED TRIAL # 1	GRADED TRIAL # 2	NOTES
1. ✦	Assemble all equipment and supplies.				
2. ✦	Perform proper hand hygiene. Apply gloves and personal protective equipment, as needed.				
3. ✦	Using a medicine dropper or pipette, place 5 drops of urine in a clean test tube.				
4. ✦	Add 10 drops of distilled water. Use pipette to mix water and urine, being careful not to splash the liquid.				
5. ✶	Drop 1 Clinitest tablet into the urine/water solution. Observe the solution as it reacts in the test tube; do not shake the tube. Do not touch the bottom of the tube during the chemical process.				
6. ✦	Wait 15 seconds after the reaction (boiling) stops. Gently shake the tube to mix the contents; avoid spilling.				
7. ✶	Immediately compare the color of the liquid against the color chart on the side of the Clinitest container by matching the color in the tube with one on the chart. Disregard any color change after the 15-second period. *Note:* Do not touch the test tube to the Clinitest bottle; this will contaminate the outside of the bottle.				
8. ✦	Discard the urine according to OSHA guidelines.				

Name: ______________________

Date: ______________________

POINT VALUE
✦ = 3–6 points
✶ = 7–9 points

		PRACTICE TRIAL	GRADED TRIAL # 1	GRADED TRIAL # 2	NOTES
9. ✦	Remove and dispose of gloves and PPE properly. Perform proper hand hygiene.				
10. ✶	Document the finding in the patient's record.				
11. ✦	Clean and sanitize the work area and equipment according to OSHA guidelines.				

Name: ____________________

Date: ____________________

Document: Enter the appropriate information in the chart below.

Grading

Points Earned	______		
Points Possible	______	75	75
Percent Grade (Points Earned/Points Possible)	______		
PASS:	______	❑ YES ❑ NO ❑ N/A	❑ YES ❑ NO ❑ N/A

Instructor Sign-Off

Instructor: ______________________________ **Date:** ____________________

Name: ______________________________

Date: ______________________________

Procedure 46-7:

Preparing a Urine Specimen for Microscopic Examination

Objective: Perform microscopic examination of urine sediment for casts and cells.

Supplies: Biohazard container; PPE; gloves; capillary pipette; centrifuge; centrifuge tube; microscope; microscope slide; paper and pen; Sedi-stain (optional); urine specimen

Affective Behaviors: Affective behaviors provide a professional approach to a skill that enhances the patient encounter. These behaviors may also display sensitivity to a patient's rights and enhance communication. Pay close attention to these skills, which will be in ***bold, italicized*** font.

Notes to the Student

____

____

____

____

____

____

Skills Assessment Requirements

Read and familiarize yourself with the procedure; complete the minimum practice requirements. Document each MPR using proper charting technique. Complete each procedure within a reasonable amount of time, with a minimum of 85% accuracy.

Name: ______________________________

Date: ______________________________

POINT VALUE
✦ = 3–6 points
∗ = 7–9 points

		PRACTICE TRIAL	GRADED TRIAL # 1	GRADED TRIAL # 2	NOTES
1. ✦	Assemble all equipment and supplies.				
2. ✦	Perform proper hand hygiene. Apply gloves and personal protective equipment, as needed.				
3. ✦	Mix specimen gently to stir up sediment that has settled to the bottom.				
4. ✦	Place 10 mL of urine into a centrifuge tube and cap the tube. Place 10 ml of water in a centrifuge tube and cap the tube. Place both tubes in centrifuge to balance each other.				
5. ✦	Set centrifuge timer for 5 minutes.				
6. ✦	After centrifuge has stopped, remove the tube and pour off the supernatant fluid.				
7. ✦	Mix sediment by holding the top of the tube and tapping the bottom with a finger, mixing well to ensure correct reading.				
8. ✦	Use capillary pipette to transfer one drop of sediment to a clean slide.				
9. ✦	Cover drop of sediment with a cover slip.				
10. ✦	Place slide on microscope stage.				
11. ✦	Focus under low power and reduced light for casts and epithelial cells.				

Name: ____________________

Date: ____________________

POINT VALUE
✦ = 3–6 points
✶ = 7–9 points

		PRACTICE TRIAL	GRADED TRIAL # 1	GRADED TRIAL # 2	NOTES
12. ✦	Carefully examine for anything abnormal, paying close attention to the edges, which are where casts are seen if they are present.				
13. ✶	Examine 10–15 fields using low power. Count the number of casts or other abnormalities seen in each field. If there is nothing in one field, record as zero. Average the count from the fields for a final result.				
14. ✶	Use the high-power magnification and adjust more light, reviewing the 10–15 fields. Identify casts if they are present. Count RBCs, WBCs, and round, transitional, and squamous epithelial cells. Average the count for all fields for each formed element seen. Record appropriately.				
15. ✶	Observe for crystals and identify. Observe for bacteria, sperm, yeast, and parasites. Report them as few, moderate, or many.				
16. ✦	Discard urine according to OSHA guidelines.				
17. ✦	Remove and dispose of gloves and PPE appropriately.				
18. ✦	Clean and sanitize work area and equipment according to OSHA guidelines.				
19. ✦	Perform proper hand hygiene.				
20. ✶	Document findings in the patient's record.				

Name: ____________________

Date: ____________________

Document: Enter the appropriate information in the chart below.

Grading

Points Earned	_______		
Points Possible	_______	132	132
Percent Grade (Points Earned/Points Possible)	_______		
PASS:	_______	❑ YES ❑ NO ❑ N/A	❑ YES ❑ NO ❑ N/A

Instructor Sign-Off

Instructor: ______________________________ **Date:** ____________________

Name: ______________________________

Date: ______________________________

Procedure 46-8:

Performing a Urine Pregnancy Test Using the Enzyme Immunoassay Method

Objective: Perform urine pregnancy testing of hCG using an EIA test. Correctly interpret the test results.

Supplies: Patient's first morning urine specimen, EIA test kit for hCG, timer, gloves, laboratory report

Affective Behaviors: Affective behaviors provide a professional approach to a skill that enhances the patient encounter. These behaviors may also display sensitivity to a patient's rights and enhance communication. Pay close attention to these skills, which will be in ***bold, italicized*** font.

Notes to the Student

____

____

____

____

____

____

Skills Assessment Requirements

Read and familiarize yourself with the procedure; complete the minimum practice requirements. Document each MPR using proper charting technique. Complete each procedure within a reasonable amount of time, with a minimum of 85% accuracy.

Name: ______________________________

Date: ______________________________

POINT VALUE
✦ = 3–6 points
✶ = 7–9 points

		PRACTICE TRIAL	GRADED TRIAL # 1	GRADED TRIAL # 2	NOTES
1. ✦	Assemble all equipment and materials.				
2. ✦	Perform proper hand hygiene. Apply gloves.				
3. ✦	Allow the urine specimen and testing materials to reach room temperature.				
4. ✶	Label the test with the patient's name or ID number.				
5. ✦	Label one area positive (+) and one area negative (−) for controls.				
6. ✦	Place the patient's urine in the test chamber following the manufacturer's directions.				
7. ✦	Place positive and negative controls in the correct area.				
8. ✦	Time the test according to the manufacturer's directions.				
9. ✦	Interpret the results correctly.				
10. ✶	Record the results on the patient's laboratory slip.				
11. ✦	Record positive and negative controls in the quality control log book according to office policy.				
12. ✦	Dispose of gloves and equipment. Perform proper hand hygiene.				

Name: ______________________________

Date: ______________________________

Document: Enter the appropriate information in the chart below.

Grading

Points Earned	_______		
Points Possible	_______	78	78
Percent Grade (Points Earned/Points Possible)	_______		
PASS:	_______	❑ YES ❑ NO ❑ N/A	❑ YES ❑ NO ❑ N/A

Instructor Sign-Off

Instructor: ______________________________ **Date:** ____________________

Name: ______________________________

Date: ______________________________

Procedure 47-1:

Quality Control for Collecting a Blood Specimen

Objective: Perform quality control procedure without error while collecting a blood specimen.

Supplies: Antiseptic cleaner; biohazard waste container; necessary sterile equipment; specimen collection container; disposable alcohol wipe; disposable gloves; appropriate requisition or paperwork; patient's record; pen

Affective Behaviors: Affective behaviors provide a professional approach to a skill that enhances the patient encounter. These behaviors may also display sensitivity to a patient's rights and enhance communication. Pay close attention to these skills, which will be in ***bold, italicized*** font.

Notes to the Student

____

____

____

____

____

____

Skills Assessment Requirements

Read and familiarize yourself with the procedure; complete the minimum practice requirements. Document each MPR using proper charting technique. Complete each procedure within a reasonable amount of time, with a minimum of 85% accuracy.

Name: ______________________________

Date: ______________________________

POINT VALUE ✦ = 3–6 points ✶ = 7–9 points		PRACTICE TRIAL	GRADED TRIAL # 1	GRADED TRIAL # 2	NOTES
1. ✦	Review request and verify test ordered.				
2. ✦	Prepare necessary equipment and work area.				
3. ✦	Perform proper hand hygiene and don gloves.				
4. ✶	***Identify the patient and explain the procedure.***				
5. ✦	***Confirm that patient has followed any pretest preparation requirements.***				
6. ✦	Collect the specimen properly, using the appropriate equipment and technique.				
7. ✦	Use the appropriate collection container and right preservative.				
8. ✶	Immediately label the specimen with the patient's name, date, and time of collection; test's name; and the name of the person collecting the specimen.				
9. ✦	Follow correct procedure for disposing of hazardous specimen waste. Decontaminate work area according to OSHA guidelines.				
10. ✦	Remove and dispose of gloves. Perform proper hand hygiene. Dispose of all used needles and equipment in biohazard waste container.				
11. ✦	***Thank the patient, and observe for any signs or symptoms of inappropriate response to the procedure.***				

Name: ______________________________

Date: ______________________________

POINT VALUE
✦ = 3–6 points
✶ = 7–9 points

		PRACTICE TRIAL	GRADED TRIAL # 1	GRADED TRIAL # 2	NOTES
12. ✶	Document the procedure in the patient record.				
13. ✦	If necessary, prepare specimen for transport to outside laboratory with all information according to OSHA guidelines.				

Name: ______________________________

Date: ______________________________

Document: Enter the appropriate information in the chart below.

Grading

Points Earned	______		
Points Possible	______	87	87
Percent Grade (Points Earned/Points Possible)	______		
PASS:	______	❑ YES ❑ NO ❑ N/A	❑ YES ❑ NO ❑ N/A

Instructor Sign-Off

Instructor: ______________________________ **Date:** ______________

Name: ____________________

Date: ____________________

Procedure 47-2:

Obtaining Venous Blood with a Sterile Syringe and Needle

Objective: Perform venipuncture without error using the syringe and needle method.

Supplies: Sterile needle and syringe; appropriate vacuum specimen tubes for tests ordered; tourniquet; gloves; alcohol sponge; cotton balls or dry gauze squares; adhesive bandage; patient record; pen; lab coat; biohazard waste container

Affective Behaviors: Affective behaviors provide a professional approach to a skill that enhances the patient encounter. These behaviors may also display sensitivity to a patient's rights and enhance communication. Pay close attention to these skills, which will be in ***bold, italicized*** font.

Notes to the Student

Skills Assessment Requirements

Read and familiarize yourself with the procedure; complete the minimum practice requirements. Document each MPR using proper charting technique. Complete each procedure within a reasonable amount of time, with a minimum of 85% accuracy.

Name: ______________________

Date: ______________________

POINT VALUE
✦ = 3–6 points
✶ = 7–9 points

		PRACTICE TRIAL	GRADED TRIAL # 1	GRADED TRIAL # 2	NOTES
1. ✦	Assemble all equipment and supplies.				
2. ✦	Perform proper hand hygiene and apply gloves.				
3. ✦	***Identify the patient and explain the procedure.***				
4. ✦	Securely attach the sterile needle to the syringe.				
5. ✦	Apply a tourniquet 3–4 inches above the tourniquet site.				
6. ✶	Palpate the vein. Clean the venipuncture site with an alcohol sponge and dry with clean gauze.				
7. ✦	***Ask the patient to make a fist and hold it shut until instructed to release it.***				
8. ✶	Be sure that the needle is securely attached to the syringe. Push the plunger all the way down, making sure that no air is in the syringe.				
9. ✦	Remove the needle guard and insert the needle into the vein.				
10. ✶	Slowly pull back on the plunger until the proper amount of blood has been obtained.				
11. ✦	***Instruct the patient to release the fist***.				
12. ✶	Release the tourniquet and withdraw the needle quickly at the same angle of insertion. Using cotton or gauze, ***instruct the patient to hold pressure on the site and raise the arm***.				

Name: ______________________________

Date: ______________________________

POINT VALUE
✦ = 3–6 points
✶ = 7–9 points

		PRACTICE TRIAL	GRADED TRIAL # 1	GRADED TRIAL # 2	NOTES
13. ✦ 14. ✦	Using the tube rack, fill the vacuum tubes to the proper level. Discard the needle and syringe in a biohazard sharps container.				
15. ✦	Remove the cotton ball and inspect the injection site. Apply a bandage to the puncture site.				
16. ✦	Remove your gloves and discard them appropriately.				
17. ✦	Perform proper hand hygiene.				
18. ✶	Document the procedure in the patient's record.				
19. ✦	Label all tubes accurately and send them to the lab.				

Name: ______________________________

Date: ______________________________

Document: Enter the appropriate information in the chart below.

Grading

Points Earned	______		
Points Possible	______	129	129
Percent Grade (Points Earned/Points Possible)	______		
PASS:	______	❑ YES ❑ NO ❑ N/A	❑ YES ❑ NO ❑ N/A

Instructor Sign-Off

Instructor: ______________________________ **Date:** ____________________

Name: ______________________________

Date: ______________________________

Procedure 47-3:

Performing a Venipuncture Using the Vacutainer Method

Objective: Perform venipuncture by correctly assembling, locating, and entering a vein, and withdrawing a blood sample.

Supplies: Biohazard sharps container, Vacutainer tubes, multisample needle, gauze squares, alcohol pads, gloves, Vacutainer sleeve, tourniquet, bandage, cotton balls, adhesive, pen, lab coat, patient record, ammonia ampules

Affective Behaviors: Affective behaviors provide a professional approach to a skill that enhances the patient encounter. These behaviors may also display sensitivity to a patient's rights and enhance communication. Pay close attention to these skills, which will be in ***bold, italicized*** font.

Notes to the Student

Follow standard precautions and safety guidelines when working with blood samples. Use care to avoid splashing or spilling blood. Wipe up all spills using guidelines established by OSHA.

____

____

____

____

____

____

Skills Assessment Requirements

Read and familiarize yourself with the procedure; complete the minimum practice requirements. Document each MPR using proper charting technique. Complete each procedure within a reasonable amount of time, with a minimum of 85% accuracy.

Name: ____________________

Date: ____________________

POINT VALUE
✦ = 3–6 points
✶ = 7–9 points

		PRACTICE TRIAL	GRADED TRIAL # 1	GRADED TRIAL # 2	NOTES
1. ✦	Assemble all equipment and materials.				
2. ✦	Perform proper hand hygiene.				
3. ✶	***Identify the patient and explain the procedure. Position the patient either sitting or lying down.***				
4. ✦	Apply gloves.				
5. ✦	Screw the Vacutainer needle into the plastic sleeve. Insert the tube into the other end of the sleeve; be sure not to puncture the tube.				
6. ✦	Apply the tourniquet 2 inches above the antecubital space tight enough to engorge the vein with blood.				
7. ✦	***Place the patient's arm in an extended position with the palm facing up and comfortably resting.***				
8. ✦	Palpate the vein with your fingertips.				
9. ✶	Cleanse the chosen venipuncture site with an alcohol sponge in a circular pattern. Allow alcohol to dry.				
10. ✦	Anchor the vein properly.				
11. ✶	Insert the needle smoothly and rapidly at a 15-degree angle with the bevel of the needle up. Insert the needle only past the bevel. Keep the needle in line with the vein.				
12. ✦	While stabilizing the sleeve, push the tube into the sleeve. Allow the tube to fill.				

Name: ______________________________

Date: ______________________________

POINT VALUE
✦ = 3–6 points
✶ = 7–9 points

		PRACTICE TRIAL	GRADED TRIAL # 1	GRADED TRIAL # 2	NOTES
13. ✦	Carefully remove the tube from the sleeve without moving the needle and insert a second tube, if needed.				
14. ✦	Gently invert the tube five or six times after removing it to allow the blood to mix with the additive. *Note:* If both a red and purple tube are needed, first collect blood in the red tube with no additive.				
15. ✶	Release the tourniquet once the last tube has been inserted into the adaptor. After filling, invert the tube to mix the additives.				
16. ✦	Remove the needle while covering the site with a gauze sponge. Immediately have the patient apply firm, continuous pressure.				
17. ✶	Discard the needle in the biohazard sharps container.				
18. ✦	Gently invert all tubes collected eight to ten times in a figure-eight pattern.				
19. ✦	***Assess the patient.*** Check the venipuncture site for bleeding. Apply cotton and a strip of adhesive.				
20. ✶	Label the tubes accurately. Fill out a laboratory requisition form.				
21. ✦	Remove and dispose of gloves. Perform proper hand hygiene.				
22. ✶	Document the procedure in the patient's record.				

Name: ______________________

Date: ______________________

Document: Enter the appropriate information in the chart below.

Grading

Points Earned	______		
Points Possible	______	153	153
Percent Grade (Points Earned/Points Possible)	______		
PASS:	______	❑ YES ❑ NO ❑ N/A	❑ YES ❑ NO ❑ N/A

Instructor Sign-Off

Instructor: ______________________ **Date:** ______________

Name: ______________________________

Date: ______________________________

Procedure 47-4:

Performing a Capillary Puncture (Manual)

Objective: Perform a capillary stick using a lancet or spring-loaded lancet following correct aseptic technique and obtaining an adequate sample without error.

Supplies: Biohazard sharps container; gloves; alcohol sponge; 2 × 2 gauze squares or cotton balls; lancet or spring-loaded lancet; capillary tubes; sealing clay; ammonia ampules; bandage; lab coat

Affective Behaviors: Affective behaviors provide a professional approach to a skill that enhances the patient encounter. These behaviors may also display sensitivity to a patient's rights and enhance communication. Pay close attention to these skills, which will be in ***bold, italicized*** font.

Notes to the Student

Follow standard precautions and safety guidelines when working with blood samples. Wipe up all spills using guidelines established by OSHA.

____

____

____

____

____

Skills Assessment Requirements

Read and familiarize yourself with the procedure; complete the minimum practice requirements. Document each MPR using proper charting technique. Complete each procedure within a reasonable amount of time, with a minimum of 85% accuracy.

Name: ______________________

Date: ______________________

POINT VALUE
✦ = 3–6 points
✶ = 7–9 points

		PRACTICE TRIAL	GRADED TRIAL # 1	GRADED TRIAL # 2	NOTES
1. ✦	Assemble all equipment and supplies.				
2. ✦	Perform proper hand hygiene.				
3. ✶	***Identify the patient and explain the procedure. Position the patient either sitting or lying down.***				
4. ✦	Apply gloves.				
5. ✦	***Select either the ring or great finger of the patient's nondominant hand.*** Cleanse the site with an alcohol sponge. Allow the alcohol to dry.				
6. ✦	Remove the plastic cover from the lancet.				
7. ✦	Grasp the patient's hand and gently squeeze the finger 1 inch below the puncture site.				
8. ✶	Puncture the finger with a quick jabbing motion (or release the spring-loaded lancet). Do not puncture the site in the direct center of the finger pad.				
9. ✦	Immediately discard the lancet.				
10. ✶	Wipe away the first drop of blood with a gauze square or cotton ball.				
11. ✦	Obtain the sample using a capillary tube. Seal one end of the tube in a clay sealer. *Note:* The finger may be gently massaged to increase blood flow.				
12. ✦	Apply clean gauze over the site and instruct the patient to apply firm pressure until the bleeding stops.				

Name: ____________________

Date: ____________________

POINT VALUE
✦ = 3–6 points
✶ = 7–9 points

		PRACTICE TRIAL	GRADED TRIAL # 1	GRADED TRIAL # 2	NOTES
13. ✦	***Assess the patent.*** Apply a bandage to the site, if needed.				
14. ✦	Remove and dispose of gloves. Perform proper hand hygiene.				
15. ✶	Document the procedure in the patient's record.				

Name: ______________________________

Date: ______________________________

Document: Enter the appropriate information in the chart below.

Grading

Points Earned	______		
Points Possible	______	102	102
Percent Grade (Points Earned/Points Possible)	______		
PASS:	______	❑ YES ❑ NO ❑ N/A	❑ YES ❑ NO ❑ N/A

Instructor Sign-Off

Instructor: ______________________________ **Date:** ______________

Name: ______________________________

Date: ______________________________

Procedure 47-5:

Monitoring Blood Glucose Levels

Objective: Accurately determine blood glucose level using a glucometer.

Supplies: Sterile lancet, testing strips, glucometer, gloves, cotton balls, alcohol sponges, gauze squares, pen lab coat, patient record

Affective Behaviors: Affective behaviors provide a professional approach to a skill that enhances the patient encounter. These behaviors may also display sensitivity to a patient's rights and enhance communication. Pay close attention to these skills, which will be in ***bold, italicized*** font.

Notes to the Student

____

____

____

____

____

____

Skills Assessment Requirements

Read and familiarize yourself with the procedure; complete the minimum practice requirements. Document each MPR using proper charting technique. Complete each procedure within a reasonable amount of time, with a minimum of 85% accuracy.

Name: ______________________

Date: ______________________

POINT VALUE
✦ = 3–6 points
✶ = 7–9 points

		PRACTICE TRIAL	GRADED TRIAL # 1	GRADED TRIAL # 2	NOTES
1. ✦	***Identify the patient and explain the procedure. Make sure the patient is fasting, if required.***				
2. ✦	Assemble equipment and supplies.				
3. ✦	Perform proper hand hygiene and apply gloves.				
4. ✶	Be sure that the glucometer is calibrated and ready for use.				
5. ✦	Remove a plastic strip from the container and place it in the designated slot on the glucometer. Ensure the "Apply Blood" message appears on the screen.				
6. ✦	Perform a capillary puncture using a sterile lancet.				
7. ✶	Apply a large drop of blood from the capillary puncture site to the test strip, ensuring that it is completely covered. *Note:* Be sure to wipe away the first drop of blood with cotton or gauze. Touch the test strip to the second drop of blood. The glucometer should automatically start the timer.				
8. ✦	***Provide the patient with cotton or a gauze square to hold over the puncture site.***				
9. ✦	When the glucometer alerts you, look at the reading, and immediately remove the test strip and discard all used equipment. *Note:* The blood glucose reading will remain on the glucometer until the unit is turned off.				

Name: ______________________________

Date: ______________________________

POINT VALUE
✦ = 3–6 points
✶ = 7–9 points

		PRACTICE TRIAL	GRADED TRIAL # 1	GRADED TRIAL # 2	NOTES
10. ✦	Remove and dispose of gloves. Perform proper hand hygiene.				
11. ✶	Record in patient record as number of mg (milligrams) of glucose per deciliter (mg/dL) displayed on glucometer screen.				

Name: ______________________

Date: ______________________

Document: Enter the appropriate information in the chart below.

Grading

Points Earned	______		
Points Possible	______	75	75
Percent Grade (Points Earned/Points Possible)	______		
PASS:	______	❑ YES ❑ NO ❑ N/A	❑ YES ❑ NO ❑ N/A

Instructor Sign-Off

Instructor: ______________________ **Date:** ______________________

Name: ______________________________

Date: ______________________________

Procedure 47-6:

Performing a Microhematocrit

Objective: Perform a microhematocrit on a capillary blood sample using proper aseptic technique without error.

Supplies: Biohazard sharps container; gloves; capillary tubes; sealing clay; microhematocrit centrifuge; whole blood; hematocrit card or other reader

Affective Behaviors: Affective behaviors provide a professional approach to a skill that enhances the patient encounter. These behaviors may also display sensitivity to a patient's rights and enhance communication. Pay close attention to these skills, which will be in ***bold, italicized*** font.

Notes to the Student

____

____

____

____

____

____

Skills Assessment Requirements

Read and familiarize yourself with the procedure; complete the minimum practice requirements. Document each MPR using proper charting technique. Complete each procedure within a reasonable amount of time, with a minimum of 85% accuracy.

Name: ______________________________

Date: ______________________________

POINT VALUE
✦ = 3–6 points
✶ = 7–9 points

		PRACTICE TRIAL	GRADED TRIAL # 1	GRADED TRIAL # 2	NOTES
1. ✦	Assemble all equipment and materials.				
2. ✦	Use proper hand hygiene and apply gloves.				
3. ✶	Fill two capillary tubes three-quarters full. Obtain a blood specimen from a vacuum tube of anticoagulated blood using a plain capillary tube or directly from a finger stick using a heparinized capillary tube. Seal one end with sealing clay.				
4. ✦	Place the capillary tube in a centrifuge with the sealed ends against the rubber gaskets. Write down the slot number the patient tube is in. Spin for 3 to 5 minutes at 10,000 rpm. *Note:* Always check manufacturer's recommendations for proper time and speed.				
5. ✦	Remove the tube immediately after the centrifuge stops.				
6. ✶	Determine the results. Use the hematocrit card by placing the sealing clay just below the zero line on both tubes. Then, on both tubes, match the top of the plasma with the 100 line. Read the results on both tubes directly below the buffy coat; add those results together and divide by 2.				
7. ✦	Discard the tubes in the sharps container.				
8. ✦	Remove and dispose of gloves. Perform proper hand hygiene.				
9. ✶	Document the value as a percentage in the patient's record.				

Name: ______________________________

Date: ______________________________

Document: Enter the appropriate information in the chart below.

Grading

Points Earned	_______		
Points Possible	_______	63	63
Percent Grade (Points Earned/Points Possible)	_______		
PASS:	_______	❑ YES ❑ NO ❑ N/A	❑ YES ❑ NO ❑ N/A

Instructor Sign-Off

Instructor: ______________________________ **Date:** ____________________

Name: ____________________

Date: ____________________

Procedure 47-7:

Determining Hemoglobin Using the Hemoglobinometer

Objective: Perform a blood test to determine hemoglobin levels using the hemoglobinometer.

Supplies: Hemoglobinometer; glass slide chamber; hemolysis applicator; sterile manual or spring-loaded lancet; cotton balls; dry gauze squares; alcohol sponges; gloves; patient's record; lab coat; biohazard sharps container

Affective Behaviors: Affective behaviors provide a professional approach to a skill that enhances the patient encounter. These behaviors may also display sensitivity to a patient's rights and enhance communication. Pay close attention to these skills, which will be in ***bold, italicized*** font.

Notes to the Student

____

____

____

____

____

____

Skills Assessment Requirements

Read and familiarize yourself with the procedure; complete the minimum practice requirements. Document each MPR using proper charting technique. Complete each procedure within a reasonable amount of time, with a minimum of 85% accuracy.

Name: ______________________________

Date: ______________________________

POINT VALUE
✦ = 3–6 points
✶ = 7–9 points

		PRACTICE TRIAL	GRADED TRIAL # 1	GRADED TRIAL # 2	NOTES
1. ✦	Gather necessary equipment and supplies.				
2. ✦	Perform proper hand hygiene and apply gloves.				
3. ✦	Clean the puncture site with an alcohol sponge.				
4. ✶	Obtain capillary blood using a sterile lancet.				
5. ✦	Pull the glass chamber out of the hemoglobinometer and position the lower part of the slide so that it is slightly offset.				
6. ✦	Place a large drop of blood onto the slide.				
7. ✦	Wipe the patient's puncture site with a cotton ball and provide the patient with a dry gauze square to apply mild pressure to the puncture.				
8. ✶	Mix blood with hemolysis applicator until the blood becomes clear.				
9. ✦	Push glass chamber into the clip and place into the slot on the left side of the hemoglobinometer.				
10. ✦	Hold the machine at eye level while turning on the light by depressing the bottom button. Look into the instrument to see a split green field.				
11. ✦	Slide the button on the right side of the meter while looking into the meter until a matching green field occurs. Leave the sliding scale on the calibrated line where the solid green field appeared.				

Name: ______________________________

Date: ______________________________

POINT VALUE
✦ = 3–6 points
✶ = 7–9 points

		PRACTICE TRIAL	GRADED TRIAL # 1	GRADED TRIAL # 2	NOTES
12. ✦	Read the hemoglobin value at the top of the scale. The results are read as grams of hemoglobin per 100 mL of blood (g/dL).				
13. ✦	Wash chamber and reusable hemolysis applicator with a detergent solution. Rinse, dry, and return hemolysis applicator to the appropriate area.				
14. ✦	Remove and dispose of gloves and supplies. Perform proper hand hygiene.				
15. ✶	Record the results in the patient's record.				

Name: ______________________

Date: ______________________

Document: Enter the appropriate information in the chart below.

Grading

Points Earned	______		
Points Possible	______	99	99
Percent Grade (Points Earned/Points Possible)	______		
PASS:	______	❑ YES ❑ NO ❑ N/A	❑ YES ❑ NO ❑ N/A

Instructor Sign-Off

Instructor: ______________________ **Date:** ______________________

Name: ____________________

Date: ____________________

Procedure 47-8:

Preparing Slides

Objective: Prepare a slide for a differential white blood cell count using correct aseptic procedure without error.

Supplies: Clean glass slides, whole blood (EDTA), gloves, biohazard waste container, eye dropper, Wright's stain, lab coat, pen, patient record

Affective Behaviors: Affective behaviors provide a professional approach to a skill that enhances the patient encounter. These behaviors may also display sensitivity to a patient's rights and enhance communication. Pay close attention to these skills, which will be in ***bold, italicized*** font.

Notes to the Student

____

____

____

____

____

____

Skills Assessment Requirements

Read and familiarize yourself with the procedure; complete the minimum practice requirements. Document each MPR using proper charting technique. Complete each procedure within a reasonable amount of time, with a minimum of 85% accuracy.

Name: ____________________

Date: ____________________

POINT VALUE
✦ = 3–6 points
✶ = 7–9 points

		PRACTICE TRIAL	GRADED TRIAL # 1	GRADED TRIAL # 2	NOTES
1. ✦	Assemble all equipment and materials.				
2. ✦	Perform proper hand hygiene and apply gloves.				
3. ✦	Obtain a whole blood sample using EDTA as the anti-coagulant of choice. *Note:* Blood must be thoroughly mixed before use.				
4. ✦	Using a dropper, place 1 drop of room-temperature blood on the end of a clean glass slide.				
5. ✶	Using the short side of another clean glass slide, back the slide to the drop of blood, allowing the blood to spread across the short side of the slide. Holding the spreader slide at a 30 degree angle, spread the blood across the length of the slide using gentle, continuous pressure and a smooth gliding motion to create a smear.				
6. ✦	Allow the slide to air dry on the rack.				
7. ✶	Label the frosted edge of the slide with the patient's name and the date.				
8. ✶	Stain the slide using Wright's staining method. Flood the slide with the stain for exactly 45 seconds.				
9. ✦	Rinse the slide with distilled water until the water runs clear.				
10. ✦	Allow the slide to dry before examining it under the microscope.				
11. ✶	Document the results in the patient's record.				

Name: ______________________________

Date: ______________________________

Document: Enter the appropriate information in the chart below.

Grading

Points Earned	______		
Points Possible	______	78	78
Percent Grade (Points Earned/Points Possible)	______		
PASS:	______	❑ YES ❑ NO ❑ N/A	❑ YES ❑ NO ❑ N/A

Instructor Sign-Off

Instructor: ______________________________ **Date:** ______________________

Name: ______________________________

Date: ______________________________

Procedure 47-9:

Performing an Erythrocyte Sedimentation Rate Test Using the Wintrobe Tube Method

Objective: Perform an ESR (erythrocyte sedimentation rate) using the Wintrobe tube method and aseptic technique without error.

Supplies: Gloves, whole blood (EDTA), Wintrobe tube, Wintrobe rack, pen, patient record, lab coat, biohazard sharps container

Affective Behaviors: Affective behaviors provide a professional approach to a skill that enhances the patient encounter. These behaviors may also display sensitivity to a patient's rights and enhance communication. Pay close attention to these skills, which will be in ***bold, italicized*** font.

Notes to the Student

____

____

____

____

____

____

Skills Assessment Requirements

Read and familiarize yourself with the procedure; complete the minimum practice requirements. Document each MPR using proper charting technique. Complete each procedure within a reasonable amount of time, with a minimum of 85% accuracy.

Name: ______________________________

Date: ______________________________

POINT VALUE
✦ = 3–6 points
✶ = 7–9 points

		PRACTICE TRIAL	GRADED TRIAL # 1	GRADED TRIAL # 2	NOTES
1. ✦	Assemble all equipment and materials.				
2. ✦	Use proper hand hygiene and apply gloves.				
3. ✦	Obtain a whole blood sample using a purple-top tube. Mix well. EDTA is the anti-coagulant of choice.				
4. ✦	Slowly fill the Wintrobe tube with the blood, avoiding air bubbles.				
5. ✶	Adjust the meniscus of the specimen to the zero line at the bottom of the tube.				
6. ✦	Maintain the tube in an upright vertical position for 1 hour.				
7. ✶	After 1 hour has lapsed, record the number of red blood cells that settle. Read the ESR on the same side of the tube as the zero line at the top.				
8. ✦	Discard tube in the sharps container.				
9. ✦	Remove and dispose of gloves. Perform proper hand hygiene.				
10. ✶	Document the procedure in the patient's record.				

Name: ______________________________

Date: ______________________________

Document: Enter the appropriate information in the chart below.

Grading

Points Earned	_______		
Points Possible	_______	69	69
Percent Grade (Points Earned/Points Possible)	_______		
PASS:	_______	❑ YES ❑ NO ❑ N/A	❑ YES ❑ NO ❑ N/A

Instructor Sign-Off

Instructor: ______________________________ **Date:** ____________________

Name: ______________________

Date: ______________________

Procedure 47-10:

Performing a PKU Test

Objective: Collect blood specimen for PKU testing.

Supplies: Sterile manual or spring-loaded lancet; alcohol sponge; gloves; sterile gauze; special filter paper card

Affective Behaviors: Affective behaviors provide a professional approach to a skill that enhances the patient encounter. These behaviors may also display sensitivity to a patient's rights and enhance communication. Pay close attention to these skills, which will be in ***bold, italicized*** font.

Notes to the Student

The special filter paper cards used for this procedure are usually supplied by the state health department.

____

____

____

____

____

Skills Assessment Requirements

Read and familiarize yourself with the procedure; complete the minimum practice requirements. Document each MPR using proper charting technique. Complete each procedure within a reasonable amount of time, with a minimum of 85% accuracy.

Name: ______________________________

Date: ______________________________

POINT VALUE
✦ = 3–6 points
✶ = 7–9 points

		PRACTICE TRIAL	GRADED TRIAL # 1	GRADED TRIAL # 2	NOTES
1. ✦	Assemble all equipment and materials.				
2. ✦	Perform proper hand hygiene and apply gloves.				
3. ✶	Cleanse the infant's heel with an alcohol sponge. Allow it to dry.				
4. ✦	Puncture the back of the heel with a sterile lancet.				
5. ✶	Wipe away the first drop of blood with dry, sterile gauze.				
6. ✦	Allow a large blood droplet to form.				
7. ✦	Touch the blood droplet to the center of the circle on one side of the special filter paper.				
8. ✶	Ensure that the blood has completely soaked through the paper card by looking at the back side.				
9. ✦	Fill all required circles on the card.				
10. ✶	Do not squeeze the infant's heel too firmly to avoid collecting tissue with the blood.				
11. ✦	Place the card in an appropriate area to dry for 2 hours at room temperature.				
12. ✦	When the card is completely dry, place it in the state-provided envelope and mail it within 48 hours.				
13. ✶	Document the procedure in the patient's record.				

Name: ______________________________

Date: ______________________________

Document: Enter the appropriate information in the chart below.

Grading

Points Earned	_______		
Points Possible	_______	93	93
Percent Grade (Points Earned/Points Possible)	_______		
PASS:	_______	❑ YES ❑ NO ❑ N/A	❑ YES ❑ NO ❑ N/A

Instructor Sign-Off

Instructor: ______________________________ **Date:** ______________

Name: ______________________________

Date: ______________________________

Procedure 47-11:

Performing a Mono Test

Objective: Perform a mono test.

Supplies: Antiseptic cleaner, biohazard waste container, disposable lancet, disposable gloves, capillary tube, test tube, mono test diluent, mono test stick(s), blood specimen

Affective Behaviors: Affective behaviors provide a professional approach to a skill that enhances the patient encounter. These behaviors may also display sensitivity to a patient's rights and enhance communication. Pay close attention to these skills, which will be in ***bold, italicized*** font.

Notes to the Student

____

____

____

____

____

____

Skills Assessment Requirements

Read and familiarize yourself with the procedure; complete the minimum practice requirements. Document each MPR using proper charting technique. Complete each procedure within a reasonable amount of time, with a minimum of 85% accuracy.

Name: ______________________

Date: ______________________

POINT VALUE
✦ = 3–6 points
✶ = 7–9 points

		PRACTICE TRIAL	GRADED TRIAL # 1	GRADED TRIAL # 2	NOTES
1. ✦	Assemble all equipment and supplies.				
2. ✦	Perform proper hand hygiene and apply gloves.				
3. ✦	Perform capillary puncture on patient's finger.				
4. ✦	Fill a capillary tube end to end, dispensing all of the blood into the test tube.				
5. ✦	Slowly add 1 drop of diluent to the bottom of the test tube.				
6. ✶	Mix.				
7. ✦	Remove the test stick from the container. Immediately re-cap the container.				
8. ✦	Place the absorbent end of the test stick into the treated sample. Leave the test stick in the test tube.				
9. ✶	Read the results at 5 minutes. Positive results may be read as soon as the red control line appears.				
10. ✦	Discard used test tubes, lancet, and test sticks in the biohazard waste container.				
11. ✦	Remove and dispose of gloves. Perform proper hand hygiene.				
12. ✶	Document the results in the patient's record.				
13. ✦	Clean work area and equipment according to OSHA guidelines.				

Name: ______________________

Date: ______________________

Document: Enter the appropriate information in the chart below.

Grading

Points Earned	_____		
Points Possible	_____	87	87
Percent Grade (Points Earned/Points Possible)	_____		
PASS:	_____	❑ YES ❑ NO ❑ N/A	❑ YES ❑ NO ❑ N/A

Instructor Sign-Off

Instructor: ______________________ **Date:** ______________________

Name: ______________________________

Date: ______________________________

Procedure 48-1:

Procedure for a General X-Ray Examination

Objective: Assist with a radiologic procedure under the supervision of a physician or radiologic technologist.

Supplies: Order for x-ray examination, dosimeter badge, appropriate x-ray equipment (x-ray film, holder, machine), processing equipment drape, lead patient shield

Affective Behaviors: Affective behaviors provide a professional approach to a skill that enhances the patient encounter. These behaviors may also display sensitivity to a patient's rights and enhance communication. Pay close attention to these skills, which will be in ***bold, italicized*** font.

Notes to the Student

____

____

____

____

____

____

Skills Assessment Requirements

Read and familiarize yourself with the procedure; complete the minimum practice requirements. Document each MPR using proper charting technique. Complete each procedure within a reasonable amount of time, with a minimum of 85% accuracy.

Name: ______________________________

Date: ______________________________

POINT VALUE
✦ = 3–6 points
✶ = 7–9 points

		PRACTICE TRIAL	GRADED TRIAL # 1	GRADED TRIAL # 2	NOTES
1. ✦	Check the x-ray examination order.				
2. ✦	Check the necessary equipment, as needed.				
3. ✶	***Identify the patient.***				
4. ✦	***Determine the patient's compliance with the procedure preparation instructions.***				
5. ✦	***Explain the procedure to the patient.***				
6. ✦	***Instruct the patient to remove all clothing appropriate for the procedure.***				
7. ✶	***Ask the patient to remove all jewelry and metals as needed for the procedure.***				
8. ✦	After the radiologic technologist is finished, ***ask the patient to take a comfortable position while x-rays are processed and reviewed***.				
9. ✦	***Instruct the patient to dress if the x-rays are satisfactory.***				
10. ✦	Label the x-rays and place them in an envelope, according to facility protocol.				
11. ✶	Document in patient's record.				

Name: ______________________________

Date: ______________________________

Document: Enter the appropriate information in the chart below.

Grading

Points Earned	_______		
Points Possible	_______	75	75
Percent Grade (Points Earned/Points Possible)	_______		
PASS:	_______	❑ YES ❑ NO ❑ N/A	❑ YES ❑ NO ❑ N/A

Instructor Sign-Off

Instructor: ______________________________ **Date:** ______________

Name: ______________________________

Date: ______________________________

Procedure 49-1:

Recording a 12-Lead Electrocardiograph

Objective: Perform an ECG, obtaining a satisfactory tracing without assistance.

Supplies: ECG machine with sensors; patient cable and power cord; ECG paper; electrolyte gel (if needed); alcohol; screwdriver (for adjustments); patient gown

Affective Behaviors: Affective behaviors provide a professional approach to a skill that enhances the patient encounter. These behaviors may also display sensitivity to a patient's rights and enhance communication. Pay close attention to these skills, which will be in ***bold, italicized*** font.

Notes to the Student

____

____

____

____

____

____

Skills Assessment Requirements

Read and familiarize yourself with the procedure; complete the minimum practice requirements. Document each MPR using proper charting technique. Complete each procedure within a reasonable amount of time, with a minimum of 85% accuracy.

Name: ____________________

Date: ____________________

POINT VALUE
✦ = 3–6 points
✶ = 7–9 points

		PRACTICE TRIAL	GRADED TRIAL # 1	GRADED TRIAL # 2	NOTES
1. ✦	Perform proper hand hygiene.				
2. ✦	Assemble all necessary equipment and supplies.				
3. ✦	Attach and plug in the power cord.				
4. ✶	Verify that the machine is operational and positioned properly.				
5. ✦	***Identify and interview the patient, and explain the procedure to him or her.***				
6. ✦	***Offer female patients gowns with the opening in the front.***				
7. ✦	***Position the patient flat on the table with a pillow under head and one under knees (if needed).***				
8. ✶	Prepare the electrode sites and attach the electrodes.				
9. ✦	Connect the patient cable.				
10. ✶	***Instruct the patient to relax, breathe normally, and refrain from speaking.***				
11. ✶	Standardize the machine.				
12. ✦	Adjust the stylus to the center of the paper or the center of each channel.				
13. ✦	Record. Depress the AUTO-RUN for automatic machines. For manual machines, adjust the stylus to the center, select the leads in sequence, and use RUN-25.				

Name: ____________________

Date: ____________________

POINT VALUE
✦ = 3–6 points
✶ = 7–9 points

		PRACTICE TRIAL	GRADED TRIAL # 1	GRADED TRIAL # 2	NOTES
14. ✦	If artifacts are encountered, use problem-solving skills. Mark the leads, if necessary.				
15. ✦	***Remove the sensors. Wipe the gel from the patient's skin, if necessary.***				
16. ✦	***Assist the patient in getting up, if necessary. Instruct the patient to dress.***				
17. ✦	Perform proper hand hygiene.				
18. ✦	Clean the machine, straps, and sensors. *Note:* Always follow manufacturer's directions for cleaning.				
19. ✦	Mount the ECG, if necessary, and transfer patient information.				
20. ✶	Document in the patient record. Initial the work.				

Name: ______________________________

Date: ______________________________

Document: Enter the appropriate information in the chart below.

Grading

Points Earned	_______		
Points Possible	_______	135	135
Percent Grade (Points Earned/Points Possible)	_______		
PASS:	_______	❑ YES ❑ NO ❑ N/A	❑ YES ❑ NO ❑ N/A

Instructor Sign-Off

Instructor:______________________________ **Date:** ____________________

Name: ______________________

Date: ______________________

Procedure 49-2:

Preparing and Monitoring the Patient During a Treadmill Stress Test

Objective: Prepare the patient for a treadmill test per physician's order, including all preliminary testing of vital signs and ECGs.

Supplies: Treadmill, sensors, blood pressure monitor

Affective Behaviors: Affective behaviors provide a professional approach to a skill that enhances the patient encounter. These behaviors may also display sensitivity to a patient's rights and enhance communication. Pay close attention to these skills, which will be in ***bold, italicized*** font.

Notes to the Student

____

____

____

____

____

____

Skills Assessment Requirements

Read and familiarize yourself with the procedure; complete the minimum practice requirements. Document each MPR using proper charting technique. Complete each procedure within a reasonable amount of time, with a minimum of 85% accuracy.

Name: ____________________

Date: ____________________

POINT VALUE
✦ = 3–6 points
✶ = 7–9 points

		PRACTICE TRIAL	GRADED TRIAL # 1	GRADED TRIAL # 2	NOTES
1. ✦	Assemble all necessary equipment.				
2. ✦	Plug in the power cord and turn on the machine.				
3. ✦	Verify that the treadmill is operational.				
4. ✶	***Identify the patient and explain the procedure.***				
5. ✦	Measure vital signs and record them.				
6. ✶	Attach electrode patches securely. Attach limb leads on torso at midclavicular line and on abdomen at midclavicular line. Attach chest leads as usual.				
7. ✦	Perform a baseline, resting ECG. *Note:* Check the facility protocol for a standing ECG reading.				
8. ✦	Disconnect patient cable from ECG.				
9. ✦	Attach a sphygmomanometer to the patient's arm.				
10. ✶	***Ask the patient to walk around the room or on the slow-moving treadmill.***				
11. ✦	Connect the patient to all recording devices.				
12. ✦	Check with the physician to determine the pace and incline of the treadmill.				

Name: ______________________

Date: ______________________

POINT VALUE
✦ = 3–6 points
✶ = 7–9 points

		PRACTICE TRIAL	GRADED TRIAL # 1	GRADED TRIAL # 2	NOTES
13. ✶	Record BP, ECG, and heart and respiratory rates periodically. ***Observe the patient's face for redness, difficulty breathing, chest pain, or other signs of distress.***				
14. ✦	Allow the patient to rest, and continue monitoring vital signs and ECG, as required.				
15. ✦	When the test is complete, ***clean the patient's skin and assist with dressing, as needed.***				
16. ✦	Organize the documentation into the patient's record.				

Name: ______________________________

Date: ______________________________

Document: Enter the appropriate information in the chart below.

Grading

Points Earned	______		
Points Possible	______	108	108
Percent Grade (Points Earned/Points Possible)	______		
PASS:	______	❑ YES ❑ NO ❑ N/A	❑ YES ❑ NO ❑ N/A

Instructor Sign-Off

Instructor: ______________________________ **Date:** ____________________

Name: ______________________________

Date: ______________________________

Procedure 49-3:

Applying a Holter Monitor

Objective: Apply a Holter monitor, properly instruct the patient, and obtain a satisfactory recording.

Supplies: Holter monitor with sensors, patient cable, patient activity diary, fresh batteries, blank recording tape, adhesive tape, razor, alcohol

Affective Behaviors: Affective behaviors provide a professional approach to a skill that enhances the patient encounter. These behaviors may also display sensitivity to a patient's rights and enhance communication. Pay close attention to these skills, which will be in ***bold, italicized*** font.

Notes to the Student

____

____

____

____

____

____

Skills Assessment Requirements

Read and familiarize yourself with the procedure; complete the minimum practice requirements. Document each MPR using proper charting technique. Complete each procedure within a reasonable amount of time, with a minimum of 85% accuracy.

Name: ______________________

Date: ______________________

POINT VALUE
✦ = 3–6 points
✶ = 7–9 points

		PRACTICE TRIAL	GRADED TRIAL # 1	GRADED TRIAL # 2	NOTES
1. ✦	Assemble all necessary equipment.				
2. ✶	Install new batteries and a blank tape in the monitor.				
3. ✦	Verify that the machine is operational.				
4. ✶	***Identify, interview, and instruct the patient.***				
5. ✦	***Ask the patient to undress from the waist up***, put on a gown opened in the front, and sit on the examination table.				
6. ✦	Perform proper hand hygiene.				
7. ✦	Prepare the electrode sites and attach the electrodes. Remember to attach the sensors in the proper locations (third intercostal space 2 or 3 inches to the right of the sternum, third intercostal space 2 or 3 inches to the left of the sternum, fifth intercostal space, sixth intercostal space at the right, and sixth intercostal space at the left).				
8. ✦	Attach the wires so that they point toward the feet and connect the patient cable.				
9. ✦	Secure each sensor with adhesive tape.				
10. ✦	Connect the patient cable.				
11. ✦	***Assist the patient with dressing.*** Extend the cable between the buttons or under the hem.				

Name: ______________________________

Date: ______________________________

POINT VALUE
✦ = 3–6 points
✶ = 7–9 points

		PRACTICE TRIAL	GRADED TRIAL # 1	GRADED TRIAL # 2	NOTES
12. ✦	Place the recorder in the carrying case, or attach it to the patient's belt or shoulder strap. Be sure that there is no tension on the wires.				
13. ✦	Plug the cable into the recorder.				
14. ✶	Record the start time in the patient's diary.				
15. ✦	***Ensure that the patient understands the instructions completely.***				
16. ✦	***Confirm the time for the patient's*** return to the clinic for removal of the Holter monitor. Instruct the patient that he or she may leave.				
17. ✶	Document the information in the patient's record. Sign and initial your work.				

Name: ____________________

Date: ____________________

Document: Enter the appropriate information in the chart below.

Grading

Points Earned	______		
Points Possible	______	114	114
Percent Grade (Points Earned/Points Possible)	______		
PASS:	______	❑ YES ❑ NO ❑ N/A	❑ YES ❑ NO ❑ N/A

Instructor Sign-Off

Instructor: ____________________ **Date:** ____________________

Name: ______________________________

Date: ______________________________

Procedure 50-1:

Performing a Spirometry Test to Measure Forced Vital Capacity

Objective: Perform a spirometer test to accurately measure forced vital capacity.

Supplies: Spirometry machine; nose clip; mouthpiece; disinfectant; biohazard waste container; patient record; scale for height and weight; sphygmomanometer; stethoscope

Affective Behaviors: Affective behaviors provide a professional approach to a skill that enhances the patient encounter. These behaviors may also display sensitivity to a patient's rights and enhance communication. Pay close attention to these skills, which will be in ***bold, italicized*** font.

Notes to the Student

____

____

____

____

____

____

Skills Assessment Requirements

Read and familiarize yourself with the procedure; complete the minimum practice requirements. Document each MPR using proper charting technique. Complete each procedure within a reasonable amount of time, with a minimum of 85% accuracy.

Name: ______________________________

Date: ______________________________

POINT VALUE
✦ = 3–6 points
✶ = 7–9 points

		PRACTICE TRIAL	GRADED TRIAL # 1	GRADED TRIAL # 2	NOTES
1. ✦	Assemble all equipment and materials. Perform proper hand hygiene.				
2. ✦	Calibrate the spirometer, as necessary.				
3. ✶	***Identify the patient and inquire about his or her present general health.***				
4. ✶	***Question the patient about proper preparation for the test by not smoking or using bronchodilators for at least 6 hours.***				
5. ✦	***Explain and demonstrate the procedure.***				
6. ✦	Weigh and measure the patient, obtain vital signs, and document.				
7. ✦	Explain the proper positioning and have the patient loosen any tight clothing.				
8. ✦	Start the machine and enter data, as necessary.				
9. ✶	***Review the procedure with the patient. Make sure the patient knows to breathe forcibly several times into the spirometer.***				
10. ✦	Instruct the patient to place the mouthpiece in the mouth and tightly seal the lips around it.				
11. ✦	Apply nose clips.				
12. ✦	***Ask patient to inhale deeply.***				

Name: ______________________________

Date: ______________________________

POINT VALUE
✦ = 3–6 points
✶ = 7–9 points

		PRACTICE TRIAL	GRADED TRIAL # 1	GRADED TRIAL # 2	NOTES
13. ✦	Push the start button at the same time that you ***instruct the patient.***				
14. ✶	***Encourage or "coach" the patient to blast breath out hard, quickly, and as long as possible.***				
15. ✦	***Make recommendations to improve outcome,*** if necessary.				
16. ✦.	Obtain the second set of maneuvers.				
17. ✦	Obtain the third set of maneuvers.				
18. ✦	Continue until you have three acceptable outcomes. *Note:* You may facilitate up to eight attempts. Some computerized machines will pick the best attempt and print.				
19. ✦	Remove nose clips. ***Ask the patient to remain until the physician reviews the results.***				
20. ✦	Provide the physician with the trial information for review.				
21. ✶	Record the results in the patient's record.				
22. ✦	Clean tubing and dispose of mouthpieces using standard precautions.				

Name: ____________________

Date: ____________________

Document: Enter the appropriate information in the chart below.

Grading

Points Earned	_______		
Points Possible	_______	147	147
Percent Grade (Points Earned/Points Possible)	_______		
PASS:	_______	❑ YES ❑ NO ❑ N/A	❑ YES ❑ NO ❑ N/A

Instructor Sign-Off

Instructor: ____________________ **Date:** ____________________

Name: ______________________________

Date: ______________________________

Procedure 50-2:

Teaching Peak Flow Measurement

Objective: Instruct the patient to correctly monitor peak flow and to record results.

Supplies: Peak flow meter; documentation diary/chart; diagram of lungs and breathing processes; pen; patient record

Affective Behaviors: Affective behaviors provide a professional approach to a skill that enhances the patient encounter. These behaviors may also display sensitivity to a patient's rights and enhance communication. Pay close attention to these skills, which will be in ***bold, italicized*** font.

Notes to the Student

____

____

____

____

____

____

Skills Assessment Requirements

Read and familiarize yourself with the procedure; complete the minimum practice requirements. Document each MPR using proper charting technique. Complete each procedure within a reasonable amount of time, with a minimum of 85% accuracy.

Name: ______________________

Date: ______________________

POINT VALUE
✦ = 3–6 points
✶ = 7–9 points

		PRACTICE TRIAL	GRADED TRIAL # 1	GRADED TRIAL # 2	NOTES
1. ✦	Perform proper hand hygiene.				
2. ✦	Assemble peak flow meter with disposable mouthpiece or individual peak flow meter for patient use at home.				
3. ✶	***Identify the patient and explain the procedure:*** ***Explain breathing processes and their importance to overall health. Demonstrate how the mouthpiece fits and explain what the numbers mean. The peak flow meter should always be set at zero.***				
4. ✦	***Have the patient place the mouthpiece in the mouth and form a tight seal. Explain that better results may be obtained if the patient is standing during the test.***				
5. ✶	***Instruct the patient to stand, take deepest breath possible, position mouthpiece without biting down, and exhale completely and as forcefully as possible.***				
6. ✦	***Instruct the patient to note the number on the machine where the sliding gauge stopped and to record the results. Reset to zero. Repeat three times.***				
7. ✦	***Instruct the patient to follow the physician's orders for when and how often to perform the test each day. The "best" result is documented.***				

Name: ______________________________

Date: ______________________________

POINT VALUE
✦ = 3–6 points
✶ = 7–9 points

		PRACTICE TRIAL	GRADED TRIAL # 1	GRADED TRIAL # 2	NOTES
8. ✦	***Demonstrate how to wash the mouthpiece with soap and water without submerging the peak flow meter.***				
9. ✶	Document the instruction in the patient's record.				
10. ✦	Perform proper hand hygiene.				

Name: ______________________________

Date: ______________________________

Document: Enter the appropriate information in the chart below.

Grading

Points Earned	______		
Points Possible	______	69	69
Percent Grade (Points Earned/Points Possible)	______		
PASS:	______	❑ YES ❑ NO ❑ N/A	❑ YES ❑ NO ❑ N/A

Instructor Sign-Off

Instructor: ______________________________ **Date:** ________________

Name: ______________________________

Date: ______________________________

Procedure 50-3:

Measuring Oxygen Saturation

Objective: Attach and measure the patient's oxygen saturation.

Supplies: Pulse oximeter, nail polish remover, alcohol wipe, patient record, gloves, adhesive tape

Affective Behaviors: Affective behaviors provide a professional approach to a skill that enhances the patient encounter. These behaviors may also display sensitivity to a patient's rights and enhance communication. Pay close attention to these skills, which will be in ***bold, italicized*** font.

Notes to the Student

____

____

____

____

____

____

Skills Assessment Requirements

Read and familiarize yourself with the procedure; complete the minimum practice requirements. Document each MPR using proper charting technique. Complete each procedure within a reasonable amount of time, with a minimum of 85% accuracy.

Name: ______________________

Date: ______________________

POINT VALUE
✦ = 3–6 points
✶ = 7–9 points

		PRACTICE TRIAL	GRADED TRIAL # 1	GRADED TRIAL # 2	NOTES
1. ✦	Perform proper hand hygiene. Apply gloves.				
2. ✦	Assemble equipment based on patient's size and condition.				
3. ✦	***Identify the patient and explain the procedure.***				
4. ✶	Choose the correct size sensor for the patient.				
5. ✦	***Ask if the patient is allergic to adhesive tape.*** If so, use a clip on the oximeter.				
6. ✦	Remove nail polish, if needed.				
7. ✦	Assess patient's pulse rate.				
8. ✶	Wipe the site with an alcohol wipe. Attach the sensor. Be sure the sensors are correctly aligned opposite each other.				
9. ✦	Connect the sensor to the pulse oximeter. *Note:* Some oximeters are cordless.				
10. ✦	Turn on the machine and set the alarm as directed.				
11. ✦	Change the position of the oximeter every 4 hours or as directed.				
12. ✶	Compare the pulse previously evaluated with pulse on the oximeter. If there is a large difference between these pulse measurements, check the oximeter function.				

Name: ______________________

Date: ______________________

POINT VALUE
✦ = 3–6 points
∗ = 7–9 points

		PRACTICE TRIAL	GRADED TRIAL # 1	GRADED TRIAL # 2	NOTES
13. ✦	Record the oxygen saturation level in the patient record at the intervals ordered by the physician.				
14. ✦	If oxygen saturation level is abnormal, follow facility protocol for notifying superiors.				

Name: ______________________

Date: ______________________

Document: Enter the appropriate information in the chart below.

Grading

Points Earned	_____		
Points Possible	_____	93	93
Percent Grade (Points Earned/Points Possible)	_____		
PASS:	_____	❏ YES ❏ NO ❏ N/A	❏ YES ❏ NO ❏ N/A

Instructor Sign-Off

Instructor: ______________________ **Date:** ______________________

Name: ______________________________

Date: ______________________________

Procedure 51-1:

Application of a Hot Compress

Objective: Perform application of a hot compress and document the procedure without error.

Supplies: Sink; basin of warm water or soaking solution. as directed by the physician; bath thermometer; absorbent cloths or gauze squares; waterproof cover; pencil or pen

Affective Behaviors: Affective behaviors provide a professional approach to a skill that enhances the patient encounter. These behaviors may also display sensitivity to a patient's rights and enhance communication. Pay close attention to these skills, which will be in ***bold, italicized*** font.

Notes to the Student

____

____

____

____

____

____

Skills Assessment Requirements

Read and familiarize yourself with the procedure; complete the minimum practice requirements. Document each MPR using proper charting technique. Complete each procedure within a reasonable amount of time, with a minimum of 85% accuracy.

Name: ____________________

Date: ____________________

POINT VALUE
✦ = 3–6 points
✶ = 7–9 points

		PRACTICE TRIAL	GRADED TRIAL # 1	GRADED TRIAL # 2	NOTES
1. ✦	Perform proper hand hygiene.				
2. ✦	Assemble all equipment and materials. Use sterile equipment and standard precautions if open wound is present.				
3. ✶	Identify the patient and explain the procedure.				
4. ✦	Fill the basin half full of warm water or medicated solution prepared according to the physician's directions.				
5. ✦	Request that the patient remove any clothing; compresses must be on bare skin. ***Assist the patient, if necessary***.				
6. ✦	Check the temperature of the solution with a bath thermometer.				
7. ✦	Position the patient comfortably and in a well-supported position.				
8. ✦	Place the cloths in the basin of hot water solution. Wring out one cloth until it is wet but not dripping.				
9. ✦	Gradually place the compress on the patient's body part; ***ask the patient how the temperature feels.***				
10. ✦	Frequently test the temperature of the solution. Replace the water as the solution cools with warm water.				

Name: ____________________

Date: ____________________

POINT VALUE ✦ = 3–6 points ✶ = 7–9 points		PRACTICE TRIAL	GRADED TRIAL # 1	GRADED TRIAL # 2	NOTES
11. ✶	Time the procedure according to the physician's order, usually 15–30 minutes. Check the patient periodically for signs of increased redness, swelling, or pain.				
12. ✦	Gently dry the affected body part.				
13. ✦	***Instruct the patient on any further care, such as continuing the soaks at home.***				
14. ✦	Place towels in the laundry and clean all equipment.				
15. ✦	Perform proper hand hygiene.				
16. ✶	Document the procedure in the patient's record.				

Name: ______________________________

Date: ______________________________

Document: Enter the appropriate information in the chart below.

Grading

Points Earned	______		
Points Possible	______	105	105
Percent Grade (Points Earned/Points Possible)	______		
PASS:	______	❑ YES ❑ NO ❑ N/A	❑ YES ❑ NO ❑ N/A

Instructor Sign-Off

Instructor: ______________________________ **Date:** ______________

Name: ______________________________

Date: ______________________________

Procedure 51-2:

Application of a Hot Soak

Objective: Perform hot soak application and document the procedure without error.

Supplies: Soaking solution or water; basin or tub; bath thermometer; towels

Affective Behaviors: Affective behaviors provide a professional approach to a skill that enhances the patient encounter. These behaviors may also display sensitivity to a patient's rights and enhance communication. Pay close attention to these skills, which will be in ***bold, italicized*** font.

Notes to the Student

____

____

____

____

____

____

Skills Assessment Requirements

Read and familiarize yourself with the procedure; complete the minimum practice requirements. Document each MPR using proper charting technique. Complete each procedure within a reasonable amount of time, with a minimum of 85% accuracy.

Name: ______________________

Date: ______________________

POINT VALUE
✦ = 3–6 points
✶ = 7–9 points

		PRACTICE TRIAL	GRADED TRIAL # 1	GRADED TRIAL # 2	NOTES
1. ✦	Assemble all equipment and materials. *Note:* If an open wound is present, use sterile equipment and standard precautions.				
2. ✦	Perform proper hand hygiene.				
3. ✦	***Identify the patient and explain the procedure.***				
4. ✦	Fill the basin or tub half full of water or solution as directed by the physician.				
5. ✦	The soaks should be applied to bare skin. ***Request that the patient remove any clothing and assist, if necessary.***				
6. ✶	Check water temperature with bath thermometer. *Note:* The temperature range for an adult should be between 105° F and 107° F (41° C and 44 °C).				
7. ✦	***Position the patient in a comfortable, well-supported position.***				
8. ✦	***Pad the side of the basin or tub with a towel to prevent the patient's body from rubbing on the edge.***				
9. ✦	***Gradually place the patient's body part in the solution. Ask the patient to tell you how the temperature feels.***				

Name: ____________________

Date: ____________________

POINT VALUE
✦ = 3–6 points
✶ = 7–9 points

		PRACTICE TRIAL	GRADED TRIAL # 1	GRADED TRIAL # 2	NOTES
10. ✦	Frequently test the temperature of the solution. Using a pitcher, remove part of the liquid every 5 minutes and replace it with hot water. Pour the hot water at the edge of the basin and protect the patient by placing your hand between the patient's body part and the hot water. Swirl the water while pouring to mix the water.				
11. ✶	Time the procedure according to the physician's order, usually 15–30 minutes. ***Check the patient periodically for signs of increased redness, swelling, or pain.***				
12. ✦	Gently dry the affected body part.				
13. ✦	Instruct the patient on any further care, or on further soaks at home.				
14. ✦	Place towels in the laundry. *Note:* If an open wound is present, handle linens according to standard precautions.				
15. ✦	Clean all equipment.				
16. ✦	Perform proper hand hygiene and return equipment.				
17. ✶	Document procedure in patient's record.				

Name: ___________________________

Date: ___________________________

Document: Enter the appropriate information in the chart below.

Grading

Points Earned	_______		
Points Possible	_______	111	111
Percent Grade (Points Earned/Points Possible)	_______		
PASS:	_______	❑ YES ❑ NO ❑ N/A	❑ YES ❑ NO ❑ N/A

Instructor Sign-Off

Instructor: ___________________________ **Date:** ___________________________

Name: ____________________

Date: ____________________

Procedure 51-3:

Application of a Heating Pad

Objective: Perform a heating pad application and document the procedure without error.

Supplies: Heating pad with protective covering or pillowcase

Affective Behaviors: Affective behaviors provide a professional approach to a skill that enhances the patient encounter. These behaviors may also display sensitivity to a patient's rights and enhance communication. Pay close attention to these skills, which will be in ***bold, italicized*** font.

Notes to the Student

Perform a preliminary check of the heating pad without bending it to determine that the wires are in good condition.

Skills Assessment Requirements

Read and familiarize yourself with the procedure; complete the minimum practice requirements. Document each MPR using proper charting technique. Complete each procedure within a reasonable amount of time, with a minimum of 85% accuracy.

Name: ____________________

Date: ____________________

POINT VALUE
✦ = 3–6 points
✶ = 7–9 points

		PRACTICE TRIAL	GRADED TRIAL # 1	GRADED TRIAL # 2	NOTES
1. ✦	Assemble and test the equipment.				
2. ✦	Perform proper hand hygiene.				
3. ✶	***Identify the patient and explain the procedure. Caution against using pins, bending the heating elements within the pad, or lying on the heating pad.***				
4. ✦	Place the heating pad in a protective covering or pillow case.				
5. ✦	Connect the heating pad cord to an electrical outlet. Set the temperature at the ordered setting (low or medium).				
6. ✦	***Place the heating pad over the patient's affected area. Ask the patient how it feels.***				
7. ✦	***Instruct the patient regarding the proper temperature setting.***				
8. ✶	Leave the heating pad in place for the ordered amount of time (15 to 20 minutes). ***Check the patient periodically for any signs of redness, swelling, or pain.***				
9. ✦	Remove the heating pad when the procedure is complete. ***Instruct the patient on any after-care procedures such as further home treatment.***				
10. ✦	Place the protective covering in the laundry.				
11. ✦	Use proper hand hygiene and return all used equipment.				
12. ✶	Document the procedure in the patient's record.				

Name: ______________________________

Date: ______________________________

Document: Enter the appropriate information in the chart below.

Grading

Points Earned	______		
Points Possible	______	81	81
Percent Grade (Points Earned/Points Possible)	______		
PASS:	______	❑ YES ❑ NO ❑ N/A	❑ YES ❑ NO ❑ N/A

Instructor Sign-Off

Instructor: ______________________________ **Date:** ______________

Name: ______________________________

Date: ______________________________

Procedure 51-4:

Application of a Cold Compress

Objective: Perform a cold compress application and document the procedure without error.

Supplies: Water; absorbent cloths or gauze squares; waterproof cover or plastic wrap; basin; ice

Affective Behaviors: Affective behaviors provide a professional approach to a skill that enhances the patient encounter. These behaviors may also display sensitivity to a patient's rights and enhance communication. Pay close attention to these skills, which will be in ***bold, italicized*** font.

Notes to the Student

____

____

____

____

____

____

Skills Assessment Requirements

Read and familiarize yourself with the procedure; complete the minimum practice requirements. Document each MPR using proper charting technique. Complete each procedure within a reasonable amount of time, with a minimum of 85% accuracy.

Name: ______________________

Date: ______________________

POINT VALUE
✦ = 3–6 points
✶ = 7–9 points

		PRACTICE TRIAL	GRADED TRIAL # 1	GRADED TRIAL # 2	NOTES
1. ✦	Perform proper hand hygiene.				
2. ✦	Assemble all equipment. *Note:* If an open wound is present, use sterile equipment and standard precautions.				
3. ✦	***Identify and instruct the patient regarding the procedure.***				
4. ✦	Fill the basin half full of cold water. Add ice cubes and compress.				
5. ✶	Wring out the compress until it is wet but not dripping. Wrap the compress in a plastic or waterproof covering to prevent dripping. Gently place the compress on the patient's affected body part.				
6. ✦	Check the compress every 3–5 minutes and replace it with another cold compress when it is no longer cool. Add more ice as the water warms.				
7. ✦	Leave the compress in place for the time specified by the ordering physician (usually 15–20 minutes).				
8. ✦	Gently dry the affected body part.				
9. ✦	Place the linens in the proper container. Clean all the equipment.				
10. ✦	Perform proper hand hygiene and return all equipment.				
11. ✶	Document the procedure in the patient's record.				

Name: ______________________________

Date: ______________________________

Document: Enter the appropriate information in the chart below.

Grading

Points Earned	________		
Points Possible	________	72	72
Percent Grade (Points Earned/Points Possible)	________		
PASS:	________	❑ YES ❑ NO ❑ N/A	❑ YES ❑ NO ❑ N/A

Instructor Sign-Off

Instructor: ______________________________ **Date:** ________________

Name: ______________________

Date: ______________________

Procedure 51-5:

Application of an Ice Bag

Objective: Perform application of an ice bag and document the procedure without error.

Supplies: Ice bag with protective cover; ice chips or crushed ice

Affective Behaviors: Affective behaviors provide a professional approach to a skill that enhances the patient encounter. These behaviors may also display sensitivity to a patient's rights and enhance communication. Pay close attention to these skills, which will be in ***bold, italicized*** font.

Notes to the Student

____

____

____

____

____

____

Skills Assessment Requirements

Read and familiarize yourself with the procedure; complete the minimum practice requirements. Document each MPR using proper charting technique. Complete each procedure within a reasonable amount of time, with a minimum of 85% accuracy.

Name: ___________________________

Date: ___________________________

POINT VALUE
✦ = 3–6 points
✶ = 7–9 points

		PRACTICE TRIAL	GRADED TRIAL # 1	GRADED TRIAL # 2	NOTES
1. ✦	Perform proper hand hygiene.				
2. ✦	Assemble and test equipment.				
3. ✦	***Identify the patient and instruct the patient about the procedure.***				
4. ✦	Fill the ice bag one-half to two-thirds full of ice. Expel air by squeezing the empty portion of the ice bag. Replace the cap.				
5. ✦	Dry the bag, and place it in a protective cover or small hand towel.				
6. ✦	Place the ice bag over the patient's affected body part. ***Ask the patient how it feels.***				
7. ✶	Leave the bag in place for the time specified by the physician's order (15–20 minutes).				
8. ✦	Refill the bag with ice, as needed.				
9. ✦	Clean the equipment. Allow the bag to air dry.				
10. ✦	Perform proper hand hygiene.				
11. ✶	Document the procedure in the patient's record.				

Name: ______________________________

Date: ______________________________

Document: Enter the appropriate information in the chart below.

Grading

Points Earned	________		
Points Possible	________	72	72
Percent Grade (Points Earned/Points Possible)	________		
PASS:	________	❑ YES ❑ NO ❑ N/A	❑ YES ❑ NO ❑ N/A

Instructor Sign-Off

Instructor: ______________________________ **Date:** ______________________________

Name: ______________________________

Date: ______________________________

Procedure 51-6:

Application of a Cold Chemical Pack

Objective: Perform a cold chemical pack application and document the procedure without error.

Supplies: Cold chemical pack, soft cloth

Affective Behaviors: Affective behaviors provide a professional approach to a skill that enhances the patient encounter. These behaviors may also display sensitivity to a patient's rights and enhance communication. Pay close attention to these skills, which will be in ***bold, italicized*** font.

Notes to the Student

____

____

____

____

____

____

Skills Assessment Requirements

Read and familiarize yourself with the procedure; complete the minimum practice requirements. Document each MPR using proper charting technique. Complete each procedure within a reasonable amount of time, with a minimum of 85% accuracy.

Name: ______________________

Date: ______________________

POINT VALUE
✦ = 3–6 points
✶ = 7–9 points

		PRACTICE TRIAL	GRADED TRIAL # 1	GRADED TRIAL # 2	NOTES
1. ✦	Perform proper hand hygiene.				
2. ✦	Assemble the equipment.				
3. ✦	***Identify the patient and instruct the patient about the procedure.***				
4. ✶	Shake the bag to allow the crystals to fall to the bottom. Firmly squeeze the bag until the inner bag ruptures and mix the contents.				
5. ✦	Place the bag inside a soft cloth.				
6. ✦	Place the cloth-protected bag over the patient's affected body part.				
7. ✦	Check the patient every 3–5 minutes.				
8. ✦	Leave the cold pack in place for the specified time (15–20 minutes).				
9. ✦	Discard the ice pack in a proper waste container after use.				
10. ✦	Perform proper hand hygiene.				
11. ✶	Document the procedure in the patient's record.				

Name: ______________________

Date: ______________________

Document: Enter the appropriate information in the chart below.

Grading

Points Earned	______		
Points Possible	______	72	72
Percent Grade (Points Earned/Points Possible)	______		
PASS:	______	❑ YES ❑ NO ❑ N/A	❑ YES ❑ NO ❑ N/A

Instructor Sign-Off

Instructor: ______________________ **Date:** ______________________

Name: ___________________________

Date: ___________________________

Procedure 51-7:

Instructing a Patient to Use Crutches Correctly

Objective: Instruct a patient on the correct use of crutches.

Supplies: Crutches, gait belt

Affective Behaviors: Affective behaviors provide a professional approach to a skill that enhances the patient encounter. These behaviors may also display sensitivity to a patient's rights and enhance communication. Pay close attention to these skills, which will be in ***bold, italicized*** font.

Notes to the Student

____

____

____

____

____

____

Skills Assessment Requirements

Read and familiarize yourself with the procedure; complete the minimum practice requirements. Document each MPR using proper charting technique. Complete each procedure within a reasonable amount of time, with a minimum of 85% accuracy.

Name: ______________________________

Date: ______________________________

POINT VALUE
✦ = 3–6 points
✶ = 7–9 points

		PRACTICE TRIAL	GRADED TRIAL # 1	GRADED TRIAL # 2	NOTES
1. ✦	Assemble all equipment as ordered by the physician.				
2. ✶	Check the crutches to determine that they are in good working order and without defects.				
3. ✦	Perform proper hand hygiene.				
4. ✦	***Identify the patient and explain the procedure.***				
5. ✶	***Be sure that the patient is wearing sturdy, nonskid shoes.***				
6. ✦	***Demonstrate the correct positioning.***				
7. ✦	***Demonstrate the gait requested by the physician.***				
8. ✦	***Have the patient stand against the wall or near a chair for support.***				
9. ✶	Adjust the crutch length to the appropriate height. *Note:* The distance between the top of the crutch and axilla should be equivalent to three finger widths.				
10. ✦	***Instruct the patient to hold his or her head up and to stand straight, with the abdomen in and the feet straight, with a slight bend at the knee.***				
11. ✶	***Explain to the patient that his or her weight should be supported by the hands, not the underarms.*** *Note:* Be sure to instruct the patient to not rest his or her body weight on the axillary bars for more than 1–2 minutes.				

Name: ______________________________

Date: ______________________________

POINT VALUE
✦ = 3–6 points
✶ = 7–9 points

		PRACTICE TRIAL	GRADED TRIAL # 1	GRADED TRIAL # 2	NOTES
12. ✦	***Instruct the patient to assume the basic crutch or tripod stance to provide a firm base of support.***				
13. ✦	Crutches should always be moved forward and to the side so the feet can swing through.				
14. ✦	***Instruct the patient to take small steps and swing through when first learning to use crutches.*** *Note:* The crutches should only move about 12 inches forward with each step.				
15. ✶	***Have the patient practice the gait.***				
16. ✦	***Remind the patient to report any numbness or tingling in the arm. Pad crutch shoulders and hand bars for extra comfort, if necessary.***				
17. ✦	***Remind the patient to periodically check the nuts and wing bolts to maintain tightness, and to frequently check the rubber tips for cracks.***				
18. ✦	Make corrections on the patient's crutches, as needed.				
19. ✶	Document the procedure in the patient's record.				

Name: ______________________

Date: ______________________

Document: Enter the appropriate information in the chart below.

Grading

Points Earned	______		
Points Possible	______	132	132
Percent Grade (Points Earned/Points Possible)	______		
PASS:	______	❑ YES ❑ NO ❑ N/A	❑ YES ❑ NO ❑ N/A

Instructor Sign-Off

Instructor: ______________________ **Date:** ______________________

Name: ______________________________

Date: ______________________________

Procedure 51-8:

Instructing a Patient to Use a Cane or Single Crutch Correctly

Objective: Instruct a patient on the correct use of a cane.

Supplies: Cane suited to the patient's needs, gait belt

Affective Behaviors: Affective behaviors provide a professional approach to a skill that enhances the patient encounter. These behaviors may also display sensitivity to a patient's rights and enhance communication. Pay close attention to these skills, which will be in ***bold, italicized*** font.

Notes to the Student

____

____

____

____

____

____

Skills Assessment Requirements

Read and familiarize yourself with the procedure; complete the minimum practice requirements. Document each MPR using proper charting technique. Complete each procedure within a reasonable amount of time, with a minimum of 85% accuracy.

Name: ______________________________

Date: ______________________________

POINT VALUE
✦ = 3–6 points
✶ = 7–9 points

		PRACTICE TRIAL	GRADED TRIAL # 1	GRADED TRIAL # 2	NOTES
1. ✦	Assemble all equipment as ordered by the physician.				
2. ✶	Check the cane height and condition of the cane tip.				
3. ✦	***Identify the patient and explain the procedure.***				
4. ✦	Perform proper hand hygiene.				
5. ✶	Be sure that the patient is wearing sturdy, nonskid shoes.				
6. ✦	Demonstrate the correct position.				
7. ✦	Demonstrate the gait requested by the physician.				
8. ✦	***Instruct the patient*** to hold the cane on the unaffected side.				
9. ✶	***Instruct the patient*** to place the cane 6 inches in front and slightly to one side of the unaffected side. Make sure the cane tip is firmly on the floor and the weight is supported on the strong leg and cane. The patient's elbow should be slightly flexed during weight bearing.				
10. ✦	***Instruct the patient*** to hold his or her head up and to stand straight, not looking down at the feet.				
11. ✦	Have the patient move the cane forward 6–12 inches and bring the affected leg forward until it is even with the cane.				

Name: ______________________________

Date: ______________________________

POINT VALUE
✦ = 3–6 points
✶ = 7–9 points

		PRACTICE TRIAL	GRADED TRIAL # 1	GRADED TRIAL # 2	NOTES
12. ✶	***Instruct the patient*** to move the strong leg forward past the cane and weaker leg. As the unaffected foot moves forward, the weight is shifted to the weak or affected foot and cane. Thus the cane will provide support for weight bearing.				
13. ✦	Have the patient repeat the walking pattern, and evaluate the patient's balance and endurance.				
14. ✶	Document the procedure in the patient's record.				

Name: ______________________

Date: ______________________

Document: Enter the appropriate information in the chart below.

Grading

Points Earned	______		
Points Possible	______	99	99
Percent Grade (Points Earned/Points Possible)	______		
PASS:	______	❑ YES ❑ NO ❑ N/A	❑ YES ❑ NO ❑ N/A

Instructor Sign-Off

Instructor: ______________________ **Date:** ______________

Name: ______________________________

Date: ______________________________

Procedure 51-9:

Teaching a Patient to Correctly Use a Walker

Objective: Instruct a patient on the correct use of a walker.

Supplies: Walker suited to patient's needs, gait belt

Affective Behaviors: Affective behaviors provide a professional approach to a skill that enhances the patient encounter. These behaviors may also display sensitivity to a patient's rights and enhance communication. Pay close attention to these skills, which will be in ***bold, italicized*** font.

Notes to the Student

____

____

____

____

____

____

Skills Assessment Requirements

Read and familiarize yourself with the procedure; complete the minimum practice requirements. Document each MPR using proper charting technique. Complete each procedure within a reasonable amount of time, with a minimum of 85% accuracy.

Name: ______________________

Date: ______________________

POINT VALUE
✦ = 3–6 points
✶ = 7–9 points

		PRACTICE TRIAL	GRADED TRIAL # 1	GRADED TRIAL # 2	NOTES
1. ✦	Assemble all equipment as ordered by the physician.				
2. ✶	Check the condition of the walker.				
3. ✦	Perform proper hand hygiene.				
4. ✦	***Identify the patient and explain the procedure.***				
5. ✶	Be sure that the patient is wearing sturdy, nonskid shoes.				
6. ✦	***Demonstrate the correct stance and gait with the walker.***				
7. ✦	***Assist the patient into the walker.***				
8. ✶	***Evaluate the walker for proper height and fit.*** *Note:* The top of the walker should reach the patient's hip-bone and the patient's hands should be on the handgrip with the elbow flexed at a 30-degree angle.				
9. ✶	Instruct the patient to distribute his or her weight evenly between the walker and both legs.				
10. ✦	Have the patient move the walker 6–8 inches ahead, with all four legs of the walker hitting the floor at the same time.				
11. ✦	Instruct the patient to bring the weaker foot into the walker.				
12. ✦	Instruct the patient to bring the stronger foot forward, even with the weaker foot.				

Name: ____________________

Date: ____________________

POINT VALUE
✦ = 3–6 points
✶ = 7–9 points

		PRACTICE TRIAL	GRADED TRIAL # 1	GRADED TRIAL # 2	NOTES
13. ✦	Have the patient continue walking with the walker while you evaluate the patient's balance and endurance.				
14. ✶	Document the teaching and the patient's response in the patient's record.				

Name: ______________________________

Date: ______________________________

Document: Enter the appropriate information in the chart below.

Grading

Points Earned	_______		
Points Possible	_______	99	99
Percent Grade (Points Earned/Points Possible)	_______		
PASS:	_______	❏ YES ❏ NO ❏ N/A	❏ YES ❏ NO ❏ N/A

Instructor Sign-Off

Instructor: ______________________________ **Date:** ______________________________

Name: ____________________

Date: ____________________

Procedure 51-10:

Wheelchair Transfer to Chair or Examination Table

Objective: Move the patient from a wheelchair to a chair or examination table without error.

Supplies: Chair or examination table; gait belt; step stool

Affective Behaviors: Affective behaviors provide a professional approach to a skill that enhances the patient encounter. These behaviors may also display sensitivity to a patient's rights and enhance communication. Pay close attention to these skills, which will be in ***bold, italicized*** font.

Notes to the Student

____

____

____

____

____

____

Skills Assessment Requirements

Read and familiarize yourself with the procedure; complete the minimum practice requirements. Document each MPR using proper charting technique. Complete each procedure within a reasonable amount of time, with a minimum of 85% accuracy.

Name: ______________________

Date: ______________________

POINT VALUE
✦ = 3–6 points
✶ = 7–9 points

		PRACTICE TRIAL	GRADED TRIAL # 1	GRADED TRIAL # 2	NOTES
1. ✦	Use proper hand hygiene.				
2. ✶	***Identify the patient and introduce yourself.***				
3. ✶	***Explain what you are going to do before you start. Discuss what the patient can do to assist.***				
4. ✦	Place the wheelchair at a 45-degree angle to the chair or exam table.				
5. ✦	Apply the wheelchair brakes on both sides. Move the foot pedals up and out of the way, clearing a path for patient movement. ***Gently place the patient's feet on the floor and have the patient shift forward.***				
6. ✶	Make sure that the exam table or chair is stable before attempting to transfer the patient.				
7. ✦	***Position yourself near the patient's nonparalyzed side so you can provide support and the patient can use the unaffected side.*** *Note:* Use terms such as "stronger, weaker" or "affected, unaffected" instead of "good, bad."				
8. ✶	Place one of your feet forward to establish a firm base of support. Move down toward the patient while keeping your back straight.				

Name: ______________________________

Date: ______________________________

POINT VALUE
✦ = 3–6 points
✶ = 7–9 points

		PRACTICE TRIAL	GRADED TRIAL # 1	GRADED TRIAL # 2	NOTES
9. ✦	Have the patient place his or her hands on the arm supports of the wheelchair. Ask the patient to lean forward and push up while assisting the patient to a standing position.				
10. ✦	***Position yourself so that the patient's weak leg is between your knees.*** Support the paralyzed leg with your knees.				
11. ✦	***Place your hands in the patient's axillary areas and help the patient to stand.*** Use your leg muscles to push the patient's body upward.				
12. ✦	Allow the patient to stand for a few moments before attempting to move the patient into the chair or onto the examination table.				
13. ✦	Assist the patient to turn toward the nonparalyzed side by pivoting your own body as you hold the patient under the arms. Do not twist your body. Turn with the patient as a unit.				
14. ✶	Gently lower the patient into the chair by bending your knees and keeping your back straight.				

Name: ______________________

Date: ______________________

POINT VALUE ✦ = 3–6 points ✶ = 7–9 points		PRACTICE TRIAL	GRADED TRIAL # 1	GRADED TRIAL # 2	NOTES
15. ✦	If the patient must move onto an exam table and can assist you, then support the weak side as the patient places the stronger leg on the step stool. Pivot the patient around to sit on the edge of the table. Instruct and assist the patient to move back on the table to eliminate the risk of injury. *Note:* Never attempt to move a patient who is unable to assist. Ask for assistance from another person.				
16. ✦	***When assisting the patient into a supine position, support the paralyzed leg and ease the patient gently onto the table.***				
17. ✦	Never leave a physically challenged patient unattended.				

Name: ______________________________

Date: ______________________________

Document: Enter the appropriate information in the chart below.

Grading

Points Earned	______		
Points Possible	______	117	117
Percent Grade (Points Earned/Points Possible)	______		
PASS:	______	❑ YES ❑ NO ❑ N/A	❑ YES ❑ NO ❑ N/A

Instructor Sign-Off

Instructor: ______________________________ **Date:** ____________________

Name: ______________________

Date: ______________________

Procedure 54-1:

Administering Oral Medications

Objective: Administer oral medication.

Supplies: Medication order signed by physician; oral medication; calibrated paper cup or receptacle for medication; water in glass; patient instruction sheet; biohazard waste container; pen

Affective Behaviors: Affective behaviors provide a professional approach to a skill that enhances the patient encounter. These behaviors may also display sensitivity to a patient's rights and enhance communication. Pay close attention to these skills, which will be in ***bold, italicized*** font.

Notes to the Student

____

____

____

____

____

____

Skills Assessment Requirements

Read and familiarize yourself with the procedure; complete the minimum practice requirements. Document each MPR using proper charting technique. Complete each procedure within a reasonable amount of time, with a minimum of 85% accuracy.

Name: ____________________

Date: ____________________

POINT VALUE
✦ = 3–6 points
✶ = 7–9 points

		PRACTICE TRIAL	GRADED TRIAL # 1	GRADED TRIAL # 2	NOTES
1. ✦	Assemble equipment.				
2. ✦	Perform proper hand hygiene.				
3. ✶	Select the correct medication using the "three befores" technique. *Note:* If you are not familiar with the medication, look it up in a reference book, read the package insert, and/or consult the physician.				
4. ✶	Always double-check the label to make sure the strength is correct.				
5. ✦	Correctly calculate the dosage in writing. Double-check your calculations with someone else.				
6. ✦	Place a medicine cup or container on a flat surface.				
7. ✦	Gently shake the medication if it is in liquid form.				
8. ✶	Hold the bottle so that the label is in the palm of your hand to prevent damaging the label with liquid medication.				
9. ✶	Recheck the label.				
10. ✶	Remove the cap from the medicine container and place it upside down on a clean surface.				

Name: ______________________

Date: ______________________

POINT VALUE
✦ = 3–6 points
✶ = 7–9 points

		PRACTICE TRIAL	GRADED TRIAL # 1	GRADED TRIAL # 2	NOTES
11. ✦	**Liquid Medication:** Hold the calibrated medicine cup at eye level and pour the medication into the cup, stopping at the correct dosage line. Pour the medication away from the label side of the bottle. If too much medication is poured into the calibrated cup, do not return it to the bottle. Discard it into a sink. **Table or Capsule Medication:** Shake out the correct number of tablets or pills into the bottle cap. Then, place the tablets or pills in the medicine cup. If you accidentally pour out an extra tablet, do not return it to the medication bottle; discard it.				
12. ✦	Check the medication again to make sure the dosage is the same as the medication order.				
13. ✦	Replace the cap on the medication bottle and return the bottle to the storage shelf.				
14. ✶	Take the prepared medication and a glass of water to the patient.				
15. ✦	***Identify the patient and warmly greet the patient. Introduce yourself to the patient and ask the patient if he or she has any allergies.***				

Name: ______________________

Date: ______________________

POINT VALUE
✦ = 3–6 points
✶ = 7–9 points

		PRACTICE TRIAL	GRADED TRIAL # 1	GRADED TRIAL # 2	NOTES
16. ✦	Tell the patient the name of the medication and dosage that you are administering per the physician's order. ***Ask the patient if he or she has any questions prior to taking the medication.***				
17. ✦	***Remain with the patient until the medication has been swallowed.*** *Note:* After giving the medication to the patient, it is best to have the patient wait in the office for 30 minutes.				
18. ✦	***Provide the patient with written followup instructions if further medication is to be taken.***				
19. ✶	Document the medication administration, noting in the patient's record the time, medication name, dosage route, and your name.				

Name: ______________________________

Date: ______________________________

Document: Enter the appropriate information in the chart below.

Grading

Points Earned	_______		
Points Possible	_______	135	135
Percent Grade (Points Earned/Points Possible)	_______		
PASS:	_______	❑ YES ❑ NO ❑ N/A	❑ YES ❑ NO ❑ N/A

Instructor Sign-Off

Instructor:______________________________ **Date:** ____________________

Name: ______________________________

Date: ______________________________

Procedure 54-2:

Administering Sublingual or Buccal Medication

Objective: Administer a medication to a patient under the tongue or between the cheek and gum.

Supplies: Medication order; oral medication; paper cup or receptacle for medication; patient instruction sheet; biohazard waste container; pen; patient record

Affective Behaviors: Affective behaviors provide a professional approach to a skill that enhances the patient encounter. These behaviors may also display sensitivity to a patient's rights and enhance communication. Pay close attention to these skills, which will be in ***bold, italicized*** font.

Notes to the Student

____

____

____

____

____

____

Skills Assessment Requirements

Read and familiarize yourself with the procedure; complete the minimum practice requirements. Document each MPR using proper charting technique. Complete each procedure within a reasonable amount of time, with a minimum of 85% accuracy.

Name: ____________________

Date: ____________________

POINT VALUE
✦ = 3–6 points
✶ = 7–9 points

		PRACTICE TRIAL	GRADED TRIAL # 1	GRADED TRIAL # 2	NOTES
1. ✦	Assemble equipment.				
2. ✦	Perform proper hand hygiene.				
3. ✶	Select the correct medication using the "three befores" technique. *Note:* If you are not familiar with the medication, look it up in a reference book, read the package insert, and/or consult the physician.				
4. ✶	Always double-check the label to make sure the strength is correct.				
5. ✦	Correctly calculate the dosage in writing. Double-check your calculations with someone else.				
6. ✦	Place a medicine cup/container on a flat surface.				
7. ✦	Shake the tablet ordered into the bottle cap and then into a medication container.				
8. ✶	Check the dosage again against the medication order.				
9. ✶	Replace the cap on the medication bottle, and return the bottle to the storage shelf after reading the label *again.*				
10. ✶	***Introduce yourself, identify the patient, and warmly greet the patient. Ask the patient if he or she has any allergies.***				

Name: ______________________

Date: ______________________

POINT VALUE ✦ = 3–6 points ✶ = 7–9 points		PRACTICE TRIAL	GRADED TRIAL # 1	GRADED TRIAL # 2	NOTES
11. ✦	***Tell the patient the name of the medication and dosage you are administering per the physician's order. Ask the patient if he or she has any questions prior to taking the medication.***				
12. ✦	**Sublingual medication:** Have the patient place the tablet under the tongue. ***Instruct the patient not to swallow until the tablet has dissolved.*** **Buccal medication:** Have the patient place the tablet *between the cheek and gum area.* Instruct the patient not to swallow until the tablet is dissolved.				
13. ✦	***Tell the patient not to take fluids until the tablet is dissolved.***				
14. ✦	***Remain with the patient until the medication has dissolved.*** *Note:* After administration of the medication, it is best to have the patient wait in the office for 30 minutes.				
15. ✦	***Provide the patient with written followup instructions if further medication is to be taken.***				
16. ✶	Document the medication administration in the patient's record.				

Name: ______________________________

Date: ______________________________

Document: Enter the appropriate information in the chart below.

Grading

Points Earned	______		
Points Possible	______	114	114
Percent Grade (Points Earned/Points Possible)	______		
PASS:	______	❑ YES ❑ NO ❑ N/A	❑ YES ❑ NO ❑ N/A

Instructor Sign-Off

Instructor:______________________________ **Date:** ______________________

Name: ______________________________

Date: ______________________________

Procedure 54-3:

Administering a Rectal or Vaginal Suppository

Objective: Insert a suppository as ordered by the physician.

Supplies: Medication order; lubricant; biohazard waste container; patient instructions; vaginal suppository or cream; gloves; sanitary napkin; rectal suppository; 4 x 4 gauze square; pen; patient record

Affective Behaviors: Affective behaviors provide a professional approach to a skill that enhances the patient encounter. These behaviors may also display sensitivity to a patient's rights and enhance communication. Pay close attention to these skills, which will be in ***bold, italicized*** font.

Notes to the Student

____

____

____

____

____

____

Skills Assessment Requirements

Read and familiarize yourself with the procedure; complete the minimum practice requirements. Document each MPR using proper charting technique. Complete each procedure within a reasonable amount of time, with a minimum of 85% accuracy.

Name: ____________________

Date: ____________________

POINT VALUE
✦ = 3–6 points
✶ = 7–9 points

		PRACTICE TRIAL	GRADED TRIAL # 1	GRADED TRIAL # 2	NOTES
1. ✦	Assemble equipment.				
2. ✦	Perform proper hand hygiene.				
3. ✦	Select the medication using the "three befores." *Note:* If you are not familiar with the medication, look it up in a reference book, read the package insert, and/or consult the physician.				
4. ✶	Double-check the suppository label. Check the drug and its strength.				
5. ✦	Correctly calculate the dosage in writing. Double-check your calculations with someone else.				
6. ✶	Check the dosage again against the medication order.				
7. ✦	Replace the cap on the medication bottle and return the bottle to the storage shelf or refrigerator after reading the label again.				
8. ✦	***Identify and warmly greet the patient. Introduce yourself, and ask the patient if he or she has any allergies.***				
9. ✦	Give the patient a gown or sheet. Have the patient remove all clothing from the waist down. Assist the patient, as necessary, ***and provide reassurance if the patient seems uncomfortable with the administration of a suppository***.				

Name: ____________________

Date: ____________________

POINT VALUE
✦ = 3–6 points
✶ = 7–9 points

		PRACTICE TRIAL	GRADED TRIAL # 1	GRADED TRIAL # 2	NOTES
10. ✦	Tell the patient the name of the medication and dosage that you are administering, per the physician's order. ***Ask the patient if he or she has any questions prior to receiving the medication.***				
11. ✶	**Rectal suppository administration:** Have the patient lie on the left side, with the top leg bent. ***Drape the patient with a sheet.*** Apply gloves. Open the suppository and place it on a gauze square. Moisten the suppository with lubricant or a small amount of water. With one hand, separate the buttocks. Pick up the suppository with the other hand. ***Ask the patient to breathe slowly as you insert the suppository.*** Insert the suppository 1 to 1-and-one-half inches past the rectal sphincter. Hold the buttocks together and instruct the patient not to bear down. Wipe the anal area with the gauze square and discard the square in a biohazard waste container. Have the patient remain in the side-lying position for approximately 20 minutes.				

Name: ______________________________

Date: ______________________________

POINT VALUE ✦ = 3–6 points ✶ = 7–9 points		PRACTICE TRIAL	GRADED TRIAL # 1	GRADED TRIAL # 2	NOTES
	Vaginal suppository administration: Have the patient lie in the dorsal recumbent position with the legs apart. ***Drape the patient with a sheet***. With a gloved hand, open the suppository. If an applicator is provided, drop it on the clean surface. With a gloved hand, separate the labia minora and hold them in place. Using the other hand, insert the suppository one finger length into the vagina. If an applicator was provided, place the suppository in the applicator and insert it in the vagina in a downward direction. Instruct the patient to remain in this position for 10 minutes. Dispose of the applicator. Remove your gloves. Dispose of the items in the biohazard waste container. ***Give the patient wipes to clean with and provide the patient with a sanitary napkin.***				
12. ✶	***Remain with the patient until the medication has dissolved.***				
13. ✦	***Provide the patient with written followup instructions if further medication is to be taken.***				
14. ✶	Document the medication administration in the patient's record.				

Name: ______________________________

Date: ______________________________

Document: Enter the appropriate information in the chart below.

Grading

Points Earned	______		
Points Possible	______	99	99
Percent Grade (Points Earned/Points Possible)	______		
PASS:	______	❏ YES ❏ NO ❏ N/A	❏ YES ❏ NO ❏ N/A

Instructor Sign-Off

Instructor: ______________________________ **Date:** ______________

Name: ______________________________

Date: ______________________________

Procedure 54-4:

Withdrawing Medication from Single-Dose or Multiple-Dose Vials

Objective: Withdraw medication from single-dose and multiple-dose vials.

Supplies: Gloves, biohazard waste container, biohazard sharps container, needle, syringe, alcohol sponge, medication vial, pen, patient record

Affective Behaviors: Affective behaviors provide a professional approach to a skill that enhances the patient encounter. These behaviors may also display sensitivity to a patient's rights and enhance communication. Pay close attention to these skills, which will be in ***bold, italicized*** font.

Notes to the Student

____

____

____

____

____

____

Skills Assessment Requirements

Read and familiarize yourself with the procedure; complete the minimum practice requirements. Document each MPR using proper charting technique. Complete each procedure within a reasonable amount of time, with a minimum of 85% accuracy.

Name: ______________________________

Date: ______________________________

POINT VALUE
✦ = 3–6 points
✶ = 7–9 points

		PRACTICE TRIAL	GRADED TRIAL # 1	GRADED TRIAL # 2	NOTES
1. ✦	Check the medication using the "three befores" technique before beginning. Compare the medication vial (bottle) against the physician's order.				
2. ✶	Select the correct syringe and needle; this depends on the medication and the location of the injection site.				
3. ✦	Perform proper hand hygiene and apply gloves.				
4. ✦	Roll the vial between your hands to ensure adequate mixing. Be sure that nothing has settled at the bottom.				
5. ✶	With an alcohol sponge, wipe the rubber stopper firmly using a circular motion. Set the vial on a clean surface while preparing the syringe.				
6. ✦	Remove the protective cap from the needle on the syringe. Be sure to maintain the sterility of the inner surface of the protective cap, since it will be needed to cover the needle once the syringe is filled.				
7. ✦	Withdraw the plunger of the syringe, and allow air to enter the syringe barrel equal to the amount of medication to be withdrawn.				
8. ✦	Turning the vial upside down at eye level and, using care not to touch the rubber stopper, insert the needle into the rubber stopper and inject the air into the vial. *Note:* Be extremely cautious about contamination as you enter the multiple-dose bottle.				

Name: ____________________

Date: ____________________

POINT VALUE
✦ = 3–6 points
✶ = 7–9 points

		PRACTICE TRIAL	GRADED TRIAL # 1	GRADED TRIAL # 2	NOTES
9. ✦	Keeping the vial upside down at eye level with the needle still inserted into the rubber stopper, slowly withdraw the correct amount of medication.				
10. ✶	While the needle is still in the vial, check that the dosage is accurate. Remove any air bubbles from the syringe.				
11. ✦	Remove the needle from the vial.				
12. ✶	If too much medication was drawn into the syringe, you may discard the excess by shooting it into the sink or waste receptacle. Do not return medication to the vial.				
13. ✶	Check the vial once again to make sure that you have withdrawn the correct amount. *Note:* If a multidose vial was used, check to see if it needs to be refrigerated.				
14. ✦	Remove gloves and perform proper hand hygiene.				
15. ✶	Document the medication and procedure in the patient's record.				

Name: ______________________

Date: ______________________

Document: Enter the appropriate information in the chart below.

Grading

Points Earned	______		
Points Possible	______	108	108
Percent Grade (Points Earned/Points Possible)	______		
PASS:	______	❑ YES ❑ NO ❑ N/A	❑ YES ❑ NO ❑ N/A

Instructor Sign-Off

Instructor: ______________________ **Date:** ______________________

Name: ______________________________

Date: ______________________________

Procedure 54-5:

Withdrawing Medication from an Ampule

Objective: Open and withdraw medication from an ampule.

Supplies: Ampule containing medication, alcohol sponge, needle, syringe, gloves, biohazard waste container, pen, patient record

Affective Behaviors: Affective behaviors provide a professional approach to a skill that enhances the patient encounter. These behaviors may also display sensitivity to a patient's rights and enhance communication. Pay close attention to these skills, which will be in ***bold, italicized*** font.

Notes to the Student

____

____

____

____

____

____

Skills Assessment Requirements

Read and familiarize yourself with the procedure; complete the minimum practice requirements. Document each MPR using proper charting technique. Complete each procedure within a reasonable amount of time, with a minimum of 85% accuracy.

Name: ______________________

Date: ______________________

POINT VALUE
✦ = 3–6 points
✶ = 7–9 points

		PRACTICE TRIAL	GRADED TRIAL # 1	GRADED TRIAL # 2	NOTES
1. ✦	Check the medication against the physician's medication order, following the "three befores" technique.				
2. ✦	Do not open the ampule until you are ready to withdraw the fluid.				
3. ✦	Perform proper hand hygiene and apply gloves.				
4. ✶	Snap your thumb and middle finger gently against the tip of the ampule to move all the medication away from the neck and into the bottom of the ampule.				
5. ✦	Clean the neck of the ampule using an alcohol swab.				
6. ✶	Use gauze between ampule and thumb when breaking the ampule. With one hand holding the bottom of the vial, snap the top off with the other hand using a gauze square to prevent a cut when the glass neck breaks.				
7. ✦	If the top of the ampule does not snap off easily, you may have to use a file to create a cut or "score" the ampule at the neck. Once scored, the glass ampule should break easily.				
8. ✦	Insert a needle attached to a syringe into the ampule and withdraw the fluid without touching the sides of the ampule.				

Name: ______________________________

Date: ______________________________

POINT VALUE ✦ = 3–6 points ✶ = 7–9 points		**PRACTICE TRIAL**	**GRADED TRIAL # 1**	**GRADED TRIAL # 2**	**NOTES**
9. ✦	Withdraw all the medication from the ampule. It may be necessary to tip the ampule slightly to withdraw all of the fluid.				
10. ✦	Discard the broken ampule into a biohazard waste container.				
11. ✶	Remove the filter needle from the syringe and discard it into the sharps container. Place the correct size needle necessary for medication administration.				
12. ✦	Remove and discard gloves and perform proper hand hygiene.				

Name: ______________________

Date: ______________________

Document: Enter the appropriate information in the chart below.

Grading

Points Earned	_______		
Points Possible	_______	81	81
Percent Grade (Points Earned/Points Possible)	_______		
PASS:	_______	❑ YES ❑ NO ❑ N/A	❑ YES ❑ NO ❑ N/A

Instructor Sign-Off

Instructor: ______________________ **Date:** ______________________

Name: ______________________________

Date: ______________________________

Procedure 54-6:

Administering Parenteral, Subcutaneous, or Intramuscular Injections

Objective: Administer subcutaneous (SubQ) and intramuscular (IM) injections.

Supplies: Medication order; vial of medication; gloves; alcohol sponges; biohazard sharps container; biohazard waste container; appropriate needle and syringe, depending on type of injection; pen; patient record

Affective Behaviors: Affective behaviors provide a professional approach to a skill that enhances the patient encounter. These behaviors may also display sensitivity to a patient's rights and enhance communication. Pay close attention to these skills, which will be in ***bold, italicized*** font.

Notes to the Student

____

____

____

____

____

____

Skills Assessment Requirements

Read and familiarize yourself with the procedure; complete the minimum practice requirements. Document each MPR using proper charting technique. Complete each procedure within a reasonable amount of time, with a minimum of 85% accuracy.

Name: ______________________________

Date: ______________________________

POINT VALUE
✦ = 3–6 points
✶ = 7–9 points

		PRACTICE TRIAL	GRADED TRIAL # 1	GRADED TRIAL # 2	NOTES
1. ✦	Perform proper hand hygiene.				
2. ✦	Apply gloves, and follow universal blood and body fluid precautions.				
3. ✦	Gather supplies. Use the "three befores" technique. *Note:* If you are not familiar with the medication, look it up in a reference book, read the package insert, and/or consult the physician.				
4. ✦	Gently roll the medication between your hands to mix any medication that may have settled. Refrigerated medication can be rolled between your hands to warm it slightly.				
5. ✶	Prepare the syringe using the correct technique. Carefully carry the covered needle and syringe to the patient.				
6. ✦	***Identify and warmly greet the patient. Introduce yourself, and ask the patient if he or she has any allergies.***				
7. ✦	***Tell the patient the name of the medication and dosage. Ask the patient if he or she has any questions prior to receiving the medication.***				
8. ✦	Position the patient depending on the site you are using.				
9. ✦	Using a circular motion, cleanse the patient's skin with an alcohol sponge. Wipe the skin with a sweeping motion from the center of the area outward.				

Name: ______________________________

Date: ______________________________

POINT VALUE ✦ = 3–6 points ✶ = 7–9 points		PRACTICE TRIAL	GRADED TRIAL # 1	GRADED TRIAL # 2	NOTES
10. ✶	Again check the medication dosage against the order.				
11. ✦	Remove the protective cover from the needle, taking care not to touch the needle. *Note:* If you accidentally touch the needle, excuse yourself to the patient. Then, return to the preparation area and change the needle on the syringe. If you are using a self-contained syringe and needle unit that does not come apart, discard the entire syringe with the medication and start the process over again.				
12. ✦	When you are prepared to administer the injection, place a new alcohol sponge between two fingers of your nondominant hand so that you can easily grasp it when you are finished with the injection.				
13. ✦	Firmly grasp the syringe in your dominant hand, similar to holding a pencil.				
14. ✦	**Subcutaneous injection:** Pick up a small mass of tissue with your nondominant hand. **Intramuscular injection:** With your nondominant hand, stretch the skin tightly at the intersection site.				
15. ✦	Grasp the syringe in a dart-like fashion and insert the entire needle quickly with one swift movement.				

Name: ____________________

Date: ____________________

POINT VALUE
✦ = 3–6 points
✶ = 7–9 points

		PRACTICE TRIAL	GRADED TRIAL # 1	GRADED TRIAL # 2	NOTES
16. ✶	Be sure to insert the needle at the correct angle based on the type of injection: Subcutaneous: 45-degree angle Intramuscular: 90-degree angle				
17. ✦	Once the needle is inserted, do not move it.				
18. ✶	Aspirate to make sure that you have not punctured a blood vessel. If blood appears, discard the syringe and start over.				
19. ✦	If there is no blood return, slowly inject the medication without moving the needle. *Note:* Insert and withdraw the needle quickly to minimize pain, but administer the medication slowly.				
20. ✦	Taking the alcohol sponge (or cotton ball) from between the last two fingers of your non-dominant hand, place it over the area containing the needle. Withdraw the needle at the same angle you used for insertion, using care not to stick yourself with the needle.				
21. ✦	With one hand, place the sponge firmly over the injection site. With the other hand, discard the needle in a biohazard sharps container.				
22. ✦	***You may gently massage the injection site to assist absorption and ease the patient's pain.***				

Name: ______________________________

Date: ______________________________

POINT VALUE
✦ = 3–6 points
✶ = 7–9 points

		PRACTICE TRIAL	GRADED TRIAL # 1	GRADED TRIAL # 2	NOTES
23. ✶	***Make sure the patient is safe before leaving him or her unattended. Observe the patient for any adverse effect of the medication for at least 15 minutes.***				
24. ✦	Correctly dispose of all materials.				
25. ✦	Remove gloves and discard them into a biohazard waste bag. Perform proper hand hygiene.				
26. ✶	Record the procedure in the patient's record.				

Name: ______________________

Date: ______________________

Document: Enter the appropriate information in the chart below.

Grading

Points Earned	______		
Points Possible	______	174	174
Percent Grade (Points Earned/Points Possible)	______		
PASS:	______	❑ YES ❑ NO ❑ N/A	❑ YES ❑ NO ❑ N/A

Instructor Sign-Off

Instructor: ______________________ **Date:** ______________________

Name: ______________________________

Date: ______________________________

Procedure 54-7:

Administering a Z-Track Injection

Objective: Administer a Z-track injection using proper technique.

Supplies: Alcohol sponges; biohazard sharps container; biohazard waste container; gloves; medication order; pen; sterile needle and syringe; medication vial; patient record

Affective Behaviors: Affective behaviors provide a professional approach to a skill that enhances the patient encounter. These behaviors may also display sensitivity to a patient's rights and enhance communication. Pay close attention to these skills, which will be in ***bold, italicized*** font.

Notes to the Student

____

____

____

____

____

____

Skills Assessment Requirements

Read and familiarize yourself with the procedure; complete the minimum practice requirements. Document each MPR using proper charting technique. Complete each procedure within a reasonable amount of time, with a minimum of 85% accuracy.

Name: ______________________________

Date: ______________________________

POINT VALUE
✦ = 3–6 points
✶ = 7–9 points

		PRACTICE TRIAL	GRADED TRIAL # 1	GRADED TRIAL # 2	NOTES
1–15. ✦	Follow steps 1–15 of procedure for intramuscular injection.				
16. ✦	After withdrawing the medication from the vial, change to a fresh needle.				
17. ✦	When ready to administer the medication, pull the skin of the buttocks to one side and hold it in place with your nondominant hand. *Note:* You may wish to use a dry gauze sponge if the skin is slippery.				
18. ✶	With your dominant hand and using a dartlike grip on the syringe, insert the needle up to the hub quickly into the gluteus medius muscle. Do not move the needle once it is in place.				
19. ✦	While still maintaining a firm hold on the taut skin with your nondominant hand, pull back on the plunger of the syringe to check for blood return. To do this, simply move your fingers up the syringe, while keeping the needle steady within the patient's buttocks, until your thumb and index finger reach the top of the plunger. If blood appears in the hub of the syringe, use the correct technique to withdraw the syringe, discard it, and begin with step 1 again.				

Name: ______________________________

Date: ______________________________

POINT VALUE
✦ = 3–6 points
✶ = 7–9 points

		PRACTICE TRIAL	GRADED TRIAL # 1	GRADED TRIAL # 2	NOTES
20. ✶	If there is no blood return, very slowly inject the medication into the muscle.				
21. ✶	Wait several seconds after injecting the medication before you withdraw the needle. Cover the area with the alcohol sponge, and withdraw the needle at the same angle of insertion. Wait at least 10 seconds before releasing the skin being held by the nondominant hand.				
22. ✦	Do not massage the area. Observe the patient for at least 15 minutes for any adverse reaction. ***You may advise the patient to walk around to assist in the medication's absorption process.***				
23. ✦	Correctly dispose of all materials.				
24. ✦	Remove and discard gloves, and perform proper hand hygiene.				
25. ✦	Document the procedure in the patient's record.				

Name: ______________________

Date: ______________________

Document: Enter the appropriate information in the chart below.

Grading

Points Earned	______		
Points Possible	______	75	75
Percent Grade (Points Earned/Points Possible)	______		
PASS:	______	❑ YES ❑ NO ❑ N/A	❑ YES ❑ NO ❑ N/A

Instructor Sign-Off

Instructor: ______________________ **Date:** ______________________

Name: ______________________

Date: ______________________

Procedure 54-8:

Administering an Intradermal Injection

Objective: Administer an intradermal injection.

Supplies: Gloves, hazardous waste container, alcohol sponges, sterile needle, sterile syringe, vial of medication, medication order, pen, patient record

Affective Behaviors: Affective behaviors provide a professional approach to a skill that enhances the patient encounter. These behaviors may also display sensitivity to a patient's rights and enhance communication. Pay close attention to these skills, which will be in ***bold, italicized*** font.

Notes to the Student

____

____

____

____

____

____

Skills Assessment Requirements

Read and familiarize yourself with the procedure; complete the minimum practice requirements. Document each MPR using proper charting technique. Complete each procedure within a reasonable amount of time, with a minimum of 85% accuracy.

Name: ______________________

Date: ______________________

POINT VALUE
✦ = 3–6 points
✶ = 7–9 points

		PRACTICE TRIAL	GRADED TRIAL # 1	GRADED TRIAL # 2	NOTES
	I. Preparation				
1. ✦	Perform proper hand hygiene.				
2. ✦	Apply gloves, and follow universal blood and body fluid precautions.				
3. ✶	Select the correct medication using the "three befores" technique.				
4. ✦	Gently roll the medication between your hands to mix any medication that may have settled. Refrigerated medication can be rolled between your hands to warm it slightly.				
5. ✶	Prepare the syringe using the correct technique. Carefully carry the covered needle and syringe to the patient.				
6. ✦	***Identify and warmly greet the patient. Introduce yourself and ask the patient if he or she has any allergies.***				
7. ✦	***Tell the patient the name of the medication and dosage ordered by the physician. Explain the process of the PPD skin test. Ask the patient if he or she has any questions prior to receiving the medication.***				
8. ✦	Select the proper site (center of forearm, upper chest, or upper back) for an intradermal skin injection.				
9. ✦	Using a circular motion, clean the patient's skin with an alcohol sponge. Wipe the skin with a sweeping motion from the center of the area outward.				

Name: ______________________

Date: ______________________

POINT VALUE
✦ = 3–6 points
✶ = 7–9 points

		PRACTICE TRIAL	GRADED TRIAL # 1	GRADED TRIAL # 2	NOTES
10. ✦	Allow the antiseptic to dry.				
11. ✶	Check the medication dosage against the patient's order.				
12. ✦	Remove the protective covering from the needle, using care not to touch the needle. *Note:* If you accidentally touch the needle, excuse yourself to the patient. Return to your preparation area and change the needle on the syringe. If you are using a self-contained syringe and needle unit that does not come apart, you will have to discard the entire syringe with the medication and start the process over again.				
	II. Injection				
13. ✶	Hold the syringe between the first two fingers and thumb of your dominant hand with the palm down and the bevel of the needle up.				
14. ✦	Hold the skin taut with the fingers of your nondominant hand. If you are using the center of the forearm, place the nondominant hand under the patient's arm and pull the skin taut. This will allow the needle to slip into the skin more easily.				
15. ✶	Using a 15-degree angle, insert the needle through the skin to about one-eighth of an inch. The bevel of the needle will be facing upward and covered with skin. The needle will still show through the skin. Do not aspirate.				

Name: ______________________

Date: ______________________

POINT VALUE
✦ = 3–6 points
✶ = 7–9 points

		PRACTICE TRIAL	GRADED TRIAL # 1	GRADED TRIAL # 2	NOTES
16. ✦	Slowly inject the medication beneath the surface of the skin. A small elevation of skin, or wheal, will occur where you have injected the medication.				
17. ✶	Quickly withdraw the needle. With the other hand, discard the needle into the biohazard sharps container.				
	III. Patient followup				
18. ✦	Do not massage the area.				
19. ✶	***Make sure the patient is safe before leaving him or her unattended. Observe the patient for at least 20–30 minutes for any negative reactions to the medication. Tell the patient not to rub the area.*** ***Instruct the patient to return to the office within 48–72 hours for the reading of the skin test. Make certain that the patient understands the directions and does not have any questions.***				
20. ✦	Correctly dispose of all materials.				
21. ✦	Remove and discard gloves, and perform proper hand hygiene.				
22. ✶	Document the procedure in the patient's record.				

Name: ______________________

Date: ______________________

Document: Enter the appropriate information in the chart below.

Grading

Points Earned	_______		
Points Possible	_______	156	156
Percent Grade (Points Earned/Points Possible)	_______		
PASS:	_______	❑ YES ❑ NO ❑ N/A	❑ YES ❑ NO ❑ N/A

Instructor Sign-Off

Instructor: ______________________ **Date:** ______________________

Name: ______________________________

Date: ______________________________

Procedure 54-9:

Preparing an Intravenous Tray

Objective: Prepare an intravenous (IV) tray.

Supplies: Absorbent disposable sheet, alcohol prep pads, Betadine swabs, disposable tourniquet, IV setup (IV tubing with attached filter; IV catheter; bag of IV fluid labeled with type and patient's name, date, and time), paper tape, syringe, port cap, gloves, gauze, IV setup tray, IV pole with pump

Affective Behaviors: Affective behaviors provide a professional approach to a skill that enhances the patient encounter. These behaviors may also display sensitivity to a patient's rights and enhance communication. Pay close attention to these skills, which will be in ***bold, italicized*** font.

Notes to the Student

____

____

____

____

____

____

Skills Assessment Requirements

Read and familiarize yourself with the procedure; complete the minimum practice requirements. Document each MPR using proper charting technique. Complete each procedure within a reasonable amount of time, with a minimum of 85% accuracy.

Name: ______________________

Date: ______________________

POINT VALUE
✦ = 3–6 points
✶ = 7–9 points

		PRACTICE TRIAL	GRADED TRIAL # 1	GRADED TRIAL # 2	NOTES
1. ✦	Perform proper hand hygiene.				
2. ✦	Apply gloves.				
3. ✶	Prepare an IV fluid administration set: • Inspect fluid bag to be sure it contains desired fluid, and that the fluid is clear, free from leaks, and hasn't expired. • Select correct administration set and uncoil tubing, taking care that the ends of the tubing do not become contaminated. • Close flow regulator to the fluid bag. • Remove protective covering from the port of the fluid bag and the protective covering from the spike of the administration set. • Insert the spike of the administration set into the port of the fluid bag with a quick, twisting motion. • Squeeze the drip chamber once or twice to start flow of fluid. • Open flow regulator and allow the fluid to flush all the air from the tubing. • Turn off the flow and place the sterile cap back on the end of the administration set.				
4. ✦	Place absorbent disposable sheet on the tray.				

Name: ______________________________

Date: ______________________________

POINT VALUE
✦ = 3–6 points
✶ = 7–9 points

		PRACTICE TRIAL	GRADED TRIAL # 1	GRADED TRIAL # 2	NOTES
5. ✦	Assemble equipment and supplies on the tray in order of use.				
6. ✶	If using an IV pole or pump, hang the IV solution on the pole; *do not set it up or calculate drops in the pump.*				
7. ✦	Notify appropriate personnel that IV setup tray is ready for administration.				
8. ✦	Remove and dispose of gloves. Perform proper hand hygiene.				
9. ✶	Document the procedure.				

Name: ___________________________

Date: ___________________________

Document: Enter the appropriate information in the chart below.

Grading

Points Earned	______		
Points Possible	______	63	63
Percent Grade (Points Earned/Points Possible)	______		
PASS:	______	❑ YES ❑ NO ❑ N/A	❑ YES ❑ NO ❑ N/A

Instructor Sign-Off

Instructor: ___________________________ **Date:** ___________________________

Name: ______________________________

Date: ______________________________

Procedure 54-10:

Reconstituting a Powdered Medication for Administration

Objective: Reconstitute a powdered medication.

Supplies: Alcohol swab, disposable gloves, medication label, medication order, pen, sterile needle, biohazard sharps container, vial of medication

Affective Behaviors: Affective behaviors provide a professional approach to a skill that enhances the patient encounter. These behaviors may also display sensitivity to a patient's rights and enhance communication. Pay close attention to these skills, which will be in ***bold, italicized*** font.

Notes to the Student

____

____

____

____

____

____

Skills Assessment Requirements

Read and familiarize yourself with the procedure; complete the minimum practice requirements. Document each MPR using proper charting technique. Complete each procedure within a reasonable amount of time, with a minimum of 85% accuracy.

Name: ______________________________

Date: ______________________________

POINT VALUE
✦ = 3–6 points
✶ = 7–9 points

		PRACTICE TRIAL	GRADED TRIAL # 1	GRADED TRIAL # 2	NOTES
1. ✦	Gather supplies, perform proper hand hygiene, and apply gloves.				
2. ✦	Select the correct medication and diluent, perform the "three befores" technique, verify the dosage against the physician's order, and calculate dosage (if necessary).				
3. ✦	Remove the top from the powder medication and the top from the diluent, and then wipe the tops of both vials with separate alcohol swabs.				
4. ✶	Insert a sterile needle through the rubber stopper on the vial of diluent.				
5. ✦	Withdraw the appropriate amount of diluent and add it to the powder medication.				
6. ✦	Remove the needle from the medication vial and discard it in the sharps container.				
7. ✶	To ensure that the medication is mixed well, roll the vial between the palms of your hands.				
8. ✦	Label the mixed vial with the strength of the prepared medication, time, date, your initials, and the expiration date.				

Name: ______________________

Date: ______________________

Document: Enter the appropriate information in the chart below.

Grading

Points Earned	_______		
Points Possible	_______	54	54
Percent Grade (Points Earned/Points Possible)	_______		
PASS:	_______	❑ YES ❑ NO ❑ N/A	❑ YES ❑ NO ❑ N/A

Instructor Sign-Off

Instructor: ______________________ **Date:** ______________________

Name: ______________________________

Date: ______________________________

Procedure 55-1:

Creating a Community Resource Brochure

Objective: Create a brochure that educates patients about available community resources.

Supplies: Computer, computer program that allows the creation of a brochure, printer, pen, phone book, Internet access, newspaper

Affective Behaviors: Affective behaviors provide a professional approach to a skill that enhances the patient encounter. These behaviors may also display sensitivity to a patient's rights and enhance communication. Pay close attention to these skills, which will be in ***bold, italicized*** font.

Notes to the Student

____

____

____

____

____

____

Skills Assessment Requirements

Read and familiarize yourself with the procedure; complete the minimum practice requirements. Document each MPR using proper charting technique. Complete each procedure within a reasonable amount of time, with a minimum of 85% accuracy.

Name: ______________________________

Date: ______________________________

POINT VALUE
✦ = 3–6 points
✶ = 7–9 points

		PRACTICE TRIAL	GRADED TRIAL # 1	GRADED TRIAL # 2	NOTES
1. ✦	Identify community resources that are available to help patients with disease prevention or health promotion, such as smoking cessation or weight loss. Research information found in a phone book, newspaper, or website.				
2. ✦	Create an attractive brochure for distribution to patients that includes the names, locations, phone numbers, and services offered by the resources.				
3. ✦	Check your brochure for spelling and grammatical errors prior to printing.				
4. ✦	Print one copy, and perform another spelling and grammar check on the printed document.				
5. ✦	After the brochure has been polished, obtain approval from the office manager or physician to print and distribute the brochures in the office waiting room.				

Name: ______________________________

Date: ______________________________

Document: Enter the appropriate information in the chart below.

Grading

Points Earned	______		
Points Possible	______	30	30
Percent Grade (Points Earned/Points Possible)	______		
PASS:	______	❑ YES ❑ NO ❑ N/A	❑ YES ❑ NO ❑ N/A

Instructor Sign-Off

Instructor: ______________________________ **Date:** ______________________

Name: ______________________________

Date: ______________________________

Procedure 55-2:

Creating a Public Relations Brochure

Objective: Promote the office by creating a brochure for distribution to current and potential patients.

Supplies: Computer, printer, office information, pen

Affective Behaviors: Affective behaviors provide a professional approach to a skill that enhances the patient encounter. These behaviors may also display sensitivity to a patient's rights and enhance communication. Pay close attention to these skills, which will be in ***bold, italicized*** font.

Notes to the Student

Skills Assessment Requirements

Read and familiarize yourself with the procedure; complete the minimum practice requirements. Document each MPR using proper charting technique. Complete each procedure within a reasonable amount of time, with a minimum of 85% accuracy.

Name: ______________________

Date: ______________________

POINT VALUE
✦ = 3–6 points
✶ = 7–9 points

		PRACTICE TRIAL	GRADED TRIAL # 1	GRADED TRIAL # 2	NOTES
1. ✶	Gather the necessary data and create a brochure to advertise your office. Be sure to include the following: • Office name (e.g., Pearson Physicians Group) • Type of practice (e.g., Family Medicine) • Office hours • Office address • Names and information about physicians • Insurance plans accepted • Payment expectations (e.g., copayments are expected before visit begins; all methods of payment are acceptable except cash)				
2. ✶	Check your brochure for spelling and grammatical errors prior to printing.				
3. ✶	Print one copy, and perform another spelling and grammar check on the printed document.				
4. ✶	After the brochure has been polished, obtain approval from the office manager or physician to print and then distribute the brochures to patients.				

Name: ___________________________

Date: ___________________________

Document: Enter the appropriate information in the chart below.

Grading

Points Earned	______		
Points Possible	______	36	36
Percent Grade (Points Earned/Points Possible)	______		
PASS:	______	❑ YES ❑ NO ❑ N/A	❑ YES ❑ NO ❑ N/A

Instructor Sign-Off

Instructor: ___________________________ **Date:** ___________________

Name: ________________________________

Date: ________________________________

Procedure 55-3:

Instructing Patients According to Their Needs for Health Maintenance and Promotion

Objective: Instruct a deaf individual to prepare for outpatient surgery by creating a brochure on steps to follow in order to minimize postoperative infection.

Supplies: Computer, printer, pen, stapler

Affective Behaviors: Affective behaviors provide a professional approach to a skill that enhances the patient encounter. These behaviors may also display sensitivity to a patient's rights and enhance communication. Pay close attention to these skills, which will be in ***bold, italicized*** font.

Notes to the Student

____

____

____

____

____

____

Skills Assessment Requirements

Read and familiarize yourself with the procedure; complete the minimum practice requirements. Document each MPR using proper charting technique. Complete each procedure within a reasonable amount of time, with a minimum of 85% accuracy.

Name: ____________________

Date: ____________________

POINT VALUE
✦ = 3–6 points
✶ = 7–9 points

		PRACTICE TRIAL	GRADED TRIAL # 1	GRADED TRIAL # 2	NOTES
1. ✦	Create postoperative instructions for the deaf patient, including information about activities, medications, dressing changes, diet, and followup care. Create one copy for the client and one for the chart.				
2. ✶	***Face the patient so your lips can be read easily.***				
3. ✶	***Greet the patient, using the patient's name.***				
4. ✶	***Discuss the contents of the postoperative instructions with the patient.***				
5. ✶	***Obtain feedback from the patient to show understanding.***				
6. ✶	***Give a copy of the information to the patient.***				
7. ✶	***Have the patient sign one copy of the brochure and keep one copy for the patient chart.***				
8. ✶	Document the education.				

Name: ______________________________

Date: ______________________________

Document: Enter the appropriate information in the chart below.

Grading

Points Earned	_______		
Points Possible	_______	69	69
Percent Grade (Points Earned/Points Possible)	_______		
PASS:	_______	❑ YES ❑ NO ❑ N/A	❑ YES ❑ NO ❑ N/A

Instructor Sign-Off

Instructor: ______________________________ **Date:** ____________________

Name: ______________________________

Date: ______________________________

Procedure 57-1:

Role-Playing a Situation in Which a Patient Is from Another Culture

Objective: Learn how to communicate with patients from another culture.

Supplies: Pen or pencil; paper

Affective Behaviors: Affective behaviors provide a professional approach to a skill that enhances the patient encounter. These behaviors may also display sensitivity to a patient's rights and enhance communication. Pay close attention to these skills, which will be in ***bold, italicized*** font.

Notes to the Student

____

____

____

____

____

____

Skills Assessment Requirements

Read and familiarize yourself with the procedure; complete the minimum practice requirements. Document each MPR using proper charting technique. Complete each procedure within a reasonable amount of time, with a minimum of 85% accuracy.

Name: ____________________

Date: ____________________

POINT VALUE
✦ = 3–6 points
✶ = 7–9 points

		PRACTICE TRIAL	GRADED TRIAL # 1	GRADED TRIAL # 2	NOTES
1. ✦	Choose a classmate.				
2. ✦	Select a quiet part of the classroom to conduct the procedure.				
3. ✦	Determine who will be the medical assistant and who will be the patient.				
4. ✦	***Have the "patient" act as if he or she speaks very little English.***				
5. ✦	***Be calm, respectful, and considerate.***				
6. ✦	***Use simple and common words.***				
7. ✦	***Avoid using medical terms.***				
8. ✦	Never use slang.				
9. ✶	***Be attentive to eye contact, facial expressions, and use of hand gestures.***				
10. ✦	***Make the patient as comfortable as possible.*** ***Note: In a real-life situation, if a staff member who speaks the patient's language is available, have him or her translate the conversation, if that would make the patient feel more comfortable.***				
11. ✦	Document the interaction in the patient's chart.				

Name: ______________________________

Date: ______________________________

Document: Enter the appropriate information in the chart below.

Grading

Points Earned	______		
Points Possible	______	69	69
Percent Grade (Points Earned/Points Possible)	______		
PASS:	______	❑ YES ❑ NO ❑ N/A	❑ YES ❑ NO ❑ N/A

Instructor Sign-Off

Instructor: ______________________________ **Date:** ______________________

Name: ______________________________

Date: ______________________________

Procedure 57-2:

Role-Playing a Situation in Which a Patient Is Frightened, Angry, or Depressed

Objective: Learn how to deal with a patient who is frightened, angry, or depressed.

Supplies: Pen, medical record

Affective Behaviors: Affective behaviors provide a professional approach to a skill that enhances the patient encounter. These behaviors may also display sensitivity to a patient's rights and enhance communication. Pay close attention to these skills, which will be in ***bold, italicized*** font.

Notes to the Student

____

____

____

____

____

____

Skills Assessment Requirements

Read and familiarize yourself with the procedure; complete the minimum practice requirements. Document each MPR using proper charting technique. Complete each procedure within a reasonable amount of time, with a minimum of 85% accuracy.

Name: ______________________________

Date: ______________________________

POINT VALUE
✦ = 3–6 points
✶ = 7–9 points

		PRACTICE TRIAL	GRADED TRIAL #1	GRADED TRIAL #2	NOTES
1. ✦	Choose a classmate.				
2. ✦	Select a quiet part of the classroom to conduct the procedure.				
3. ✦	Determine who will be the medical assistant and who will be the patient.				
4. ✦	Have the "patient" express the emotion of fear, anger, or depression.				
5. ✦	***Once you recognize one of these emotions, remain calm.***				
6. ✦	If the patient is not displaying destructive behavior, ***continue to allow the patient to express his or her feelings without interruption***.				
7. ✦	***Let the patient know that you understand.***				
8. ✦	***Inquire about the issue so that you can work toward resolution of the problem.***				
9. ✶	During the conversation, ***express empathy; let the patient see that you are concerned***.				
10. ✦	Notify the physician of the conversation.				
11. ✶	Document the procedure in the patient's record.				

Name: ______________________________

Date: ______________________________

Document: Enter the appropriate information in the chart below.

Grading

Points Earned	_______		
Points Possible	_______	72	72
Percent Grade (Points Earned/Points Possible)	_______		
PASS:	_______	❑ YES ❑ NO ❑ N/A	❑ YES ❑ NO ❑ N/A

Instructor Sign-Off

Instructor: ______________________________ **Date:** ____________________

Name: ______________________________

Date: ______________________________

Procedure 57-3:

Develop a Patient Teaching Handout About Stress

Objective: Develop an appropriate teaching tool about stress.

Supplies: Computer, word processor, printer, pen, paper

Affective Behaviors: Affective behaviors provide a professional approach to a skill that enhances the patient encounter. These behaviors may also display sensitivity to a patient's rights and enhance communication. Pay close attention to these skills, which will be in ***bold, italicized*** font.

Notes to the Student

____

____

____

____

____

____

Skills Assessment Requirements

Read and familiarize yourself with the procedure; complete the minimum practice requirements. Document each MPR using proper charting technique. Complete each procedure within a reasonable amount of time, with a minimum of 85% accuracy.

Name: ______________________________

Date: ______________________________

POINT VALUE
✦ = 3–6 points
✶ = 7–9 points

		PRACTICE TRIAL	GRADED TRIAL # 1	GRADED TRIAL # 2	NOTES
1. ✦	Decide what information should be included on the patient teaching handout.				
2. ✦	Develop an outline of the information you plan to include on the patient teaching handout.				
3. ✦	Using a word-processing program, develop a patient teaching handout.				
4. ✶	Make sure your patient teaching includes at a minimum the definition, causes, and ways to cope with stress.				
5. ✦	Proofread the patient teaching handout on the computer screen.				
6. ✦	Make any necessary corrections to the patient teaching handout.				
7. ✦	Print the handout.				
8. ✶	Proofread your hard copy of the handout.				
9. ✦	Make any necessary corrections to the patient teaching handout.				
10. ✦	Turn in the handout to your instructor.				

Name: ______________________

Date: ______________________

Document: Enter the appropriate information in the chart below.

Grading

Points Earned	_______		
Points Possible	_______	66	66
Percent Grade (Points Earned/Points Possible)	_______		
PASS:	_______	❑ YES ❑ NO ❑ N/A	❑ YES ❑ NO ❑ N/A

Instructor Sign-Off

Instructor: ______________________ **Date:** ______________________

Name: ______________________________

Date: ______________________________

Procedure 59-1:

Conducting a Job Search

Objective: Conduct a job search.

Supplies: Computer; Internet access; newspaper; medical assisting publication; printer; pen; paper; dictionary; thesaurus; telephone book; job search organizer or folder; calendar; contact log

Affective Behaviors: Affective behaviors provide a professional approach to a skill that enhances the patient encounter. These behaviors may also display sensitivity to a patient's rights and enhance communication. Pay close attention to these skills, which will be in ***bold, italicized*** font.

Notes to the Student

In your journal, document how you felt about the job search.

____

____

____

____

____

Skills Assessment Requirements

Read and familiarize yourself with the procedure; complete the minimum practice requirements. Document each MPR using proper charting technique. Complete each procedure within a reasonable amount of time, with a minimum of 85% accuracy.

Name: ______________________

Date: ______________________

POINT VALUE
✦ = 3–6 points
✶ = 7–9 points

		PRACTICE TRIAL	GRADED TRIAL # 1	GRADED TRIAL # 2	NOTES
1. ✦	Determine two sources you will use to conduct a job search.				
2. ✶	Determine a plan for your job search.				
3. ✶	Prepare a list of information sources for identifying job opportunities.				
4. ✶	Update your resume.				
5. ✶	Rehearse interviewing with a close family member or friend.				
6. ✶	Plan your professional attire for the interview process.				
7. ✦	Perform a self-assessment.				
8. ✦	Develop a job search organizer or folder.				
9. ✦	Develop a contact log.				
10. ✦	Use a calendar to determine what times are available for job searching and interviewing.				
11. ✦	Select two sources you will use to conduct a job search.				
12. ✦	Conduct your job search.				
13. ✦	Turn in all information gathered during your job search, as well as a copy of your resume and contact log, to your instructor.				

Name: ____________________

Date: ____________________

Document: Enter the appropriate information in the chart below.

Grading

Points Earned	______		
Points Possible	______	93	93
Percent Grade (Points Earned/Points Possible)	______		
PASS:	______	❏ YES ❏ NO ❏ N/A	❏ YES ❏ NO ❏ N/A

Instructor Sign-Off

Instructor: ______________________________ **Date:** ____________________

Name: ______________________________

Date: ______________________________

Procedure 59-2:

Preparing Your Resume and References

Objective: Prepare a resume and references.

Supplies: Computer; printer; pen; paper; dictionary; thesaurus; telephone book; current and past employment information; current and past educational information

Affective Behaviors: Affective behaviors provide a professional approach to a skill that enhances the patient encounter. These behaviors may also display sensitivity to a patient's rights and enhance communication. Pay close attention to these skills, which will be in ***bold, italicized*** font.

Notes to the Student

____

____

____

____

____

____

Skills Assessment Requirements

Read and familiarize yourself with the procedure; complete the minimum practice requirements. Document each MPR using proper charting technique. Complete each procedure within a reasonable amount of time, with a minimum of 85% accuracy.

Name: ___________________________

Date: ___________________________

POINT VALUE
✦ = 3–6 points
✶ = 7–9 points

		PRACTICE TRIAL	GRADED TRIAL # 1	GRADED TRIAL # 2	NOTES
1. ✦	Gather equipment and supplies.				
2. ✦	Prepare your resume.				
3. ✦	Using a word-processing program, complete the standard parts of a resume: heading; objective; education; employment; professional organizations and memberships; credentials; and references.				
4. ✦	Proofread your resume.				
5. ✦	Have a close family member or friend proofread your resume.				
6. ✦	Make any corrections to errors found on the resume.				
7. ✦	Using good-quality white or off-white 8½ × 11 paper, print your resume.				
8. ✦	On a separate piece of paper, list at least three references with their addresses and phone numbers.				
9. ✦	Proofread your references.				
10. ✦	Have a close family member or friend proofread your references.				
11. ✦	Make any corrections to errors found on your references.				
12. ✦	Using good-quality white or off white 8½ × 11 paper, print your references.				

Name: ______________________________

Date: ______________________________

POINT VALUE ✦ = 3–6 points ✶ = 7–9 points		PRACTICE TRIAL	GRADED TRIAL # 1	GRADED TRIAL # 2	NOTES
13. ✦	Save your resume and list of references on a disk, USB drive, computer hard drive, or other storage device.				
14. ✦	Update your resume whenever changes occur.				
15. ✦	Turn in your resume and references to your instructor.				

Name: ____________________

Date: ____________________

Document: Enter the appropriate information in the chart below.

Grading

Points Earned	______		
Points Possible	______	90	90
Percent Grade (Points Earned/Points Possible)	______		
PASS:	______	❑ YES ❑ NO ❑ N/A	❑ YES ❑ NO ❑ N/A

Instructor Sign-Off

Instructor: ____________________ **Date:** ____________________

Name: ______________________________

Date: ______________________________

Procedure 59-3:

Preparing a Cover Letter

Objective: Prepare a cover letter.

Supplies: Computer, printer, pen, paper, dictionary, thesaurus, telephone book

Affective Behaviors: Affective behaviors provide a professional approach to a skill that enhances the patient encounter. These behaviors may also display sensitivity to a patient's rights and enhance communication. Pay close attention to these skills, which will be in ***bold, italicized*** font.

Notes to the Student

____

____

____

____

____

____

Skills Assessment Requirements

Read and familiarize yourself with the procedure; complete the minimum practice requirements. Document each MPR using proper charting technique. Complete each procedure within a reasonable amount of time, with a minimum of 85% accuracy.

Name: ______________________________

Date: ______________________________

POINT VALUE
✦ = 3–6 points
✶ = 7–9 points

		PRACTICE TRIAL	GRADED TRIAL # 1	GRADED TRIAL # 2	NOTES
1. ✦	Gather equipment and supplies.				
2. ✶	Prepare a cover letter using a word-processing program.				
3. ✶	Proofread your cover letter.				
4. ✶	Have a close family member or friend proofread your cover letter.				
5. ✶	Make any corrections to errors found on the cover letter.				
6. ✶	Using good-quality, white or off-white 8½ × 11 paper, print your cover letter.				
7. ✶	Turn your cover letter in to your instructor.				

Name: ______________________________

Date: ______________________________

Document: Enter the appropriate information in the chart below.

Grading

Points Earned	_______		
Points Possible	_______	60	60
Percent Grade (Points Earned/Points Possible)	_______		
PASS:	_______	❑ YES ❑ NO ❑ N/A	❑ YES ❑ NO ❑ N/A

Instructor Sign-Off

Instructor: ______________________________ **Date:** ____________________

Name: ______________________________

Date: ______________________________

Procedure 59-4:

Role-Playing an Interview

Objective: Successfully role-play a job interview

Supplies: None

Affective Behaviors: Affective behaviors provide a professional approach to a skill that enhances the patient encounter. These behaviors may also display sensitivity to a patient's rights and enhance communication. Pay close attention to these skills, which will be in ***bold, italicized*** font.

Notes to the Student

Skills Assessment Requirements

Read and familiarize yourself with the procedure; complete the minimum practice requirements. Document each MPR using proper charting technique. Complete each procedure within a reasonable amount of time, with a minimum of 85% accuracy.

Name: ______________________________

Date: ______________________________

POINT VALUE
✦ = 3–6 points
✶ = 7–9 points

		PRACTICE TRIAL	GRADED TRIAL # 1	GRADED TRIAL # 2	NOTES
1. ✦	Determine five questions that may be asked during a job interview.				
2. ✦	Choose a classmate.				
3. ✦	Select a quiet part of the classroom to conduct the interview.				
4. ✦	Determine who will be the interviewer and who will be the interviewee.				
5. ✦	The interviewer will begin the interview process by giving the interviewee a general idea about the medical office and the employees who work there.				
6. ✦	The interviewer will ask the interviewee the five questions he or she selected in Step 1.				
7. ✦	The interviewer will gather information about the interviewee's past work experience.				
8. ✦	The interviewer will gather information about the interviewee's educational experience.				
9. ✦	The interviewee will answer the interviewer's questions.				
10. ✦	The interviewee will ask the interviewer questions about the medical office and the position.				
11. ✦	The interviewer will answer the interviewee's questions.				
12. ✦	Repeat the process, with students reversing roles. (Each student should play the part of the interviewer and the interviewee once.)				

Name: ______________________________

Date: ______________________________

POINT VALUE
✦ = 3–6 points
✶ = 7–9 points

		PRACTICE TRIAL	GRADED TRIAL # 1	GRADED TRIAL # 2	NOTES
13. ✦	Now the students should discuss the ten most common mistakes made in an interview. Did either student make any of these mistakes?				
14. ✦	Each student will assess his or her own interviewing skills.				
15. ✦	Each student will discuss the appropriate attire to wear to a job interview.				
16. ✦	Each student will discuss the successful interviewing guide-lines outlined in the textbook.				

Name: ______________________

Date: ______________________

Document: Enter the appropriate information in the chart below.

Grading

Points Earned	______		
Points Possible	______	96	96
Percent Grade (Points Earned/Points Possible)	______		
PASS:	______	❑ YES ❑ NO ❑ N/A	❑ YES ❑ NO ❑ N/A

Instructor Sign-Off

Instructor: ______________________ **Date:** ______________

Name: ______________________________

Date: ______________________________

Procedure 59-5:

Preparing a Follow-up Letter

Objective: Prepare an interview follow-up letter.

Supplies: Computer, printer, pen, paper, dictionary, thesaurus, telephone book

Affective Behaviors: Affective behaviors provide a professional approach to a skill that enhances the patient encounter. These behaviors may also display sensitivity to a patient's rights and enhance communication. Pay close attention to these skills, which will be in ***bold, italicized*** font.

Notes to the Student

____

____

____

____

____

____

Skills Assessment Requirements

Read and familiarize yourself with the procedure; complete the minimum practice requirements. Document each MPR using proper charting technique. Complete each procedure within a reasonable amount of time, with a minimum of 85% accuracy.

Name: ______________________________

Date: ______________________________

POINT VALUE
✦ = 3–6 points
✶ = 7–9 points

		PRACTICE TRIAL	GRADED TRIAL # 1	GRADED TRIAL # 2	NOTES
1. ✦	Prepare a follow-up letter.				
2. ✦	Proofread your follow-up letter.				
3. ✦	Have a close family member or friend proofread your follow-up letter.				
4. ✦	Make any corrections to errors found on the follow-up letter.				
5. ✦	Using good-quality, white or off-white 8½ × 11 paper, print your follow-up letter.				
6. ✦	Turn in your follow-up letter to your instructor.				

Name: ______________________________

Date: ______________________________

Document: Enter the appropriate information in the chart below.

Grading

Points Earned	_______		
Points Possible	_______	36	36
Percent Grade (Points Earned/Points Possible)	_______		
PASS:	_______	❑ YES ❑ NO ❑ N/A	❑ YES ❑ NO ❑ N/A

Instructor Sign-Off

Instructor: ______________________________ **Date:** ____________________

Notes

Notes

Notes

Notes

Notes

Notes

Notes

Notes

Notes

Notes

Notes

Notes

Notes